Mosby's
Comprehensive Review for
VETERINARY TECHNICIANS

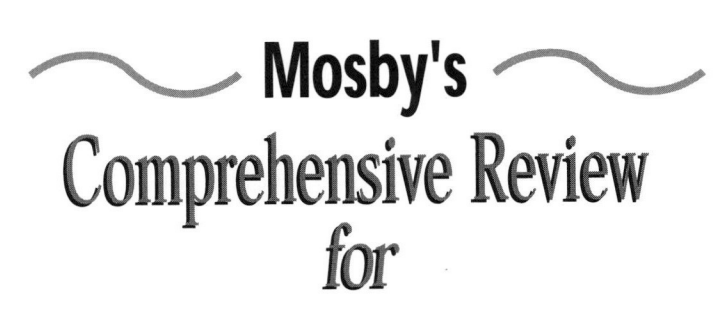

Mosby's
Comprehensive Review
for
VETERINARY
TECHNICIANS

Edited by

Monica M. Tighe, RVT, BA
Professor, Veterinary Technician Program
St. Clair College of Applied Arts and Technology
Windsor, Ontario
Canada

Marg Brown, RVT
Professor, Veterinary Technician Program
Seneca College, King Campus
King City, Ontario
Canada

Based on an original study guide published by the Ontario Association of Veterinary Technicians

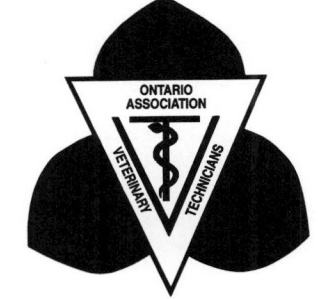

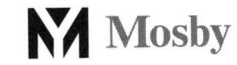 Mosby

An Affiliate of Elsevier Science

St. Louis   London   Philadelphia   Sydney   Toronto

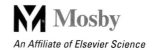

An Affiliate of Elsevier Science

Printed in the United States of America

Mosby, Inc.
11830 Westline Industrial Drive
St. Louis, Missouri 64146

ISBN 0-8151-9044-1

9 8 7 6

To **Dove, Becky, Mr. Beans, Mum, Phil, Jacquie, Tucker,**
*and the staff and students of the Veterinary Technician Programs
at Seneca and St. Clair College*

Preface

In 1990 the Ontario Association of Veterinary Technicians (OAVT) began using an examination to register its members. A study guide was compiled by the registration committee, written as an aid for both practicing and student veterinary technicians. Since its original publication, the OAVT study guide has been re-edited, duplicated many times, and used extensively across Canada.

Building on the strong foundation of the original study guide, this new, completely reformatted, and comprehensive review was written collectively by Canadian and American veterinary technicians for veterinary technicians and students. Very basic subjects, as well as some advanced areas for future reference, are included. This text cannot possibly cover all areas of veterinary technology to the degree desired; however, it is an excellent primary overall review guide that can be used in conjunction with specific-area textbooks.

The text is written in outline format for easy review of material. Each chapter also includes learning outcomes, multiple-choice questions, and a list of current references for further information. The appendices contain addresses and contacts of provincial and state associations and a current list of veterinary technology programs in Canada and the United States.

Our thanks to Janet Russell and Linda Duncan, Mosby Publishing, for helping us make decisions and keep a clear focus.

Special recognition is extended to the contributors who wrote these chapters—and thanks also to their families and employers for their support.

Finally, thanks to all technicians who continue to learn and grow on the pathway to professionalism.

Monica M. Tighe
Marg Brown

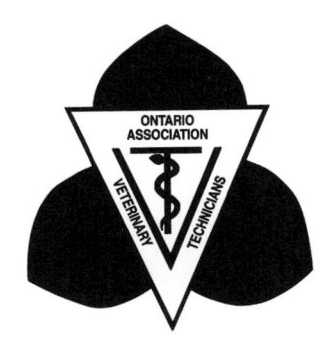

Contributors

Sandy Agla, AHT, BA
Lecturer
Ridgetown College
University of Guelph
Ridgetown, Ontario
Canada

Rebecca Atkinson, BSc, RVT
Head Avian and Exotic Veterinary Technician
Veterinary Teaching Hospital
Ontario Veterinary College
University of Guelph
Guelph, Ontario
Canada

Julie M. Ball-Karn, RVT
Intensive Care Unit Technician
Small Animal Intensive Care Unit
Ontario Veterinary College
University of Guelph
Guelph, Ontario
Canada

Patricia L. Bell, RVT, BSc
Instructor
Veterinary Technology & Biotechnology Programs
Saskatchewan Institute of Applied Sciences &
    Technologies-Kelsey Institute
Saskatoon, Saskatchewan
Canada

Marg Brown, RVT
Professor
Veterinary Technician Program
Seneca College, King Campus
King City, Ontario
Canada

Linda Campbell, AHT
Laboratory Technician
Natural Science Department
Vanier College
Montreal, Quebec
Canada

Susan Cornwell, RVT
Veterinary Technician
Large Animal Clinic
Veterinary Teaching Hospital
University of Guelph
Guelph, Ontario
Canada

Patricia Cutler, RAHT
Instructor
Animal Health Technology
University College of the Cariboo
Kamloops, British Columbia
Canada

Carlene A. Decker, BS, CVT
Associate Professor
Veterinary Technology
Parkland College
Champaign, Illinois, USA

Barb Donaldson, BA, BEd, MEd, RVT, VDT
Professor
Veterinary Technology
St. Lawrence College
Kingston, Ontario
Canada

Frances Federbush-Cheslo, RVT
Dietary Management Consultant
Hills Pet Nutrition, Canada
Mississauga, Ontario
Canada

Cathy J. Foulkes, RVT
Veterinary Technician
Veterinary Hospital
Dallas Zoo
Dallas, Texas, USA

Betty Gregan, AHT
Theriogenology
Veterinary Teaching Hospital
Atlantic Veterinary College
Charlottetown, Prince Edward Island
Canada

Joanne M. Hamel, VT, MLT, BA
Program Coordinator
Veterinary Technology
School of Health Sciences
St. Lawrence College
Kingston, Ontario
Canada

Melanie K. Harris, CVT, ASVT
Technician Supervisor, Surgery
Tampa Bay Veterinary Referral, Inc.
Largo, Florida
USA

Sandy Hass, VT
Past President
Canadian Association of Animal Health Technologists
and Technicians
Grandora, Saskatchewan
Canada

Amanda Hathway, RVT, RLATR
Veterinary Technician
Department of Clinical Studies
Ontario Veterinary College
University of Guelph
Guelph, Ontario
Canada

Colleen Hill, RVT
Veterinary Technician
Large Animal Clinic
Veterinary Teaching Hospital
University of Guelph
Guelph, Ontario
Canada

Pierry Kuskis, RVT
Radiology and Ultrasound Division
Veterinary Teaching Hospital
Ontario Veterinary College
University of Guelph
Guelph, Ontario
Canada

Mary Lake, RVT
Research Technician, Pathobiology
Ontario Veterinary College
University of Guelph
Guelph, Ontario
Canada

A. Patrick Navarre, BS, RVT
Professional Assistant
Veterinary Clinical Sciences
Purdue University
West Lafayette, Indiana
Executive Director
North American Veterinary Technician Association
Battle Ground, Indiana
USA

Elisa A. Petrollini, CVT
Emergency Service
University of Pennsylvania
Philadelphia, Pennsylvania
USA

Barbara Pinker, CVT
Former President
North American Veterinary Technician Association
Reading, Pennsylvania
USA

Jodilynn Pitcher, RVT
Manager, Animal Care
Department of Zoology
University of Western Ontario
Past President
Ontario Association of Veterinary Technicians
London, Ontario
Canada

**Sally R. Powell CVT, VTS-Emergency
and Critical Care**
Supervisor of Nursing, Emergency Services
University of Pennsylvania Veterinary Hospital
Philadelphia, Pennsylvania
USA

Penny Rivait, RVT, BA, RLAT
Professor
Veterinary Technician Program
St. Clair College
Windsor, Ontario
Canada

Sandra Skeba, CVT
Veterinary Lab Technician
Veterinary Department
Philadelphia Zoological Society
Philadelphia, Pennsylvania
USA

Teresa F. Sonsthagen, BS, LVT
Research Specialist II
Veterinary & Microbiological Sciences
North Dakota State University
Fargo, North Dakota
USA

Cynthia Stoate, AHT, RVT
Anesthesia Division
Veterinary Teaching Hospital
Ontario Veterinary College
University of Guelph
Guelph, Ontario
Canada

Katherine Taylor, RVT
Intensive Care Unit Technician
Small Animal Intensive Care Unit
Ontario Veterinary College
University of Guelph
Guelph, Ontario
Canada

Monica M. Tighe, RVT, BA
Professor
Veterinary Technician Program
St. Clair College of Applied Arts and Technology
Windsor, Ontario
Canada

William L. Wade, LVT, LATG
Supervisor, Veterinary Laboratory Animal Care
School of Veterinary Medicine
Purdue University
West Lafayette, Indiana
Immediate Past President
North American Veterinary Technician Association
Battle Ground, Indiana
USA

Kisha L. White-Farrar, RVT, BS
Veterinary Technologist
Veterinary Department
Dallas Zoo
Dallas, Texas
USA

CONSULTANTS

Gary P. Campbell, PhD
Associate Professor,
Veterinary Science Technology
Suffolk Community College
Brentwood, New York

Beth Harries, MEd, LVT
Wayne County Community College
Veterinary Technology Program
Wayne State University
Detroit, Michigan

Kathleen Rider, LVT, AAS, BA
LaGuardia Community College
Long Island City, New York

Contents

1 **Animal Anatomy and Physiology** 1
Penny Rivait

2 **Genetics** 18
Monica M. Tighe

3 **Breeding, Reproduction, and Neonatal Care** 25
Betty Gregan

4 **Restraint and Handling** 32
Teresa F. Sonsthagen

5 **Companion Animal Behavior** 48
Linda Campbell

6 **Pharmacology** 57
Cathy J. Foulkes

7 **Pharmaceutical Calculations and Metric Conversion** 70
Monica M. Tighe

8 **Small Animal Nursing** 76
Julie M. Ball-Karn, Kathy Taylor, and Monica M. Tighe

9 **Equine Nursing and Surgery** 94
Susan Cornwell and Colleen Hill

10 **Ruminant and Swine Nursing, Surgery, and Anesthesia** 104
Sandy Agla

11 **Veterinary Dentistry** 116
Barbara Donaldson

12 **Radiography** 126
Marg Brown

13 **Ultrasonography** 147
Pierry Kuskis

14   Sanitation, Sterilization, and Disinfection 155
Patricia Cutler

15   Surgical Preparation and Instrument Care 164
Melanie K. Harris

16   Anesthesia 176
Cynthia Stoate

17   Parasitology 194
Mary Lake

18   Diagnostic Microbioloby and Mycology 220
Sandra Skeba

19   Urinalysis, Hematology, Cytology 231
William L. Wade and Marg Brown

20   Clinical Chemistry 249
Joanne M. Hamel

21   Virology 263
Patricia L. Bell

22   Immunology 271
Patricia L. Bell

23   Zoonoses 282
Kisha L. White-Farrar

24   Small Animal Nutrition 294
Frances Federbush-Cheslo

25   Large Animal Nutrition and Feeding 312
Sandy Hass

26   Emergency and First Aid 327
Sally R. Powell and Elisa A. Petrollini

27   Laboratory Animal Medicine 338
Amanda Hathaway and Jodilynn Pitcher

28   Avian and Reptile Medicine 353
Rebecca M. Atkinson

29   Personal and Professional Management Skills 365
Carlene A. Decker and A. Patrick Navarre

APPENDIXES

A   The Veterinary Technician Profession, Legislation, Associations, and Colleges 381

B   Medical Terminology 389

C   Normal Values 392

D   Table of Species Names 393

E   Abbreviations and Symbols 394

F   The Metric System and Equivalents 399

ANSWER KEY 400

Mosby's
Comprehensive Review
for
VETERINARY
TECHNICIANS

CHAPTER 1

Animal Anatomy and Physiology

Penny Rivait

OUTLINE

Definitions
Cell Structure and Physiology
  Prokaryote
  Eukaryote
Movement In and Out of Cells
  Definitions
  Passive Processes
  Active Processes
  Hypotonic, Hypertonic, and Iso-
    tonic
Tissues
  Epithelia

Connective
Muscle
Nervous
Directional Terminology
Body Systems
  Skeletal
  Muscular
  Nervous
  Cardiovascular
  Central Vascular
  Digestive
  Lymphatic

Respiratory
Excretory
Reproductive—Male
Reproductive—Female
Endocrine
Integumentary
Senses

LEARNING OUTCOMES

After reading this chapter you should be able to:

1. Explain the various processes that enable substances to move in and out of cells.
2. List the structural and functional characteristics of the four primary body tissues and their subtypes.
3. Define and be able to use all directional terms.
4. List and explain six classes of bones according to their gross appearance.
5. Identify the parts of a long bone.
6. State the three structural and three functional classifications of joints.
7. List the three types of muscle and state the distinct characteristics of each.
8. Describe the divisions of the nervous system and state how they relate to each other.
9. Describe the protective coverings on the brain and spinal cord.
10. List the parts of the brain and state their functions.

11. List the parts of the cardiovascular system and state their functions.
12. Compare and contrast systemic, coronary, and pulmonary circulation.
13. Explain the cardiac cycle.
14. Identify the components of a typical ECG tracing.
15. Compare and contrast the structure and function of arteries and veins.
16. Explain the process of digestion.
17. Define: herbivore, carnivore, omnivore.
18. Name the parts and their functions of the ruminant stomach.
19. Describe the structure and function of lymph vessels, lymph nodes, and lymphatic organs.
20. Name and state the function of all parts of the respiratory system.
21. Describe the three basic processes of respiration.
22. Define: tidal volume, residual volume, dead space, apnea, eupnea, dyspnea.
23. Explain the anatomy and functions of the excretory system.

24. Explain the three phases of urine production.
25. Explain the anatomy and physiology of the male and female reproductive system.
26. Explain the estrous cycle.
27. List the embryonic membranes and state their location and function.
28. Describe the process of parturition and lactation.
29. List the endocrine glands; state the hormones they release and their functions.
30. Describe the structure and function of skin.
31. Describe the structure and function of the eye and ear.

Anatomy and physiology are the essential foundations of many aspects of veterinary technology. Many clinical procedures such as positioning of a patient for a radiograph, preparing for a surgical procedure, or simply placing a catheter, involve a working knowledge of anatomy and physiology.

DEFINITIONS

I. **Anatomy:** the science that studies the body's form and structure
II. **Physiology:** the study of how the body functions

CELL STRUCTURE AND PHYSIOLOGY

Cells are the basic unit of life. Cells are prokaryotes or eukaryotes.

Prokaryote: "before nucleus"

I. A cell that lacks a true membrane-bound nucleus
II. All bacteria are prokaryotes

Eukaryote: "true nucleus"

I. A cell that has a membrane-bound nucleus and contains many different membrane-bound organelles
II. All multicellular organisms are comprised of eukaryotic cells
III. Composition of eukaryotic cells
Three major parts: cell membrane, cytoplasm, nucleus
   A. Cell membrane (plasma membrane)
      1. Consists of a double phospholipid layer with proteins interspersed (fluid-mosaic model)
      2. Contains carbohydrate chains and cholesterol; semipermeable, therefore allows various substances in and out of the cell
      3. Some cells have hairlike projections known as cilia used for surface movement; others may have a single, longer projection, known as a flagellum, for cellular movement
   B. Cytoplasm
   Consists of everything within the cell except the nucleus—organelles
      1. Ribosomes
         a. Found free-floating in the cytoplasm or attached to the endoplasmic reticulum
         b. Composed of protein and ribosomal RNA
         c. Site of protein synthesis
      2. Mitochondria
         a. Powerhouse of the cell
         b. Contains mitochondrial DNA and protein
         c. Smooth outer membrane and an inner membrane that extends into folds called cristae
         d. Cristae increase surface area for ATP (adenosine triphosphate) production
         e. ATP is produced through the process of cellular respiration (Krebs cycle, citric-acid cycle, tricarboxylic-acid cycle)
         f. Cells that use large amounts of energy (e.g., muscle) would have large numbers of mitochondria
      3. Endoplasmic reticulum
         a. Rough endoplasmic reticulum (RER)
            (1) Hollow system of membranous channels with ribosomes attached
            (2) Acts as transportation network for proteins
         b. Smooth endoplasmic reticulum (SER)
            (1) Hollow system of membranous channels without ribosomes attached
            (2) Not involved in protein synthesis
            (3) Transports and synthesizes carbohydrates, fats, cholesterol; important in detoxification
            (4) Organs important in detoxifying substances have large amounts of SER
      4. Golgi complex (Golgi apparatus)
         a. Saucer-shaped membranes with secretory vesicles

b. Receives protein, fat, or steroids from the RER and SER

c. Modifies these molecules and then transports them to the cell membrane (for release from the cell), another Golgi complex, or storage

d. Functions as a receiving, packaging, and distributing center

e. Produces lysosomes

5. Lysosomes

a. Known as "suicide sacs," since if their digestive enzymes were released the cell would be digested

b. Large numbers found in phagocytic cells

6. Peroxisomes

a. Membrane-bound organelles that contain strong oxidative enzymes

b. Important in detoxification and fat digestion

7. Cytoskeleton

a. Consists of microtubules, microfilaments, and intermediate filaments that are made of proteins

b. Provides an internal system that gives the cells form, structure, support, and intracellular movement

8. Centrioles

a. Bodies responsible for forming the spindle during mitosis

C. Nucleus

1. Control center of the cell

2. Contains DNA (deoxyribonucleic acid), which governs heredity and protein synthesis

3. DNA is in the form of chromatin in the nondividing cell and in the form of chromosomes in the dividing cell

4. Has a double, semipermeable nuclear envelope

5. Contains one or more nucleoli composed of ribosomal RNA and protein

MOVEMENT IN AND OUT OF CELLS ▬▬▬

Definitions

I. **Solute:** a substance that can be dissolved

II. **Solvent:** a substance that does the dissolving

III. **Solution:** when the solute has dissolved and is no longer distinguishable from the solvent (a uniform mixture)

IV. **Intracellular:** within a cell

V. **Extracellular:** outside of a cell

VI. **Intercellular:** (interstitial) between cells

Passive Processes: No Energy is Expended by the Cell

I. Diffusion

A. Movement of molecules from a high concentration to a low concentration

B. Oxygen can pass into a cell while carbon dioxide passes out of cells by simple diffusion

II. Osmosis

A. Movement of water through a semipermeable membrane from a region of low solute (high solvent) to a region of high solute (low solvent)

B. Water constantly moves in and out of the cell by osmosis

III. Facilitative diffusion

A. Diffusion with the aid of carrier proteins

B. Glucose enters the cell by this method

IV. Filtration

A. Substances are forced through a membrane by hydrostatic pressure; small solutes will pass through; larger molecules will not

B. Important in kidney function

Active Processes: Energy is Expended by the Cell

I. Endocytosis: taking into the cell

A. **Phagocytosis:** cell membrane extends around solid particles, "cell eating"

B. Some white blood cells are phagocytic

C. **Pinocytosis:** cell membrane extends around fluid droplets, "cell drinking"

II. Exocytosis: materials are expelled by a cell

III. Active transport

A. Movement of molecules from a low concentration to a high concentration

B. The sodium-potassium pump is an active transport pump

Hypotonic, Hypertonic, Isotonic

I. **Hypotonic:** red blood cells placed in a hypotonic solution due to osmosis will gain water and burst (hemolysis)

II. **Hypertonic:** red blood cells placed in a hypertonic solution due to osmosis will lose water and crenate (shrivel)

III. **Isotonic:** red blood cells placed in an isotonic solution will remain unchanged due to equal osmotic pressures

TISSUES ▬▬▬

I. Definition: a group of cells with similar functions

II. Four primary types of tissue

A. Epithelial

B. Connective

    C. Muscle
    D. Nervous

Epithelia

  I. Covers body surface, lines body cavities, and forms the active part of glands
  II. May form simple (one cell layer) or stratified (more than one cell layer) tissue
  III. Subtypes
    A. Squamous
      1. Flat, platelike shape
      2. Simple squamous lines blood vessels
      3. Stratified squamous lines the mouth
    B. Cuboidal
      1. Cube shaped
      2. Simple cuboidal forms the active part of glands and their ducts
    C. Columnar
      1. Rectangular shape
      2. Often contains mucus secreting goblet cells
      3. Often ciliated, found in respiratory tract
      4. Simple columnar lines the gut
    D. Pseudostratified
      1. Appears to be more than one layer but all cells touch the basal membrane
      2. Usually ciliated, as found in the respiratory tract
    E. Transitional
      1. May have a combination of shapes but will be found in areas where a great degree of distention is needed (e.g., urinary bladder)
    F. Glandular
      1. Highly specialized epithelial cells with the ability to secrete various products
      2. Classified as endocrine or exocrine
        a. Endocrine: ductless, secrete hormones directly into the blood stream (e.g., ovaries—estrogen)
        b. Exocrine: have ducts and secrete onto an epithelial surface (e.g., sweat glands)

Connective

  I. Connects and supports tissue
  II. Widely distributed throughout the body
  III. Subtypes
    A. Loose (areolar)
      1. Most widely distributed
      2. Supports organs and provides flexibility (e.g., under skin, surrounding blood vessels)

    B. Dense (collagenous)
      1. Predominately collagen fibers
      2. May be regularly arranged (e.g., tendons [connect muscle to bone], ligaments [connect bone to bone], or irregularly arranged, [for example, dermis])
    C. Reticular
      1. Interwoven reticular fibers
      2. Forms frame for several organs (e.g., spleen, lymph nodes)
    D. Adipose
      1. Fat cell storage
      2. Major food reserve, insulates
    E. Cartilage
      1. Provides strength and flexibility
      2. Mix of collagen and elastic fibers
      3. Principal cell chondrocyte
      4. Three types
        a. Hyaline (e.g., nose, larynx)
        b. Fibrocartilage (e.g., pubic symphysis)
        c. Elastic (e.g., pinna)
    F. Blood
      1. Consists of plasma (fluid portion), red cells, and white cells
    G. Bone
      1. Two types: compact and spongy (cancellous)

Muscle

  I. Skeletal
    A. Under voluntary control
    B. Contraction causes movement of bone
  II. Smooth
    A. Involuntary control
    B. Found in intestines, blood vessels
  III. Cardiac
    A. Involuntary control
    B. Myocardium

Nervous

  I. Specialized for conduction of electrical impulses
  II. Neurons conduct impulses, neuroglial cells are connective

DIRECTIONAL TERMINOLOGY

  I. **Cranial:** toward the head (e.g., the thoracic vertebrae are cranial to the sacral vertebrae)
  II. **Caudal:** toward the tail (e.g., the lumbar vertebrae are caudal to cervical vertebrae)
  III. **Dorsal:** toward the backbone (e.g., the thoracic vertebrae are dorsal to the sternum)
  IV. **Ventral:** away from the backbone (e.g., the umbilicus is on the ventral surface of the cat)

V. **Medial:** closest to the median plane (e.g., the tibia is medial to the fibula)

VI. **Lateral:** furthest from the medial plane (e.g., the ribs are lateral to the sternum)

VII. **Proximal:** the point closest to the backbone, used especially in reference to bones (e.g., the greater trochanter is on the proximal end of the femur)

VIII. **Distal:** the point furthest away from the backbone, used especially in reference to bones (e.g., the patella is located at the distal end of the femur)

IX. **Anterior:** toward the head, used especially in reference to limbs (e.g., the patella [knee cap] is on the anterior aspect of the rear leg)

X. **Posterior:** toward the tail, used especially in reference to limbs (e.g., the hock joint is on the posterior aspect of the rear leg)

BODY SYSTEMS

Skeletal System

In addition to reading the following, review all bones on a diagram or model.

I. Osteology: study of bones that make up the skeleton

II. Divisions
   A. Axial skeleton
      1. Bones found on the midline or attached to it (excludes the limbs)
      2. Examples: ribs, skull, vertebral column, sternum
   B. Appendicular skeleton
      1. All bones comprising the limbs (e.g., femur, humerus)

III. Function
   A. To support soft tissues of the body
   B. Protect vital organs (e.g., heart)
   C. Act as levers for muscle attachment
   D. Storage for minerals
   E. Blood cell production

IV. Types
   A. Compact (dense)
      1. Has very few spaces, provides strength and support
      2. Made of Haversian systems; each system is composed of:
         a. Central Haversian canal
         b. Canaliculi: canals that radiate out from central Haversian canal
         c. Lamellae: concentric rings of bone
         d. Lacunae: small spaces that house osteocytes (mature bone cells)
   B. Spongy (cancellous)
      1. No Haversian systems
      2. Large spaces between lattice-like pieces of bone
      3. Spaces are filled with marrow

V. Classification
   A. Long
      1. Consist of shaft (diaphysis), two ends (epiphyses), and a marrow cavity (e.g., radius, femur)
      2. Parts of a long bone
         a. **Diaphysis:** shaft
         b. **Epiphysis:** proximal or distal end of the bone
         c. **Articular cartilage** covers epiphyses
         d. **Periosteum:** fibrous membrane covering outside of bone
         e. **Endosteum:** lines the marrow cavity
         f. **Medullary** (marrow) **cavity:** space within the bone that contains marrow (red or yellow)
         g. **Epiphyseal cartilage:** region between diaphysis and epiphysis where bone grows in length; becomes epiphyseal line in mature animals
   B. Short
      1. Cube shaped
      2. No marrow cavity, filled with spongy bone
      3. Function as shock absorbers (e.g., carpus)
   C. Flat
      1. Thin, flat bones
      2. Protective function (e.g., pelvis)
   D. Pneumatic
      1. Contain sinuses (e.g., frontal)
   E. Irregular
      1. Unpaired bones (e.g., vertebra)
   F. Sesamoid
      1. Small bones attached to tendons
      2. Reduce friction along a joint (e.g., patella)

VI. Osteogenesis (ossification)—formation of bone
   A. Types
      1. Endochondral
         a. Bones formed from cartilage bars laid down in the embryo
      2. Intramembranous
         a. Bones formed from fibrous membranes laid down in the embryo
         b. Osteoblasts produce new bone and become mature osteocytes
      3. Bone becomes calcified

VII. Vertebral formula—consists of a letter symbol for each region followed by the number of vertebrae in that region
   A. The following letters are used to designate regions of the vertebral column
      C: Cervical vertebrae—neck region
      T: Thoracic or dorsal—chest region
      L: Lumbar—loin region
      S: Sacral—(in region of pelvis), fused or false vertebrae
      LS: Fused lumbar and sacral
      Cd: Caudal (coccygeal)—located in tail
   B. Examples
      1. Horse: C-7, T-18, L-6, S-5, Cd-15-20
      2. Dog and Cat: C-7, T-13, L-7, S-3, Cd-20-23
      3. Chicken: C-14, T-7, LS-14, Cd-6
VIII. Skeletal species differences
   A. The cat has a clavicle; the dog does not
   B. Male dogs have a bone (os penis) in the penis
IX. Articulations (joints)
   A. Formed when two or more bones are united by fibrous, elastic, or cartilagenous tissue
   B. Classification by function
      1. Synarthrosis—immovable joint (e.g., skull sutures)
      2. Amphiarthrosis—Slightly moveable joint (e.g., pubic symphysis)
      3. Diarthrosis—freely moveable joint (e.g., stifle)
   C. Classification by structure
      1. Fibrous: united by fibrous tissue, no joint cavity
      2. Cartilagenous: united by cartilage, no joint cavity
      3. Synovial: joint cavity and synovial fluid present

Muscular System

I. Function
   A. Movement of entire body or parts
      1. Maintains posture
      2. Heat production
II. Types
   A. Skeletal muscle (somatic, striated, voluntary striated)
      1. Skeletal muscle is multinucleated cells with cross-striations
      2. Run parallel to each other
      3. Functional unit is a sarcomere
      4. Each muscle fiber is a muscle cell consisting of many myofibrils
      5. Myofibrils are composed of myofilaments (i.e., actin and myosin)

6. Contracts by means of the sliding-filament theory
      7. Myosin and actin bind together during muscle contraction
      8. ATP provides the necessary energy; calcium is also required
      9. All-or-none principle states that muscle fibers will contract completely or not at all
   B. Smooth muscle (visceral, plain, unstriped, involuntary)
      1. Smooth muscle cells are spindle shaped with one centrally located nucleus and no striations
      2. Responsible for involuntary movement (e.g., digestion)
   C. Cardiac muscle
      1. Involuntary, striated muscle
      2. Similar to skeletal but cardiac muscle fibers join together, forming a network
      3. Cells are joined by intercalated disks, which aid in conduction of the nervous impulse
III. Skeletal muscle actions
   A. **Flexor:** usually decreases the angle of a joint
   B. **Extensor:** usually increases the angle of a joint
   C. **Abductor:** moves a bone away from the midline
   D. **Adductor:** moves a bone toward the midline
   E. **Levator:** produces a dorsally directed movement
   F. **Depressor:** produces a ventrally directed movement
   G. **Sphincter:** decreases the size of an opening

Nervous System

ORGANIZATION

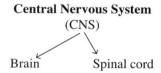

Central Nervous System
(CNS)

Brain   Spinal cord

Peripheral Nervous System
(PNS)

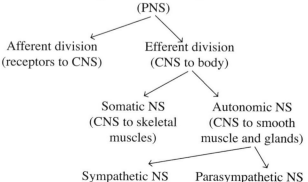

Afferent division   Efferent division
(receptors to CNS)   (CNS to body)

Somatic NS   Autonomic NS
(CNS to skeletal   (CNS to smooth
muscles)   muscle and glands)

Sympathetic NS   Parasympathetic NS

The central nervous system consists of brain and spinal cord.

I. Brain
A. Cerebrum
1. Site of motor control, interpretation of sensory impulses, and areas of association
2. Surface area increased by gyri (elevations) and sulci (fissures)
B. Diencephalon
1. Region of thalamus and hypothalamus
2. The thalamus acts as a relay station for sensory impulses and interprets some sensations such as temperature and pain
3. Hypothalamus controls body temperature, fluid balance, sexual drives, and influences the pituitary
C. Brain stem
1. Consists of midbrain, pons, and medulla oblongata
2. The midbrain serves as a connecting link
3. The pons contains important respiratory centers
4. In the medulla oblongata, nerve fibers cross from left to right and vice versa
5. The medulla also influences respiration, heart rate, vomiting, coughing, and sneezing
6. Throughout the brain stem is the reticular activating system (RAS), which is responsible for sleep/wake cycles
D. Cerebellum
1. Responsible for coordination and balance
II. Spinal cord
A. Runs through the vertebral foramen
B. Contains ascending and descending nerve tracts
C. Major function is to convey sensory (afferent) nerve impulses from the periphery to the brain and conduct motor (efferent) nerve impulses from the brain to the periphery
D. The brain and spinal cord are protected by bone and meninges
III. Meninges
A. **Dura mater:** dense fibrous connective tissue
B. **Arachnoid** (arachnoidea mater): very delicate connective tissue
C. **Pia mater:** transparent fibrous membrane that contains blood vessels and adheres to the surface of the brain and spinal cord
D. **Epidural space** is between bone and dura mater
E. **Subarachnoid space** contains cerebrospinal fluid

IV. Cerebrospinal fluid (CSF)
A. Colorless fluid of watery consistency, contains protein, glucose, ions, and other substances
B. pH and pressure are particularly important
C. A lumbar tap is used for CSF sampling
V. Blood-Brain barrier
A. A protective barrier in the brain; separates blood from nerve cells
B. Consists of selectively permeable capillaries
C. Substances such as oxygen, glucose, and fat soluble substances enter the brain easily; many waste products and drugs are blocked by the barrier
VI. Principle cells of the nervous system
A. Neuron (nerve cell)
1. Dendrites, cell body, axon
2. Conducts nerve impulses by generation of action potentials
3. An action potential is depolarization followed by repolarization; the electrical charge of the cell is changed
4. Impulses travel in one direction
B. Neuroglial cells (glial)
1. Connective tissue cells of central nervous system
a. Function: phagocytic, produce myelin, insulate, form part of blood-brain barrier

Cardiovascular System

I. Function
A. The heart provides the force to circulate blood to all parts of the body
II. Structure
A. The myocardium is the heart (cardiac) muscle
B. Muscle is striated and cells are connected by intercalated disks
C. Intercalated disks have a low electrical resistance; therefore the impulse spreads very quickly and all cells seem to function as one
III. Protective layers
A. Pericardium: a double-walled membranous sac covering the myocardium
1. Visceral pericardium (epicardium): the inner layer of the pericardium
2. Parietal pericardium: the outer layer of the pericardium
B. Endocardium: a serous membrane lining the inner chambers of the heart
IV. Pulmonary circulation
A. Consists of the precava (cranial vena cava or superior vena cava) and postcava (caudal

vena cava or inferior vena cava) emptying into the right atrium through the tricuspid valve into the right ventricle, through the pulmonary artery (passes pulmonary semilunar valve) to the lungs where it is oxygenated and returned to the heart by pulmonary veins

V. Systemic circulation (somatic circulation)
  A. Oxygenated blood in the left atrium flows through the bicuspid (mitral) valve to the left ventricle, out the aorta (passes aortic semilunar valve) to all parts of the body
  B. Two branches off the aortic arch
    1. The first is the innominate artery (brachiocephalic), which branches into the right subclavian artery and right and left common carotid arteries
    2. The second branch is the left subclavian artery
VI. Coronary circulation
  A. Coronary arteries provide nutrients and oxygen to the myocardium; coronary veins drain waste and carbon dioxide from the myocardium
VII. Cardiac cycle
  A. One complete cycle: as atria contract (systole) the ventricles relax (diastole) and as ventricles contract the atria relax
  B. Atrial diastole: atria are at rest
    1. The right atrium is receiving blood from the precava and postcava while the left atrium is receiving blood from the pulmonary veins
  C. Atrial systole: atria are contracting
    1. The sinoatrial (SA) node fires, causing contraction of the atria; blood is pushed through the tricuspid and bicuspid valves into the right and left ventricles
  D. Ventricular diastole
    1. The ventricles receive blood from the atria
  E. Ventricular systole
    1. The impulse from the SA node has been conducted to the AV node, which conducts the impulse down the bundle of HIS (AV bundle) to the Purkinje fibers
    2. The ventricles are now stimulated to contract and blood is forced through the semilunar valves into the pulmonary artery and aorta
VIII. Heart sounds
  A. Auscultation (listening to heart sounds)
  B. Lubb, dupp, pause
  C. Lubb is the first sound; it is a long sound made when the AV valves close
  D. Dupp is the second sound; it is a short, sharp sound made when the semilunar valves close
IX. Heart rate
  A. Dogs' heart rates vary with age, size, breed, health, and fitness
  B. Dog: 70-140 beats per minute
  C. Cat: 110-140 beats per minute
  D. Heart rate may be affected also by chemicals, hormones, temperature, behavior, and respiration
X. ECG/EKG
  A. Electrocardiogram records the electrical activity of the heart
  B. The first wave is the P wave, which represents the electrical events during atrial systole
  C. The large QRS complex represents the electrical events of ventricular systole
  D. The T wave represents the electrical events during ventricular diastole
  E. Atrial diastole occurs during ventricular systole; therefore it is masked by the QRS complex

Central Vascular System

I. Blood vessels
  A. Arteries
    1. Carry blood away from the heart
    2. Carry oxygenated blood (except for pulmonary artery)
    3. Thicker and stronger than veins
    4. Pressure within is greater than in veins
  B. Arteriole
    1. Small arteries
    2. Leads to capillaries and regulates the blood flow into them
  C. Capillaries
    1. Consist of one layer of endothelium
    2. Microscopic in size
    3. Exchange of oxygen and carbon dioxide takes place here
  D. Venules
    1. Emerge from capillaries and enlarge into veins
  E. Veins
    1. Larger than arteries and thinner walled
    2. Low blood pressure; therefore have valves to prevent the backflow of blood
    3. Carry blood back to the heart
II. Fetal circulation
  A. Lungs, kidneys, and digestive tract are nonfunctional in fetus but must be nourished by oxygen

B. Exchange of nutrients and waste takes place within the placenta

C. Oxygenated blood enters the fetus via one umbilical vein

D. Vein ascends toward the fetal liver and divides into two: one branch joins the hepatic portal vein and enters the liver while the majority of blood flows into the ductus venosus, which connects to the postcava

E. The postcava enters the right atrium. The precava from the head enters the right atrium as well

F. Most of the blood goes directly through the foramen ovale to the left atrium into the left ventricle and out the aorta to all parts of the fetus

G. Blood that goes into the right ventricle passes into the pulmonary artery; most is diverted through the ductus arteriosus into the aorta (a small amount will go to the lungs)

H. Blood in the descending aorta will branch into the iliac arteries; the two umbilical arteries branch off and return deoxygenated blood to the placenta

Digestive System

I. Process
  A. The digestive system uses five basic processes to prepare the food for utilization by the body
    1. Ingestion of food
    2. Peristalsis: moving food through the digestive tract
    3. Mechanical and chemical digestion
    4. Absorption
    5. Defecation
II. Types
  A. **Herbivore:** plant eating animal
  B. **Carnivore:** meat eating animal
  C. **Omnivore:** plant and meat eating animal
  D. Ruminant
    1. Regurgitates food (bolus), remasticates (rechews), and swallows (deglutition) it again
    2. All ruminants are herbivores but all herbivores are not ruminants
III. Structures
  A. Mouth
    1. Receives food and mixes food with saliva during mastication
    2. Bolus is formed
  B. Pharynx
    1. Common passageway for digestive and respiratory systems

C. Esophagus
  1. Muscular tube running from the pharynx to the stomach
  2. Food moves through the esophagus by peristalsis
  3. Caudal region contains a sphincter
D. Stomach
  1. Simple stomach
    a. Found, for example, in man, pig, horse, and dogs
    b. Four regions (i.e., esophageal, cardiac, fundic, pyloric)
    c. Inner folds known as rugae
    d. Food is mixed in the stomach with secretions from the digestive glands until it is reduced to a liquid known as chyme
    e. pH of stomach is acidic
  2. Ruminant stomach
    a. Found in cattle, sheep, goats, and llama
    b. Very large organ
    c. Composed of four compartments: rumen, reticulum, omasum, abomasum
      (1) Rumen: called "fermentation vat"
        (a) The largest compartment
        (b) Food is mixed and churned in a favorable environment (i.e., proper pH, temperature, bacteria and anerobic conditions)
      (2) Reticulum: called "hardware" compartment
        (a) Most cranial compartment that is not completely separate from the rumen
        (b) Also called the honeycomb
        (c) Acts as a passageway for food, paces the contraction of the rumen, and is the usual site for ingested foreign objects
      (3) Omasum
        (a) Grinds up the food, absorbs water and bicarbonate
        (b) Composed of many layers of laminae, which resemble leaves
      (4) Abomasum
        (a) The true glandular stomach
        (b) Mixes the food with enzymes, initiating chemical digestion

E. Small intestine
1. Divided into three regions: duodenum, jejunum, ileum
2. Major site of absorption via intestinal villi
F. Large intestine
1. Three regions
a. Cecum (where the small intestine meets the large intestine)
b. Colon (ascending, transverse, descending)
c. Rectum
2. Absorbs water, produces vitamins B and K, and propels waste toward the rectum
G. Other organs involved
1. Pancreas: releases digestive enzymes
2. Liver: produces bile, which emulsifies fats
3. Gallbladder: stores bile, absent in the rat and horse
IV. Digestive process (simple stomach)
A. Food enters the mouth and is mixed with salivary amylase (from salivary glands, i.e., parotid, sublingual, mandibular, and zygomatic)
B. Amylase begins to break down starch
C. Saliva in the ruminant neutralizes acidity from the rumen
D. Food entering the stomach is mixed with gastric juice (protein digesting enzymes, hydrochloric acid, mucus)
E. Rennin is also present in the young to coagulate milk
F. In the small intestine the chyme is acted upon by pancreatic enzymes
1. Pancreatic amylase to act on starch
2. Trypsin to act on proteins
3. Chymotrypsin to act on proteins
4. Elastase to act on elastin
5. Peptidases to act on large peptides (proteins)
6. Lipase to act on fats
7. Nucleases to act on nucleic acids
G. The pancreatic enzymes are delivered in an alkaline fluid to help neutralize the acidic chyme
H. The small intestine also secretes enzymes
1. Trypsin to act on dipeptides
2. Maltase, sucrase, lactase to act on disaccharides
3. Nuclease to act on nucleic acids
4. Nutrients are absorbed through the intestinal villi

I. Large intestine moves solid waste to the rectum for defecation, water is absorbed here, and vitamins B and K are produced

Lymphatic System
I. Function
A. Absorbs protein-containing tissue fluid that escapes from capillaries and returns it to the venous system
B. Transports fats from digestive tract to blood
C. Produces lymphocytes
D. Develops immunity
II. Structure
A. Lymph vessels
1. Blind end tubes running parallel to venous system, which eventually empty into precava
2. Resemble veins but have thinner walls and more valves; lymph fluid is filtered through the lymph nodes
B. Lymph nodes (glands)
1. Oval-shaped structures
2. Filter lymph fluid
3. Produce lymphocytes
C. Lymph organs
1. Tonsils
a. Mass of lymphoid tissue embedded in mucous membrane
b. Supplied with reticuloendothelial cells
2. Spleen
a. Largest mass of lymphoid tissue
b. Phagocytic function
c. Produces lymphocytes
d. Stores and releases blood as needed
3. Thymus
a. Important in developing immune response in the young
b. Eventually replaced by fat in the adult, depending on the species

Respiratory System
I. Structures
A. Nostrils (nares)
1. External openings
B. Nasal cavity
1. Lined with mucous membrane
2. Houses turbinate bones
3. Air is warmed by capillaries, moistened and filtered
C. Pharynx
1. Nasopharynx: from posterior nares to the soft palate

2. Oropharynx: from soft palate to the hyoid bone
3. Laryngopharynx: from hyoid bone to the larynx
4. Eustachian tube: from the middle ear to the nasopharynx

D. Larynx (voice box)
   1. Consists of cartilage (e.g., thyroid, cricoid, arytenoid, and epiglottis)
   2. Epiglottis covers the glottis during swallowing
   3. Vocal folds attach to arytenoid cartilage

E. Trachea
   1. Consists of noncollapsible, C-shaped, cartilagenous rings
   2. Lined with ciliated columnar cells
   3. Divides into bronchi at the tracheal bifurcation

F. Bronchi
   1. Right and left cartilagenous bronchi enter the lungs
   2. Passageways get progressively smaller and the amount of cartilage diminishes

G. Bronchiole
   1. Consists of smooth muscle, no cartilage
   2. Lead to the alveoli

H. Lungs
   1. Varying number of lobes, depending on species
   2. Covered with visceral pleura
   3. House microscopic air sacs known as alveoli, where exchange of oxygen and carbon dioxide takes place

II. Physiology
A. Respiration of mammals—three basic processes
   1. **Ventilation:** movement of air between the atmosphere and the lungs
   2. **External respiration:** exchange of gases between the atmosphere and the blood
   3. **Internal respiration:** exchange of gases between the blood and the cells

B. Ventilation
   1. Inspiration (inhalation)
      a. A stimulus from the brain causes the diaphragm and external intercostal muscles to contract
      b. The diaphragm moves caudally and the chest moves ventrally; therefore the size of the thoracic cavity is increased, causing a decrease in intrathoracic pressure and a decrease in intraalveolar pressure
      c. Since intraalveolar pressure is now less than atmospheric pressure, air moves into the lungs
   2. Expiration (exhalation)
      a. The diaphragm and external intercostal muscles relax
      b. The diaphragm moves cranially and the chest moves dorsally; this decreases the size of the thoracic cavity, therefore causing an increase in intrathoracic pressure and an increase in intraalveolar pressure
      c. Since intraalveolar pressure is now greater than atmospheric pressure air moves out of the lungs

III. Lung volumes
A. **Tidal volume:** the volume of air exchanged during normal breathing
B. **Inspiratory reserve volume:** the amount of air inspired over the tidal volume
C. **Expiratory reserve volume:** the amount of air expired over the tidal volume
D. **Residual volume:** air remaining in the lungs after a forced expiration
E. **Dead space:** air in the pathways of the respiratory system

IV. Respiratory rate
A. Dog: 10-30 breaths/min
B. Cat: 24-42 breaths/min
C. Horse: 8-16 breaths/min

V. Control of respiration
A. Medullary rhythmicity center in the medulla oblongata, a region that has inspiratory and expiratory neurons
B. Apneustic area in the pons, which prolongs inspiration
C. Pneumotaxic area in the pons, which inhibits the apneustic area and causes expiration
D. Hering-Breuer reflex: stretch receptors in the lungs that prevent the lungs from overinflating
E. Carbon dioxide: an increase in CO_2 will cause an increase in respirations
F. Other factors may affect the rate of respiration (i.e., pain, cold, blood pressure, pH, oxygen, stress)

VI. Terminology
A. **Pneumothorax:** air in the thoracic cavity
B. **Atelectasis:** collapsed lungs
C. **Pleuritis** (pleurisy): inflammation of the pleural membranes
D. **Pneumonia:** inflammation of the lungs caused primarily by bacteria, viruses, or chemical irritants

E. **Eupnea:** normal, quiet respiration

F. **Dyspnea:** difficult breathing

G. **Apnea:** no breathing

Excretory System

I. Anatomy

A. Kidneys

1. Extract and remove waste products from the blood

2. Size and shape vary according to the species; majority are bean shaped

3. Right kidney is more firmly attached and cranial to the left kidney

4. Microscopic unit is the nephron

5. Outer cortex: contains the glomerulus, Bowman's capsule, proximal convoluted tubules (PCT), and distal convoluted tubules (DCT)

6. Medulla: contains the loop of Henle and most of collecting tubules

7. The medulla is arranged into various numbers of pyramids

8. The apex of the pyramid is the papilla, which opens into the minor calyx, major calyx, and renal pelvis

B. Ureters

1. Consist of smooth muscle

2. Capable of peristalsis to move urine to the urinary bladder

C. Urinary bladder

1. Consists of smooth muscle

2. Lined with transitional cell epithelium

D. Urethra

1. Tube of smooth muscle to transport urine from the urinary bladder to the exterior

II. Physiology—There are three phases to urine production

A. Filtration

1. Blood enters glomerulus by the afferent arteriole

2. Due to various pressures, water, salt, and small molecules move out of the glomerulus into the Bowman's capsule

3. It is now called the glomerular filtrate

B. Reabsorption

1. Occurs in the PCT and loop of Henle; substances needed by the body will be reabsorbed from the glomerular filtrate into the peritubular capillaries

C. Secretion

1. Substances are selectively secreted from the peritubular capillaries into the distal convoluted tubule

III. Urination (micturition)

A. To void urine

B. Filtrate flows into collecting ducts, renal pelvis, ureter, urinary bladder, and urethra and is voided as urine

C. Urine is water plus waste products (e.g., urea, excess ions)

IV. Hormonal influence

A. ADH (antidiuretic hormone, vasopressin)

1. An increase in ADH will increase the reabsorption of water within the kidney

B. Aldosterone

1. Stimulates sodium (Na) reabsorption in the kidney

Reproductive System—Male

I. Male anatomy

A. Testicles

1. Two oval-shaped glands in a skin-covered scrotum

2. Seminiferous tubules produce sperm

3. Cells of Leydig produce testosterone

4. The epididymis adheres to the side of the testicle; it connects the seminiferous tubules to the vas deferens and provides storage for sperm and a place of maturation

5. Testicles develop inside the abdomen but descend into the scrotum (after birth in dogs and cats) where the body temperature is more favorable for sperm development

B. Vas deferens (ductus deferens)

1. Connects from the epididymis to the urethra

2. Is a part of the spermatic cord along with blood vessels and nerves

3. The spermatic cord passes through the inguinal ring; at this point the vas deferens separates and joins the urethra

C. Accessory sex glands

1. These glands produce semen

2. Semen provides a transport medium for sperm, protects the sperm against the acidity in the female genital tract, and provides a source of nutrition

3. Glands vary with the species

4. Dogs have a prostate only

5. Cats have a prostate and bulbourethral (or Cowper's) glands

6. Stallions have seminal vesicles, prostate, bulbourethral, and ampulla

D. Penis

1. Houses the urethra, which transports sperm into the female genital tract

2. Consists of a shaft and the tip known as the glans penis
3. Erectile tissue surrounds the urethra; with sexual excitement the tissue becomes engorged with blood, leading to an erection, followed by the release of sperm during ejaculation
   a. The penis of the dog and stallion is composed of almost all erectile tissue and a small amount of connective tissue
   b. The penis of the bull, ram, and boar is composed of almost all connective tissue and very little erectile tissue
      (1) These animals achieve erection by the straightening of the sigmoid flexure (S-shaped)
4. The dog penis is unique in that it has a very long glans penis and a bone (os penis)
5. The cat penis is retracted and covered with spiny epithelial projections

II. Male physiology
A. Follicle stimulating hormone (FSH) is secreted from the pituitary, causing spermatogenesis to begin
B. Spermatogonia in the testicle will undergo meiosis; each cell will give rise to four mature sperm with the haploid number
C. Interstitial cell stimulating hormone (ICSH) is secreted from the pituitary, causing the cells of Leydig to produce testosterone

Reproductive System—Female

I. Female Anatomy
A. Ovaries
   1. Paired oval organs found in the abdomen
   2. Produces ova and hormones
B. Oviduct
   1. Conduct ova from ovary to uterine horn or uterus (depending on the species)
C. Uterus
   1. Consists of uterine horns, body, and a cervix
   2. The presence or absence of uterine horns varies with the species; they are largest in polytocous animals
   3. In dogs and cats, young develop within the uterine horns
   4. In monotocous animals, young develop in the body of the uterus
   5. The opening to the uterus is the cervix; some species may have a double cervix
   6. Uterine horns and uterus have three layers
      a. Endometrium: epithelial cells and mucous membrane
         (1) Varies in thickness with the cycle
         (2) Is reabsorbed in animals with an estrous cycle and sloughed in animals with a menstrual cycle
      b. Myometrium: smooth muscle
      c. Perimetrium: serous covering, which is continuous with peritoneum
D. Vagina (birth canal)
   1. Muscular tube from the cervix to the urethral orifice
E. Vulva
   1. Internally from the urethral opening to the external genitalia
   2. Many female animals have a common urogenital pathway

II. Female physiology
A. Estrous cycle
   1. **Monestrous:** one cycle per year, usually seasonal breeders
   2. **Polyestrous:** more than one cycle per year
   3. Nonbred females may have recurring estrous cycles regardless of the season (e.g., mice, rats, cat; seasonally polyestrous)
   4. Reflex or induced ovulators: ovulate after being bred (e.g., cat, rabbit, mink, ferret)
   5. Spontaneous ovulator: ovulation occurs naturally regardless of coitus

III. Estrus cycle
A. Proestrus
   1. Period of preparation
   2. Under influence of follicle stimulating hormone (FSH) from the pituitary
   3. New ovarian follicles grow and release estrogen, which builds up the uterus and uterine horns
B. Estrus (standing heat)
   1. Female is sexually receptive
   2. Uterus and uterine horns are ready to receive an embryo
   3. Release of luteinizing hormone (LH) from the pituitary causes ovulation
   4. May have a bloody discharge
C. Metestrus
   1. Short post-ovulatory phase
   2. Each ruptured follicle develops into a corpus luteum

3. Corpus luteum produces progesterone, which puts final maturation on uterine horns and/or uterus and inhibits development of new follicles
4. If pregnancy does not occur the corpus luteum will degenerate
5. If pregnancy occurs the corpus luteum will be maintained and continue to secrete hormones

D. Diestrus
   1. Polyestrous animals go through this short stage of inactivity then enter proestrus
E. Anestrus
   1. Long period of inactivity

IV. Pregnancy
   A. Fertilization begins with the union of sperm and egg during estrus within the oviduct
   B. The zygote undergoes mitotic divisions as it is propelled through the uterine tubes and will then implant in the uterine horns or uterus, depending on the species
   C. The placenta forms to allow the exchange of nutrients and waste products between mother and fetus (fetal and maternal blood do not mix)
   D. Fetal membranes form around the developing embryo for protection
   E. As the embryo grows it develops a placenta and attaches to the endometrial lining of the uterus
   F. After implantation until parturition, the developing organism is called a fetus
   G. Protective fetal membranes
      1. **Amnion:** forms a fluid-filled sac closest to the fetus; this is filled with amniotic fluid
      2. **Allantois:** a two-layered membrane: one layer adheres to the amnion, the other layer to the chorion; fluid fills this cavity
      3. **Chorion:** outermost layer, which attaches to the endometrium
         a. Different species have various types of fetal attachment

V. Parturition: act of giving birth
   A. Labor
      1. Under the influence of oxytocin from the pituitary the uterus and/or uterine horns begin contracting
      2. Delivery of fetus: fetus is pushed through the cervix and vagina
      3. Delivery of placenta: placenta (afterbirth) is delivered after the birth of each fetus

VI. Gestation periods: length of time from fertilization to birth
   A. Feline and canine: average 63 days
   B. Horse: average 336 days
   C. Bovine: average 285 days

VII. Dystocia: difficult birth
   A. May result in a caesarean section

VIII. Lactation: milk production
   A. First milk is colostrum, contains antibodies, proteins, vitamins, and is important for the neonate
   B. Milk production is under the influence of prolactin from the pituitary

Endocrine System

Endocrine glands (Table 1-1) are ductless and produce chemical substances (hormones) that have a specific effect on a target area. The hormones are secreted directly into the blood stream.

I. Characteristics
   A. Hormones may
      1. Change the permeability of a cell
      2. Change the permeability of an organelle
      3. Activate or inactivate an enzyme system
      4. Change the rate of enzyme production

II. Control
   A. Hormone secretion is regulated through a feedback system—as the hormone levels rise their secretion is inhibited
   B. Only the adrenal medulla is under neural control

INTEGUMENTARY SYSTEM
Anatomy

I. Skin: consists of two layers
   A. Epidermis
      1. Superficial layer is the stratum corneum; this is a nonvascular, cornified layer
      2. Constantly being shed and replaced
      3. Below this is the actively growing stratum germinativum
      4. Melanocytes (pigment cells) produce melanin, giving skin its color, and are found in this region
   B. Dermis (corium)
      1. Deep to the epidermis
      2. Contains arteries, veins, capillaries, lymphatics, and nerve fibers

Function

I. Protective barrier, sense organ, site for vitamin D synthesis
II. Contains many glands and nerve receptors, e.g., Meissner's corpuscle (touch receptor), sweat glands, Ruffini endings (heat), Pacinian corpuscles (pressure), sebaceous glands

Table 1-1 Endocrine glands

Gland	Hormone	Action
Thyroid	Thyroxin	Accelerates metabolism
	Calcitonin	Regulates calcium levels
Parathyroid	Parathormone	Regulates Ca and P levels
Adrenal cortex	Glucocorticoids, mineralcorticoids, gonadocorticoids	Protein and carbohydrate metabolism, stress resistance, antiinflammatory, regulates Na and K levels, male and female sex hormones
Adrenal medulla	Epinephrine, norepinephrine	Stimulate sympathetic nervous system; "fight or flight"
Pituitary	Growth hormone	Stimulates growth
(master gland)	Thyrotropic	Stimulates thyroid gland
	Adrenocorticotropic,	Stimulates adrenal cortex
	Follicle stimulating	Growth of ovarian follicle
	Luteinizing, interstitial cell-stimulating hormone	Causes ovulation, stimulates testosterone production
	Prolactin	Stimulates lactation
	Oxytocin	Causes uterine contractions
	Antidiuretic	Causes water reabsorption
Pancreas	Insulin	Decreases blood glucose
	Glucagon	Increases blood glucose
Ovary	Estrogen	Female sex characteristics
	Progesterone	Prepare uterus and uterine horns
Testes	Testosterone	Male sex characteristics

Hair

I. Hair contains an inner medulla, which is covered by the thicker cortex followed by a keratinized layer called the cuticle

II. Hair is produced within a follicle with growth originating in the bulb region

III. Hair below the skin is known as the root; the region above the skin is the shaft

IV. The numbers of hair per follicles vary

V. Each hair follicle is supplied with sebaceous glands and an arrector pili muscle

VI. Contraction of this muscle is responsible for the hair raising seen in frightened cats

VII. Types

   A. Normal guard or cover hair: usually accompanied by shorter wool hair in the same follicle

   B. Wool hair: shorter, wavy, no medulla (e.g., sheep)

   C. Tactile hairs (sinus hairs) (e.g., whiskers) are used as feelers; very sensitive to movement

Specialized Integument

I. Horns, claws, hooves grow from a specialized dermis and consist of cornified epidermal cells

Senses

I. Vision

   A. Anatomy—eye

     1. **Sclera:** outermost fibrous coat (white of the eye)

     2. **Choroid:** vascular coat between the sclera and retina

     3. **Retina:** nervous coat housing photoreceptors (i.e., rods and cones)

     4. **Vitreous humor:** clear, watery fluid filling the vitreous body

     5. **Lens:** focuses light onto the retina

     6. **Iris:** colored, contractile membrane between the lens and the cornea; regulates amount of light passing through the pupil

     7. **Pupil:** opening in the center of the iris

     8. **Aqueous humor:** clear, watery fluid filling the anterior and posterior chambers

     9. **Cornea:** clear, transparent covering on the eye

    10. **Conjunctiva:** mucous membrane that lines the eyelids

    11. **Nictitating membrane:** third eyelid

   B. Lacrimal apparatus

     1. Tears from the lacrimal gland located in the upper eyelids flow onto the eyeball to flush debris from the eye, moisten, and lubricate

     2. Tears drain out a lacrimal duct located in the medial canthi of the upper and lower lids into the nasal cavity via the nasolacrimal duct

   C. Physiology

     1. Light passes through the pupil, is refracted by the lens and hits the photore-

ceptors (i.e., rods and cones of the retina)

2. Rods respond to dim light and occur in greater numbers in nocturnal animals
3. Cones respond to bright light and color
4. The nervous impulse is passed via the optic nerve to the brain

II. Hearing
   A. Anatomy—ear (consists of three regions)
      1. Outer ear
         a. From the pinna up to and including the tympanic membrane
         b. Air filled
      2. Middle ear
         a. Houses three ossicles: malleus (hammer), incus (anvil), stapes (stirrup)
         b. Air filled, communicates with the nasopharynx by way of the eustachian tube
      3. Inner ear
         a. Houses the cochlea and semicircular canals
         b. Fluid filled
         c. The cochlea houses the organ of Corti (hearing receptors)
         d. The semicircular canals contain nerve receptors that respond to balance
   B. Physiology
      1. Sound waves are transmitted through the outer ear and strike the tympanic membrane
      2. Sound is concentrated and conducted through the three ossicles to the round window of the cochlea
      3. The cochlea houses the organ of Corti, which when stimulated conducts a nervous impulse along the auditory nerve to the brain
   C. Deafness
      1. Nerve deafness
         a. Results from malfunction of receptors or auditory nerve
         b. Most common in white, blue-eyed cats, Sealyham terriers, Scotch terriers, Border collies, and fox terriers
      2. Transmission deafness
         a. Results from malfunction in transmission of sound waves from outer to inner ear

III. Smell
   A. Associated with the olfactory bulb
   B. Receptors lie in the mucous membranes of the nasal cavity

   C. Odor is dissolved in receptors and transmitted to the brain

IV. Taste
   A. Taste receptors enclosed in papillae on the tongue
   B. Four types of papillae: fungiform, filiform, foliate, and vallate
   C. Majority of taste occurs through fungiform and vallate papillae

Glossary

anatomy The study of form and structure

apnea No breathing

articulation Where two or more bones meet, also called a joint

canthi (singular, canthus) The junction of the upper and lower eyelids at either corner of the eyes

carnivore Meat-eating animal

conjunctiva Mucous membrane that lines the eyelids

cornea Clear, transparent covering on the eye

coronary circulation Blood circulation that nourishes the myocardium

dead space Air found in the respiratory passageways

dyspnea Difficult breathing

dystocia Difficult birth

endocrine glands Secrete hormones directly into the bloodstream

estrus Time of the female's cycle when she is receptive to a male

eupnea Normal respiration

exocrine glands Secretions are through ducts, usually onto an epithelial surface

extracellular Outside a cell

herbivore Plant-eating animal

hormone Chemical substance that has an effect on specific target areas of the body

hypertonic Having a higher osmotic pressure than another solution

hypotonic Having a lower osmotic pressure than another solution

intercellular Between the cells

intracellular Within a cell

isotonic Having equal osmotic pressures

lacrimal apparatus Lacrimal duct conducts tears from the medial corners to the nasal cavity

lactation Milk production

laminae (singular, lamina) A thin, flat layer or membrane

meninges Protective coverings of the brain and spinal cord

monestrous One estrous cycle per year

monotocous Producing one offspring at birth

myocardium Heart muscle

nonspontaneous ovulator Ovulation occurs only when bred

omnivore Eats meat and plants

osteology The study of bones

parturition Act of giving birth

physiology The study of body functions

polyestrous More than one estrous cycle per year

polytocous Giving birth to several offspring at one time

residual volume Air remaining in the lungs after a forced expiration

ruminant Animal with a four chambered stomach; animal that commonly chews its cud

spontaneous ovulator Ovulation occurs naturally within the cycle

tidal volume The volume of air exchanged during eupnea

Review Questions

1 The process by which bone is formed from cartilage bars is known as:
   a. Intramembranous ossification
   b. Endochondral ossification
   c. Heteroplastic osteogenesis
   d. Chondrabar osteogenesis

2 Skeletal muscle is:
   a. Parallel, multinucleated fibers
   b. Interconnected, uninucleated fibers
   c. Spindle shaped, uninucleate fibers
   d. Parallel, uninucleate fibers

3 The scientific discipline that studies the functions of living things is:
   a. Anatomy
   b. Systemic anatomy
   c. Physomy
   d. Physiology

4 The canine foreleg is composed of the following bones:
   a. Tibia, radius, ulna
   b. Humerus, radius, ulna
   c. Humerus, radius, fibula
   d. Femur, tibia, fibula

5 A canine who has had a major hemorrhage accidentally receives a large transfusion of distilled water into the cephalic vein. This would probably have:
   a. no result as long as the water was sterile
   b. serious, perhaps fatal, results because the red blood cells would shrink
   c. no effect since the dog was dehydrated
   d. serious, perhaps fatal, results because the red blood cells would burst

6 In the digestive tract the three histological layers of the mucosa are:
   a. Epiglottis, soft palate, and larynx
   b. Epithelium, muscularis mucosa, lamina propria
   c. Submucosa, muscularis externa, serosa
   d. Columnar, squamous, cuboidal

7 In the canine, the sinoatrial node is located in the:
   a. Left auricle
   b. Right atrium
   c. Left ventricle
   d. Right ventricle

8 Which one of the following hormones is not secreted by the pituitary:
   a. FSH
   b. ACTH
   c. Cortisone
   d. Growth hormone

9 All of the following are major sites of lymphatic tissue except:
   a. Tonsils
   b. Thymus
   c. Spleen
   d. Kidneys

10 Choose the false statement about the middle ear:
   a. Contains three ossicles
   b. Infection in the middle ear is called otitis media
   c. Communicates with the nasopharynx by means of the eustachian tube
   d. The cochlea is located here

BIBLIOGRAPHY

Bone JF: *Animal anatomy and physiology,* ed 3, Virginia, 1988, Reston Publishing Co.

Frandson RD: *Anatomy and physiology of farm animals,* ed 5, Philadelphia, 1992, Lea & Febiger.

Marieb E: *Human anatomy and physiology,* ed. 2, 1992, California, Benjamin Cummings Publishing Co.

McBride DF: *Learning veterinary terminology,* St. Louis, 1996, Mosby-Year Book Inc.

Miller ME, Christensen GC, Evans HE: *Anatomy of the dog,* 1964, Pennsylvania, W.B. Saunders.

Ruckebusch Y, Phaneuf L-P, Dunlop R: *Physiology of small & large animals,* 1991, Ontario, Mosby Inc.

Genetics

Monica Tighe

OUTLINE

Genes and Variations
  Monohybrid Cross
  Dihybrid Cross
X-linked Inheritance
  Definitions

Identification of Autosomal and
  X-linked Genes
Example X-linked Heredity in
  Cats
Breeding Genetics

Chromosomal Abnormalities
  Definitions
  Lethal Genes

LEARNING OUTCOMES

After reading this chapter you should be able to:

1. Understand the basic definitions associated with inheritance.
2. Define monohybrid and dihybrid cross and complete a Punnett square for each type.
3. Describe the difference between outbreeding, back cross, inbreeding, and line breeding.
4. Describe the characteristics of X-linked genes.
5. Describe chromosomal abnormalities.
6. Define lethal gene and its consequences.

This chapter contains the basics of genetics and animal breeding. Students often find genetics difficult. The difficulty could be due to the terminology that students must learn to understand the subject or because genetics cause instant panic to most people. Approach this chapter one step at a time and understand the definitions before continuing on to the next section.

GENES AND VARIATIONS

The monohybrid cross or the crossing of a single gene is obviously the most simple cross. Note that, in most cases, multiple genes are usually the case in inheritance.

Monohybrid Cross

Defining homozygous and heterozygous.

  I. Example: the punnett square for the cross between cattle. Two black individuals are crossed. Their genotype is Bb (heterozygous). "B" represents the dominant allele of black. "b" represents the recessive allele of red

Punnett square for
the cross Bb × Bb

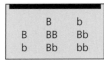

	B	b
B	BB	Bb
b	Bb	bb

  II. According to the Punnett square, the F_1 generation will be made up of 25% genotype BB, 50% will have genotype Bb, and 25% will have the genotype bb
  III. The ratio is 1:2:1

IV. However, 75% of the F_1 generation will have the phenotype or physical trait of black color since the B allele is dominant over the recessive allele b
   A. There are 2 Bb (heterozygous) individuals produced who will be black and 1 BB (homozygous) individual produced who will also be black in color. Only 25% of the F_1 generation will be red or bb
V. This 3:1 ratio (3 black to 1 red) is used to trace the heterozygous and homozygous genes of the parents
VI. The following matings are possible:
   A. Homozygous black to homozygous black will produce only black offspring
   B. Homozygous black to heterozygous black will produce all black: 50% of the offspring will be homozygous and 50% will be heterozygous
   C. Homozygous black to homozygous red will produce all heterozygous black
   D. Heterozygous black to heterozygous black will produce 25% homozygous black, 50% heterozygous black, and 25% red
   E. Heterozygous black to red will produce 50% heterozygous black and 50% red
   F. Red to red will produce only red, since all genes are recessive

Dihybrid Cross

The crossing of two independent alleles
I. Example: bantam chickens
   A. R (rose comb), r (single comb), B (black), b (white)
   B. The cross of a rose comb, black and a single comb, white produces only rose comb, black chickens (F_1 generation)
      1. RRBB × rrbb will produce only RrBb (the F_1 generation)
      2. If two of the F_1 generation are crossed, they will produce the ratio of approximately 9 rose comb, black : 3 rose comb, white : 3 single, black : 1 single, white

		RrBb			
		RB	Rb	rB	rb
	RB	RRBB	RRBb	RrBB	RrBb
	Rb	RRBb	RRBb	RrBb	Rrbb
RrBb	rB	RrBB	RrBb	rrBB	rrBb
	rb	RrBb	Rrbb	rrBb	rrbb

C. The F_2 generation is produced from the breeding of the F_1 generation or RrBb × RrBb
D. This ratio is the standard ratio in any F_2 generation when two independent pair of alleles are involved
II. Variable expressivity—traits that show continuous variation
   A. Example: orange tabby cats that display the phenotype of light ginger to deep red in color
   B. Example: some dogs are 80% spotted and 20% white; other dogs of the same breed are 20% spotted and 80% white
III. Polygenic traits—traits that are due to the interaction of several gene pairs. Polygene inheritances produce phenotypes that vary quantitatively over a wide range
   A. Example: IQ, height, or eye color
   B. These traits are due to a polygenic effect or many genes acting collectively to produce variations
IV. Incomplete dominance or intermediate inheritance—a cross where both genes are expressed equally
   A. The heterozygote has a phenotype in between those of the homozygous dominant and homozygous recessive individual
   B. Example: roan cattle
      1. Roan cattle are produced by breeding a red shorthorn and a white shorthorn
         a. When these two colors are crossed they produce a red and white haired individual
   C. Other examples include merle color in collies, foxes, great danes, and sheepdogs that have a characteristic black/grey color
      1. The color is irregular blotches of dark pigment against a lighter background of the same pigment
V. Co-dominance: A cross where each allele makes a comparable contribution to the phenotype
   A. Example: human blood type AB. This blood grouping contains the antigen A and B equally
VI. Epistasis: a masking of one allele over the genes on another locus
   A. Epistasis is different than dominance, since epistasis masks independently inherited genes
   B. Example: black cats still carry tabby stripes. The stripes are visible at certain ages of development in specific lights. The striping is masked by the black color allele

C. Example: an agouti mouse (AACC) crossed with an albino mouse (aacc)
  1. A (agouti), a (nonagouti), C (full color), c (albino)
  2. (_) designates the dominant or recessive form of the gene
  3. The resulting F_1 generation is AaCc or an agouti mouse with full color
  4. If the F_1 generation is crossed, the F_2 generation consists of 16 animals in the following color combinations:
       9 A_C_, agouti
       3 A_cc, albino
       3 aaC_, nonagouti
       1 aacc, albino
D. In this case c, or the albino gene, masks any and all other pigment genes

X-LINKED INHERITANCE (ALSO CALLED SEX-LINKED INHERITANCE)

Definitions

I. Sex chromosomes
  A. Females have the designation XX, meaning two X chromosomes
  B. Males have the designation XY meaning one X chromosome and one Y chromosome
  C. When a male inherits an X-linked recessive allele, it is always expressed, since there is no corresponding allele (even though it is a single dose)
  D. Females must have X-linked recessive alleles to express the trait
  E. X-linked traits are usually passed from mothers to sons; fathers do not pass an X chromosome to their sons, thus only a Y chromosome is passed from father to son
  F. X-linked: the gene in question is located only on the X chromosome
  G. Autosomal: Refers to chromosomes not involved with sex determination

Identification of Autosomal or X-linked Genes

I. X-linked dominant familial characteristics
  A. A normal female will have two X-linked chromosomes and males have only one X-linked gene
  B. Since the X chromosome of the male is always transmitted to daughters, affected males will pass the trait to daughters but not to sons
  C. Carrier females are heterozygous for a recessive X-linked gene and therefore will pass it

on to 50% of their sons and 50% of their daughters (who will be normal but carriers)
  D. Example: color blindness in humans
II. X-linked recessive
  A. The disease appears in males whose mothers are unaffected but are heterozygous carriers of the mutant recessive allele
  B. Each son of a carrier female has a 1:1 chance of being affected
  C. An affected male never transmits the gene to his sons; however, he will transmit to all his daughters, who will be carriers
  D. Unaffected males never transmit the gene
III. Autosomal dominant
  A. Dominant alleles will transmit disease from one affected individual to their offspring; there will be no skipping of generations unless penetrance is reduced
  B. There will be approximately an equal number of each sex affected with the disease
  C. Fifty percent of the progeny of each affected individual will be affected (due to Aa × aa matings)
  D. The dominant allele will be transmitted by mother or father
IV. Autosomal recessive
  A. Parents and remote relatives of an affected individual will not be affected (often skips generations)
  B. In matings producing an affected offspring, approximately 25% of the progeny will be affected
  C. There should be an equal number of females and males with the defect or trait
  D. If both parents are affected, offspring will most likely be affected

Example X-linked Heredity in Cats

I. The tortoiseshell pattern in cats is an example of X-linked genetics
II. There are very few male tortoiseshell cats; nearly all tortoiseshell cats are female
III. G symbolizes the ginger or orange coat color, which is carried on the X chromosome
IV. Male cats have only one X chromosome, so their genotype can be only G (yellow) or g (nonyellow)
V. Female cats have two X chromosomes; therefore females can be three genotypes
  A. GG (yellow), Gg (tortoiseshell), or gg (nonyellow)

VI. Therefore the tortoiseshell is heterozygous and has a unique coat color

VII. The color variation is due to the influence of both the G and g gene in different parts of the animal at the same time

VIII. The important point to remember is that a male can transmit only one gene (G or g) in 50% of the gamete; the other 50% carries a Y chromosome that does not possess a G locus

| | | Gametes from tortoiseshell female Gg | |
		X_G	X_g
Gametes from yellow male GY	X_G	$X_G X_G$ Yellow female	$X_G X_g$ Tortoiseshell female
	Y	$X_G Y$ Yellow male	$X_g Y$ Black male

BREEDING GENETICS ▰▰▰▰▰

I. Definitions

A. Pedigree chart: a chart that shows the ancestry of a particular family

1. Specific symbols are used to designate different individual characteristics

a. Open symbols indicate the individual does not possess the trait

b. Solid symbols indicate the presence of a trait under study or an individual having the trait

c. Half of a solid symbol indicates the individual is a carrier of the trait

d. Male—symbolized by a square

e. Female—symbolized by a circle

f. Unknown sex—symbolized by a diamond

g. A number in the symbol indicates the number of individuals

h. Two symbols joined by a line means marriage or mating

2. By constructing a pedigree, recessive allele carriers may be identified and eventually culled from the stock, depending on the trait in question

II. Test cross: This cross is used to determine the genotype of a particular phenotype

A. Usually the unknown phenotype is crossed with a homozygous recessive individual

B. Example: is a black Doberman pinscher phenotype of BB or Bb?

1. The genotype B represents black color and the genotype b represents brown color

2. The cross will be B _ × bb (a homozygous recessive individual)

3. If the dog is Bb, the cross will produce 50% bb (brown Dobermans) and 50% Bb (black Dobermans)

4. If the dog is BB all of the offspring will be black or Bb

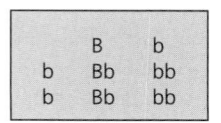

	B	b
b	Bb	bb
b	Bb	bb

III. Heterosis, or hybrid vigor

A. An F_1 generation is produced by crossing two different inbred strains

B. Heterosis usually results in increases in size and weight gain; reproductive ability and resistance to disease are also increased

C. Two individuals from the F_1 generation cannot be bred, since this breeding will produce variables in the phenotype

IV. Outbreeding, or random breeding: This type of breeding is considered to keep the gene pool as large as possible; matings to other strains maintain an increasing amount of heterozygous genes

A. This type of breeding keeps all fitness traits such as resistance to disease at high levels

B. In general, this type of breeding is between two animals who are unrelated

V. Back cross: the pairing of an F_1 generation hybrid with an organism whose genotype is identical to the parental strain

VI. Inbreeding: breeding together of closely related individuals to produce ever increasing similarities in the offspring

A. This breeding will produce as many homozygote individuals as possible

B. Advantages: the breeding will be "true" and it is possible to fix mutant alleles into a line or strain of animals

C. Disadvantage: recessive alleles may be revealed, such as lethal genes

VII. Line breeding: breeding of related individuals to guarantee similar traits in the offspring

A. Types
   1. Brother × half sister
   2. Parent × offspring
VIII. Inbreeding depression: relates to traits of fitness such as early growth, resistance to disease, or fertility, which are all multifunctional traits
   A. If an individual becomes homozygous, inbreeding depression occurs
   B. To reduce inbreeding depression
      1. Inbreed slowly and be stringent in selection of mating
      2. Do not breed poor phenotypes
   C. If inbreeding depression occurs
      1. Introduce a new sire or male with as many desirable traits as possible
      2. Outcross within your population to minimize inbreeding
      3. Always select healthy animals with good reproductive ability
IX. Harem mating: a mating where one male is mated to five females
   A. Generally used in some lab animal colonies

CHROMOSOMAL ABNORMALITIES

Definitions

A. **Translocation:** the breakage of two chromosomes, resulting in repair in an abnormal arrangement
B. **Deletion:** a part or all of a chromosome is missing
C. **Duplication:** an allele is duplicated, for example, human Trisomy 21 or Down's syndrome—there are three chromosomes rather than two at location 21 in the karyotype
D. **Anomalies:** deviations from normal
   1. There are many examples of anomalies in small animal breeding
   2. Examples: malocclusions, hip dysplasia, collie eye, Perthe's disease, hemophilia, diabetes mellitus, microphthalmia, deafness, entropion or dwarfism

Lethal Genes

A gene that will cause the death of the embryo or cause serious impairment or death sometime after birth (sometimes called a delayed lethal)
A. A semilethal gene causes the individual to have abnormal traits
B. A lethal gene is expressed as a homozygous recessive, usually in the F_2 generation
C. The genotype will be in the ratio of 1:2 instead of 1:2:1 (one individual will die)
D. A dominant lethal gene is usually expressed only once and cannot be proven to be inherited genetically

	M	m
M	MM	Mm
m	Mm	mm

   1. However there are some dominant disorders in which the individual is only impaired and is still able to reproduce
   2. Example: achondroplasia (dwarfism)
E. Most lethal genes are recessive
F. An incomplete dominance lethal gene: homozygous dominant individuals will die but heterozygous individuals will show clinical signs, such as the manx cat and many human lethal genes
   1. Example: Manx cat
   2. MM (lethal), Mn (tailless or Manx), mm (normal tail)
   3. The resulting ratio of the cross Mm × Mm is 25% of the kittens will die (MM), 50% will be the genotype Manx (Mm), and 25% will have genotype normal tail (mm)

Glossary

agouti Brown/grey coat color found in mice and wolves
allele An alternate form of a gene at the same site on a chromosome that determines different traits in an individual. Alleles may code for the same or for alternate forms of the trait
autosomal Used to describe nonsex chromosomes
back cross Pairing of an F_1 generation hybrid with an organism whose genotype is identical to the parental strain
chromosome Contains DNA (deoxyribonucleic acid), which transfers genetic information
codominance: A cross where each allele makes a comparable contribution to the phenotype
dihybrid cross The crossing of two traits
diploid Two copies of a chromosome in each cell or nucleus
dominant gene A gene that produces an effect in an organism regardless of the corresponding allele. A dominant gene masks or suppresses the expression of its corresponding allele. The dominant allele is usually written as a capital 22letter
epistasis A masking of one allele over the genes on another locus
F_1, F_2 Family or familial generation
gene A unit of inheritance
genetics The study of similarities and differences that are passed from parent to offspring
genotype The genetic makeup of an individual
haploid Having one copy of each chromosome per cell or nucleus

harem mating A mating where one male is mated to five females

heterosis Same as hybrid vigor; a cross performed to produce a better quality genotype and phenotype

heterozygous Different alleles, for example, Bb

homozygous Identical alleles, for example, BB

hybrid Offspring that are different than the parents

inbreeding Mating of closely related individuals to produce ever increasing similarities in the offspring

inbreeding depression Relates to traits of fitness such as early growth, resistance to disease, or fertility, which are multifunctional traits

incomplete dominance A cross in which both genes are expressed equally

intermediate inheritance The same as incomplete dominance

karyotype A photomicrograph of a single cell in the metaphase stage (meiosis) of division that displays chromosomes in descending order and describes the number and morphology of the chromosomes. It is similar to a blueprint or fingerprint. Karyotype is also called diploid chromosome complement

lethal gene A gene that will cause the death of the embryo or cause serious impairment or death sometime after birth

line breeding Breeding of related individuals to guarantee similar traits in the offspring

locus Specific site or location of a gene on a chromosome

meiosis Sex cell division that results in haploid cells and independent assortment of chromosomes

mitosis A method of cell replication that creates cells identical to the parent cells

monohybrid cross The crossing of one trait

outbreeding Same as random breeding; matings to other strains to increase the amount of heterozygous genes

pedigree chart A chart that shows the ancestry of a particular family

penetrance Refers to the appearance in the phenotype of traits determined by the genotype

phenotype Physical characteristics of an individual and/or performance of an individual that is expressed

polygenic traits Traits that are due to the interaction of several gene pairs

Punnett square A chart used by geneticists to show possible outcomes of specific breeding. Also called a checkerboard

recessive gene A gene that produces an effect only when it is inherited from both parents. Usually written in small case letters

sex chromosomes X and Y chromosomes determine the genetic sex of the individual

test cross A cross performed to determine the genotype of a particular phenotype

variable expressivity Traits that show continuous variation

Review Questions

1 A hybrid is:
   a. An offspring that is different from the parents
   b. An offspring that is identical to the parents
   c. A cross between genetically identical parents
   d. A cross between physically identical parents

2 The cross between a black doberman pincher (BB) and a red Doberman pincher (rr) would yield:
   a. Homozygous red Doberman pinchers
   b. Two homozygous red Doberman pinchers and two black heterozygous Doberman pinchers
   c. Heterozygous black Doberman pinchers
   d. Two heterozygous red Doberman pinchers and one black heterozygous Doberman pincher

3 The Manx cat is considered to be an example of:
   a. Translocation of chromosomes
   b. The expression of a lethal gene
   c. A sex-linked anomaly
   d. A homozygous individual

4 Suppose that gene b is sex-linked, recessive, and lethal. A dog is mated to a bitch who is heterozygous for this gene. If this mating produces normal offspring, what would the predicted sex ratio of the offspring be?
   a. 2 female : 1 male
   b. 2 male : 2 female
   c. 2 male : 1 female
   d. None of the offspring would survive

5 A homozygous animal with progressive retinal atrophy is mated to a heterozygote carrier. What is this breeding called?
   a. Inbreeding
   b. Heterosis
   c. Test cross
   d. Back cross

6 Hen-feathered (H), in fowl, is dominant to cock-feather (h). Hen feather is expressed in both sexes but cock-feathering is sex-limited to the male. What ratios of feather pattern would be expected among the offspring of a cock and hen both heterozygous for hen-feather?
   a. Male offspring: 3 hen-feathered : 1 cock-feathered
      Female offspring: all hen-feathered
   b. Male offspring: 4 hen-feathered
      Female: 4 hen-feathered
   c. Male offspring: 3 cock-feathered : 1 hen-feathered
      Female offspring: all cock feathered
   d. Male offspring: 4 cock-feathered
      Female offspring: 4 hen-feathered

7 A dominant X-linked gene, *B*, in the mouse, results in a short, crooked tail; its recessive allele, *b*, represents a normal tail. If a normal-tailed female is mated to a bent-tailed male, what phenotypic ratio should occur in F$_1$?
   a. 3 bent tail females : 1 normal tail male
   b. All mice will have a bent tail
   c. 2 normal tail female : 2 bent tail male
   d. 2 bent tail female : 2 normal tail male

8 A karyotype is a picture of chromosomes:
   a. In mitosis phase of division
   b. In meiosis phase of division
   c. In metaphase of meiosis
   d. In metaphase of mitosis
9 Are all genes always expressed?
   a. Yes
   b. No, the range of penetrance is variable
   c. Yes, to some degree
   d. No, some traits are polygenic and therefore require specific partners to express a phenotype
10 Tortoiseshell cats are usually females due to:
   a. Autosomal inheritance
   b. X-linked inheritance
   c. Polygenic inheritance
   d. Chromosomal abnormalities

BIBLIOGRAPHY

Hutt FB: *Genetics for dog breeders,* San Francisco, 1979, W.H. Freeman & Co.

Nicholas FW: *Veterinary genetics,* Oxford, 1987, Clarendon Press.

Robinson R: *Genetics for cat breeders,* Oxford, 1973, Pergamon Press.

Tamarin R: *Principles of Genetics,* ed 3, Dubuque, Iowa, 1991, Wm. C. Brown.

West G, editor: *Black's veterinary dictionary,* ed 16, New Jersey, 1988, Barnes & Noble Books.

CHAPTER 3

Breeding, Reproduction, and Neonatal Care

Betty Gregan

OUTLINE

Feline
  Puberty
  Semen Characteristics
  Estrous Cycle
  Signs of Estrus
  Gestation/Parturition
  Pregnancy Diagnosis
  Neonatal Care
Canine
  Puberty
  Semen Characteristics
  Estrous Cycle
  Gestation/Parturition
  Pregnancy Diagnosis
  Neonatal Care
Equine
  Puberty
  Semen Characteristics
  Estrous Cycle

Signs of Estrus
Gestation/Parturition
Pregnancy Diagnosis
Neonatal Care
Bovine
  Puberty
  Semen Characteristics
  Estrous Cycle
  Signs of Estrus
  Gestation/Parturition
  Pregnancy Diagnosis
  Neonatal Care
Caprine
  Puberty
  Semen Characteristics
  Estrous Cycle
  Signs of Estrus
  Gestation/Parturition

Pregnancy Diagnosis
Neonatal Care
Ovine
  Puberty
  Semen Characteristics
  Estrous Cycle
  Signs of Estrus
  Gestation/Parturition
  Pregnancy Diagnosis
  Neonatal Care
Porcine
  Puberty
  Semen Characteristics
  Estrous Cycle
  Signs of Estrus
  Gestation/Parturition
  Pregnancy Diagnosis
  Neonatal Care

LEARNING OUTCOMES

After reading this chapter you should be able to:

1. Define the basic reproductive characteristics in the bovine, canine, caprine, equine, feline, ovine, and porcine.
2. Define the nursing requirements of a neonatal bovine, canine, caprine, equine, feline, ovine, and porcine.

This chapter briefly describes the reproductive cycles of small and large animals. It includes information such as puberty onset, estrous cycles, semen evaluation, gestation/parturition, and pregnancy diagnosis. Also included under each species heading is a small section on neonatal care.

FELINE

Puberty

  I. Queen
    A. Average age 5 to 9 months
    B. Long-haired cats reach puberty later than short-haired breeds

II. Tom
   A. Sexual maturity about 9 months

Semen Characteristics

I. Volume: 0.01 to 0.7 mL
II. Concentration: 50 to 60 million/mL
III. Motility: 80% progressively motile

Estrous Cycle

I. First estrous cycle is usually around 9 months
II. Polyestrus
III. Estrus periods may last 3 to 6 days although they may last up to 10 days if mating does not occur
IV. Ovulation is not spontaneous; it is "induced" or "reflex"
V. Ovulation occurs only when a cat is mated or the cervix is stimulated by an instrument such as a glass rod
VI. Ovulation can be induced by treatments of hCG, LH, or GnRH

Signs of Estrus

I. Vocalization
II. Crouching and rolling on the floor, called "lordosis"
III. Tail deflection

Gestation/Parturition

I. Gestation is approximately 63 days
II. Zonary placentation
III. Mammary gland develops during the last week
IV. Last day or two, milk can usually be expressed from the nipples
V. First stage of parturition
   A. Restlessness
   B. Vocalization
   C. Nesting behavior

Pregnancy Diagnosis

I. Abdominal palpation: 3 to 4 weeks postbreeding
II. Ultrasound
   A. 11 to 16 days gestational sacs
   B. 16 to 32 days fetal heartbeats
   C. 21 days postbreeding
III. Radiographs: 45 day gestation

Neonatal Care

I. Temperature: 38 to 39°C (100-102°F), pulse: 140 to 170/min., respiration: 30 to 50/min.
II. Tomcats should be kept away from kittens
III. Handfed kittens should be fed 15% to 20% of their body weight divided into three daily feedings

CANINE ▬▬▬▬▬▬▬▬
Puberty

I. Bitch
   A. Average 8 months
   B. Puberty varies by breed and size from 6 to 18 months of age
   C. Smaller breeds reach puberty earlier than larger breeds
   D. The bitch should not be bred during her first estrus—she may be sexually mature but not as yet anatomically mature
II. Dog
   A. Approximately 9 months

Semen Characteristics

I. Volume: total volume about 20 mL but may vary from as little as 2 mL to 60 mL
II. Concentration: 200 to 3000 $\times$ 10^6/ejaculate
III. Motility: 60% to 90% motile sperm

Estrous Cycle

I. Nonseasonal
II. Phases of estrous cycle
   A. Proestrus: usually lasts 5 to 9 days
      1. Hemorrhagic vulvar discharge
      2. Vulva is swollen
   B. Estrus: usually lasts about 9 days
      1. Receptive to the male
      2. Usually ovulates 24 to 48 hours after the LH surge
      3. Clear serous discharge
   C. Metestrus: average 90 days
      1. Occurs in unmated bitches
   D. Anestrus: sexual inactivity between cycles
III. Signs of estrus
   A. Clear serous discharge
   B. Receptive to male

Gestation/Parturition

I. Average gestation 63 days
II. Zonary placentation
III. Drop in body temperature to less than 37°C (98.6°F) when parturition is imminent
IV. At 12 to 24 hours before whelping, milk can normally be expressed
V. Produce colostrum for up to 3 days
VI. First stage parturition
   A. Nervous anorexia
   B. May vomit occasionally
   C. Decrease in body temperature (other animals have elevated body temperatures)

VII. Dark green discharge the first 12 to 24 hours after parturition

Pregnancy Diagnosis

I. Abdominal palpation: 3 to 4 weeks postbreeding
II. Ultrasound: 24 to 28 days postbreeding
III. Transabdominal ultrasound: 24 to 28 days postbreeding

Neonatal Care

I. Temperature: 38 to 39°C (100-102°F), pulse: 120 to 150/min., respiration: 25 to 50/min.
II. Should be suckling by 3 hours post whelping to receive optimum amounts of colostrum
III. Pups can be handfed three times a day
IV. Newborns can take 10 to 20 mL/feeding, depending on the breed

EQUINE ▬▬▬▬▬▬▬▬▬▬▬▬▬
Puberty

I. Mare
   A. Approximately 12 months
   B. Low energy intake may delay puberty
II. Stallion
   A. Seldom used for breeding before 2 years of age
   B. Approximately 12 to 18 months
   C. Libido decreases during winter months

Semen Characteristics

I. Volume: gel free, volumes vary from 20 to 250 mL/ejaculate
II. Concentration: 30 to 600 million/mL; average 120 million/mL
III. Motility: at least 60% progressively motile sperm is desirable

Estrous Cycle

I. Generally seasonally polyestrus
II. Estrus activity can be induced by increasing the exposure to light (natural or artificial)
III. Estrous cycle is usually 21 to 22 days with estrus being 5 to 6 days
IV. Estrus cycle is divided into two phases
   A. Follicular phase: 5 to 6 days
   B. Luteal phase: about 16 days
V. Most ovulate 1 to 2 days before the end of estrus
VI. Approximately 9 days postfoaling, mares will have a fertile heat, also called "foal heat"

Signs of Estrus

I. Squatting, vulvar winking, raising tail, and urination

II. Usually show signs only in presence of a stallion

Gestation/Parturition

I. Gestation length is around 336 days (11 months)
II. Diffuse and microcotyledonary placentation
III. Corpus luteum maintains pregnancy 90 to 100 days, then the placenta produces progesterone
IV. Waxing of teats and possible discharge of milk
V. First stage of parturition
   A. Pacing in stall
   B. Abdominal discomfort
   C. Sweating
   D. Pawing

Pregnancy Diagnosis

I. Rectal palpation
II. Transrectal ultrasound: as early as 14 days postbreeding
III. Progesterone assay: 18 to 21 days postbreeding
IV. Estrone sulfate: after 80 days postbreeding

Neonatal Care

I. The foal should be standing and suckling within 3 hours
II. If not suckling by 4 to 5 hours, colostrum should be administered 250 to 500 mL
III. Physical examination of the foal
IV. Navel should be dipped with 7% tincture of iodine several times
V. A blood sample should be taken at 18 to 24 hours of age to measure IgG to make sure there is sufficient immunoglobulin absorption
VI. Temperature: 37.5 to 38.5°C (99.5-101°F), pulse: 80 to 120/min., respiration: 14 to 15/min.

BOVINE ▬▬▬▬▬▬▬▬▬▬▬▬▬
Puberty

I. Heifer
   A. Approximately 9 to 10 months
   B. Age of puberty is directly related to body weight
   C. Breed heifer at 15 months of age or 1000 lbs of body weight
   D. A female is not called a "cow" until she drops her first calf, at approximately 2 years of age
II. Bull
   A. Scrotal circumference is correlated with fertility

Semen Characteristics

I. Volume: 2 to 15 mL
II. Concentration: 300 to 2500 million spermatozoa/mL
III. Motility: rapid vigorous wave motion

Estrous Cycle

I. 21 day estrous cycle
II. Estrus 18 to 24 hours
III. Ovulates 10 to 11 hours after the end of estrus, unlike other farm animals who all ovulate during estrus
IV. Breeding should occur approximately 12 hours after the first signs of estrus or standing heat
V. Metestral bleeding occurs about 24 hours after ovulation

Signs of Estrus

I. Stands still while being mounted by other cows
II. Bawling
III. Clear mucus discharge from the vulva (bull stringing)

Gestation/Parturition

I. Gestation 278 days (9 months)
II. Cotyledonary placentation: a combination of maternal caruncles and fetal cotyledons
III. Four to five days before calving a clear mucus discharge from the vulva can be seen
IV. Vulva enlarges the last week of gestation and sacrosciatic ligaments relax and cause the gluteal muscles to sink

Pregnancy Diagnosis

I. Rectal palpation: 30 to 40 days postbreeding
II. Progesterone assay: 19 to 24 days postbreeding
III. Rectal ultrasound: after 25 days postbreeding
IV. Abdominal ballottement: after 5 months postbreeding

Neonatal Care

I. Temperature: 37.5 to 39.5°C (99.5-103°F), pulse: 100 to 150/min., respiration: 30 to 60/min.
II. Clear mucus from the upper airway
III. Sneezing can be stimulated by tickling the nostrils with straw
IV. Calf should be suckling 2 to 5 hours after birth
V. Colostrum may be administered if calf has not suckled (5%-8% of its body weight)
VI. Dip umbilical stump in tincture of iodine to prevent navel ill or omphalitis

CAPRINE

Puberty

I. Doe
  A. Average age 6 to 7 months (pygmy goats could reach puberty as early as 3 months)
II. Buck
  A. Fertile at 6 to 7 months

Semen Characteristics

I. Volume: low, approximately 1 mL/ejaculate
II. Concentration: very high
III. Motility: swirling masses of spermatozoa are seen
  A. This swirling mass is called the wave motion

Estrous Cycle

I. Estrous cycle is approximately 21 days and is divided into two phases
  A. Follicular phase: 3 to 4 days
  B. Luteal phase: 17 days
II. Estrus (heat) is 30 to 40 hours and ovulation occurs near the end of estrus
III. Optimal breeding time is 12 to 24 hours after the onset of estrus
IV. Seasonally polyestrous
  A. Estrous cycle is limited to the fall and winter under natural conditions
  B. Manipulations of light cycles offers year-round breeding capability of does and bucks

Signs of Estrus

I. Restlessness
II. Vocalization
III. Rapid tail wagging
IV. A "buck jar": jar containing a rag that has been rubbed on the scent glands of the buck's horns; may be used to enhance the signs of estrus

Gestation/Parturition

I. Gestation length: 149 days
II. Maintenance of pregnancy depends on luteal progesterone rather than placental progesterone
III. Cotyledonary placentation

Pregnancy Diagnosis

I. Progesterone assay: 21 days postbreeding
  A. Serum should be used instead of milk (milk gives false negatives)
II. Estrone sulphate: 50 or more days postbreeding
III. External transabdominal ultrasound: 40 or more days postbreeding

Neonatal Care

I. Temperature: 38.5 to 40.5°C (101-105°F), pulse: 80 to 120/min., respiration: 12 to 20/min.

II. The umbilicus should be dipped several times in 7% tincture of iodine

OVINE

Puberty

I. Ewe
  A. Average age 6 to 7 months
  B. Minimum of 60% of their adult body weight
  C. Nutrition is important in puberty
  D. Mutton breeds tend to reach puberty earlier than wool breeds
  E. Age of puberty in ewes can be influenced by selecting a ram with a large scrotal circumference

II. Ram
  A. Fertile as early as 7.5 to 9 months, but should not be considered to have adult capacity until they are at least 2 years old

Semen Characteristics

I. Volume: low, approximately 1 mL/ejaculate

II. Concentration: very high

III. Motility: swirling masses of spermatozoa are seen and are called the wave motion

Estrous Cycle

I. Estrous cycle is approximately 17 days long and is divided into two phases
  A. Follicular phase (3-4 days)
  B. Luteal phase (13 days)

II. Estrus (heat) is 10 to 30 hours and ovulation occurs near the end of estrus

III. Optimal breeding time is 12 to 18 hours after the first signs of estrus

IV. Ewes tend to cycle only during periods of short daylight; breeding season is usually from September to December
  A. Most breeds of sheep are seasonally polyestrous; they undergo a series of estrous cycles only during the fall

V. Shortly before or at the onset of breeding season, a ram is introduced to the ewes and the ewes will begin cycling 5 to 6 days later. This is known as the "Whitten effect"

Signs of Estrus

I. Ewes will seek out the ram and remain immobile while being investigated

II. Tail wagging

III. Without a ram present, it is almost impossible to tell if a ewe is cycling

Gestation/Parturition

I. Gestation length 145-155 days (5 months)

II. Nutrition should be increased by 50% in the last trimester

III. First third of pregnancy depends on the corpus luteum for progesterone; after 50 days progesterone is mainly produced by the placenta

IV. Cotyledonary placentation

V. Mammary development the last 2 weeks of gestation

VI. Colostrum can be expressed 2 to 3 days before lambing

VII. Body temperature drops 0.5°C (1-2°F) during the last 48 hours

VIII. Signs of the first stage of parturition
  A. Restlessness
  B. Decreased appetite
  C. Swollen vulva

Pregnancy Diagnosis

I. Use a teaser ram (castrated male) to detect ewes returning to estrus

II. Progesterone assay: 17 to 18 days postbreeding

III. Rectal ultrasound: 30 or more days postbreeding

IV. External transabdominal ultrasound: 40 or more days postbreeding

V. Estrone sulphate: 50 or more days postbreeding

Neonatal Care

I. Temperature: 37.5 to 39.5°C (99.5-103°F), pulse: 100 to 150/min., respiration: 30 to 60/min.

II. Lambs should be given a complete physical examination

III. Common defects are
  A. Cleft palate
  B. Umbilical herniation
  C. Entropion

IV. The umbilicus should be dipped in 7% tincture of iodine

V. If lambs have not suckled within 3 hours after being born they should be given 30 mL of colostrum

PORCINE

Puberty

I. Sows
  A. Gilts normally reach puberty around 250 pounds (114 kg) or about 200 days (6-7 months) in most breeds

II. Boars
  A. Reach puberty about 5 to 7 months
  B. They are mature about 2 years of age

Semen Characteristics

I. Volume: 8 to 12 months of age, 150 mL ejaculate
II. Older boars 250 mL of ejaculate
III. Concentration: 150×10^6/mL
IV. Motility: 70% to 90% progressively motile sperm

Estrous Cycle

I. Polyestrus
II. Estrus cycle is approximately 21 days in duration
III. Standing estrus 48 to 55 hours
IV. Return to estrus 4 to 7 days after weaning
V. Should be bred 24 hours after the onset of estrus and every 24 hours
VI. Gilts should be bred 12 hours after the onset of estrus and repeated at 12 hour intervals

Signs of Estrus

I. Vulvar swelling
II. Restlessness
III. Alertness
IV. Receptivity to the boar
V. Stationary stance (apply moderate pressure over the loin area with the flat of your hand)

Gestation/Parturition

I. Length of gestation: 114 days (3 months, 3 weeks, 3 days)
II. Diffuse placentation
III. Main source of progesterone is from the corpus luteum
IV. Abdominal and mammary development as early as 2.5 months gestation
V. Three to four hours before parturition sows become restless and attempt to nest
VI. Respiratory rate peaks about 6 hours before birth of the first piglet

Pregnancy Diagnosis

I. Teasing sow 18 to 24 days postbreeding
II. Ultrasound 23 days postbreeding
III. Progesterone assay: 17 to 20 days postbreeding
IV. Estrone sulphate: 25 to 29 days postbreeding

Neonatal Care

I. Temperature: 36.8 to 39°C (98-102°F), pulse: 200 to 250/min., respiration: 50 to 60/min.
II. Piglets should be placed under a heat lamp and kept warm until all piglets are born; then all are placed with the dam to suckle
III. Usually weaned at 3 to 5 weeks of age

IV. Dip umbilicus in 7% tincture of iodine
V. Clip needle teeth
VI. Notch ears
VII. 1.0 mL injection of iron dextran
VIII. Castrate young boars not being retained for breeding
IX. Dock tails

Glossary

abdominal ballottement Palpation of the fetal head by pushing the fist or fingertips into the abdominal wall, causing the fetus to move away from and then return to the fist or fingers

colostrum Immunoglobulin-rich milk secreted from the mammary gland shortly after parturition; "first milk"

corpus luteum Formed in the ovary after ovulation and produces progesterone

cotyledonary placentation Attachment of fetal membranes to the endometrium occurring only at projections from the endometrium, as in ruminants

diffuse placenta When attachment of the fetal membranes of the endometrium are continuous throughout the entire surface of the fetal membrane, as in the horse and pig

gestation Pregnancy

GnRH Gonadotropin releasing hormone, a type of hormone that causes gonads to mature to adult state

hCG Human chorionic gonadotropin, a hormone found in the urine after implantation of the ovum that is used to diagnose pregnancy

IgG Type of antibody in plasma that can cross placental barriers

monestrus Experiencing one estrus cycle each year

neonatal New born

ovulation Release of the egg (ovum) from the ovarian follicle

parturition The act of giving birth

polyestrous More than one estrus cycle in each year

puberty The physical stage at which sexual reproduction is possible

seasonally polyestrus Occurs in an animal that has several estrous cycles within a breeding season, followed by anestrus until the following breeding season, as in the cat

spermatozoa Sperm

whelping The birthing process

zonary placentation The fetus is attached to the endometrium by a band that encircles the placenta, as in the dog and cat

Review Questions

1 Piglets are normally weaned at the age of:
   a. 2-4 weeks
   b. 3-5 weeks
   c. 6-8 weeks
   d. 8-12 weeks

2 Colostrum is:
a. The immunoglobulin-rich milk secreted from the mammary gland shortly after parturition
b. Formed in the ovary after ovulation and produces progesterone
c. The act of artificial insemination
d. The period of ovulation

3 Which species is seasonally polyestrus?
a. Ovine
b. Porcine
c. Canine
d. Feline

4 The order of the stages of the estrous cycle are:
a. Estrus, anestrus, proestrus, metestrus
b. Estrus proestrus, anestrus, metestrus
c. Proestrus, anestrus, metestrus, estrus
d. Proestrus, estrus, metestrus, anestrus

5 The three main characteristics of semen evaluation are:
a. Volume, mobility, and characteristics
b. Volume, motility, and characteristics
c. Volume, motility, and concentration
d. Volume, parts per million, and concentration

6 In which animal is the age of puberty directly related to body weight?
a. Feline
b. Canine
c. Bovine
d. Caprine

7 Shortly before breeding season a ram is introduced to the ewes and the ewes will begin cycling 5 to 6 days later. This is known as the:
a. Whitten effect
b. Proestrus cycle
c. Breeding season
d. Optimum breeding time

8 On a radiograph, the skeleton of a canine fetus can first be noted at:
a. 45 days gestation
b. 30 days gestation
c. 10 days gestation
d. 62 days gestation

9 A boar is mature at approximately:
a. 2 years of age
b. 9 months of age
c. 1 year of age
d. 6 months of age

10 Scrotal circumference is correlated with fertility in which animal?
a. Dog
b. Bull
c. Tom
d. Ram

BIBLIOGRAPHY

Compendium of animal reproduction, ISBN Publisher, 1987, International B. V.

Christiansen IJ: *Reproduction in the dog and cat,* Toronto, W.B. Saunders.

Hafez ESE: *Reproduction in farm animals,* ed 5, Philadelphia, 1993, Lea & Febiger.

Lofstedt RM: *Reproductive physiology of the domestic species,* ed 1, P.E.I., 1987.

Lofstedt RM, Richardson GF: *A manual for theriogenology,* ed 6, P.E.I., U.P.E.I Audio Visual Services.

McKinnon, Voss: *Equine reproduction,* Philadelphia, 1993, Lea & Febiger.

Reece WO: *Physiology of domestic animals,* Philadelphia, 1991, Lea & Febiger.

West G, editor: *Black's veterinary dictionary,* ed 16, New Jersey, 1988, Barnes & Noble Books.

CHAPTER 4

Restraint and Handling

Teresa Sonsthagen

OUTLINE

Canine Restraint
    Danger Potential
    Behavioral Characteristics
    Considerations for Restraint
    Restraint Equipment
Feline Restraint
    Danger Potential
    Behavioral Characteristics
    Considerations for Restraint
    Restraint Equipment
Horse Restraint
    Danger Potential
    Behavioral Characteristics
    Approaching a Horse
    Capturing a Horse

Leading a Horse
Tying
Restraint for General Examinations
Restraint for Dental Procedures
Distraction Techniques
Tail Tie
Picking up Feet
Foals
Cattle Restraint
    Danger Potential
    Behavioral Characteristics
    Restraint
Sheep Restraint
    Danger Potential

Behavioral Characteristics
Anatomy/Physiology
Restraint
Goat Restraint
    Danger Potential
    Behavioral Characteristics
    Anatomy
    Restraint
Porcine Restraint
    Danger Potential
    Behavioral Characteristics
    Anatomy/Physiology
    Restraint

LEARNING OUTCOMES

After reading this chapter you should be able to:

1. Know the danger potential of each species so that your safety is kept in mind when restraining successfully.
2. Predict the common behavioral characteristics so that the most successful method of restraint will be used.
3. Keep in mind the considerations of restraint so that the animal is handled safely and will recover as soon as possible after the restraint procedure.
4. Be comfortable with the restraint equipment available for the species and use the proper tool for the procedure.

This chapter will reacquaint you with some of the basic restraint techniques taught in most veterinary technology programs. Without good basic knowledge of behavior, safety measures, and proper restraint techniques the veterinary technician, veterinarian, and the owner could be injured by the patient or injury could occur to the patient. Restraint should be safe and firm, yet gentle. Restraint should be safe for the animal, safe for the person performing the restraint, and safe for the person performing the technique.

This chapter will cover the restraint of felines, canines, equines, bovines, ovines, caprines, and porcines and is designed to refresh your memory on how the basic restraint techniques are performed, how most animals behave, and some safety measures that should be used to ensure no one is injured. Restraint of rabbits and rodents will be covered in the laboratory animal section.

CANINE RESTRAINT

Danger Potential

I. Canine teeth are a main means of defense

II. Toenail scratches are painful but not usually serious

Behavioral Characteristics

I. Determined by breed, training, previous experiences, and human association

A. The normal dog is a well-cared-for social animal

1. The pet or working dog is recognized by a happy attitude

2. It has been taught definite social behaviors

3. Clients with new puppies should be advised on how to teach social behavior

4. About 90% clients will fall into this category

5. Canines are usually docile but can be pushed into biting

B. Nervous, frightened dogs are recognized by anxious expression, rapid head movement, white around eyes, grimacing, trembling lips, avoidance of eye contact, and shivering. They may cower or they may be boisterous

1. Let them come to you, never push them into a corner

2. Some nervous dogs nip out of excitement

3. Expect these dogs to bite

a. Approach them slowly, let them come to you

b. After they allow you to touch them, quickly restrain them

C. Vicious or aggressive dogs

1. Recognized by head held low, hackles raised, tail straight out

2. These dogs will stare at you. If they look away it usually means they have backed off; the best action on your part is to slowly back away. Avoid eye contact

3. Small and large dogs are capable of inflicting serious damage

a. Small dogs can be more aggressive than large but keep in mind that a large dog can cause more damage

4. Dogs will bite, especially if challenged

a. Challenge definition: looking the dog in the eye, body faced forward

b. To avoid challenging keep body sideways to the dog, look out the corner of your eye, and don't crouch

5. Dogs do not always exhibit aggressiveness; some will attack without warning

Considerations for Restraint

Look at the type of animal, behavior, and past treatment received from humans to determine what type of restraint will be needed. Keep in mind the following seven points while restraining:

I. Rough handling will always provoke retaliation; if pushed too far you will cause the animal to defend itself

A. Minimal restraint is sometimes the best restraint

II. If injured and in pain, a canine will usually be confused and disoriented, which makes determining its behavior unpredictable

A. Always **muzzle** these dogs; the exception is a dog with head injuries

1. Apply the muzzle tightly or not at all

2. The muzzle should not be left on longer than 20 minutes

B. Avoid putting pressure on injured area; pressure can cause more damage to the injured area or more pain, which in turn can cause the animal to go into shock

III. Aggression/hostility

A. Don't take chances with aggressive/hostile dogs; use restraint tools necessary to keep yourself safe. These tools include:

1. Capture poles or rabies stick

2. Gauntlets

3. Blanket if the dog is small

4. Doorways

IV. Fear and/or nervousness

A. Attempt to reason and soothe the dog but exercise caution

1. Use muzzles or rope leashes

2. Sometimes you have to sedate these animals before they are brought into the clinic

V. Old/young

A. Special care is required when dealing with the very old and the very young

1. Geriatric animals have to be handled with care and consideration

a. If hospitalized, they will miss human contact; visits by the owners should be encouraged

b. They are sensitive to stress

c. They are most likely arthritic so manipulation and pressure placed on joints can be very painful

d. Comfort measures such as a soothing voice, blankets or pads, and treats are a must

2. Puppies are difficult to hold onto because they are full of boundless energy and curiosity
   a. You must always maintain contact with them
   b. A fall from the examination table can cause fractures or dislocations
   c. When carrying them, keep a tight hold

VI. Pregnant animals should be treated the same as a geriatric patient
   A. Pregnant animals are prone to injury from increased weight, which puts pressure on hips, spine, and shoulders
   B. Pressure to the abdomen can be traumatic also and should be avoided
   C. Stress and physiological changes may cause the bitch to abort

VII. Pets that are dominant are usually difficult to handle if their owners are present, because the pets have not learned to be submissive to people
   A. Owners may be asked to leave the room
      1. Most dogs calm down because they don't know what to expect from strangers
      2. If the owner refuses to leave, explain that the dog will have to be muzzled to protect the staff and the owner and that a muzzle will also have a calming effect on the dog
   B. When the owner is not present and the dog is still misbehaving
      1. Speak to the dog in a commanding voice
      2. It may be necessary to rap it under the chin or use a choker collar
      3. Be firm, consistent, and very persistent in getting the dog to behave
      4. If the dog wins the first battle, you will lose the war

Restraint Equipment

I. Choker collars are used only as a restraint tool
   A. The correct use is to sharply snap the collar closed and then release
   B. If not placed on the neck correctly, pressure will not be released
   C. Don't pull and tug continuously on the choker collar because the dog will get used to the stimulus and not react
   D. Never use a choker collar as an everyday collar

1. Many animals have gotten caught on fences and have hanged themselves

II. Two types of leashes
   A. Leather leash should be at least 6 feet long
   B. Nylon, flat or round, rope leashes are made of soft material and are usually 4 to 5 feet in length. They have a sliding loop that will loosen when the standing part is released. They are used in several ways
      1. A nervous or vicious dog can be removed from a cage by using the rope leash
         a. A large noose is made and is flipped over the dog's head; pull the dog to the edge of the cage, keep the leash taut, grab a back leg, and quickly lower the dog to the floor
         b. Never just drag the dog out of the cage and let it drop to the floor; this can cause injury to the neck, back, and legs
      2. For vicious dogs, rope leashes can be used to crosstie them
         a. Two leashes are placed around the dog's neck and held taut in two different directions. This allows you to handle the back end for various procedures
   C. Chain or hard rope leashes will cause injuries to the hands
   D. Avoid allowing the animal to chew the leash

III. Capture pole or rabies pole is a long pole with a rope or covered wire protruding from the end to form a noose. The noose is slipped over the head
   A. Slide the noose in and out several times before using to make sure it is working correctly and can be quickly released in an emergency

IV. There are two types of muzzles
   A. The commercially prepared muzzle should be fitted to the dog at the store
   B. The gauze muzzle is a temporary muzzle constructed of roll gauze
      1. Tear off enough gauze to go around the nose of the dog twice and up behind the ears
      2. Make the first loop by tying a double loose overhand knot in the center of the gauze; quickly slip this loop over the dog's nose
      3. Crisscross the gauze under the muzzle

4. Bring the ends up behind the ears and tie with a bow
5. If the dog is a brachycephalic breed, like a boxer, tie the ends behind the ears with an overhand knot. Bring one end between the eyes, then under the loop around the nose, and tie to the other end in a bow, which will be between the eyes. This prevents the loops from slipping off
   a. This same method is used to muzzle cats

V. A harness works extremely well for small dogs
   A. They can't slip out of them
   B. If necessary you can lift them out of harm's way

VI. Fortunately, of all the animals we have to deal with the dog will respond the most to the human voice
   A. A soft crooning voice comforts and calms
   B. The tone should not be high pitched
      1. A high pitched voice tone simulates the dominant yelps and barks of littermates
   C. A sharp, commanding voice tone gets the dog's attention
      1. Avoid a yelling tone, which can frighten or cause aggression
   D. Always be consistent with your vocal tones

FELINE RESTRAINT

Danger Potential

Of all domestic animals, the cat is one of the most difficult to handle because of its agility and formidable weaponry

I. Teeth are capable of inflicting serious wounds that often become infected
II. Claws are razor sharp; all four feet can be used simultaneously and are the main means of defense

Behavioral Characteristics

I. Normal behavior
   A. Cats are aloof independent creatures; they are *not* pack animals and do not have the pack instinct like a dog
   B. They are, however, social animals and will live peacefully with an established pecking order in a group of cats
   C. They are highly intelligent and curious creatures
   D. Cats are extremely territorial and mark their territory by spraying urine and rubbing scent glands (found by the commissure of the lips

and at the base of the tail) on furniture, the boundaries of their yard, and the owner
      1. New places are thoroughly investigated; cats will explore everything and mark it as their territory
      2. When confined to a small space like a cage or small room a cat's first instinct is to escape
         a. If escape is impossible the cat will defend the area as its own territory
   E. Most cats are placid and friendly in general, especially if well treated

II. Depressed behavior
   A. A depressed cat may stop eating and drinking
   B. The cat may be depressed as a result of boarding or removal from a familiar environment
      1. Depression results from lack of freedom and interaction with people
   C. It may sit in the litter box or huddle in the corner under newspapers or a towel
   D. If depression continues, the cat can become weak and could turn hostile if pushed
   E. These cats can sometimes recover if handled gently and often

III. If hostile, pound for pound, cats are among the most fearsome animals alive
   A. Hostile cats are difficult to handle—they don't respond or submit to restraint, and if they escape they are very difficult to capture
   B. They will fight until they are too weak to fight anymore. You should handle these cats with restraint tools such as, gloves, towels, nets, or capture poles

Considerations for Restraint

Cats in general are not difficult to handle if you understand their actions. Observe each cat to determine the best method to use.

I. Begin with the least amount of restraint and become firmer as the situation demands
II. Don't begin restraint until all participants are ready to begin
III. Stay calm but firm and consistent with your voice and the restraint techniques chosen
IV. Make sure all doors and windows are locked. Cats can squeeze through very small openings and are extremely difficult to catch when they are on the floor and running
V. Cornered cats will attempt to escape and if unable to do so will fight

VI. Few cats attack without warning
  A. Attack signals include growling, crouching low, ears laid back, hissing, spitting, and batting with front paws
VII. If one is aware of the instinctive territorial trait, many problems can be avoided
  A. Allow the cat to leave its territory by walking out of the cage under its own power or quickly reach in with rope leash, capture pole, or gloved hands and remove it
VIII. Distraction techniques work very well on the cat, including inflicting mild pain to a certain area so the cat doesn't pay attention to what is going on elsewhere:
  A. "Caveman" pets, vigorous pats on the head or body
  B. Tapping or blowing on the nose
  C. Vigorous rubbing on top of the head

Restraint Equipment

  I. A rope leash as the one described in canine restraint is used in the same manner
    A. You occasionally capture one or both front legs, along with the neck
    B. The cat can slip out of this fairly easily
  II. A towel, pillowcase, or small blanket can be used to surround a hostile cat
  III. Gauntlets/gloves are made of thick leather that should cover your arms up to the elbow
    A. Disadvantages of gauntlets
      1. The loss of tactile sense, which may result in applying too much pressure
      2. They will not protect you from bites but do reduce the number of scratches you receive
    B. Use of gauntlets:
      1. Place your hand partially in one gauntlet
      2. Offer that hand to the cat while it is trying to bite or scratch
      3. Reach in with your other hand, fully encased in a gauntlet, and grab the animal by the scruff of the neck
  IV. Feline restraint bag (cat bag) is usually made of canvas or thick nylon. This bag completely encloses the body of the cat. The head is held in place and there are access zippers or Velcro strips to allow the legs to be brought out. Never leave the cat unattended
    A. Advantages to using a cat bag
      1. It usually has a calming effect; after a cat realizes it can't escape it will calm down
      2. The feet are taken out of action for use against you

  B. Disadvantages
    1. The cat can still bite
    2. You must be careful not to get the fur and skin caught in the zipper
    3. Large and/or angry cats are difficult to place into the bag
    4. The jugular vein is not easily accessible
    5. To prevent spread of disease and ectoparasites, the bag should be disinfected after each use
  V. If you are alone and need to do a simple/painless procedure, floral tape or Vet wrap works well to bind the legs together
    A. First tape front legs together; then tape rear legs together
    B. When removing tape do back legs first then front legs
    C. Never leave cat with legs bound like this alone on top of a table because they could roll off and severely injure themselves
    D. The use of adhesive tape could pull and remove hair
  VI. Muzzles such as leather/nylon or gauze muzzles work well and protect the handler from bites
    A. Reusable muzzles should be disinfected to prevent spread of respiratory diseases
  VII. An Elizabethan collar can also be effective

HORSE RESTRAINT
Danger Potential

  I. Rear feet
    A. The kicking range of the hind feet is 6 to 8 feet straight out with the furthest extension of the foot the most dangerous
    B. The aim is usually very accurate
    C. To pass behind a horse
      1. Stay at least 10 to 12 feet behind or to the side
      2. Stay in direct physical contact by placing a hand on the rump
  II. Front feet
    A. If a horse rears it can knock a person to the ground
    B. It can strike a handler's head and arms with or without rearing
  III. Teeth
    A. Front incisors can cause major injuries
    B. Discipline is a must if a horse bites

Behavioral Characteristics

  I. The horse is nervous and suspicious by nature. It is quick to detect threats and react to them in a manner that may be dangerous to humans

A. As part of its flight instinct, if suddenly frightened or hurt, reaction may include rearing, biting, kicking, or running away; all without obvious warning

B. Keep alert and never treat a horse complacently

C. Always move slowly and deliberately. Quick motions and loud noises will almost always frighten a horse into evasive action

II. Horses often show some warning signals that should be heeded to prevent possible injuries

III. The most expressive parts of a horse are the ears; however the tail, eyes, and mouth are also useful indicators of behavior

  A. Ears

    1. If the horse is alert, the ears are pricked forward

    2. If the horse is nervous or uncertain, the ears are constantly moving back and forth

    3. If the horse is angry or fearful, the ears are pinned back

    4. If the horse is concentrating, the ears are pinned back (out to the sides)

  B. Tail

    1. Nervousness is indicated by wringing or circling

    2. When in pain or sleeping the tail is straight down

    3. Fear is shown by the tail being clamped tight between gluteals

Approaching a Horse

I. Approach from the front and slightly to the left side

  A. Horses are accustomed to being handled from this near (left) side

  B. The right side is referred to as the far side

II. Move slowly without sudden movements or noise

  A. If the horse moves away, stop. If you do not stop the horse will think it's being chased and will flee

III. Talk to the horse and maybe offer it some grain

IV. Some horses will need to be put in a smaller pen in order to catch them

  A. Luring them into the pen with grain is a much better method than chasing them

V. When approaching a horse from the rear

  A. Begin talking to them before you get close. A startled horse may kick or jump forward and injure itself or you

Capturing a Horse

I. Check the halter and lead rope for splits or fraying

A. A horse can easily break a defective lead rope and/or halter

II. Slip the lead rope around the horse's neck and tie a single overhand knot to keep the rope from slipping off. Never release hold until the halter is placed on the horse

  A. Most horses will think they are caught and stand still

III. Hold the neck strap of the halter in the left hand, reach under the horse's neck and hold the head still so the right hand can bring the halter over the horse's neck

IV. Slide the nose band of the halter onto the nose and buckle the neck strap behind the ears

  A. Keep your movements slow and deliberate

V. Check to make sure the halter is settled correctly on the horse's face

VI. Attach the lead chain to the center ring of the halter under the chin

Leading a Horse

I. Always walk on the left side of the horse

II. Stay close to the shoulder

  A. Don't get too far in front of the horse because it can rear up and strike with a front foot or it can accidentally step on the back of your heels as it walks. It can also bite you on the shoulder or back

  B. When stopping, stand facing the same direction as the horse

III. Hold the lead rope with your right hand at the base of the halter

IV. The left hand should hold the loose end of the rope in neat loops with the entire rope held in front of you

  A. Never wrap the loose end of the lead rope around your hand

  B. Never have the rope loose behind you

Tying

I. A horse should always be tied to a sturdy, vertical object with a well fitting halter and suitable lead rope

II. The knot used to tie the lead rope should be a quick release knot such as the halter tie

  A. The horse can be released quickly if it gets into trouble

III. Allow about 2 to 3 feet of lead rope so it can adjust the angle of its neck and shift its position as it desires

  A. The horse may tangle its front feet in the rope if a longer rope is used

  B. A shorter rope may frustrate the horse enough to cause it to attempt to free itself

IV. Check the area around your tied horse for possible hazards that could cause serious injuries

V. Never pass under the neck of a tied horse to get to the other side. This is a very dangerous practice that could result in serious injuries if the horse is startled

Restraint for General Examinations

I. Stand on same side of horse as the person who is working on the animal

   A. By standing on the same side, the horse has the option of moving away from both of you to escape

     1. If there are people on both sides, the animal will pick the smallest of the barriers and try to move over that. Unfortunately, that may be a person bending or kneeling

II. Never stand directly in front of the horse

   A. It can rear up and come down on top of you

   B. It can strike out with its front feet

   C. It can run you over in an effort to escape

III. Hold head level with the withers. If held higher the horse has an advantage and can easily escape

IV. Cross tying

   A. Used to prevent a horse from rearing and from moving its forequarters from side to side

   B. The horse can still strike with its front feet and move its rear quarters

     1. Snap a lead rope onto the cheek piece ring on each side of the halter. Tie each lead rope to the side of the stanchion, to stocks, or beam

     2. Tie the ropes high enough to prevent the horse from rearing and entangling its feet in the ropes

     3. Use a quick release knot such as the halter tie or use a quick release buckle

V. Stocks

   A. A narrow stall with removable or semiopen sides and a gate at both ends

     1. Lead the horse through the back gate and close the front after it is in the stocks

     2. Do not go into the stocks with the horse; pass the rope around the bars as needed to keep the horse moving

VI. Blindfolds

   A. Can be used to control an obstinate horse

   B. The horse will usually calm down and depend on you to guide it wherever you want it to go

   C. Work slowly and talk constantly to reassure the horse

Restraint for Dental Procedures

I. Place your left hand on the bridge of the horse's nose with your thumb under the nose band of the halter and the right hand placed on the nape of the neck, push head down

II. To hold the tongue, reach in at the commissure of the lips, grasp the tongue, and slowly pull it out to the side through the bar (diastema) of the lower jaw

Distraction Techniques

I. Twitches

   A. Through the release of endorphins, which mask the pain, twitches are used to distract the horse from other procedures by applying a mild pain to the upper muzzle

   B. Of the three types (chain, humane, and rope) the chain is most common

     1. Place the loop of chain over your left hand, catching one side of the loop between your little finger and ring finger

     2. Grasp as much of the horse's upper lip with your left hand as possible, press the bottom edges together to protect the delicate inner surface, and quickly slide the handle up so the chain loop rests high up around the lip

     3. Tighten the chain by twisting the handle until the twitch is fitted snugly on the lip so lip curls upward

     4. Tighten and loosen the chain on the muzzle to keep the twitch effective. If steady pressure is applied the muzzle would lose circulation, thereby reducing sensitivity of the muzzle and rendering the twitch ineffective

     5. Many horses will attempt to get away or resist the twitch when it is first applied; stay with them by moving with their motions. If they shake you off the first time it will be more difficult to place the twitch again

     6. After the twitch is removed, massage the muzzle to restore circulation

   C. A humane twitch is a hinged pair of long handles that squeeze over the sides of the lip and then can be secured at the bottom

     1. Once applied it need not be held

     2. The pressure is mild and may be ignored by horses

II. Lead shank is a long leather strap with about 2 feet of flat chain attached to it with a snap on the end

   A. It is used as a distraction device, or if more restraint than just a halter is needed

B. There are several ways to use a chain shank
   1. With the halter in place, pass the chain end through the ring on the cheek piece
   2. Pull it across the bridge of the nose to the ring on the other side of the head
   3. Pull it under the jaw. This method is not ideal because this may cause the horse to throw its head up
   4. Place it under the top lip over the upper gum. This is very effective in directing the horse's attention away from other procedures, but it's painful and may inflict injury
   5. Put the chain in the mouth like the bit of a bridle and clip it to the ring on the other side
C. Be careful not to jerk excessively on the chain shank because injury may result

III. Eyelid press involves gently placing fingers on the upper eyelid and pressing down

IV. Shoulder roll is done by grasping a large fold of skin with both hands just over the shoulder and wiggling or moving it from side to side or up and down

V. "Caveman pets" or somewhat heavy swats

VI. Pick up or tie up the opposite foot from the one being radiographed or bandaged

VII. Grasp the base of the ear with the heel of your hand touching the head. Squeeze or rotate the ear in a small circle
A. It is best to use this only as a last resort
B. Do not apply so much pressure to the ear that damage occurs to the cartilage, which can result in the ear flopping over
   1. It may make the horse afraid to have its ears touched, which can cause the owner of a show animal a lot of frustration when the hair on the ears needs to be trimmed

VIII. A cradle is a device that is placed around a horse's neck to prevent it from chewing or licking at wounds; it prevents the horse from bending or turning the neck

Tail Tie

I. Always tie the tail to the animal's own body

II. Secure a cord or rope to the hair on the tail using a "sheet bend" or "tail tie" knot, which is a quick release knot

III. Pull the tail over the buttocks and pass the rope to the opposite front leg

IV. Use a quick release knot to secure the other part of the rope to the neck or front leg

Picking up Feet

I. Front feet
A. Stand lateral to the shoulder and parallel to the horse, facing the caudal end
B. Place one hand on the shoulder, gently but firmly running it down to the fetlock
C. Grasp the fetlock by placing your palm on the underside of the fetlock and wrapping your fingers around the joint
D. Squeeze and lift the foot; at the same time lean into the horse to make it shift its weight to the other three legs
E. After raising the foot up, bring it slightly out to the side. Position your body close to the horse's body so that your knees are slightly bent. Place the foot between your legs so it rests on top of your knees, allowing both hands to be free. Flex fetlock and hoof toward your self

II. Rear feet
A. Approach in the same manner as the front feet
B. After you have lifted the foot, extend the leg out to the rear and place it on top of your bent knee closest to the horse

Foals

I. Capture and restraint
A. Place the mother in a large box stall (the mare often needs to be restrained as well)
B. Grasp the foal around the front of the chest with one arm and around the rump with the other arm, or grasp the tail. Quickly move the foal clear of the dam
C. Use your arms to form a "mini corral" and keep the foal encircled with your arms
D. Do not lift the foal off its feet; this makes it very nervous and it will struggle
E. Keep the foal in sight of the mare
F. Always talk to and comfort a foal when handling it

CATTLE RESTRAINT
Danger Potential

I. Head
A. Horned animals can fatally gore a handler by quick thrusts sideways and forward
B. Be constantly aware of the swinging arc and the extent of reach from side to side and forward
C. Butting is done by polled and horned animals
   1. This can be a rushing motion, pinning you against a fence, wall, or ground

2. It can be a swing of the head, knocking you down
II. Body
  A. Cattle can pin restrainers against a wall (dairy cows in stanchions)
  B. The restrainer can be knocked against a fence or wall
III. Feet
  A. Front feet are seldom used as weapons
    1. Cattle do paw the ground
    2. The split toe can cause serious damage to human toes and feet
  B. Hind feet are very dangerous and very accurate
    1. Cattle usually kick by bringing the foot forward, arching out to the side and then backward (cow kicking)
    2. They can kick straight back, like a horse, but seldom do
    3. Usually kick one legged; not the two-legged kick like horses
  C. The safest place to stand is at the shoulder but remember a bovine can kick past its shoulder
IV. Tail
  A. The tail is useful to the bovine for swatting flies and for other twitches
  B. The tail is an annoyance and can cause injury to the restrainer's eyes during restraint procedures
    1. To prevent injury, remove awns or burrs by dipping the tail in mineral oil. Melt frozen ice and feces by dipping the tail in a warm bucket of water
  C. The tail is very fragile
    1. Never tie the tail to anything but the animal's body
V. Cattle seldom bite because they lack upper incisors
  A. If they do bite it is more of a pinch than a bite and is usually an accident

Behavioral Characteristics

Cattle differ markedly in their reactions to manipulations and the presence of humans as a result of the breed, handling, and gender.
I. Dairy cows are accustomed to being handled and are the most docile of the bovine breeds
  A. Restraint is usually done in stanchions or by tying to a fence. Talk to and treat dairy cows gently
  B. They may become nervous and vigorously resist handling if not treated gently
II. More so than any other animal, dairy bulls require special restraint techniques because they are extremely unpredictable
  A. If handled correctly, the unpredictability can be minimized
  B. Nose rings are often used in bulls for capturing and leading
    1. Do not tie the bull fast by the nose ring
III. Beef cows are easily frightened because of little association with people
  A. Restraint involves chutes (with head gates) and alley ways
IV. Beef bulls are handled the same as females; be careful around beef bulls when the females are in heat

Restraint

I. Approach
  A. Avoid quick movements so as not to startle the animals; use slow deliberate actions
  B. Talk to them so they are aware of your presence
    1. A low command to move is much preferred over sharp yelling
  C. Do not approach from the front because it is a natural instinct for cattle to charge. Cattle can not charge if they are in a squeeze chute and head gate or tied in a stanchion
    1. Remember they can still stretch their necks and butt you if you are too close
II. Head
  A. If using chutes, always check the operation of the chute before use
    1. Familiarize yourself with the operation
    2. Repair if necessary
  B. Rope halters are the basic tool of restraint
    1. The part that tightens is placed around the nose, with the loop down. The lead rope should be on the left side of the cow's head
    2. The head then can be tied to a post, fence, or part of the chute
    3. The position of the head is generally up and to the side
    4. Tie the end of the rope with a snubbing hitch or halter tie
  C. Cattle have a sensitive nasal septum that can be used to produce a mild pain that acts as a distraction technique. Pressure can be applied manually or with instruments
    1. Thumb and index finger can be used for very short periods of time (your fingers will tire quickly)

2. Nose leads (tongs) are commercially manufactured
   a. Make sure that the balls on the tongs are smooth
   b. Close tong handles together to adequately hold onto the nose without pinching too much
   c. Have a holder grasp the tongs or secure to halter
   D. Examination of eye requires the head to be rotated so that the afflicted eye is parallel with the ceiling
      1. This is usually accomplished with a halter or nose tong
   E. Passing a stomach tube requires application of a halter and a mouth speculum (such as a Frick's speculum) to hold the jaws apart while passing the stomach tube into the esophagus
      1. If the speculum is not used the cow may clamp down on the tube
III. Hobbles
   A. Used to prevent kicking
   B. Place on the back legs—the leg opposite you first then the one closest to you
      1. Keep the legs "square" so the cow can maintain its balance
IV. Feet and legs
   A. Examination of hind legs or trimming hooves can be performed
      1. Cast the cow in lateral recumbency by using the burley or double half hitch method
      2. A hydraulic lift table can be used to place in lateral recumbency
         a. Lead the animal in front of the table, strap on, and then lower the table to a lateral recumbency
      3. The legs can be raised by the use of ropes and pulleys also
V. Tail
   A. "Jacking" the tail up acts as a distraction technique
      1. This relaxes the animal as it ignores manipulation elsewhere
      2. Make sure that the animal is secured
   B. The jacking should not be done for more than a few minutes because fracture of coccygeal vertebrae is possible if done improperly
VI. Flank restraint
   A. A lariat can be tightened around the flank area just cranial to the tuber coxae to prevent kicking. Avoid excess pressure; otherwise the animal may fall
   B. A metal clamp often known as an "anti-kicker" can be placed over the dorsum, and along the sides in the same location
VII. Calf restraint
   A. Newborns are guided from place to place by placing one hand under the neck and grasping the tail head or placing the other hand around the hindquarters
   B. Calves up to 200 lbs. can be put into lateral recumbency by "flanking or legging" the calf down. After it is down, apply a three-legged tie, place one knee on its neck and the other knee in front of the closest hind leg to hold it down

SHEEP RESTRAINT
Danger Potential

I. Head is used as a battering ram with most injuries consisting of serious bruises

Behavioral Characteristics

I. Sheep are allelomimetic (strong flocking instincts) causing them to move as a group and making them easy to handle
II. Move slowly when working with sheep; one of their survival instincts is to flee

Anatomy/Physiology

I. Sheep are not the jumpers that goats are, although they can jump up to 1.2 m (4 feet)
   A. Exceptions are range sheep and cheviots (harder to handle)
II. Sheep can have problems when worked in hot weather; normal body temperature can be as high as 104°F (40°C)
   A. Running, struggling, and crowding, plus their heavy wool, can very quickly result in hyperthermia
III. **Never** grab the wool when restraining sheep because it pulls out easily. Damage to the fleece, the skin, and subcutaneous layers can result

Restraint

I. Trained sheepdogs are your best tool; they save a lot of steps when herding the sheep to specific spots
II. Crowding the flock into a small pen or area, along with portable gates, is usually the best way to capture a single sheep or to medicate it
   A. Mark the sheep with a wax crayon so that double dosing doesn't occur

III. To capture a single sheep
   A. Approach slowly, quietly, and deliberately
   B. Reach down and limit the forward movement with a hand under the chin
   C. Quickly reach for the dock or flank fold with the other hand to stop backward motion
   D. Move wherever you wish by applying pressure on the chin or dock
   E. Further control can be done by grasping the muzzle and turning the head toward the shoulder
IV. A shepherd's crook is a handy tool for catching a sheep
   A. It is used to "snare" a hind leg proximal to the stifle (hock)
V. "Setting-up" (also referred to as "rumping" or "docking") a sheep allows you to examine the underside of the sheep, shear, vaccinate, or trim the hooves of the sheep
   A. Move the sheep so it is standing sideways in front of your legs
   B. Plant your left leg by the sheep's shoulder
   C. Grasp the chin with one hand and the flank with the other
   D. Lift up on the flank, turn, and push the sheep's head into its shoulder, pivot on your right leg and move your left leg back. This throws the sheep off balance and onto its dock
   E. Lean the sheep's back between your legs and release your hands
   F. Make sure the hocks are off the ground
   G. If done properly the sheep will not be able to get to its feet. Your hands are free to do whatever procedure you choose
VI. Halters can be used but the sheep's short nose makes it difficult to prevent the nose piece from sliding down and occluding the nares
VII. Lambs are held by supporting them beneath their chest with your forearm between their front legs
   A. For castrations and tail docks the lamb can be held by grasping a front and back leg in one hand and the opposite front and back leg in the other hand, resting the lamb's back against your chest

GOAT RESTRAINT
Danger Potential
I. Goats use their heads as battering rams
   A. If annoyed they will rear up on their hind legs and slam into you with their heads
II. Most goats are disbudded or dehorned at a young age

A. Horned goats do not like to have their horns held and will swing their heads back and forth viciously if held
B. The horns add power to the butt and can cause injury

Behavioral Characteristics
I. Goats are very vocal
   A. The kids sound like human babies when handled and the entire herd will come to investigate any fuss
   B. The herd may try to protect the kid or other members of the herd in danger
II. They respond to gentle treatment and become quite tame if handled a lot
   A. Rough handling may make them nasty
III. Intact males have scent glands at the base of the horns that secrete a very disagreeable long lasting odor that attracts females during breeding season
   A. When in rut, intact males will mark their territory by urinating on their beards, legs, neck, and body and then rubbing those parts on objects around the farmyard. This odor lasts throughout the breeding season
IV. Goats are good escape artists and will work knots and chains loose
   A. Make sure all gates are properly locked

Anatomy
I. Their delicate bones are easily fractured and dislocated if grasped incorrectly
II. Goats are very sturdy animals that can take a lot of stress
III. They are very good jumpers but will rarely be able to jump over 6 feet (2 m)
   A. If they try to jump over you, you may be hit at chest or shoulder height

Restraint
I. Capture
   A. To capture a single goat it is best to place the entire herd in a small pen
      1. Since goats don't have the strong flocking instinct of sheep, it is best to lure them in with grain
      2. After the goats are in the small pen, move slowly and deliberately toward your intended patient
      3. Grasp around the neck or catch by the collar with the other hand on the goat's dock to move it
         a. If unable to grasp as above, try capturing by the front leg, but be careful.

Once caught, grasp the head behind the ears and under the chin and back the goat to a corner

4. If you are using chain collars make sure they are the flat chains to prevent the goat getting caught

5. It is best to use plastic link "breakaway" collars

II. Head

A. To restrain the head with no "neck" wear, you can place both hands on either side of the cheeks and wrap your fingers around the lower jaw

B. The handler can straddle the goat by stepping over its shoulders and securing the head by holding the jaws firmly

C. The beard can be grasped with one hand with the other hand placed on top of the head

III. Goats cannot be set on their haunches because they are much more agile than sheep and will struggle

A. They can be flanked similar to a calf or be placed against a fence and have their legs lifted similar to a horse

B. Dairy goats can be placed in a milking stanchion for restraint or secured to a fence using a quick release knot

IV. Dehorning and castration

A. To disbud kids, hold them like a lamb, then sit down, folding the kid's legs under its body and cradling its head in both hands so the thumbs hold down the ears

B. To castrate, hold the kid the same as described for lambs

V. Pick feet up as you would pick up a horse's hoof

PORCINE RESTRAINT
Danger Potential

I. Teeth

A. Newborn piglets have sharp needlelike deciduous teeth (canines and third incisors, called "needle teeth") that can damage the sow's udder and handlers

B. Clipping of the teeth, along with other management techniques, is done soon after birth

1. Wounds made by the canines (called tusks) are almost always septic

C. Adults have very strong jaws and can tear flesh easily. A male with tusks is quite dangerous

II. Adult pigs can push and knock the restrainer with its head and body

Behavioral Characteristics

I. Herding instincts are virtually nonexistent but the entire herd will converge to the rescue of a screaming mate. Sows reacting to perceived danger to their piglets are extremely dangerous

II. Pigs are stubborn and contrary but you can use this behavior to your advantage during restraint procedures

III. They are unpredictable and can become aggressive without warning

IV. They enjoy being talked to and petted or scratched gently. Simple procedures can sometimes be done while gently rubbing the ventral abdomen and while they are laying down, but be careful

V. They are extremely vocal

Anatomy/Physiology

I. Pigs have streamlined bodies that were designed to run through underbrush, making it very easy for them to slide under objects such as fences or between your legs

II. Strong neck muscles developed by rooting enables the pig to lift with considerable force such items as fencing panels or even a handler

III. Thin legs can easily be fractured or dislocated if held in the wrong manner

IV. Because of a thick layer of subcutaneous fat, pigs overheat easily

Restraint

I. Small enclosures are the easiest way to handle large numbers of smaller pigs for injections

A. Each pig is marked with a wax crayon as the injection is given

II. Squeeze pens and farrowing crates are ideal **but they can be extremely dangerous.** Never get into a small pen with a pig (especially a sow and litter) without checking for an escape route with an easy access

III. Moving

A. A cane, light plastic pipe, leather or canvas straps, or flat sticks can be used to move or direct the pig

1. A gentle slap on the rear will make a pig move forward; a tap on the side of the head will turn it in the opposite direction

2. Sound, more than pain, is what makes a pig move. Never use any of the objects to inflict pain because it can anger the pig and the pig may attack you

B. A bucket placed over the pig's head will cause the pig to back up

1. By grabbing the tail you can direct it

C. Hog panels or hurdles/shields/barriers are made of solid sheets of plywood, plastic, or aluminum and are used to move and direct pigs
  1. The hurdles have to be solid because a pig can raise it
  2. To move pigs using a hurdle, place it between you and the pig and start walking
  3. To turn the pig, set the barrier down on the opposite side of the pig's head
  4. If a pig charges, set the barrier between you and the pig and tilt the top of it toward you
  5. A tap on the snout with a cane or strap may stop a charging pig

IV. Hog snare
A. This is the restraint tool of choice when working with pigs
B. Use of the snare is easy
  1. Place the loop in front of the pig's snout
  2. Allow the pig to mouth the loop and then quickly slip the noose over the top jaw all the way back to the commissure of the lips
  3. Pull back on the handle, applying pressure to the nose; the pig's response will be to pull back in the opposite direction and squeal. The pig is immobilized by its own stubbornness
C. The snare can be used for restraint when vaccinating, drawing blood samples, or examining pigs
D. Length of time used should be 15 to 20 minutes maximum because it can have a tourniquet effect on the upper jaw
E. Release of the snare should be quick; if the snare gets caught on a tusk the pig will jerk the snare out of your hands and start swinging its head until the snare comes loose

V. Lifting
A. Lift newborns less than 15 pounds by a back leg then hold with a hand under the chest and abdomen
  1. They will squeal when picked up so you should move them quickly to your hand or out of the hearing range of the sow
B. Larger pigs under 60 pounds can be grasped by a hind leg to capture them. Once caught the other hind leg is held, the pig is held upside down with your legs supporting their back. They can then be examined or transported

C. Use the same method for pigs up to 125 pounds as for the 50 to 60 pounders, but two people are necessary with each holding one leg

VI. Recumbency
A. You can cast a pig a number of ways with the use of ropes
  1. Capture pig with hog snare
  2. Place a rope on a front and back leg on the same side of the pig
  3. Pass the ropes under the abdomen to the opposite side of the pig, moving to that side of the pig
  4. Pull the ropes toward you, pulling the legs out from under the pig; the person controlling the hog snare will have to move with the pig so the snare doesn't injure the upper jaw
  5. Use the ropes to tie three of the pig's legs together
  6. If the procedure is prolonged, every attempt should be made to make the pig comfortable to prevent nerve and muscle damage
B. V-troughs are made of wood and are V shaped
  1. Depending on the size of the trough a 50 to 70 pound pig can be placed in the trough on its back, where it will remain until you are finished
  2. This may be used for castrations or umbilical hernias

Glossary

balling gun A metal or plastic device used to pill large animals such as sheep and cattle

casting Laying an animal down on its side for restraint purposes

"caveman pets" Heavy swats usually around the shoulder region of an animal to provide minor distractions

cradle A device placed around a horse's neck to inhibit bending of the neck or turning of the head to prevent the horse from licking or chewing at its wounds

cross tying A method of securing a horse to two sides of a stanchion or stocks by use of two lead ropes, one attached to each side of the halter. This is used to prevent rearing or movement of the front quarters from side to side

disbudding The process of removing horn tissue of young goats or cattle with caustic paste or the use of a hot iron

dry An animal that is not lactating; usually in reference to the last 60 days of gestation of dairy cattle

far side The opposite or right side of the horse

farrowing The act of giving birth in swine

headgate Mechanical device at the end of a chute that secures an animal's head on both sides of the neck between the jaws and shoulder

hog snare A device made out of rope, cable, or wire and placed around the pig's upper snout so that the head can be secured

hobble A device placed on caudal aspects of the hocks of large animals to restrain hind legs

jacking A term used in reference to grasping a bovine tail at the base and elevating it dorsally to distract the animal from painful procedures elsewhere on the body

lactation Period of time during which an animal is producing milk

lead shank A lead rope with a snap of some sort attached to the halter of an animal such as a horse

near side The left side of the horse, from which it is accustomed to being handled

needle teeth A term applied to the eight deciduous teeth (canines and third incisors) that pigs are born with and that are removed within 1 to 2 days of birth

setting up Also referred to as docking or rumping and applied to sheep. Sheep are set up into a sitting position on their hind legs so that they lean against the restrainer's legs

squeeze chute An enclosed device into which large animals are individually restrained; these chutes often have various attachments to effectively restrain the head and give access to other body parts

stanchion An area in a barn usually used to tie dairy cattle or goats

twitch Used in horses; a handle with a loop of rope or chain on one end that is tightened over the upper lip or muzzle for restraint

Review Questions

1 Which of these behaviors is *not* a normal behavior for cats?
   a. Hiding under the papers in a cage
   b. Investigating a new room
   c. Being fairly aloof and independent
   d. Rubbing on the leg of a chair

2 To restrain a cat it is important to:
   a. Immediately apply the maximum restraint possible
   b. Make friends first and then apply the maximum restraint
   c. Make friends first and apply the least restrictive technique
   d. Immediately apply the least restraint possible

3 Which of these is *not* a sign of warning from a cat?
   a. Hissing
   b. Ears lowered
   c. Swiping at you with a paw
   d. Looking the other way

4 As a restraint tool, a towel is used to:
   a. Wrap up an angry cat
   b. Let the cat curl up and go to sleep
   c. Let the cat hide under
   d. Protect you from bites and scratches

5 White around the eyes, sharp movements of the head and ears, trembling lips, and boisterous behavior indicate a dog is:
   a. Nervous/frightened
   b. Happy
   c. Normal acting
   d. Hostile

6 If suspecting aggressive behavior, which dog would it most likely be?
   a. Large dog like a Newfoundland
   b. A medium size dog like a beagle
   c. A small dog like a Chihuahua
   d. All dogs can be equally aggressive

7 Always muzzle an injured, conscious dog *except* if it has:
   a. Huge gaping wounds on the neck
   b. A spinal injury
   c. A leg injury
   d. A head injury

8 Horses show many emotions through body language. Which ear movement can mean concentration or anger?
   a. Pricked forward
   b. Constantly moving back and forth
   c. Held erect
   d. Pinned back

9 Serious injury is most likely to occur from a kick if you are within this range while standing behind a horse:
   a. 1-2 feet
   b. 3-5 feet
   c. 6-8 feet
   d. 10-12 feet

10 Which tool is considered the main tool(s) of restraint on a horse?
   a. Halter and lead rope
   b. Stanchion
   c. Stocks
   d. Lariat

11 A chain twitch is best applied to the:
   a. Upper muzzle
   b. Lower muzzle
   c. Ear
   d. Tongue

12 A lead shank is used when you need:
   a. More restraint
   b. A distraction technique
   c. To discipline a horse
   d. All of the above

13 Where is the safest place to stand when you are next to a cow?
   a. Slightly in front and to the left of the head
   b. Slightly in front of the shoulder
   c. Next to the abdomen
   d. Slightly in front of the back leg

14 A nose lead or tongs is applied to the:
   a. Left nostril
   b. Right nostril
   c. Upper muzzle
   d. Nasal septum

15 "Jacking" the tail is:
 a. Twisting it to the side
 b. Bending it straight up
 c. Holding it straight out
 d. Kinking the end of it

16 To move a newborn calf from one spot to another:
 a. Place a halter on its head and neck and lead it
 b. Place your arms around its neck and rump and guide it
 c. Place a lariat around its shoulder and drag it
 d. Use a whip against its lumbar region and herd it

17 What is the sheep's main means of defense?
 a. Speed and flocking instinct
 b. Hooves and head
 c. Teeth and hooves
 d. Speed and head

18 The best way to get a herd of goats into a pen is to:
 a. Lure them in with grain
 b. Chase them in
 c. Use a hurdle and walk toward them
 d. Herd them with a well trained dog

19 Where is a hog snare placed?
 a. Bottom jaw
 b. Top jaw
 c. Around neck
 d. Around back leg

20 What method works best to move a pig from one place to another?
 a. Yelling and shouting
 b. Get a large group of people to herd them
 c. Use a dog to chase them
 d. Use a barrier or plastic pipe

21 A hog snare has an optimum effect of:
 a. 3-5 minutes
 b. 8-10 minutes
 c. 15-20 minutes
 d. 25 minutes

22 When moving a 40 lb pig it is best held by:
 a. A front leg
 b. A back leg
 c. Both front legs
 d. Both back legs

23 With swine, V-troughs are used for holding:
 a. Pigs in dorsal recumbency
 b. Pigs in ventral recumbency
 c. Water additives
 d. Feed supplements

BIBLIOGRAPHY

Aanes WA: Restraint of cattle: head restraint. In *Modern Veterinary Practice,* 5:498-501, 1987.

AVMA: *Medication and force feeding a cat at home,* Client Information Series, 1985.

Blanchard S: Here's how to read your horse's body language, In *Pet Health News,* Mission Viejo, California, 5:25, 1989, Fancy Publication Inc.

Brooks DL: Care and handling of dogs. In *Animal health technology,* ed 2 Catcott EJ, editor, Santa Barbara, 1977, pp 98-101. American Veterinary Publications, Inc.

Crow SE, Sally WO: *Restraint of dogs and cats: manual of clinical procedures in the dog and cat,* Philadelphia, 1987, J.B. Lippincott Company.

Edwards LM: Behavior and diseases of the dairy goat, In *Veterinary Technician.* 4(5):294-300, 1983.

Evans JM: Developing canine social skills, *Dogs U.S.A.* Annual, 3(1):64-65, 1988.

Faler K, Faler K: Restraint of sheep, In *Modern veterinary practice,* 6:562-563, 1987.

Fowler ME: *Restraint and handling of wild and domestic animals,* Ames 1978, Iowa State University Press.

Gilbert SG: *Pictorial anatomy of the cat,* New York, 1984, Crescent Books.

Kazmierczak K: Bandage management in small animals, *Continuing education* Article #2, 3(6):309-315, 1982.

Kocab JM: Restraint of pigs, In *New methods the journal of animal health technology,* 2(2):12-13, 1983.

Leahy JR, Barrow P: *Restraint of animals,* Ithaca, 1953, Cornell Campus Store, Inc.

McBride DF: *Learning veterinary terminology,* St. Louis, 1996, Mosby.

Moran HC et al: Basic cat handling techniques, *Lab Animal,* 3:29-34, 1988.

Neil DH, Kese ML: Restraint and handling of animals. In *Clinical textbook for veterinary technicians,* McCurnin DM, editor, Philadelphia, 1985, W.B. Saunders.

Nelson B: Restraining horses, In *Western horseman,* 10:89-94, 1980.

Sayer A: *The complete book of the cat,* New York, 1984, Crescent Books.

Sonsthagen T: *Restraint of domestic animals,* American Veterinary Publications, 1991, pp 65-84.

Stansbury RL: Care and handling of Cats. In *Animal health technology,* Catcott EJ, editor, Santa Barbara, American Veterinary Publications, Inc. 1977.

Strickland C: How to tie your horse safely and securely. In *Horse Illustrated,* 5:39-43, 1988.

Vail C: Tips on equine dentistry. In *Nordon news,* Summer: 15-17, 1980.

Vanderhurst SR: Equine practice. In *Animal health technology,* Catcott EJ, editor, Santa Barbara, 1977, American Veterinary Publications, Inc.

Vanderhurst SR, Hunter RL: Livestock Practice. In *Animal health technology,* Catcott EJ, editor, Santa Barbara, 1977, American Veterinary Publications, Inc.

Vaughan JT, Allen R Jr.: Restraint of horses: Part I—Head restraint. In *Modern veterinary practice,* 6:373-383, 1987.

CHAPTER 5

Companion Animal Behavior

Linda Campbell

OUTLINE

Normal Canine Behavior
  Behavioral Development of the
    Canine
  Social Behavior of the Canine
Normal Feline Behavior
  Behavioral Development of the
    Feline
  Social Behavior of the Feline
Applied Animal Behavior
  Preventing Behavior Problems
  Intervention Techniques

Common Behavior Problems in the
  Canine
  Aggression
  House Soiling
Common Behavior Problems in the
  Feline
  Spraying Characteristics

Elimination Problems
Furniture Scratching
Abnormal Behavior Problems
  Obsessive/Compulsive Disorders
    and Stereotypical Behaviors

LEARNING OUTCOMES

After reading this chapter you should be able to:

1. Describe in chronological order the behavioral development of the canine and the feline.
2. Describe the social behavior of the canine and the feline.
3. Describe various methods of preventing behavior problems.
4. Identify intervention techniques that may be used to eliminate or modify abnormal behavior.
5. Describe some common behavior problems in the canine and the feline.
6. Identify abnormal behavior problems.

The study of contemporary animal behavior is based on objective information. The veterinary technician uses a nonverbal, interspecies communication system each time an animal is efficiently manipulated. Accurate knowledge about a species' typical behavior has applications for all animal related fields.

The primary role of the veterinary technician in behavior counseling is to educate pet owners about normal animal behavior and to provide accurate information about the cause and resolution of behavior problems. The goal of this chapter is to review behavioral theories and provide some understanding of normal companion animal behavior.

NORMAL CANINE BEHAVIOR

Dogs are highly social animals and it is well documented that varying degrees of social isolation during critical developmental periods results in various abnormal behavior patterns.

Behavioral Development of the Canine

I. Characterized by five major phases
  A. **Neonate period** (0-14 days): completely dependent on mother for survival
  B. **Transitional period** (14-21 days): rapid development

C. **Socialization period** (3-12 weeks): critical period in the formation of social relationships
   1. During weeks 3 to 8, dogs socialize best to other dogs
   2. During weeks 5 to 7 through 12, dogs socialize best to humans
   3. During weeks 5 to 12 through 16, dogs adapt best to novel environments
   4. At approximately 8.5 weeks, substrate preferences for elimination are developed
   5. At 8 to 10 weeks, a fear period is observed where painful or traumatic situations should be avoided
D. **Juvenile period** (10 weeks to sexual maturity): learning capacities develop
E. **Adult period** (after sexual maturity): continues to learn about environment and adds new behaviors

Social Behavior of the Canine

The domestic dog spends much of its time solely in the company of humans and views its human family as its own pack. Dogs use elements of their normal social behavior to communicate with their pack.
   I. A complex social system relies on effective communication through vision, olfaction, auditory means, and physical contact
   A. Visual communication: body postures important
      1. Dominance gestures: tail held high, head up, ears erect, direct eye contact
      2. Subordinate gestures: tail low and wagging, dog rolling on back and presenting inguinal area, nuzzling and licking face of other animal
      3. Display of ritualized gestures: threat, bluff attack, and play-soliciting behavior
   B. Olfactory communication
      1. Via deposition of signals in the environment
         a. Feces and urine or the particular odor of the animal itself
            (1) 'Inspection' of the head and anal regions
   C. Vocal communication
      1. Bark (most common): used in defense, in play, as a greeting, or as a general call for attention
      2. Growl: used in defense, warning, or as a threat
      3. Whimpering/whining: used in submission, greeting, or pain

   4. Howl: used primarily when alone—probably for seeking social contact

NORMAL FELINE BEHAVIOR

The domestic cat is a very adaptable, territorial animal that is usually described as asocial. Cats also experience sensitive periods in their development but these periods are not as well defined as in dogs. Much of a kitten's basic personality is inherited, with a distinct portion influenced by the sire.

Behavioral Development of the Feline

   I. Characterized by five major phases
   A. **Neonate period** (0-14 days): complete dependence on mother for survival
   B. **Transitional period** (14-21 days): increasing independence
   C. **Socialization period** (3-14 weeks): all primary social bonds are formed
      1. During weeks 3-5, predatory behavior develops
      2. During weeks 3-14, play behavior develops
         a. Locomotory play may be solitary or social, includes running, rolling, jumping, and climbing
         b. Object play may be solitary or social
         c. Social play, with conspecifics, includes wrestling, rolling, and biting
         d. Critical period for socialization to humans begins at 2 to 3 weeks and tapers off by 7 weeks
         e. Critical period for socialization to other cats is 3-6 weeks; cats raised in isolation may never adapt to another cat
   D. **Juvenile period** (14 weeks to sexual maturity): no significant behavioral changes
      1. Improved motor skills and coordination
   E. **Adult period** (after sexual maturity): behavior can change; may become increasingly independent

Social Behavior of the Feline

Although the cat may prefer solitude, small social groups may be formed. The social order of cats is influenced by place, time of day, presence of food, and population density. The maintenance of social systems relies on the transmission of information between individuals and groups to minimize close interactions.
   I. Vocal communication
   A. Cats can vocalize many sounds and tones
   B. Vocalization is learned and instinctive behavior, for example, kittens can hiss before their eyes open

II. Olfactory communication
   A. Provides information regarding individual sexual identity, time spent at location, and reproductive stage
      1. Urine spraying is commonly used for scent marking, particularly by intact males
      2. Feces is seldom used as scent markers; cats often cover feces; however, territorial cats may leave feces uncovered in conspicuous areas
      3. Rubbing behavior: cats may deposit secretions from large sebaceous glands onto objects or individuals
III. Visual communication
   A. Facial features reflect a cat's mood (Figure 5-1)
      1. An undisturbed cat has erect ears, relaxed whiskers in an outward position, normal pupils
      2. A disturbed cat has
         a. Flattened ears
         b. Whiskers flat (defensive) or pulled forward (offensive)
         c. Pupils constricted (offensive) or dilated (defensive)
         d. Lips pulled back baring the teeth; nose wrinkled
   B. Clawing or scratching
      1. Secondary olfactory cues may be left by sweat glands on the paws after scratching objects
   C. Body postures also reflect a cat's mood (Figure 5-2)
      1. Friendly cat: carries tail in an upright position
      2. Frightened cat: exhibits a defensive threat posture (body arched laterally, piloerection, tail held close to body or erect)
      3. Angry cat: exhibits an offensive threat posture (hindquarters elevated, tail held straight out from body then abruptly bending downward, tail tip twitching from side to side)
      4. Play: solicitation postures include rolling over to expose abdominal area, an inverted U-shaped tail position

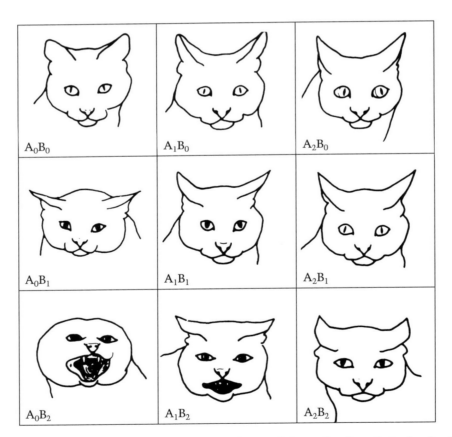

Figure 5-1 Facial expressions of the cat. Aggressiveness is increasing from A_0 to A_2, fearfulness from B_0 to B_2. (From Leyhausen P: *Cat behavior: the predatory and social behavior of domestic and wild cats,* New York, 1979, Garland STPM Press.)

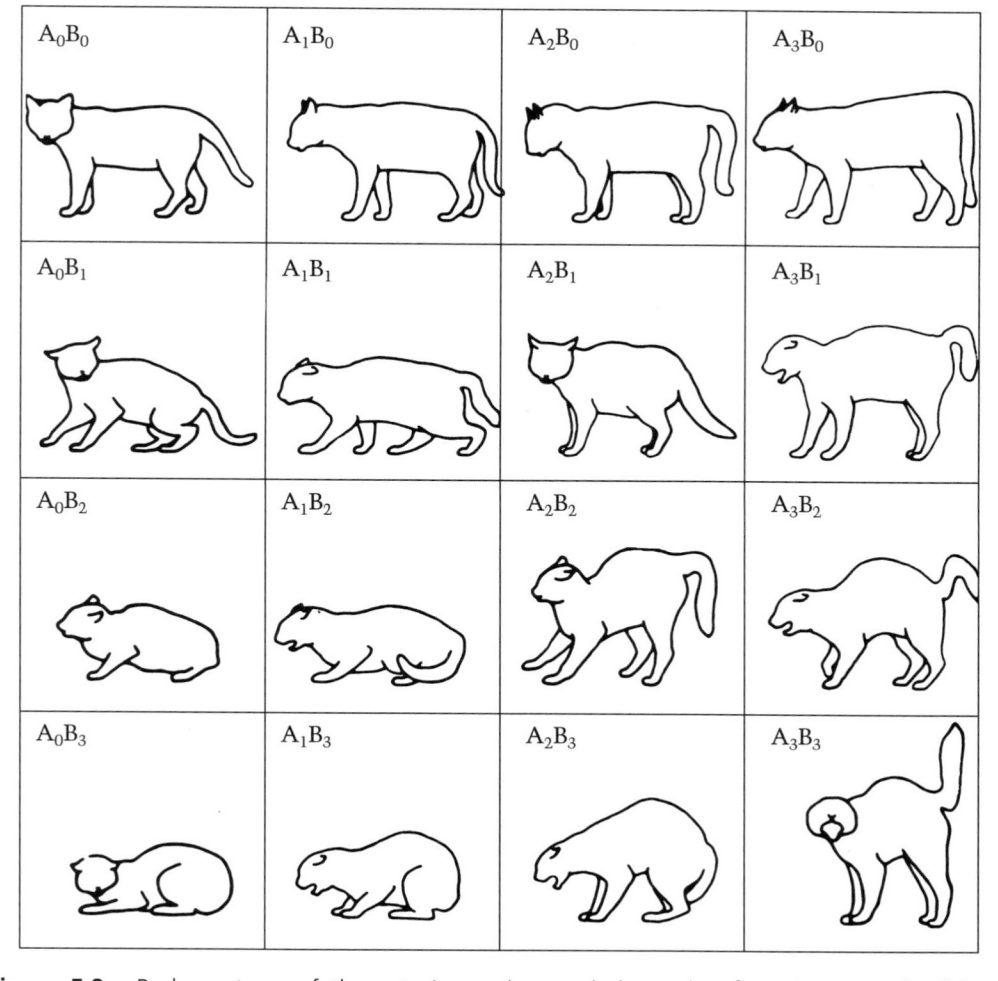

Figure 5-2 Body postures of the cat. Aggressiveness is increasing from A_0 to A_3, fearfulness from B_0 to B_3. (From Leyhausen P: *Cat behavior: the predatory and social behavior of domestic and wild cats,* New York, 1979, Garland STPM Press.)

APPLIED ANIMAL BEHAVIOR ▬▬▬▬

Behavior problems are the biggest threat to the human–animal bond. Most of the behavioral complaints of pet owners are management related problems that can be prevented or modified by early intervention. Correcting a problem may save an animal's life.

Preventing Behavior Problems

Behavior can be influenced by a multitude of variables: environment, physiology, experience, learning, and genetic predisposition.

   I. Pet selection

     A. Many pet owners choose animals that are unsuitable for their lifestyles

     B. Before acquiring a pet, clients should be advised to research species, breed, grooming and exercise needs, required medical care, and reliable sources

     C. Many dog breeders use puppy aptitude (temperament) testing as a general guide for matching pets to people

       1. This test attempts to predict a puppy's future temperament and suitability for a specific task such as obedience trial competition

       2. Because environment has a major role in behavior, the test cannot guarantee that a dog will not develop behavior problems in the future

     D. Kittens that come from known sources and have been well socialized by early and extensive handling are more likely to become calm, tractable pets

     E. Dog obedience classes can provide an excellent opportunity for interaction between pet and owner and serve to socialize pets to other dogs

1. A qualified instructor teaches owners to implement leash manners and basic verbal commands
2. Owners learn about variability in response to training and may be alerted to a potential behavior problem
3. Obedience training alone will not remedy all behavioral complaints

Intervention Techniques

The veterinary technician must be able to interpret canine and feline behavior and provide pet owners with sound information on the early recognition of potential problem behavior. Patients with extreme behavior problems are best referred to a professional animal behaviorist.

I. Before any intervention for a behavior problem is begun a thorough behavioral history must be obtained
II. All possible medical causes of a behavior problem should be evaluated by a veterinarian
III. Major areas of intervention
   A. A combination of techniques is often necessary to solve a problem successfully
      1. Environmental manipulation
         a. Example: reducing the number of cats in a household may reduce spraying behavior
      2. Physiologic intervention
         a. Castration may eliminate roaming, urine marking, and intermale aggression
         b. Drug therapy: rarely curative alone; very few psychoactive drugs are approved for use in companion animals
         c. Disease alters physiologic status of animals and consequently effects behavior
      3. Behavior modification
         Through behavior modification techniques, veterinary technicians can assist pet owners with behavior problems. All techniques use the principles of learning.
         a. Operant conditioning (positive reinforcement): a pleasant stimulus (e.g., food) after a behavior increases the probability of a behavior being repeated
            (1) To be effective, a reinforcement must immediately follow the desired behavior
            (2) Repetition: response will be stronger the more often a behavior is reinforced
            (3) After a behavior is learned, intermittent reinforcement results in a persistent response
         b. Negative reinforcement: occurs when an animal performs a behavior to avoid an aversive stimulus
            (1) Also serves to increase the probability of that behavior being repeated
         c. Shaping: reinforcement of a behavior that is different but similar to the desired response
            (1) By selectively reinforcing successive approximations of a desired behavior a new behavior can eventually develop
      4. Procedures for decreasing behavior
         a. Punishment: application of an aversive stimulus immediately after a behavior serves to decrease the probability the behavior will be repeated
            (1) Most misused behavioral modification technique
            (2) Insufficient by itself (it only teaches an animal what not to do) because it does not teach appropriate behavior
         b. Extinction: withholding or removing a reinforcement for a previously reinforced behavior that causes the behavior to cease
            (1) Difficult to implement
         c. Counter conditioning: conditioning an animal to engage in behavior that is incompatible with the undesirable behavior
         d. Systematic desensitization: process of exposing an animal to a stimulus beginning at an intensity that does not evoke the undesirable response and increasing the intensity in small increments so that the stimulus eventually loses its ability to evoke the undesirable response
            (1) Frequently used to eliminate anxiety or fear response
            (2) Systematic desensitization and counter conditioning (usually implemented simultaneously)
         e. Habituation: when no consequences follow an animal's response to a stimulus that response habituates or diminishes

COMMON BEHAVIOR PROBLEMS IN THE CANINE

Most behavior problems considered undesirable by pet owners are manifestations of normal behavior.

Aggression

The most common behavioral complaint of pet owners (Figure 5-3).
  I. Aggressive behavior is classified according to the stimulus or circumstances: dominance, possessive, territorial, predatory, fear induced, pain induced, intermale, maternal, and redirected
  II. Factors affecting the development of aggression are inheritability, hormonal, and learning
  III. Aggression is not the result of a single cause
  IV. Early warning signs usually can be recognizable
  V. Not uncommon for a dog to develop more than one type of aggressive behavior problem
  VI. Intervention procedures
    A. Castration: especially helpful in intermale dominance and territorial aggression
    B. Drugs: short-term progestin therapy
    C. Castration and drug therapy: of limited use unless combined with behavioral modification
    D. Counter conditioning and desensitization: most effective
    E. Punishment: (except in young puppies) almost never effective and should be avoided, since it may elicit further aggression
  VII. Note: problems involving aggression are controlled, never cured

House Soiling

Must differentiate cause with behavioral history.
  I. House soiling due to territorial marking
    A. Usually male dogs after reaching sexual maturity
    B. Unrelated to presence/absence of owner
    C. Small numerous spots of urine are evident
    D. Intervention procedures
      1. Castration
      2. Short-term progestin therapy in conjunction with behavior modification
      3. Punishment may be partially effective
      4. Aversive condition: association of an aversive stimulus with a particular location
  II. House soiling due to separation anxiety
    A. Urination and/or defecation combined with other behaviors such as vocalization and destruction
    B. Occurs consistently and only when the dog is left alone—usually within 30 minutes after the owner's departure
    C. Factors correlating with the development of the problem
      1. Excessive greeting behaviors
      2. Strong attachment to owner
      3. Change in routine
    D. Intervention procedures
      1. Behavior modification program of counter conditioning and desensitization or habituation techniques
      2. Antianxiety drug therapy
      3. Cage training is not a solution because it does not address the anxiety; the behavior may manifest in another area (e.g., self-trauma)
  III. House soiling due to submissive or excitement motivated urination
    A. Urination accompanied by excited greeting and submissive body postures
    B. Most often seen in puppies
    C. Intervention procedures
      1. Avoid dominant gestures (e.g., direct eye contact)
      2. Control greeting: keep low key
      3. Counter conditioning where calm behavior and nonsubmissive postures are rewarded

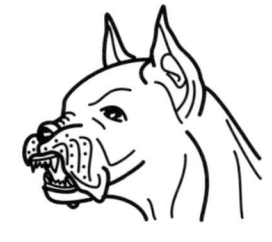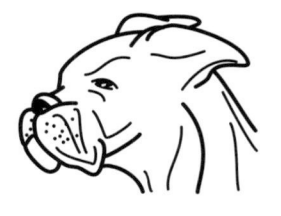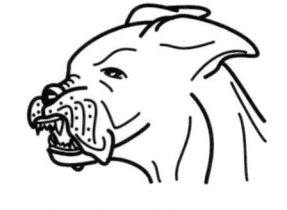

Figure 5-3 A dog's expression at strong aggression *(left)* and pronounced fear *(middle)*, and a mood that contains aggression and fear *(right)*.

4. Punishment will exacerbate the problem
   D. Problem may resolve as puppies mature
IV. House soiling due to fear or phobia
   A. Urination or defecation as a consequence of a fear induced stimuli (e.g., thunderstorm)
   B. Intervention procedures
      1. Source of fear must be identified
      2. Counter conditioning and desensitization program
V. House soiling due to lack of or ineffective house training
   A. Urination and/or defecation usually unrelated to the presence/absence of the owner
   B. Large pools of urine often in one or a few locations
   C. Intervention procedures
      1. Environmental management
      2. Temporary confinement (cage train)
      3. Appropriate punishment (if caught in the act)
      4. Reward appropriate behavior

COMMON BEHAVIOR PROBLEMS IN THE FELINE

The most common behavior problem reported by cat owners is elimination: urination or defecation outside the litter box. This is distinct from spraying, a territorial marking behavior.

Spraying Characteristics

I. Cat assuming standing posture
II. Backing up against a vertical object
III. Releasing urine several inches above the ground
IV. Tail typically aquiver
V. Occurs more frequently in intact males; however, castrated males and spayed females can spray urine
VI. Associated with social conflict and competitive or sexual behavior
VII. Direct relationship exists between the number of cats in a household and the probability of spraying
VIII. May become a habit even if initiating stimulus is no longer present
IX. Intervention procedures
   A. Difficult to resolve because it is difficult to identify the eliciting stimulus
   B. Neutering always recommended
   C. Modify locations
      1. Make marking areas aversive with unpleasant odors (e.g., muscle rubs) or uncomfortable substrate (e.g., aluminum foil)

2. Change significance of the area by placing food, toys, or catnip
3. Punishment or aversive conditioning may be successful
   D. Resolve conflicts with other cats
      1. Increase space available per cat (e.g., cat condos, allowing an indoor cat outdoors)
      2. Barricade windows to prevent indoor cats from viewing neighboring cats
      3. Antianxiety drug therapy

Elimination Problems

I. Many elimination problems can be resolved by changing various components of the litter box and/or making inappropriate areas less attractive
II. Common causes for elimination outside the litter box are surface preferences, location preferences, and/or fear associated with the litter box
III. Intervention procedures
   A. Techniques to increase litter box attractiveness
      1. Change style of litter box (e.g., change covered) box to an open box
      2. Keep litter box clean: remove feces daily
      3. Provide at least one litter box per cat
      4. Respect privacy: litter box should not be in high traffic, noisy area
      5. Odors associated with certain litter may be offensive to cat (e.g., chlorophyll)
      6. Changes to litter type, if necessary, should be gradual
      7. Plastic litter boxes should be replaced periodically
      8. Cats favor fine-ground clumping litters
   B. Techniques to decrease elimination at inappropriate locations
      1. Clean area and remove odor of elimination
      2. Repel cat with aversive odors (e.g., mothballs)
      3. Change significance of the area: place food, toys, or catnip in the area
   C. Other factors involved in elimination problems
      1. Learned preference for scratching on a nonlitter substrate (e.g., carpet under the litter box)
      2. Learned location preferences or aversions
         a. An aversion to the litter box can develop if pain or something unpleasant is associated with the litter box

b. May require a new litter box, different substrate, a new location, and/or counter conditioning and desensitization techniques

Furniture Scratching

I. Scratching is a normal inherited behavior of cats that serves to condition claws

II. It is also a means of visual and olfactory marking and stretching for the front limbs

III. Early learning, genetic variability, and the cat's physical environment have a profound effect on the severity and intensity of scratching behavior within a household

IV. Household scratching can be prevented by providing a suitable scratching post in a prominent location, preferably near the kitten's sleeping area

V. Intervention procedures

    A. Minimize damage to furniture by keeping claws trimmed

    B. Behavior modification

        1. Positive reinforcement (e.g., food, toys, catnip) can make a scratching post more appealing

    C. Punishment (e.g., loud noise, water squirt, a tin can filled with rocks and thrown near the cat when caught scratching)

    D. Modify environment by moving or covering furniture

    E. Restrict access to scratching area

    F. Allow cat outdoors

    G. Declawing: alternative if owner is unwilling to use retraining techniques

ABNORMAL BEHAVIOR PROBLEMS ■■■■
Obsessive/Compulsive Disorders and Stereotypical Behaviors

I. Usually described as maladaptive, inappropriate, and sometimes self-destructive

II. Often expressions of normal species—typical behaviors such as grooming, vocalization, and locomotion

III. Etiology

    A. Strong genetic influence

    B. Disease

    C. Conflict induced by environment

IV. Intervention procedures

    A. Environmental management

    B. Drug therapy

    C. Counter conditioning behavioral therapy

V. Examples of stereotypical behavior in the dog

    A. Acral-like dermatitis (lick granuloma)

    B. Flank sucking (usually Doberman pinchers)

    C. Tail chasing, circling, and whirling

    D. Fly catching

VI. Examples of stereotypical behavior in the cat

    A. Excessive self-licking and hair chewing

    B. Wool sucking (usually Siamese cats)

    C. Tail biting

Glossary

auditory Pertaining to the ear or sense of hearing

aversive Unpleasant

conspecifics Members of the same species

olfaction The act of smelling

piloerection Erection of hair

psychoactive drugs Drugs that modify mental activity

successive approximation Consecutively reinforce a close estimate of the desired behavior

Review Questions

1 Castration of a male dog will help to eliminate which type of aggressive behavior?

    a. Territorial aggression

    b. Fear induced aggression

    c. Predatory aggression

    d. Redirected aggression

2 Which of the following criteria cannot be modified to affect an animal's behavior?

    a. Heritability

    b. Physical condition

    c. Environment

    d. Training

3 In an attempt to shape a new behavior in a dog, which of the following criteria would be least appropriate?

    a. Persistence

    b. Patience

    c. Timing of reward

    d. Punishment when dog makes a mistake

4 A 2-year-old dog has developed an intense fear of the vacuum cleaner. Which behavior modification technique would most likely be successful?

    a. Punishment

    b. Counter conditioning and desensitization

    c. Confinement

    d. Drug therapy—tranquillize the dog

5 A family wishes to adopt a 4-month-old puppy from a breeder. Which question is least significant?

    a. What is the puppy's choice of substance for elimination?

    b. Has the puppy been socialized to other dogs and different people?

    c. Has the puppy been exposed to novel environments?

    d. Do the parents show signs of dominant aggressive behavior?

6 When trying to remove a frightened cat from a kennel, which body postures are you least likely to see?
a. Tail carried upright
b. Pupils dilated
c. Ears flattened against head
d. Crouched position

7 Marking behavior in cats is indicative of:
a. Poor nutrition
b. Dirty environment
c. Conflict
d. Lack of attention

8 A young cat that was bottle-fed as an orphan exhibits excessively rough and persistent play with its family. What is a possible developmental cause for this type of play aggression?
a. Lack of socialization to humans
b. Lack of social play
c. Lack of maternal bond
d. Not enough environmental enrichment

9 A 1-year-old neutered male cat attacks his neutered litter mate after watching a strange cat through the window. This is an example of:
a. Intermale aggression
b. Territorial aggression
c. Redirected aggression
d. Dominance aggression

10 A 5-year-old spayed dog suddenly starts to urinate on the carpet overnight. The first step an owner should take is
a. Punish the dog
b. Confine the dog overnight
c. Have the dog examined by a veterinarian
d. Enroll the dog in obedience classes

BIBLIOGRAPHY

Beaver V: *Feline behavior: a guide for veterinarians,* Philadelphia, 1992, W.B. Saunders.

Borchelt PL: *Cat elimination behavior problems,* Marder A, Voith V, editors, Advances in companion animal behavior, The Veterinary Clinics of North America, *Small Animal Practice* 21(2):257-264, 1991, W.B. Saunders.

Burghardt WF: *Behavioral medicine as a part of a comprehensive small animal medical program,* Marder A, Voith V, editors, Advances in companion animal behavior, The Veterinary Clinics of North America, *Small Animal Practice,* 21(2):343-352, 1991, W.B. Saunders.

Campbell WE: *Behavior problems in dogs,* ed 2, Golita, California, 1992, American Veterinary Publications, Inc.

Fox, MW: *The dog its domestication and behavior,* Malabar, Florida, 1978, Krieger Publishing Company.

Hart BK: *The behavior of domestic animals,* New York, 1985, W.H. Freeman and Company.

Hetts S: *Animal Behavior,* McCurnis DM, editor, *Clinical textbook for veterinary technicians,* ed 3, Philadelphia, 1994, W.B. Saunders.

Landsberg GM: *Feline scratching and destruction and the effects of declawing;* Marder A, Voith V, editors, Advances in companion animal behavior, The Veterinary Clinics of North America, *Small Animal Practice* 21(2):265-279, 1991, W.B. Saunders.

Luesher WA, McKeown DB, Halip J: *Stereotypic or obsessive-compulsive disorders in dogs and cats,* Marder A, Voith V, editors, Advances in companion animal behavior, The Veterinary Clinics of North America, *Small Animal Practice,* 21(2):401-413, 1991, W.B. Saunders.

Overall KL: *Prevention of and early intervention for canine and feline behavioral problems,* Veterinary Technician Proceedings, 9:59-66, 1995, The North American Veterinary Conference.

Overall KL: *The technician's role in dealing with management related behavioral problems in cats,* Veterinary Technician Proceedings, 9:55-56, 1995, The North American Veterinary Conference.

Pedersen NC: *Feline husbandry, disease and management in the multiple cat environment,* Goleth, California, 1991, American Veterinary Publications, Inc.

Spreat S, Rogers-Spreat S: *Learning principles,* Voith V, Borchelt P, editors, Symposium on animal behavior, The Veterinary Clinics of North America, *Small Animal Practice* 12(4):593-606, 1982, W.B. Saunders.

Thorne C, editor: *The Waltham book of dog and cat behavior,* New York, 1992, Pergamon Press.

Voith V, Borchelt PL: *Introduction to Animal behavior therapy,* Voith V, Borchelt P, editors, Symposium on animal behavior, The Veterinary Clinics of North America, *Small Animal Practice* 12(4):565-570, 1982. W.B. Saunders.

Wolski TR: *Social behavior of the cat,* Voith V, Borchett P, editors, Symposium on animal behavior, The Veterinary Clinics of North America, *Small Animal Practice,* 12(4):693-706, 1982, W.B. Saunders.

Pharmacology

Cathy Foulkes

OUTLINE

Definitions
Basic Terminology
Pharmacokinetics
Classes of Drugs
Antibiotics
Analgesics/Sedatives

General Anesthetics
Cardiovascular Drugs
Respiratory Drugs
Gastrointestinal Drugs
Anthelmintics
Hormones and Endocrine Drugs

Vaccines (Biologicals)
Topical Drugs
Oncological Agents
Euthanizing Agents

LEARNING OUTCOMES

After reading this chapter you should be able to:

1. Understand basic classifications of drugs and general characteristics of each.
2. Understand importance of proper drug administration and problems associated with incorrect administration.
3. Be aware of common, yet potentially serious errors that can occur with certain drugs.
4. Explain the process of drug degradation to excretion.
5. Be aware of potential human health hazards associated with drugs.

Pharmacology is a science that deals with the origin, nature, chemistry, effects, and uses of drugs. This chapter will address the basic concepts of pharmacology by exploring definitions, pharmacokinetics, and distinctive characteristics of common drugs. Veterinary technicians cannot by law prescribe drugs; however, there is still a need for technicians to recognize and understand drug therapy. In many practices, the veterinary technician is the first and the last contact with the client/patient and therefore should be a source of current drug information.

This chapter contains the basics for a review of veterinary pharmacology. The tables contain examples of common drugs in use in veterinary practice. For supplementary information, consult a formulary, which contains complete lists of drugs, their major effects, contraindication, and dosages.

DEFINITIONS

I. A drug is "any chemical compound that may be used on or administered to humans or animals as an aid in diagnosis, treatment, or prevention of disease or other abnormal conditions, for the relief of pain or suffering, or to control or improve any physiologic or pathologic condition."[1]

II. A poison is "a substance that, on ingestion, inhalation, absorption, application, injection, or development within the body, in relatively small amounts, may cause structural damage or functional disturbance."[2]

   A. The drugs we use in veterinary medicine to help our patients could very easily fit the definition of a poison if given incorrectly

---

[1]From Taylor EJ, editor: *Dorland's illustrated medical dictionary*, ed 27, Philadelphia, 1988, W.B. Saunders.
[2]From O'Toole M, editor: *Miller-Keane encyclopedia and dictionary of medicine, nursing, and allied health*, ed 5, Philadelphia, 1992, W.B. Saunders.

BASIC TERMINOLOGY

I. All drugs have a generic name. This is derived from the chemical structure of the drug. A single generic drug can have several trade names
   A. For example, the drug neomycin is the active ingredient in the brand name products Biosol, Tritop, Panalog, and Tresaderm
II. All drugs have specific animal species for which they are approved. However, many of these drugs are commonly used for species not listed on the label. This is termed *extra-label usage* and is allowed only if a veterinarian/client/patient relationship exists and when it is a "generally accepted alternate use"
III. Drugs are manufactured in many forms. It is left to the veterinary practitioner to choose the best form for a given situation
   A. Capsules, tablets, solutions, suspensions, ointments, semisolids, and extracts are all examples of dosage forms
   B. Some drugs, particularly suspensions, are labeled "shake well"; it is a good idea to gently rotate all solutions, injectable and oral, before administration to ensure proper distribution of the drug particles. This rule applies unless otherwise specified by the manufacturer
IV. Drugs that have the potential to be addictive are termed *controlled drugs*
   A. These drugs are classified by the United States Drug Enforcement Administration (DEA) according to their abuse potential. They are denoted by the symbols C-I through C-V. The lowest Roman numerals are the most addictive
   B. The Canadian Food and Drug Act Schedules specify which drugs are over the counter (OTC), prescription, control, and narcotics
V. Drug withdrawal times are important in food animal medicine
   A. Any drug given to a food animal can potentially be transferred to people through ingestion of animal products
   B. It is legally required that a drug dispensed for food animals have the withdrawal time listed on the label
   C. Many books listing withdrawal times are available to the practitioner

PHARMACOKINETICS

I. A drug must reach its target organ or tissue to exert an effect

II. Proper administration of a drug is the initial step and must include administering the correct drug, at the right time, by the correct route, in the proper amount, to the correct patient
   A. Some drug companies use look alike vials for different drugs and different concentrations of the same drug. It is best to use the "three checks" system when preparing drugs
      1. Look at the drug name and concentration as you pull the bottle off the shelf
      2. Look again as you are drawing it into the syringe
      3. Check a third time as you are returning the drug to the shelf
   B. Watch concentrations carefully. Many drugs come in small animal and large animal concentrations. A mistake in this area can be fatal to the patient
   C. Some drugs must be administered more frequently than others to remain at a therapeutic level
      1. Ingesta interferes with the absorption of some drugs so timing doses around mealtimes becomes important
   D. Drugs labeled for IM administration may not be absorbed if administered via other routes. Likewise, an oral drug injected IV could have serious or fatal consequences
   E. When preparing an injectable drug use the largest syringe that will measure the drug accurately
III. The therapeutic index (TI) is a calculation used to define the amount of toxicity of a drug
   A. The TI is the comparison between a drug's ability to reach the desired effect and its tendency to produce toxic effects
      1. The TI is expressed as a ratio between the LD_{50} and the ED_{50}
         a. LD_{50} is the dose of a drug that is lethal to 50% of the animals in a dose related drug trial
         b. ED_{50} is the dose of a drug that produces the effective dose in 50% of the animals in a dose related drug trial
      2. The calculation is:

$$TI = \frac{LD_{50}}{ED_{50}}$$

      3. The larger the number for the TI, the safer the drug. Drugs with lower TI numbers tend to be more toxic

4. Drugs used to treat cancer have low TI

IV. After administration a drug must make its way to the bloodstream and then into the intended tissues. This is known as absorption

A. Absorption depends on several factors in the body and the drug itself, including pKa of the drug, pH of the tissues, and ionization status of the drug

1. The pKa determines in what form the drug will exist (ionized or un-ionized) at any given pH

B. The body has its own defenses against drug invasion such as the "blood-brain barrier"

C. Orally administered drugs pass through the liver before reaching systemic circulation. This reduces the amount of drug available systemically in most cases and is known as the "first pass effect"

V. When a drug reaches its target tissues it may exert an effect in three ways:

A. Bind to a receptor site and cause the cell to react

B. Interact with ions in the body to create a chemical reaction

C. Physical presence of the drug facilitates a reaction

VI. The process of eliminating a drug from the body is termed *excretion*

A. Changes in the chemical structure of drugs are caused by the liver and, to a lesser degree, other organs. This process is termed *metabolization* and the resulting drug components are termed *metabolites*

B. Circulating metabolites are usually excreted in the urine when they pass through the kidneys

1. Occasionally the metabolites of a drug will be more active than the parent compound

2. In some instances the metabolites may be toxic to the animal

3. Monitoring hydration status becomes critical with drugs such as aminoglycosides, which are nephrotoxic and excreted by the kidneys

4. Patients with decreased liver or kidney function may not be able to eliminate drugs efficiently

C. Oral drugs that are not absorbed pass through the intestine unchanged and are excreted in the feces

CLASSES OF DRUGS

I. Drugs are divided into different classes according to the effect they have on the body

II. One drug may have multiple indications for use. For example, diazepam (Valium) is used as a sedative, a preanesthetic, and for short-term seizure control

ANTIBIOTICS

I. Antibiotics are drugs that are toxic to bacteria (Table 6-1)

II. Antibiotics are the most commonly prescribed drugs in veterinary medicine

A. Bacterial resistance to antibiotics is a major problem in human and veterinary medicine

B. The least resistant bacteria will be the first to die when a dose of antibiotic is given. If only 5 days of a 7-day antibiotic treatment is administered, bacteria that were resistant enough to survive are left to reproduce

C. Technicians need to explain to clients the importance of giving the full course of antibiotics

III. Antibiotics are bacteriocidal (they kill the bacteria) or bacteriostatic (bacteria reproduction or development is inhibited). This is accomplished by five different means

A. Disruption of the bacterial cell wall

1. Penicillins exert this mechanism of action

2. Loss of cell wall integrity causes the cell to lyse

3. This method works on bacteria in the growth stage only. Therefore giving a bacteriostatic antibiotic (thus stopping bacterial growth) concurrently with a penicillin will antagonize the effects of the penicillin

B. Change in permeability of bacterial cell membrane

1. Polymyxins utilize this mechanism

2. Change in permeability allows (1) drugs to diffuse into the bacterial cell and (2) bacterial structures to diffuse out

C. Interference with bacteria's protein synthesis

1. Aminoglycosides are bacteriocidal. They make their way into the bacteria and attach to the ribosomes, rendering the bacteria unable to produce vital proteins

2. Tetracyclines, lincosamides, chloramphenicol, and macrolides use the same method but are bacteriostatic

Table 6-1 Antibiotics

Generic	Trade name	Routes	Class	Notes
amikacin	Amiglyde-V Amikin	IV IM—stings SC—stings intrauterine	aminoglycoside	Keep animal well hydrated and use extra caution with animals trained to guide handicapped persons due to nephrotoxic and ototoxic effects
amoxicillin	Amoxi-Tabs Biomox Robamox-V	IV IM SC PO	penicillin	May be given with or without food; if GI upset is probable give with a meal
ampicillin	Polyflex Amcill Amp-Equine Princillin	IV—slowly IM PO	penicillin	Do not give orally to rabbits: can interfere with normal intestinal flora and could result in death
cefazolin sodium	Kefsol Ancef Zolicef	IV—slowly IM SC	cephalosporin	First generation cephalosporin; good activity against gram-positive and anaerobic bacteria
chloramphenicol	Amphicol	IV IM SC PO	chloramphenicol	Do not give before pentobarbital anesthesia: may increase recovery time; penetrates CNS; may cause aplastic anemia in humans; Do not give to food animals
clindamycin	Antirobe	IM—stings SC PO	lincosamide	Do not administer to rabbits, hamsters, guinea pigs, and horses
enrofloxacin	Baytril	IV (not approved, however enrofloxacin is given IV over 20 minutes when mixed 1:2 with sterile water for injection) IM PO	quinolone	Do not give to puppies up to 28 weeks of age: it may cause hindquarter weakness and abnormal carpal joint formation
erythromycin	Erythro-100 Erythro-200	IV—very slowly IM—stings PO teat infusion	macrolide	Enters prostate but not the CNS
griseofulvin	Fulvicin-U/F Grisactin Grifulvin	PO	antifungal	Known teratogen in cats
gentamicin	Gentocin Garasol Garacin	IV IM—stings SC—stings PO	aminoglycoside	Ototoxic, nephrotoxic, and neurotoxic; make sure animal is well hydrated to reduce nephrotoxicity
lincomycin	Lincocin	IV—infusion only IM PO	lincosamide	Do not administer to guinea pigs, rabbits, horses, or hamsters Do not give to patients with existing Candidiasis infections: yeast overgrowth can occur
metronidazole	Flagyl	IV PO	antiprotozoal	Carcinogenic in rats
neomycin	Biosol	IV IM SC PO topical	aminoglycoside	Usually given orally for treatment of diarrhea: not absorbed very well systemically Extremely nephrotoxic when given parenterally
potentiated amoxicillin	Clavamox	PO	penicillin	Clavulanic acid is a β-lactamase inhibitor Works well for bacteria that have developed resistance to amoxicillin
potentiated sulfa	Di-trim Tribrissen	IV IM SC PO	sulfonamide	Can precipitate in the kidneys of dehydrated patients; can cause KCS (keratoconjunctivitis sicca)
tetracycline	Panmycin Achromycin-V	IV—slowly IM PO	tetracycline	May cause tooth discolorization in prenatal (if given to mother), neonatal, and early postnatal patients

D. Inhibition of nucleic acid production
 1. Because this method interferes with DNA and/or RNA the potential exists for mutations and birth defects to occur in patients receiving these drugs
 2. Griseofulvin, ketoconazole, and metronidazole are drugs that use this mechanism
 3. Enrofloxin (Baytril) uses this method but is selective for bacterial DNA
E. Disruption of bacteria's normal metabolic activity
 1. Sulfa drugs are included in this category
 2. This usually results in bacteria being unable to divide. Therefore drugs using this method are bacteriostatic

ANALGESICS/SEDATIVES (Table 6-2)

I. These drugs are two separate classes but most show effects of both categories. They can reduce pain, be used as a preanesthetic, ease positioning for radiographs, and reduce patient anxiety
II. Examples are phenothiazine tranquilizers, alpha$_2$-agonists, anticonvulsants, opioid (narcotic) analgesics, corticosteroids, and nonsteroidal antiinflammatory drugs

A. Phenothiazines/promazines
 1. Can be used as preanesthetic drugs to agonize anesthesia
 2. Some can be used as antiemetics
 3. Can lower the seizure threshold in dogs and cause penile prolapse in horses, sometimes leading to injury and paralysis of the penis retractor muscle
B. Alpha$_2$-agonists include xylazine and detomidine
 1. Cattle are extremely sensitive to xylazine
 2. Detomidine is stronger than xylazine and used mostly in the horse
C. Anticonvulsants include diazepam and phenobarbital
 1. Diazepam is used most frequently for short-term seizure control
 2. Phenobarbital is used orally for long-term seizure control and IV for treatment of status epilepticus
D. Opioid analgesics include morphine, meperidine, oxymorphone, butorphanol, and codeine
 1. Narcotics are competitively antagonized by naloxone (Narcan) and naltrexone (Trexan)

Table 6-2 Analgesics/sedatives

Generic	Trade name	Routes	Class	Notes
acepromazine maleate	Promace Acepromazine Tranquazine	IV IM—stings SC PO	phenothiazine; tranquilizer	Do not use in conjunction with organophosphates
acetaminophen	Tylenol	PO	analgesic; antipyretic	Contraindicated in cats: the metabolites cause a toxicity reaction known as methemoglobinuria
aspirin		PO	NSAID	Avoid using in pregnant animals due to possibility of teratogenic effects
butorphanol tartrate	Torbugesic	IV IM SC	opiate	Butorphanol is available in 0.5 mg/mL and 10 mg/mL concentrations: watch carefully Naloxone antagonizes butorphanol
detomidine hydrochloride	Dormosedan	IV IM	alpha$_2$ agonist	Used mostly in horses Do not use with IV potentiated sulfa drugs: fatal dysrythmias can occur
fentanyl citrate/ droperidol C-II	Innovar-vet Innovar (human product)	IV—slowly IM—stings SC—stings	fentanyl-opiate droperidol-butyrophenone	Antagonized by Naloxone If given too rapidly IV, thoracic muscles may become rigid, causing respiratory arrest
flunixin meglumine	Banamine	IV IM PO	NSAID	Only labeled for use in horses in the U.S. Extra-label usage is common
xylazine HCl	Rompun Anased Geminis Solvazines Xyla-ject	IV IM SC	alpha$_2$ agonist	Available in 20 and 100 mg/mL concentrations, check carefully before administering Antagonized by yohimbine (Yobine, Antagonil) Respiratory depression and vomiting are common side effects

2. Used frequently as preanesthetic agents
3. A common side effect is respiratory depression, although panting may be seen initially

E. Dexamethazone and prednisone are two commonly used corticosteroids
   1. Corticosteroids act as analgesics by reducing tissue swelling
   2. Corticosteroid drugs are synthetic reproductions of naturally occurring hormones; therefore extra care must be taken with their use
   3. Gradual reduction in dosage is critical with corticosteroid therapy

F. Phenylbutazone, aspirin, ibuprofen, and flunixin meglumine (Banamine) are nonsteroidal antiinflammatory drugs (NSAIDs)
   1. NSAIDs will not produce sufficient analgesia to counteract pain associated with organs or broken bones

2. Most NSAIDs work by blocking prostaglandin production

GENERAL ANESTHETICS (Table 6-3) ▬▬▬

I. General anesthetics cause the loss of all sensation
II. General anesthetics are available as injectables and inhalants
III. Overdoses of some general anesthetics are used for euthanasia
IV. Any general anesthetic can be fatal if overdose occurs

CARDIOVASCULAR DRUGS (Table 6-4) ▬▬▬

Cardiovascular drugs effect the heart. They include antiarrhythmics, diuretics, positive inotropic drugs, catecholamines, and vasodilators
   I. Antiarrhythmics
      A. Antiarrhythmics include lidocaine, propranolol, and verapamil

Table 6-3   General anesthetics

Generic	Trade name	Routes	Class	Notes
halothane	Halothane, USP Fluothane, Somnothane	inhalation	inhalant	Increases cerebrospinal fluid pressure; can cause condition called malignant hyperthermia, where body temperatures increase rapidly; hepatoxic
isoflurane	Aerrane Forane	inhalation	inhalant	Rapid induction and recovery Can allow too rapid a recovery in horses, which will stand before they are fully alert
ketamine hydrochloride	Ketaset Vetalar	IV—bolus IM	dissociative anesthetic	Corneal, pedal, cough, and swallowing reflexes are not eliminated
methoxyflurane	Metofane	inhalation	inhalant	Soluble in plastic Do not use if solution is discolored Not considered as safe as isoflurane and halothane
oxymorphone hydrochloride C-II	P/M Oxymorphone HCl injection Numorphan	IV IM SC rectal	opiate	Oxymorphone is antagonized by Naloxone
pentobarbital sodium C-II	Euthanyl, Euthansol	IV—slowly to effect	barbiturate	Pentobarbital may cause precipitation when added to acidic solutions
propofol	Rapinovet	IV only—to effect	sedative/hypnotic	Facilitates rapid induction and recovery
sodium thiopental C-III	Pentothal-Kit	IV only	thiobarbiturate	May adsorb to plastic IV tubing and bags
sodium thiamylal	Anestatal	IV only	barbiturate	Disagreeable odor is normal Reconstitute with sterile water; LRS can cause precipitation If further dilution is needed use 5% dextrose or isotonic saline
tiletamine hydrochloride/ zolazepam hydrochloride C-III	Telazol	IV IM	tiletamine-dissociative anesthetic zolazepam-diazepinone tranquilizer	Corneal, pedal, cough, and swallowing reflexes remain Not for use in tigers

B. When arrhythmias occur in the heart, antiarrhythmics restore normal electrical activity

II. Diuretics

    A. Furosemide and mannitol are examples of diuretics

    B. Diuretics create an osmotic force in the renal tubules, thus drawing in water and increasing urine output

       1. Removing water decreases cardiac workload

       2. Use cautiously in hypovolemic or hypotensive animals

III. Positive inotropes and catecholamines

    A. These drugs increase the strength of contraction of the heart

       1. Positive inotropes are used for long-term maintenance of contractility by increasing the amount of calcium available to the myocardial cells

       2. Digoxin is the most commonly prescribed positive inotrope

       3. Catecholamines are used when short-term contractility is needed; they act by mimicking the sympathetic nervous system

       4. Epinephrine and dobutamine are catecholamines

IV. Vasodilators

    A. Nitroglycerin and enalapril are vasodilators

    B. Vasodilators cause an expansion in the diameter of blood vessels. This increase in diameter allows blood to flow more easily, which in turn reduces the heart's workload

RESPIRATORY DRUGS (Table 6-5)

I. Antitussives suppress the cough reflex

    A. Codeine and butorphanol are antitussives

    B. Antitussives may be contraindicated with productive coughs

II. Expectorants increase the amount of fluid in respiratory mucus

    A. Guaifenesin and volatile oils are expectorants

    B. Nebulization and humidification can also increase mucus fluidity

III. Bronchodilators: expand the bronchioles in the lungs, making it easier to breathe

    A. Terbutaline, albuterol, and metaproterenol stimulate beta-2 receptors in the lung, which in turn cause bronchodilation

    B. Theophylline and aminophylline cause relaxation of smooth muscles in the lungs and, in turn, bronchodilation

Table 6-4 Cardiovascular drugs

Generic	Trade name	Routes	Class	Notes
digoxin	Lanoxin Cardoxin	IV—rapidly PO	positive inotrope	Toxic and therapeutic doses may overlap Dobermans tend to be sensitive to digoxin
dobutamine HCl	Dobutrex	IV	synthetic inotropic agent	Give as an infusion only; use diluted solutions within 24 hours

enalapril
  maleate
enalaprilat
	Enacard
	Vasotec
		IV
		PO
			angiotensin-converting
			  enzyme (ACE) inhibitor
				Give on an empty stomach

epinephrine	Adrenalin chloride	IV IM SC	catecholamine	Epinephrine is available in 1 mg/mL and 0.1 g/mL concentrations; watch concentrations carefully
furosemide	Lasix Disal Diuride	IV IM PO	diuretic	Veterinary furosemide (50 mg/mL) concentration normally is slightly yellow; if the human product (10 mg/mL) turns yellow do not use it

lidocaine	Xylocaine	IV
		IM—in canines,
		  if necessary
			antiarrhythmic local
			  anesthetic
				Lidocaine is also available in combination with epinephrine: this preparation is *not* to be used in IV solutions

nitroglycerin	Nitro-bid Nitrol Nitrong Nitrostat	topical	vasodilator	Wear gloves when applying nitroglycerin ointment
propranolol HCl	Inderal	IV—slowly PO	beta-blocker antiarrhythmic	Sympathomimetic drug effects can be blocked by propranolol
verapamil	Calan Isoptin	IV	calcium channel blocker; indicated for supraventricular tachycardia	Verapamil has a high first-pass effect; watch for overdose in animals with hepatic disease

Table 6-5 Respiratory drugs

Generic	Trade name	Routes	Use	Notes
aminophylline		IV IM—very painful PO	bronchodilator	CO_2 causes aminophylline to precipitate *Do not* inject air into multiuse vials
butorphanol tartrate	Torbutrol Torbugesic	IV IM SC PO	cough suppressant analgesic preanesthetic antiemetic: used before cisplatin treatment	Package insert approves its use for relief of the nonproductive cough in dogs For other uses see Table 6-2
codeine phosphate C-II		PO IV IM SC	antitussive antidiarrheal analgesic	Codeine is an opiate agonist; products con- taining codeine such as Tylenol with codeine and cough syrups containing codeine range from C-III to C-V
diphenhydramine	Benadryl	IV IM PO	antihistamine antipruritic antiemetic	IV product used to counteract anaphylactic reactions
guaifenesin (GG, glycerol guaiacolate)	Guailaxin Gecolate	IV PO	expectorant muscle relaxant	Guaifenesin causes skeletal, pharyngeal, and laryngeal muscle relaxation
terbutaline sulfate	Brethine Bricanyl	IV SC PO	bronchodilator	CNS excitation has been reported in horses given this drug

Some references recommend injecting air into multiuse vials to facilitate drug withdrawal. However, air is not sterile; therefore injecting air into any multidose vial of otherwise sterile drug does not seem appropriate.

IV. Antihistamines: also cause bronchodilation if given prophylactically. Antihistamines do not reverse the bronchoconstriction that histamine causes

GASTROINTESTINAL DRUGS (Table 6-6)

I. Emetics cause vomiting
  A. Used when noncaustic poisons are eaten or as preanesthetic
  B. Emetics are locally acting (cause irritation to the GI tract) or centrally acting (stimulate vomiting center in CNS)
II. Antiemetics prevent vomiting
  A. Used when vomiting is not beneficial to the animal
  B. Sooth GI tract or block impulses to CNS vomiting center
III. Antidiarrheals treat diarrhea
  A. These drugs work by modifying intestinal motility; adsorbing enterotoxins, thus protecting intestinal wall; and preventing intestinal hypersecretions
IV. Laxatives are used to relieve constipation and to clear the lower intestinal tract
V. Antacids increase gastric pH, reducing irritation
  A. Nonsystemic antacids directly neutralize acid
  B. Systemic antacids block gastric acid production

VI. Antiulcer medications are used to treat gastric ulcers

ANTHELMINTICS (Table 6-7)

I. Anthelmintics kill or inactivate parasites
II. Rotating anthelmintics use can help prevent parasite resistance

HORMONES AND ENDOCRINE DRUGS

I. Most reproductive drugs are hormones. These include the estrogens, progestins, prostaglandins, and oxytocin
  A. Estrogens
    1. Commonly used in "mis-mating" injections
    2. Interfere with ova by not letting them reach the uterus
    3. Aplastic anemia is one of many serious side effects
  B. Progestins
    1. Used for estrous cycle regulation
      a. If a mare is in transitional anestrus, progestins can return the animal to proestrus
      b. If an animal is in proestrus, progestins can prevent estrus
    2. Liquid progestins can be absorbed through skin, therefore use caution and

Table 6-6   Gastrointestinal drugs

Generic	Trade name	Routes	Use	Notes
activated charcoal	SuperChar Toxiband	PO	adsorbant	See "notes" for syrup of ipecac
aminopentamide hydrogen sulfate	Centrine	IM SC PO	antispasmotic	If urine retention is noted stop administration of this drug
antacids	Amphogel Magnalax Basalgel Maalox Tums	PO	neutralize acid	Antacids can reduce, or in some instances increase, the absorption of other drugs
apomorphine		IV IM SC Topically in conjunctiva of eye	emetic	If apomorpine does not cause animal to vomit in a timely manner, further administration will probably be ineffective and could cause toxicity
bismuth subsalicylate	Corrective mixture Pepto-Bismol	PO	antidiarrheal	Can decrease absorption of tetracyclines; if giving both drugs, separate doses by at least 2 hours
cimetidine	Tagamet	IV IM—stings SC PO	antiulcer	Do not refrigerate injectable form: precipitate may develop
dioctyl sodium sulfosuccinate (docusate sodium and DDS)	Disposaject Colace	PO enema	stool softener	Watch hydration status carefully; if giving with mineral oil separate administration by a minimum of 2 hours
kaolin/pectin	Kaopectolin Kao-Forte K-P-Sol	PO	antidiarreal	If giving with lincomycin separate doses by at least 2 hours
laxatives	Carmilax Milk of Magnesia Laxatone	PO	laxatives	Laxatives soften stools, stimulate peristaltic motion, and distend the lumen of the intestine
metoclopramide	Reglan	IV—slowly IM SC PO	GI stimulatory antiemetic	Inhibits gastroesophageal reflux
poloxalene	Therabloat	PO	antibloat agent	Resolves early stages of bloat in cattle
prochlorperazine isopropamide	Darbazine	IM SC PO	antiemetic antidiarrheal	May cause urine to turn pink or red-brown
ranitidine HCl	Zantac	IV—slowly IM—stings SC PO	antiulcer	Reduces gastric acid output; more potent than cimetidine
sucralfate	Carafate	PO	antiulcer	Forms a protective barrier at the ulcer site; if giving with antacids give sucralfate one half hour before the other drug is introduced
syrup of ipecac		PO	emetic	Extract of ipecac is much stronger than syrup of ipecac: watch doses carefully If given in conjunction with activated charcoal, give ipecac first, then wait for vomiting to occur before administering charcoal

Table 6-7 Anthelmintics

Generic	Trade name	Routes	Efficacy	Notes
benzimidazoles mebendazole fenbendazole	Panacur	PO	Ascarids, *Trichuris* spp., hookworms, cestodes (except *Diplidium caninum*), some lungworms, some trichostrongyles, large and small strongyles, and oxyurids	Must follow recommended treatment schedule or fenbendazole is ineffective
diethylcarbamazine (DEC)	Difil Tabs Filaribits Nemacide Dirocide	PO	Heartworm preventive; also effective against ascarids at a higher dose	Do not give to heartworm positive animals: the degeneration of microfilaria can cause fatal anaphylactic reactions
epsiprantel	Cestex	PO	cestodes	Not absorbed systemically to a significant degree
ivermectin	Ivomec Eqvalan Liquid Heartguard Zimectrin paste	IM (birds and reptiles) SC PO topical	Effective against most parasites, except cestodes and liver flukes	Collies and similar breeds may be sensitive to ivermectin: monitor these dogs closely for adverse reactions
lufenuron	Program	PO	Interrupts flea life-cycle	Does not kill adult fleas Inhibits chitin development
melarsomine	Immiticide	IM only—stings	Heartworm adulticide	Swelling at injection site is common; can see post-treatment thromboembolism, as with thiacetarsemide
metronidazole	Flagyl	IV PO	Antiprotozoal; also bacteriocidal to many anaerobes	Has shown to be teratogenic in laboratory animals
milbemycin oxime	Interceptor	PO	Heartworm preventive; also effective against hookworms, *Trichuris*, and ascarids	May cause shocklike syndrome in dogs with high numbers of microfilaria
organophosphates*	Dursban products Task Atgard Equigard ComBot Dyrex Baymix Pro-spot Proban	PO Topical Commonly used in lawn and gardening products as powders and sprays	ectoparasites, internal parasites, including fleas, ticks, mites, and bots	Use of more than one organophosphate at a time (even those used for gardening, etc.) greatly increases the possibility of organophosphate toxicity Signs of toxicity include salivation, lacrimation, urination, defecation, dyspnea, emesis (SLUDDE), and miosis
piperazine	Pipa-Tabs† Purina liquid wormer†	PO	ascarids	Frequently used in combination with other antihelminics to increase efficacy
praziquantel	Droncit	IM—stings SC—stings PO	cestodes	Almost completely absorbed systemically after administration
pyrantel pamoate pyrantel tartrate	Nemex Strongid	PO	ascarids, hookworms, *Physaloptera* spp., trichostrongyles, and small strongyles	Piperazine antagonizes the action of pyrantel
pyrethrins	common ingredient in insect sprays	topical	insects	Very safe product; Exhibits rapid "knockdown" but does not necessarily kill insects
thiacetarsemide sodium	Carparsolate	IV	heartworm adulticide	Derived from arsenic; may cause extensive sloughing if given perivascularly; post-treatment thromboembolism can occur: minimize exercise to reduce this potential risk

*Organophosphates is the name of a group of chemicals, including chlorpyrifos, cythioate, dichlorvos, fenthion, and malathion
†These are over-the-counter products

wear gloves when preparing and administering
C. Prostaglandins
1. Lyse the corpus luteum
   a. Can initiate a new estrous cycle for animals in diestrus
   b. May cause abortion in pregnant animals and humans
2. Prostaglandins are easily absorbed through skin; use caution and wear protective apparel
D. Oxytocin
1. Causes uterine contraction and milk letdown
2. Contraindicated if cervix is not dilated
II. Examples of commonly used endocrine drugs are insulin and thyroid supplements
A. Insulin
1. Insulin is measured as international units (IU) per milliliter
2. Only insulin syringes should be used to measure insulin
3. Each mark on an insulin syringe is equal to one IU
4. Insulin is available in U-100 and U-40 concentrations. Each concentration has a syringe type associated with it that must be used to measure that particular concentration. If U-100 insulin is measured in a U-40 syringe the animal will be overdosed by a factor of 2.5
5. Insulin removes glucose from circulation and stores it in tissues
6. Insulin is available in three forms
   a. Regular insulin (short acting) is used when a rapid drop in blood sugar is needed
   b. NPH insulin (intermediate acting) is used to control diabetes mellitus on a daily basis
   c. Protamine zinc insulin (long-acting) is used in animals, usually cats, that need a slower release of insulin to carry them through 24 hours
B. Thyroid supplements
1. The pituitary gland secretes TSH (thyroid stimulating hormone), which tells the thyroid gland to produce and secrete the hormones T_3 (triiodothyronine) and T_4 (thyroxine)
2. These hormones regulate the metabolic rate for the rest of the body

3. Two common conditions associated with the thyroid gland are hypothyroidism (usually seen in dogs) and hyperthyroidism (usually seen in cats)
4. Hypothyroidism occurs when thyroid function is decreased. This can happen when the thyroid gland is diseased (primary hypothyroidism) or when the pituitary gland is diseased (secondary hypothyroidism). Hypothyroidism slows metabolic processes
   a. Thyroid supplementation is the treatment of choice for hypothyroidism
   b. Synthetic T_3, synthetic T_4, and thyroid extract are the supplementation choices available
      (1) Thyroid extract is highly variable in its effectiveness
      (2) Oversupplementation is common with T_3 administration
      (3) T_4 supplements are usually indicated in animals
5. Hyperthyroidism occurs when thyroid function is increased, thus speeding up metabolic processes
   a. Thyroidectomy is usually indicated for hyperthyroid treatment
   b. Two other courses of treatment are also available
      (1) Methimazol (Tapazole), which interferes with production of T_3 and T_4
      (2) Introduction of radioactive iodine, which is taken up by the thyroid gland and destroys any tumor cells (and most of the normal thyroid cells) that are present

VACCINES (BIOLOGICALS)

I. The sheer number of vaccines available limits their discussion in this chapter to general characteristics
II. Vaccines are used to prevent disease or to reduce the virulence of diseases that animals may contract
A. Vaccines cannot cure a disease process that is present before vaccination
III. Vaccines stimulate an animal's immune system by introducing antigen derived from pathogenic agents and encouraging an anamnestic response
A. Vaccines are described as live, modified live, or killed

B. Killed vaccines are safest but tend to be less effective than the other forms

IV. Vaccines are available in many forms, including injections, intranasal solutions, powdered feed additives, aerosol sprays, and water additives

V. Vaccine efficacy depends on several factors, including dose given, route of administration, age of animal, storage conditions, health/immune status of animal, and breed/species of animal

VI. It is not known exactly when passive immunity via maternal antibodies ceases to protect neonates; therefore multiple doses of vaccine are required at regular intervals to optimize protection for young animals

VII. Most vaccines are not effective immediately after administration. Some take 2 weeks or more to reach maximum efficacy

VIII. Warming vaccines just before use reduces pain of administration

TOPICAL DRUGS

I. Topical drugs are applied to the skin surface, including mucous membranes, otically, optically, intranasal, sublingual, and intravaginal

A. Generally, topical drugs are not absorbed well systemically

B. Because veterinary patients tend to "lick their wounds," read package instructions carefully. Extra caution is warranted when using human products because they are more likely to be toxic if consumed

C. Wear proper protective clothing when applying topical drugs that are meant to be absorbed systemically (e.g., nitroglycerin and "pour-on" preparations)

ONCOLOGICAL AGENTS

I. Oncological agents kill cells. They do not discriminate between "good" cells and "bad" cells or animal cells and human cells. Therefore it is of utmost importance to wear protective clothing when administering or preparing these agents

II. These drugs target rapidly dividing cells such as cancer, bone marrow, and GI cells

III. Doses are administered according to body surface in meters squared *not* body weight

IV. Oncological agents and all equipment that contacts the agents must be disposed of in chemotherapeutic waste bags with warning labels

EUTHANIZING AGENTS

I. An overdose of any anesthetic can be used to euthanize an animal

II. Pentobarbital sodium is the most common euthanizing agent

A. Pentobarbital sodium by itself is a C-II drug (US-DEA); controlled drug (Canada)

B. Some products include additives such as phenytoin in Beuthanasia-D special or lidocaine in FP-3. These additives act as cardiac depressives and change the pentobarbital sodium to a C-III (US-DEA) drug

1. Pentobarbital sodium can cause necrosis if injected perivascularly into a human

2. Perivascular injection into an animal will delay or inhibit death

3. Animals in pain may require a tranquilizer before pentobarbital sodium administration

4. These products must not be used in animals to be used for human or animal consumption

Pharmacology is an inexact science. Any given drug may affect different animal species, or even individual animals within one species, unpredictably. Remember to treat each patient as an individual and pay attention to any abnormal behavior displayed by an animal being treated with any pharmaceutical. Used correctly, drugs are a great benefit to veterinary medicine; used incorrectly they can be equally detrimental.

Review Questions

1 Insulin is dosed in what units of measurement?
a. mL
b. tsp
c. IU
d. g

2 In what class of drugs is nephrotoxicity, nuerotoxicity, and ototoxicity a problem?
a. Barbiturates
b. Aminoglycosides
c. Phenothiazine tranquilizers
d. Dissociative anesthetics

3 With what group of animals is withdrawal time especially important?
a. Food animals
b. Exotics
c. Equids
d. Pets

4 What is the primary organ involved in excretion of drugs?
a. Liver
b. Intestine
c. Kidney
d. Spleen

5 A cow is accidentally dosed with an equine dose of xylazine. What drug should be immediately administered?
  a. None: the cow cannot survive that amount of xylazine
  b. Epinephrine followed by naloxone
  c. Yohimbine
  d. Do nothing

6 The therapeutic index is:
  a. The comparison between a drugs's ability to reach the desired effect and its tendency to produce toxic effects
  b. The dose of a drug that produces the lethal dose in 50% of the animals tested
  c. The comparison between a drug's ability to reach a toxic effect and a lethal effect
  d. The dose of a drug that produces the effective dose in 50% of the animals tested

7 The "first pass effect" is:
  a. Blood-brain barrier
  b. The metabolization of drugs containing proteins
  c. The reduction of drugs reaching the systemic circulation by the liver
  d. The ionization of drugs

8 Name a drug that requires protective clothing when handled:
  a. Xylazine
  b. Torbugesic
  c. Prostaglandin
  d. Lidocaine

9 Vaccines may fail because:
  a. Animal is too young for the vaccine to be effective
  b. The vaccine was improperly stored
  c. The animal was febrile at the time of administration
  d. All of the above

10 A dog is seen eating battery acid:
  a. Emesis should be induced as soon as possible
  b. Emesis should not be induced
  c. The veterinarian may prescribe a laxative to relieve the dog of the GI upset
  d. The veterinarian may prescribe an antacid such as Magnalax or Maalox

BIBLIOGRAPHY

Bill R: *Pharmacology for veterinary technicians,* ed 2, St Louis, 1997, Mosby.

Fraser CM, editor: *The Merck veterinary manual,* ed 7, Rathway, New Jersey, 1991, Merck & CO., Inc.

Ko J, Pablo L, Bailey J, Heaton-Jones T: Propofol: a new intravenous anesthetic, *Vet Tech* 16(11):734-736, 1995.

McCurnin DM: *Clinical textbook for veterinary technicians,* ed. 3, Philadelphia, 1994, W.B. Saunders.

Muir W, Hubbell J: *Handbook of veterinary anesthesia,* St. Louis, 1989, Mosby.

O'Toole M, editor: *Miller-Keane encyclopedia and dictionary of medicine, nursing, and allied health,* ed. 5, Philadelphia, 1992, W.B. Saunders.

Plumb D: *Veterinary drug handbook,* ed. 2, Ames, Iowa, 1995, Iowa State University Press.

Pratt PW: *Medical, surgical and anesthetic nursing,* ed 2, Goleta, California, 1994, American Veterinary Publications Inc.

Rawlings CA, McCall JW: Melarsomine: a new heartworm adulticide, *The Compendium* April:373-379, 1996.

Taylor EJ, editor: *Dorland's illustrated medical dictionary,* ed. 27, Philadelphia, 1988, W.B. Saunders.

Wanamaker B, Pettes CL: *Applied pharmacology for the veterinary technician,* Philadelphia, 1996, W.B. Saunders.

CHAPTER 7

Pharmaceutical Calculations and Metric Conversion

Monica Tighe

OUTLINE

Metric System
  Units
  Time
  Date
  Length
  Volume
  Area

Temperature
Mass
Quantity
  Electrical Current
Metric Conversions
Dosage Calculations
Dilutions/Solutions

Drip Rates
Prescription Labels
Metric, Apothecary, and Household
  Equivalents
Abbreviations and Definitions

LEARNING OUTCOMES

After reading this chapter you should be able to:

1. Describe the rules for writing metric numbers, dates, and symbols.
2. Perform conversion of numbers to various metric units.
3. Calculate dosages.
4. Calculate dilutions.
5. Calculate concentrations of solutions.
6. Calculate drip rates.
7. Define information that must be included on a prescription label.

This chapter contains basic information on the metric system, including rules for writing metric numbers and conversion of metric units. Formulas for calculating dosages, preparing solutions, dilutions, and estimating drip rates are also included with examples. This chapter also includes a brief section on prescription labels, an abbreviations list, and an equivalent chart. Please note that the use of calculators during the North American veterinary technician examination is not permitted.

METRIC SYSTEM

The metric system can be referred to also as the SI System or Le Systeme International d'Unites.

Units

I. There are specific rules for writing metric units
  A. Lowercase letters are used for all units—except for the symbol for liter (L) or if units are named after a person
  B. Symbols are not pluralized
  C. There should be a space between the number and the symbol
  D. Always place a zero before the decimal point when the number is less than zero
    1. The placing of a marker (0) before a decimal also prevents misreading a dosage less than 1 on a medical record

2. EXAMPLE: .8 mL should be written 0.8 mL
E. The comma is not used when writing numbers with more than three digits. A space is left instead.
   1. EXAMPLE: 987,098.098098 should be written 987 098.098 098
F. Decimals are used instead of fractions

Time

I. Measured in hours, minutes, and seconds using a 24-hour clock
A. The 24-hour clock expresses the time in four digits beginning at midnight with 00:00 or 24:00. The first two digits express the number of hours since midnight, and the second two digits express the number of minutes in that hour
B. EXAMPLE
   1. The time at 2:53 p.m. is written 14:53
   2. There is no need to write a.m. or p.m., since it is expressed in the value of time

Date

I. The date is written in the following form: year/month/day/time (24-hour clock)
A. EXAMPLE: January 24, 1996, 5:50 p.m. is written 96/01/24 17:50
II. There may be a slash, dot, or space between the numbers
III. In the United States the date is written day/month/year
A. EXAMPLE: 24/01/96

Length

I. Measured in meters (m)
II. In terms of nonmetric units, 1 inch = 0.0254 m

Volume

I. Measured in liters (L)
II. Volume is derived by length × length × length = m^3, or 1 cubic meter
III. 1 millilitre (mL) = 1 cubic centimeter (cc)
IV. Parts per million (ppm) = 1 mg of solute in 1 kg or 1 L of solvent

Area

I. Length × length = m^2, or 1 square meter
II. An angstrom (Å) = 10^{-10} m

Temperature

I. Celsius or C (capital C)
   Freezing point = 0° C at 1 atmospheric pressure

Boiling point = 100° C at 1 atmospheric pressure
II. Fahrenheit or F
   Freezing point = 32° F at 1 atmospheric pressure
   Boiling point = 212° F at 1 atmospheric pressure
III. To convert from C to F use the formula:

$$°F = °C × 1.8 + 32$$

IV. To convert from F to C use the formula:

$$°C = °F − 32 ÷ 1.8$$

V. EXAMPLES
A. To convert 10° C to Farenheit using the formula:

$$°F = 10 × 1.8 + 32$$
$$= 50° F$$

B. To convert 50° F to Celsius using the formula:

$$°C = 50 − 32 ÷ 1.8$$
$$= 10° C$$

Mass

I. Gram (g) is the standard unit
II. Nonmetric unit is the pound (lb)
III. 1 kg = 2.204 lb
IV. To convert lb to kg, kg = lb/2.204
V. To convert kg to lb, lb = kg × 2.204
VI. 1 ton = 1 000 kg or 2,204 lb

Quantity

I. Standard unit = Mole
II. A mole of any chemical has a mass equal to its molecular weight
III. Chemistry results are reported in moles
A. Example: insulin: 30 − 170 pmol/L, or 30 − 170 picomoles/liter

Electrical Current

I. Standard unit = Ampere (A)
II. Kilovolt (kV)
III. mAs = milliampere × seconds
   = mA × s

METRIC CONVERSIONS ▬▬▬▬▬▬

I. Abbreviations of commonly used units are shown in Table 7-1. The prefix and a base unit are also shown.
II. Metric unit conversion methods
A. #1: The step method
   1. Move the decimal place to the right if converting to a smaller unit, or to the left if converting to a larger unit

Table 7-1 Prefix, abbreviation, and a base unit for metric units

Prefix	Symbol	Value	
Giga	G	base unit $\times 10^9$	Largest unit
Mega	M	base unit $\times 10^6$	
Kilo	k	base unit $\times 10^3$	
Hecto	h	base unit $\times 10^2$	
Deca	da	base unit $\times 10$	
(Base unit)			
Gram	g		
Meter	m	1	
Liter	L		
Deci	d	base unit $\times 10^{-1}$	
Centi	c	base unit $\times 10^{-2}$	
Milli	m	base unit $\times 10^{-3}$	
Micro	u	base unit $\times 10^{-6}$	
Nano	n	base unit $\times 10^{-9}$	
Pico	p	base unit $\times 10^{-12}$	Smallest unit

Table 7-2 Common medical units and conversions

Unit	Value
liter (L) to milliliter (mL)	1 L = 1 000 mL
gram (g) to milligram (mg)	1 g = 1 000 mg
milliliter (mL) to microliter (uL)	1 mL = 1 000 uL
meter (m) to centimeter (cm)	1 m = 100 cm
kilometer (km) to meter (m)	1 km = 1 000 m
microgram (ug) to milligram	1 ug = 0.001 mg

2. EXAMPLE: to convert 500 mg to g
   a. As shown in Table 7-2, 1 mg = 1/1 000 of a gram
   b. Therefore the decimal must move 3 decimal places.
   c. Also a gram is larger than a milligram—therefore the decimal place must move to the left
   d. The answer is 0.5 g
B. #2: Proportion equation
   (1) EXAMPLE: to convert 500 mg to g
      (a) According to the chart 1 g = 1 000 mg
      (b) Therefore
         X g:500 mg = 1 g:1 000 mg
      (c) (X = the unknown number)

$$\frac{X\ g}{500\ mg} = \frac{1\ g}{1\ 000\ mg}$$

$$X\ g \times 1\ 000\ mg = 500\ mg \times 1\ g$$

$$X = \frac{500\ mg \times 1\ g}{1\ 000\ mg}$$

$$X = \frac{500\ g}{1\ 000}$$

$$X = 0.5\ g$$

DOSAGE CALCULATIONS

I. To calculate the dosage in mg use the formula:

mg = weight (kg) $\times$ the dose rate (mg/kg)

   A. EXAMPLE: a dog weighs 30 kg; dose rate is 10 mg/kg. The dose is calculated by multiplying the weight or 30 kg $\times$ 10 mg/kg or the dose rate. Therefore the dose = 300 mg

II. To calculate the dosage in mL (the amount to be administered) use the formula:

   A. $mL = \dfrac{dose\ (mg)}{concentration\ (mg/mL)}$

   The concentration of a drug is generally expressed in mg/mL or, in the case of tablets, mg/tablet
      1. EXAMPLE: what is the dosage of a drug if the dose is 300 mg and the concentration of the drug is 50 mg/mL? The mL dose is calculated by dividing the mg dose by the concentration, or

$$\frac{300\ mg}{50\ mg/mL} = 6\ mL$$

III. Because drugs are manufactured in various concentrations, the mg dose of a drug should always be recorded on the patient file (rather than the administered dose or mL/tablets)
   A. EXAMPLE: 1 mL of acepromazine maleate is administered to a patient. The concentration is 10 mg/mL; therefore the patient received 10 mg of the drug. However, if the concentration of the drug was 25 mg/mL the patient would have received 25 mg, or 2.5 times the prescribed amount

DILUTIONS/SOLUTIONS

I. Definitions
   A. **Solution:** mixture of substances made by dissolving solids in liquid or liquids in liquids
   B. **Solvent:** solution capable of dissolving other substances
   C. **Solute:** substance that is dissolved in a liquid
II. When working with solutions/dilutions, the concentration of the substance is the amount of solute dissolved in the solvent
III. Concentrations may be expressed as:
   A. Volume per volume (or v/v) for liquids, the most common

B. Weight per volume (or w/v) for liquids, the most common for medications

C. Weight per weight (or w/w) for solids

IV. The term *percent concentration* may be used to describe a solution

A. Percent w/v means the grams of solute in 100 mL of solution

1. EXAMPLE: 5% (w/v) solution = 5 g of solute in 100 mL of solution
2. A pure solution is assumed to be 100%

V. Formula for dilutions (volume/volume)

A. $\dfrac{\text{Desired strength}}{\text{Available strength}} = \dfrac{\text{Amount to use}}{\text{Amount to be made}}$

(Amount to use = the amount of concentrate)

(Amount to be made = the amount of final solution)

B. EXAMPLE: how would you prepare 1 L of 5% dextrose solution, given only a 50% solution and sterile water?

Using the above formula

$$\frac{5\%}{50\%} = \frac{X}{1\ L}$$

X = the unknown amount to use

$$X \times 50\% = 5\% \times 1\ 000\ \text{mL}$$

$$X = \frac{5\% \times 1\ 000\ \text{mL}}{50\%}$$

$$X = \frac{5\ 000\ \text{mL}}{50}$$

$$X = 100\ \text{mL}$$

To calculate amount of normal saline: The amount to be made − the amount to use. 1 000 mL − 100 mL = 900 mL of saline. Thus 100 mL of 50% solution is added to 900 mL of saline to make 1 000 mL of 5% solution

VI. Concentration of a solution can also be expressed as a ratio

A. 1:3 is 1 part to 3 parts

B. EXAMPLE: 10 parts of dextrose and 90 parts of saline make 100 parts of dextrose solution

Written as a percentage: 10% dextrose

Written as a ratio: 10:100 or 1:10

VII. If a pure drug is dissolved in a solution the result is a stock solution. A weaker solution can be made by diluting it with solvent; however, a stronger solution requires the preparation of a new solution

VIII. Solutions (weight/volume)

A. To determine the amount of solute needed to make a desired amount of solution

$$\frac{\text{grams of solute}}{\text{desired volume}} = \frac{\%\ \text{of desired solution}}{100}$$

1. EXAMPLE: how would you prepare a 4% solution given 125 mL of sterile water and only the powder form of a drug? What would be the concentration of the prepared solution?

X = powder form of drug

$$\frac{Xg}{125\ \text{mL}} = \frac{4\%}{100}$$

$$X \times 100 = 4\% \times 125\ \text{mL}$$

$$X = \frac{4\% \times 125\ \text{mL}}{100}$$

$$X = 5\ g$$

Therefore the solution would be prepared by adding 5 g of solute to 125 mL of sterile water. The concentration of a 4% w/v solution = 4 g/100 mL, or 4 000 mg/100 mL or 40 mg/mL

DRIP RATES

I. The drip rate $= \dfrac{\text{volume of solution (mL)} \times \text{drop/mL}}{\text{time (seconds)}}$

A. Drop/mL is the calibrated amount of an administration set

B. EXAMPLE: what is the drip rate, if the volume of the solution is 1 000 mL, or 1 L, the drop/mL = 20, and the time is 4 hours?

Drip rate $= \dfrac{1\ 000\ \text{mL} \times 20\ \text{drops/mL}}{4\ \text{hours or 14 400 seconds}}$

$= \dfrac{20\ 000\ \text{drops}}{14\ 400\ \text{seconds}}$

= 1.388 drops/sec or 13.88 drops/10 seconds or 83.3 drops/min

PRESCRIPTION LABELS

Even though most prescription labels are now generated by a computer, the label should be checked for accuracy before dispensing the drug

I. The label should contain the following information

A. Name, address, and phone number of clinic

B. Veterinarian's name

C. Name of patient and client's last name

D. Name of drug

E. Concentration of drug and amount of drug dispensed

F. Date

G. In some provinces/states, the drug identification number (DIN)

H. Refills should be noted

I. The vial may also need additional labels such as
1. For veterinary use only
2. Keep refrigerated
3. Keep out of reach of children
4. Withdrawal time
J. Specific instructions
1. No abbreviations should be used
a. EXAMPLE: b.i.d. should be written two times a day
2. If the medication is for the left or right eye, it should be noted on the label
3. If the drug should be administered with food or without food it should also be noted
4. The instructions should be clearly typed, not handwritten

METRIC, APOTHECARY, AND HOUSEHOLD EQUIVALENTS

Volume (Liquid) Measurements

1 cup = 8 ounces
2 cups = 1 pint = 16 ounces
2 pints = 1 quart = 32 ounces
4 quarts = 1 gallon = 128 ounce
1 gallon = 128 ounces

4 000 mL = 1 gallon
943.3 mL = 1 quart
500 mL = 1 pint
250 mL = 1 cup
30 mL = 1 ounce = 8 drams
15 mL = 1 tablespoon = 3 teaspoons
5 mL = 1 teaspoons = 60 drops (approx.)
1 mL = 1/ 1 000 L = 12 drops (approx.)

Weight Measurements

1 ounce = 28.5 g
16 ounces = 1 pound

30 g = 1 ounce = 8 drams
4 g = 60 grains
1 g = 15 grains = 0.03527 ounces
60 mg = 1 grain

Length Measurements

1 cm = 0.3937 inches
1 m = 39.37 inches = 1 000 mm = 100 cm
1 km = 0.6214 mile = 1 000 m
1 mm = 0.03937 inches = 1/1 000 m
1 inch = 2.54 cm
1 foot = 30.48 cm
1 yard = 0.9144 m
1 mile = 1.609 km

ABBREVIATIONS AND DEFINITIONS

Table 7-3 Abbreviations commonly used in veterinary medicine

Abbreviations	Definition
ad lib.	freely; as much as is wanted
$\overline{aa}$	of each
a.c.	before meals
aqua	water
aqua dist.	distilled water
at diet.	as directed
b.i.d.	twice daily
caps	capsules
chart.	powder
$\overline{c}$	with
cc	cubic centimeter
d.t.d.	give such doses
D5W	5% dextrose in water
gtt	a drop; drops
h	hour
h.s.	hour of sleep; at bedtime
IM	intramuscular
IV	intravenous
K	potassium
M	mix
non. rep. or N.R.	do not repeat
No.	number
o.h.	every hour
O.D.	right eye
O.S.	left eye
os	mouth
per os	oral
pil.	pill
p	after
p.c.	after meals
p.o.	by mouth
p.r.n.	according to circumstances; occasionally
q.2h	every 2 hours
q.s.	a sufficient amount
q.i.d.	four times a day
Q.R.	quantity required
Rx	dispense
sc	subcutaneous
sq	subcutaneous
ss	one-half
s.i.d.	once daily
sig.	write on label
s	without
Sx	surgery
stat	immediately
Tx	treatment
tab	tablet
t.i.d.	three times a day
Tr.	tincture
Ung.	ointment

NOTE: sometimes these abbreviations are written without periods; for example bid or po.

Review Questions

1 How much sterile water is needed to make a 4% solution using 1 gram of drug?
   a. 25 mL
   b. 400 mL
   c. 100 mL
   d. 50 mL

2 Convert 6 μm to m
   a. 0.006 m
   b. 0.000 006 m
   c. 6 000 m
   d. 600 m

3 Given a 45% solution and sterile diluent, how would you prepare 3 L of 15% solution?
   a. Take 200 mL of 45% and add 2 000 mL of sterile diluent
   b. Take 1 000 mL of sterile diluent and add 2 L of 45% solution
   c. Take 1000 mL of 45% solution and add 2 L of sterile diluent
   d. Take 2 L of water and add 4.5 L of 45% solution

4 Convert 10 g to kg
   a. 0.01 kg
   b. 0.10 kg
   c. 1 000 kg
   d. 100 kg

5 Given the following information: 1 L, 15 drops/mL over an 8-hour period, the approximate drip rate should be:
   a. 5.2/10 sec
   b. 52.0/10 sec
   c. 20/10 sec
   d. 1.92/sec

6 Given a pure solution, how would you make 500 mL of 50% solution?
   a. Take 250 mL of pure solution and add 250 mL of sterile water
   b. Add 100 mL of sterile water to 400 mL of pure solution
   c. Add 5 000 mL of sterile water to 500 mL of 50% solution
   d. Add 500 mL of 100% solution to 500 mL of water

7 Convert 15 lb to kg
   a. 23.0 kg
   b. 6.75 kg
   c. 5 kg
   d. 30 kg

8 What is the concentration (mg/mL) and percentage of the following solution (w/v)? 5 g added to 200 mL of sterile water
   a. 25 mg/mL, 2.5%
   b. 250 mg/mL, 2.5%
   c. 50 mg/mL, 5%
   d. 4 mg/mL, 40%

9 What is the percentage of the final solution (v/v) if 30 mL of solution is added to 70 mL of water?
   a. 30%
   b. 100%
   c. 10%
   d. 3%

10 A dog weighs 20 kg, the dose rate = 5 mg/kg and the tablet size = 50 mg. The prescription reads "℞ 100 mg BID for 10 days". How many tablets are needed for 1 dose and for a 24 hour period?
   a. 2 tablets, 4 tablets
   b. 1 tablet, 2 tablets
   c. 4 tablets, 2 tablets
   d. 4 tablets, 8 tablets

BIBLIOGRAPHY

1. Pratt PW: *Medical surgery and anesthesia nursing,* ed 2, St. Louis, 1994, Mosby.

CHAPTER 8

Small Animal Nursing

Julie Ball-Karn   Kathy Taylor   Monica Tighe

OUTLINE

Physical Examination
 Introduction
 General Appearance
 Examination by System
Drug Administration
 Introduction
 Oral Route
 Parenteral Route
 Topical Route
Fluid Therapy
 Introduction
 Normal Fluid Balance
 Abnormal Fluid Losses
 Signs of Dehydration
 Estimating Degree of Dehydration
 Calculation of Fluid Replacement
  Volume
 Contraindications for Fluid
  Therapy

Routes of Fluid Administration
 Types of Fluid
Blood Collection and Transfusion
 Canine Blood Collection
 Feline Blood Collection
 Indications for Use of Blood
  Component Therapy
 Shelf Life
 Transfusions
Electrocardiograph
 Definition
 Supplies
 Procedure
 Normal ECG Interpretation
 Abnormal Rhythms
Anal Sac Expression
 Definition
 Indications
 Procedure

Complications
Enemas
 Definition
 Indications
 Procedure
 Complications
Bandaging
 Materials
 Head and Neck
 Thorax
 Abdomen
 Limbs
 Paw
 Tail
 Specialized Bandaging Tech-
  niques
 Casting Material
 Aftercare of Bandaging, Slings,
  and Casts

LEARNING OUTCOMES

After reading this chapter you should be able to:

1. Explain how to perform a basic physical examination.
2. Define the importance of fluid therapy and why and how patient requirements may change.
3. Explain and identify the signs and degrees of dehydration.
4. Describe the various routes of fluid administration and why a specific route may be used.
5. Describe various routes of drug administration.
6. Define contraindications of certain routes of drug administration.

7. Describe the collection and transfusion of blood in the canine and the feline patient.
8. Define ECG.
9. Describe the equipment needed and procedure for producing an ECG.
10. Describe various abnormal ECG tracings and their etiology.
11. Describe the indications, equipment, procedure, and complications involved in anal sac expression.
11. Describe the indications, equipment, procedure, and complications involved in enema administration.
12. Define the indications and complications in bandaging various areas in small animals.

As a paraprofessional, the veterinary technician works with the veterinarian and performs many diagnostic and technical procedures to aid the veterinary patient. Veterinary technicians are very versatile and perform numerous technical skills. This chapter outlines many basic clinical techniques.

PHYSICAL EXAMINATION

Introduction

I. Under the supervision of a veterinarian, veterinary technicians may conduct physical examinations
  A. To provide information to assess a patient's anesthetic risk and prepare an anesthetic plan
  B. To obtain a status or progress report for monitoring an animal's recovery
  C. To verify medical record entries
  D. To evaluate abnormalities or conditions that should be brought to the attention of the veterinarian

II. A physical examination is the first step in assessing a patient and may indicate possible health problems

III. All body systems should be checked

IV. A consistent routine should be followed to ensure that each area is thoroughly examined
  A. EXAMPLE: evaluating from the nose to tail, or system by system

General Appearance

I. Note the animal's general appearance, gait and behavior, temperament and attitude

II. The environment of the animal should be noted
  A. Vomiting/diarrhea, urination, defecation in the cage

III. An accurate weight should be recorded, as well as temperature, pulse, and respiratory rate

Examination by System

The detection of physical problems is usually due to observing the animal and palpating, smelling, and listening. The description of what is detected is also important. Size, color, rate, and appearance should also be included in the record. For the following systems various clinical signs should be noted on the patient's file.

I. Skin/Coat
  A. Examine the skin and coat
    1. Shiny or dull
    2. Skin turgor
      a. Normal skin pliability depends on hydration of the tissues
      b. To assess turgor: tent the skin at the thoracic-lumbar junction
      c. Avoid cervical area due to the extra skin in this area
      d. If the skin returns rapidly to normal position it is normal
      e. If the skin remains tented or returns slowly to normal resting position it is a sign of dehydration
      f. Mild, moderate, and severe dehydration are graded at 6%-8%, 10%-12%, and 12%-15%, respectively
    3. Alopecia or dryness
    4. Lesions or obvious parasites such as fleas, lice, mites, or ticks
  B. Palpate the entire animal, note any lumps, swelling, or painful reactions to palpation

II. Eyes, ears, and nares
  A. Examine the eyes and note the following
    1. Reflexes and response to visual stimuli
    2. Discharge from the eyes
      a. Clear or purulent
    3. Corneal changes
    4. Color of conjunctiva
  B. Manipulate the ear and note the following
    1. Response to auditory stimuli
    2. Debris in the ear canal or unusual or excessive odor
    3. If the animal is shaking or tilting its head to one side
  C. Nares
    1. Discharge: color and consistency
    2. Sneezing and patency

III. Gastrointestinal
  A. Examine mouth, teeth and gums
    1. Signs of periodontal disease and halitosis
    2. Fractured, missing, or discolored teeth
    3. Verify age in young animals
    4. Check tonsils for enlargement
    5. Excessive salivation or difficulty swallowing
    6. Signs of malocclusion
  B. Note color of mucous membrane
    1. Mucous membranes should be a pale pink color
      a. Abnormal colors are blue-purple (cyanotic), yellow (jaundice), pale, bright red, or muddy brown
  C. Capillary refill time
    1. Press on gums and note when the color returns
    2. If color returns in less than 1 second capillary refill time is normal

3. If color returns in greater than 1 second capillary refill time is increased and abnormal

D. Palpate the abdomen gently
1. Check symmetry from side to side
2. Distention
3. Signs of discomfort during palpation
4. Bladder size

E. Examine the anal area for any abnormalities
1. Color
2. Anal gland abscesses, discharge, or inflammation

IV. Respiratory
A. Auscultate the chest
1. Using a stethoscope, auscultate the thorax dorsally and laterally
2. Listen for abnormal sounds such as crackles, wheezes, and rales
3. Be aware of referral sounds from the upper airway
    a. Listen to the trachea to rule out this source
4. Be aware of a decrease or lack of breath sounds

B. Note pattern, rate, depth, and effort of breathing
1. Hyper or hypoventilation
2. Panting or shallow breathing
3. Open mouth breathing or panting in cats is especially abnormal
4. Watch for dyspnea

V. Musculoskeletal
A. Observe the animal's gait
1. Lameness, dysplasia, or pain
B. Note obvious signs of joint swelling or displacement of joints
C. Flex the limbs
1. Painful reactions
2. Range of motion

VI. Cardiovascular
A. Palpate femoral and dorsal pedal pulses
1. Strength and rate of pulses
B. Auscultate the heart and check pulses at the same time
1. Note irregularities between pulse rate and heart rate, which can indicate pulse deficits

VII. Reproductive and urinary
A. Examine external genitalia
1. Redness or irritation
2. Abnormal discharge

VIII. Lymphatic
A. Lymph nodes may or may not be palpable
1. Lymph nodes should not be painful when palpated
2. Note any signs of enlargement

B. Major lymph nodes and locations
1. Submandibular: located cranial to the angle of the mandible
2. Prescapular: cranial to the shoulder joint
3. Axillary: where the forelimb meets the body
4. Popliteal: dorsal stifle
5. Inguinal: in the inguinal area near the femoral artery and vein, where the hind limb meets the body

IX. Neurological
A. Bright and alert
B. Check pupil size
1. Response to light
2. Pupils are of equal size
3. Nystagmus
C. Look for signs of ataxia or weakness
D. Check tail response and/or if there is anal tone
E. Response in all four limbs to painful stimuli
F. Knuckling when walking

DRUG ADMINISTRATION ▬▬▬▬▬

Introduction

I. Drugs are administered in several ways
II. The route depends on type of medication and health status of the animal
III. Most common routes: oral, parenteral, and topical
IV. Whichever method is used it is important to verify correct drug, patient, dosage, time, and route

Oral Route

I. It is important to note that oral medications are contraindicated in the following situations
A. If patient is vomiting
B. Injuries to the oral cavity or esophagus
C. Decreased swallowing reflex
D. Any disease process that prohibits oral intake such as pancreatitis

II. Medication can be a liquid, semisolid, tablet, or capsule
III. Liquid is administered via syringe in the cheek pouch
IV. Tablets or capsules are administered by:
A. Holding the patient's mouth open with one hand

B. Placing the pill at the base of the tongue with the opposite hand

C. Closing the mouth

D. Observing the animal swallowing

Parenteral Route

I. Includes all medications that are injected

II. These drugs are not absorbed through the gastrointestinal tract

III. Commonly includes three routes

A. Subcutaneous (SQ) or (SC)

B. Intramuscular (IM)

C. Intravenous (IV)

IV. Occasionally, drugs may also be administered

A. Intradermally (ID)

B. Intraperitoneally (IP)

C. Intracardiac (IC)

D. Intratracheal (IT)

E. Intramedullary

V. Subcutaneous injections

A. Solutions are injected under the skin

B. Usually where excess skin is available

1. Dorsally between the scapulas

2. Dorsal flank

VI. Intramuscular injections

A. Injections into the lumbar muscles or biceps femoris

B. Large volumes are not recommended

C. Multiple sites may be necessary

VII. Intravenous injections

A. Via a needle or catheter inserted into a blood vessel

B. Most common sites: cephalic, femoral, saphenous, and jugular

C. Alcohol is applied to the site before venipuncture to disinfect and part the fur

D. A restrainer or a tourniquet is used to apply proximal pressure to vein

E. By drawing blood into the syringe before injecting, correct placement may be ensured before administering medication

Topical Route

I. Medications applied directly to the skin

II. Can be applied directly on top of lesions

III. The area must be clipped and clean before applying medication

IV. Directions must be followed carefully

A. Absorption rate is variable and depends on the amount applied and how quickly it is absorbed

V. Wearing gloves as a precautionary measure is sometimes advisable for certain medications

FLUID THERAPY

Introduction

I. Fluid therapy is one of the most common procedures performed in veterinary medicine

II. It is used as supportive therapy in sick and injured patients

Normal Fluid Balance

I. The body is made up of approximately 60% water

II. This is divided into intracellular and extracellular fluids

III. The body maintains fluid balance on a constant basis

IV. Fluids are gained via

A. Oral intake

B. Metabolism in the body

V. Fluids are lost by

A. Respiration

B. Excretion

Abnormal Fluid Losses

I. Vomiting and diarrhea

II. Increased respiration (panting) in dogs

III. Disease with accompanying polyuria

IV. Any chronic or acute injury or disease that causes fluid loss

V. Any disease state or injury that prevents or decreases the oral intake of fluids

Signs of Dehydration

I. Indicators of dehydration can be found during physical examination

A. Evaluating weight

B. Skin turgor

C. Moistness of mucous membranes

D. Heart rate

E. Capillary refill time (CRT)

Estimating Degree of Dehydration

I. <5% Dehydration

A. Not detectable

II. 5%-6% Dehydration

A. Slight loss in skin turgor

III. 8% Dehydration

A. Definite increase in skin turgor

B. Slight increase in CRT

C. Possibly dry mucous membranes

IV. 10%-12% Dehydration

A. Skin turgor remains

B. Sunken eyes

C. Increased CRT

D. Dry mucous membranes

E. Increased heart and respiratory rate

F. Cold extremities

V. 12%-15% Dehydration

  A. Shock and its clinical signs

  B. Very depressed patient

  C. Imminent death

VI. Other indicators of dehydration

  A. Packed cell volume (PCV) and total plasma protein (TPP)

    1. PCV and TPP increase with all types of fluid loss, except in cases of severe hemorrhaging, when both will decrease

  B. Urine specific gravity

    1. Can be greatly increased (>1.045)

  C. Decreased urine production

    1. Normal production is 1-2 mL/kg/hr

Calculation of Fluid Replacement Volume

I. Determining volume and rate of fluid to be replaced depends on the severity and how acutely fluid losses occur

  A. To calculate the volume necessary to rehydrate an animal, the following must be added:

    1. Fluid deficit = % dehydration ÷ 100 × weight (kg) = volume (L)

    2. Ongoing losses

    3. Maintenance requirements: 50 to 70 mL/kg/day

    4. In addition, in the pyrexic animal, 10% of maintenance is added to every degree over normal

    5. An approximate guideline for initial therapy in the hypotensive shocky patient is 90 mL/kg/hr in the dog and 60 mL/kg/hr in the cat

Contraindications for Fluid Therapy

I. Patients may have existing conditions that may contraindicate the rapid replacement of fluid

II. Conditions that carry a risk of pulmonary edema from fluid shifting into the lungs necessitate the need for caution and frequent monitoring

III. Some conditions that are contraindicated for rapid fluid therapy are

  A. Pulmonary contusions

  B. Existing pulmonary edema

  C. Brain injury

  D. Congestive heart failure

IV. Signs of overhydration

  A. Restlessness

  B. Increased respiratory rate

  C. Increased lung sounds (crackles and wheezes)

  D. Increased blood pressure

  E. Chemosis (edema of ocular conjunctiva)

  F. Pitting edema

V. Subsequent weights should be taken, as well as urine production and specific gravity monitored regularly

VI. Fluid rates should be adjusted according to patient response and veterinarian orders

Routes of Fluid Administration

I. Oral

  A. Contraindicated if animal is vomiting and/or has a disease such as pancreatitis

  B. Can be given by syringe

  C. Can be given by feeding tube

    1. Nasal-esophageal tube or gastric tube directly into the stomach or intestinal tract

II. Subcutaneous

  A. Useful for mild dehydration

  B. Fluids must be isotonic; therefore cannot contain dextrose

  C. Contraindicated with patients in shock or with more severe cases of dehydration

    1. In these cases, peripheral circulation is very poor and very little absorption will take place

  D. Absorption can take up to 6-8 hours

  E. Approximate guidelines: 60 mL/kg of fluid

  F. Administration can be by large-gauge needle and syringe or needle attached to an administration set and IV bag

  G. Can be administered anywhere there is excess skin

    1. Dorsally, between the scapulas

    2. Dorsal flank area

III. Intravenous

  A. Preferred method for correction of moderate to severe dehydration and patients in shock

  B. Commonly administered via catheter through cephalic, saphenous, or jugular veins

IV. Intramedullary

  A. Useful in small or young patients where quick venous access is not possible

  B. Fluids administered directly into the bone marrow cavity, for rapid absorption

  C. Injected through the head of the femur or humerus

  D. Strict aseptic technique must be used and local anesthetic may be needed because this procedure can be painful

Types of Fluid

I. Crystalloids
   A. Isotonic electrolyte solutions
   B. Most commonly used
   C. EXAMPLES
      1. Lactated Ringer's solution (LRs)
      2. 0.9% saline
II. Colloids
   A. Solutions containing protein or starch molecules
   B. Stay in vascular space and expand volume
   C. Useful in patients with cerebral or pulmonary edema, and hypoproteinemia
   D. EXAMPLES
      1. Plasma
      2. Pentastarch

BLOOD COLLECTION AND TRANSFUSION ▬▬

Canine Blood Collection

I. Dogs have six identified red blood cell antigens
   A. They are named for specific canine erythrocyte antigen (DEA) 1.1, 1.2, and 3, 4, 5, and 7
   B. Approximately 40% of dogs have DEA 1.1, 20% have DEA 1.2, and 15% have DEA 7
   C. Universal donors are DEA 1.1 negative, DEA 1.2 negative, and DEA 7 negative
   D. A patient should not have a reaction after receiving blood from a universal donor
   E. Transfusion reactions may occur if a dog has been transfused previously or if receiving a transfusion from a donor that is DEA 1.1 positive or DEA 1.2 positive
II. Canine donor requirements
   A. Any breed or sex may be used
   B. A dog with a good temperament and easily accessible veins is a prime candidate
   C. Blood typing should be performed on each donor
   D. Ideally donors should be neutered and weigh more than 25 kg (55 lbs)
   E. Donors can be between 1 and 9 years of age
   F. Donors should be tested every 6 months for parasites, including
      1. Heartworm (and maintained on a preventive medication)
      2. Intestinal parasites
   G. Donors have yearly vaccines, which include distemper, hepatitis, leptospirosis, parainfluenza, parvovirus, and rabies
   H. Donors must be in excellent health with yearly normal blood chemistry, complete blood count, and urinalysis
   I. Donors must be free of the following infectious diseases
      1. Blood parasites: *Babesia canis, Hemobartonella canis*
      2. Rickettsial diseases: *Ehrlichia canis, Ehrlichia platus, Borrelia burgdorferi,* and *Rickettsia rickettsii*
III. Supplies
   A. Sedation depends on each individual animal
      1. Do not use acepromazine maleate since it causes hypotension
      2. The sedation of choice regularly used is Numorphon given approximately 15-20 minutes before blood collection
   B. A blood collection bag with anticoagulant added is required
      1. The most common anticoagulants are
         a. CPDA-1 (citrate, phosphate, dextrose, adenine) or
         b. ADSOL (composed of dextrose, sodium chloride, mannitol, adenine); ADSOL will preserve the blood product for a longer period of time
   C. Clippers and surgical scrub solutions for preparation of the veins
   D. All supplies for IV fluid administration should also be available
   E. A scale to measure the blood
      1. The total should be approximately 587 g: 470 g blood (450 mL) and 117 g that equals the weight of the collection bag and the anticoagulant
IV. Procedure
   A. Sedate animal
   B. Place animal in lateral recumbency with neck extended
   C. Clip a wide area around the jugular vein to be used for collection
   D. Clip and prep the cephalic vein for an intravenous catheter for fluid replacement after blood collection
   E. Place cephalic catheter
   F. Prepare jugular vein for blood collection
   G. Restrainer should be prepared to hold off the jugular vein in preparation for the blood collection
   H. Insert 16 gauge needle attached to the blood collection bag into the jugular vein in a cranial direction
   I. As blood enters the collection bag, move the bag slightly to mix the anticoagulant with the blood

J. 450 mL of blood constitutes one entire blood collection

K. Use the scale to measure the volume of blood in the collection bag so that it is not over or underfilled

　　1. Overfilling or under filling the blood collection bag results in improper ratio of anticoagulant to blood volume

L. After completion of blood collection, apply pressure to the jugular vein for 2 to 5 minutes to minimize hematoma formation

M. The amount of blood collected from a canine donor should not exceed 20 mL/kg

　　1. A dog can donate blood approximately every 3 weeks if necessary; however in general most facilities bleed a donor no more than once per month

N. Replace blood volume loss from the patient with three times the volume of replacement intravenous fluids

O. Clearly label the collection bag with the donor's name, date of collection, date of expiry, and the donor's PCV (packed cell volume), TP (total protein), and blood type

Feline Blood Collection

I. Felines have two blood group antigens: type A, and type B

A. Approximately 99% of all domestic cats are blood type A

B. Purebred cats have a much higher prevalence of type B blood

　　1. Purebred cats have a much higher risk of blood transfusion reaction. A severe life threatening reaction can occur with only a few mL of infused blood

　　　　a. Cross matching before transfusion prevents most reactions

II. Donor requirements

A. Less than 8 years of age

B. Blood typing should be performed on all donors

C. A lean body weight of no less than 4.5 kg (10 lbs)

D. Donor must be neutered

E. A good natured indoor cat makes donation smoother and less stressful

F. The donor should have yearly vaccines, which include panleukopenia, calicivirus, rhinotracheitis, and rabies

G. Excellent health must be maintained by monitoring serum biochemistry, complete blood count, and fecal tests on a yearly basis

H. All donors must be negative for feline leukemia, infectious peritonitis, immunodeficiency virus, and *Hemobartonella felis*

I. A donor may provide 20 mL/kg of blood no more than once a month

J. A complete feline blood donation is 51.5 mL of blood

III. Supplies

A. Sedation such as ketamine/diazepam IV

B. Clippers and surgical scrub solutions

C. Appropriate size catheter and butterfly

D. 8.5 mL CPDA-1 anticoagulant and 60 mL syringe

E. 150 mL of IV fluids

F. Ophthalmic ointment to prevent corneal drying from sedation

IV. Procedure

A. The area is aseptically prepared and a catheter is placed in the cephalic vein

B. Animal is sedated 'to effect'

C. Monitor vital signs, e.g., pulse, respiration, and blood pressure throughout the procedure

D. Administration of replacement fluids can begin approximately half way through the donation

E. Moisten eyes with ointment

F. Clip jugular vein and aseptically prepare the area

G. Place cat in lateral recumbency with neck extended, or place cat in sternal recumbency with neck extended and legs over the edge of the table

H. Insert 19 gauge butterfly into the jugular vein

I. Connect the butterfly to a 60 mL syringe containing 8.5 mL of anticoagulant, CPDA-1 (citrate phosphate dextrose acetate-1)

J. Always try to minimize movement of needle in the jugular vein

K. Mix anticoagulant and blood often throughout the donation

L. Blood collection from cats is a slow process; patience is a must

M. Collection is complete when the syringe reaches a volume of 60 mL

N. Remove butterfly and apply pressure to the vein to minimize hematoma formation

O. Replace fluid volume lost by donation with approximately three times the amount of fluids (150 mL)

P. Clearly label the syringe with the donor's name, PCV, TP, volume, date of collection, and donor blood type

Indications for Use of Blood Component Therapy

I. Fresh whole blood
- A. Hemorrhagic shock, anemia, excessive surgical hemorrhage, bleeding disorders (due to thrombocytopenia or clotting factor deficiencies), nonimmune mediated hemolytic anemia, and in some circumstances immune mediated hemolytic anemia

II. Stored whole blood
- A. Has the same indications as fresh whole blood with the exception of bleeding disorders

III. Packed red cells
- A. Fluid balance and oncotic pressure is maintained with crystalloid given with packed cells
- B. Hemolytic anemia and nonregenerative anemias
- C. The preservative 'ADSOL' will maintain cells without having to reconstitute them
  1. Approximately 200 mL packed red blood cells in 100 mL of ADSOL
  2. Always add ADSOL to the packed red cells
     - a. If packed red cells are added to the Adsol, the cells may be damaged in the process

IV. Plasma
- A. Volume expansion (shock and burn patients), hypoproteinemia, and clotting

Shelf Life

I. Whole blood
- A. Thirty-five days refrigerated
- B. Fresh whole blood cannot be left out at room temperature for longer than 8 to 12 hours
- C. Fresh whole blood cannot be frozen

II. Packed red cells without preservative
- A. Twenty-one days refrigerated (reconstitute with 120 mL saline)
- B. Cannot be frozen
- C. Packed red cells with ADSOL preservative
  1. Forty-two days refrigerated (no reconstitution required)
  2. Cannot be frozen

III. Fresh frozen plasma
- A. One year in $-20°$ C freezer ($-5°$ F)

Transfusions

I. Flush intravenous lines with only sodium chloride during transfusion of blood products
- A. Flushing intravenous lines with any other fluid or solution may cause red blood cell clumping, swelling, and subsequent hemolysis

II. For platelet administration, administration sets should not contain latex because platelets will adhere to the latex

III. Volume and rate of infusion
- A. Volume of blood to be transfused
  1. Example of a calculation used to determine the amount of whole blood to transfuse to the recipient:

$$\text{mL of canine donor blood} =$$
$$\text{recipient weight (kg)} \times 80 \times \frac{\text{desired PCV} - \text{patient PCV}}{\text{PCV of donor blood}}$$

$$\text{mL of feline donor blood} =$$
$$\text{recipient weight (kg)} \times 70 \times \frac{\text{desired PCV} - \text{patient PCV}}{\text{PCV of donor blood}}$$

  2. Maximum volume of 22 mL/kg/day (unless severe continuing blood loss)
- B. Initial administration rate should be slow (0.25 mL/kg) for the first 15 to 30 minutes to allow for observation of reactions
- C. Before infusion, baseline values should be recorded for temperature, pulse, respiratory rate, mucous membrane color, PCV, and total proteins
  1. These values should be monitored throughout the transfusion
- D. Avoid overload
  1. Maximum volumes of 22 mL/kg/day should be calculated unless hypovolemic blood loss
- E. The entire maximum daily requirement can be given in 1 hour if the recipient has no reaction to slow administration
- F. Plasma administration for hypoproteinemia, is 6 to 10 mL/kg two to three times per day as required
  1. Dose may be adjusted or given in conjunction with crystalloid fluids to the hypovolemic patient
- G. For active bleeding due to clotting factor deficiency, blood can be administered 6 to 10 mL/kg two to three times per day for 3 to 5 days or until bleeding stops

IV. Blood transfusion reactions
- A. Blood transfusion reactions can occur due to improper component preparation, improper storage, or incompatible blood types
- B. If a reaction occurs the blood product should be stopped immediately
- C. Clinical signs
  1. Restlessness and anxiety
  2. Urticaria/pruritus
  3. Muscle tremors
  4. Nausea, salivation, vomiting

5. Fever
6. Apnea and/or tachypnea
7. Tachycardia
8. Fecal and/or urinary incontinence
9. Anuria or renal failure
10. Convulsions
11. Anaphylaxis

ELECTROCARDIOGRAPH

Definition

I. The recording of the electrical activity on the surface of the body generated by the heart
II. Electrocardiograph: a machine that makes a recording of the bioelectrical signals on the surface of the body that arise from within the heart
   A. Electrocardiogram (ECG or EKG): a recording on heat-sensitive paper or on a monitor
III. The ECG represents amplitude (amount of electrical activity) and duration (length of time) of electrical activity
IV. Each contraction of the heart is preceded by an electrical wavefront that stimulates the heart muscle to contract (systole) and then relax (diastole) in preparation for the next heartbeat
   A. **Depolarization:** contraction of the myocardium
   B. **Repolarization:** relaxation of cells after depolarization
V. The continuous wave of electricity through the heart is organized, rhythmic, and repetitive
   A. The sinoatrial node, or pacemaker of the heart, is the point of origin of electrical activity
   B. The cells of the heart are linked closely together; therefore the depolarization spreads quickly from the sinoatrial node to the atria in a caudal direction toward the ventricles, finally reaching the atrioventricular node
   C. Electrical activity moves slowly from the atrioventricular node and into the proximal portions of the ventricular conduction system known as the bundle of His
   D. From the bundle of His, the depolarization moves to the interventricular septum, which is depolarized in a left to right direction
   E. The current then moves along the left and right bundle branches to the apex of the heart where the Purkinje fibers direct the wave of depolarization through the ventricles in a cranial direction
VI. The parts of an ECG tracing are associated with the waves of electrical activity that spread through the heart. The parts are labeled P, QRS, and T (Figure 8-1)
   A. P Wave: electrocardiographic representation of the depolarization of right and left atria
   B. PR Interval: electrocardiographic representation of the beginning of atrial depolarization into ventricular depolarization
      1. This interval is mainly a result of slow conduction through the AV node
      2. This interval is only the measurement of time
   C. QRS Complex: electrocardiographic expression of ventricular depolarization
   D. T Wave: electrocardiographic expression of repolarization of the ventricular myocardium
   E. Atrial repolarization is not seen on an ECG because it is hidden by ventricular depolarization

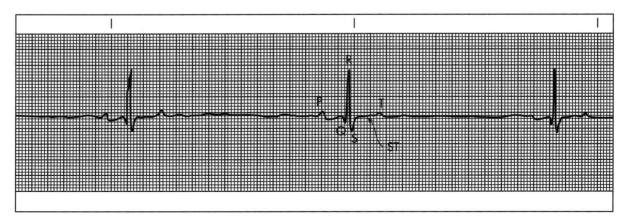

Figure 8-1 Time intervals at 50 mm/S and 1 mV standard. (Courtesy St. Clair College, Veterinary Technician Program from *Clinical Procedures Handbook*.)

Supplies

I. Protective padding, blanket, or mat for steel tables (stainless steel conducts electricity)
II. Alcohol or conducting gel or paste for increased skin contact
   A. NOTE: alcohol should not be used in an emergency situation if defibrillation is a possibility
III. ECG machines that are manufactured for human use may need to be modified
   A. Change the snap end to an alligator clip
      1. Alligator clips should be filed or bent slightly to prevent pinching and bruising
   B. For continuous monitoring, pads or wire may be used
      1. Clip fur so that pad may be applied directly to the skin
      2. For surgical wire placement, which is less painful
         a. Swab area and wire with alcohol
         b. Use a 20 gauge needle to enter and exit the skin subcutaneously
         c. The wire is then passed through the eye of the needle
         d. The needle is removed leaving the wire through the skin
         e. The ends of the wire should be twisted together and taped to prevent injury and ease retrieval in long-haired animals

Procedure

I. Ideally animal should be in right lateral recumbency during the recording of an ECG
   A. For large animals, standing position is acceptable and should be noted on the recording
   B. Cats sometimes prefer crouching on the table
      1. This is known as the 'Downey' position
II. Using manual restraint, the animal should be placed on a mat or blanket with limbs separated by paper towels or a blanket to reduce contact
III. Using alcohol or electrode gel to increase contact at the site, attach the five electrodes by alligator clips to the skin at the following locations (if using surgical wire method, attach electrodes to wire)
   A. Proximal left and right olecranons
   B. Proximal left and right stifles
   C. Chest lead: dorsal thorax near the seventh thoracic vertebra
      1. The chest lead is not universally used; however it may provide additional data

to diagnose right and left cardiac enlargement
IV. A three-lead ECG can be used
   A. The leads are labeled RA (right arm), LA (left arm), and LL (left leg)
V. Ideally the animal should be drug free and without stress; however, sedation can be given to a fractious animal
   A. If sedation is needed to perform the ECG, the drug and dosage should be recorded on the ECG, since the tracing could change
VI. Monitor the patient's color and respiration throughout the procedure because many patients have already compromised cardiac output and may have problems when in lateral recumbency or stressed
VII. ECG machine calibration and recording
   A. An mV "standard" should be recorded at the speed of 25 mm/sec on the strip prior to the ECG
      1. The mV "standard" is the measurement of the sensitivity of the machine (Figure 8-2)
   B. The paper speed should also be recorded
      1. The paper speed should be changed to 50 mm/sec for tracings
      2. A rhythm strip is run at 25 mm/sec
   C. A complete ECG consists of about 30 cm of each lead
      1. In general six leads are recorded: Lead I, II, III, AVR, AVL, and AVF
      2. A rhythm strip consisting of 30 cm of Lead II at 25 mm/sec
   D. After completing all lead tracings the following information should be recorded on the tracing
      1. Date of ECG
      2. Patient name, client name, and species
      3. Other relevant information
         a. Recumbency
         b. Drugs used
   E. The tracing may then be 'mounted' for filing purposes

Normal ECG Interpretation

I. A normal heartbeat should include a P, Q, R, S, and T segment
   A. There is a P wave for every QRS complex
   B. The PR interval is relatively constant
   C. The P wave has a positive deflection (above the baseline) in lead II
   D. The T segment can have a positive or a negative deflection

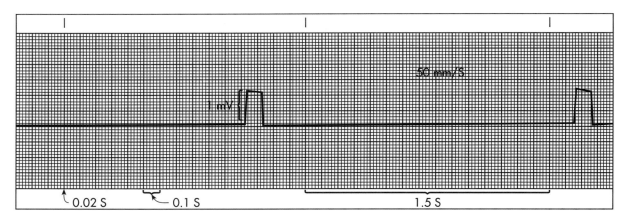

Figure 8-1 Normal Lead II complex. (Courtesy St. Clair College, Veterinary Technician Program from *Clinical Procedures Handbook.*)

II. A sinus rhythm is the normal cardiac rhythm in domestic animals
III. After completion of an ECG the veterinarian/technician can measure the complexes and compare the measurement to normal values for each species
IV. The veterinarian/technician can also calculate the heart rate by counting the complexes in a 3 second period
  A. ECG paper has specific markings for duration of time on the top of the grid

Abnormal Rhythms

I. Sinus arrhythmia
  A. An irregular ventricular rhythm, which is sinoatrial in origin
  B. On the ECG, the QRS to QRS interval varies and there is a P wave for every QRS complex
  C. Most cases of sinus arrhythmia are phasic and associated with respiration
    1. The rate increases with inspiration and decreases with expiration
    2. The sinus arrhythmia of respiratory origin occurs due to the influence of vagal tone
    3. Individuals with respiratory disease tend to have augmented sinus arrhythmia
  D. Most sinus arrhythmias are associated with slow rates
  E. Sinus arrhythmia is normal in the canine
II. Sinus bradycardia
  A. Ventricular rate is decreased
    1. <20 kg (45 lbs) canine less than 70 bpm, or >20 kg (45 lbs) canine less than 60 bpm

    2. Cat <100 bpm
  B. Profound bradycardia will cause weakness, hypotension, and syncope
  C. Etiology of sinus bradycardia
    1. Enhanced parasympathetic tone due to:
      a. Increased inspiratory effort as a result of respiratory disease
      b. Gastric irritation
      c. Increased cerebrospinal fluid pressure, hypothyroidism, hypothermia, hyperkalemia, hypoglycemia, and drug therapy
III. Sinus tachycardia
  A. Sinus rhythm with an increased ventricular rate
  B. Dog <20 kg (45 lbs) with heart rate >180 bpm, or dog >20 kg (45 lbs) with heart rate >160 bpm
  C. Puppies with heart rate >220 bpm
  D. Cat with heart rate >240 bpm
  E. Etiology of sinus tachycardia
    1. Pain
    2. Fever
    3. Anemia
    4. Reduced cardiac output
    5. Hyperthyroidism
    6. Excitement
IV. Atrial flutter
  A. Atrial flutter appears as a regular, sawtooth formation between the QRS complexes
  B. It occurs as the ventricular rate differs from the atrial rate
  C. It is the precursor to atrial fibrillation
V. Atrial fibrillation
  A. No P waves are evident and the baseline is irregular due to many erratic impulses passing through the atrial myocardium

B. The ventricular depolarization rate is also irregular and rapid

VI. Premature ventricular contractions or complexes (PVCs)
   A. Premature beats
   B. The ventricle discharges before the arrival of the next anticipated impulse from the sinoatrial node
   C. PVCs can occur at any rate but pose a greater danger when occurring with a sustained heart rate that is tachycardic
   D. The P wave is often not seen on the ECG tracing
   E. A wide distorted QRS complex is also evident
   F. The beat preceding the PVC and the beat following the PVC is equal to the time of two normal beats
   G. Etiology of premature ventricular contraction
      1. Associated with the following:
         a. Ventricular concentric hypertrophy or eccentric hypertrophy
         b. Hypoxemic states such as anemia, gastric dilation/volvulus, and heart failure
         c. Acidosis
         d. Drugs such as digitalis, barbiturates, and antiarrhythmic agents
         e. Hypokalemia
   H. Possible consequences of PVCs
      1. May initiate repetitive ventricular firing in the form of ventricular tachycardia or fibrillation
      2. Cardiac output may fall if enough premature beats are present
      3. Treatment of PVCs should occur if the patient shows signs due to dysrhythmia

VII. Atrial premature contraction
   A. The P-R interval may be short, normal, or long, depending on the area of origin of the premature beat
      1. The origin could include the sinoatrial node or ectopic locations in the atria
   B. The atrial premature contraction may or may not be conducted to the ventricles
      1. If the beat is not conducted to the ventricles and reaches the atrioventricular node before repolarization, premature P waves without QRS complexes will appear on the ECG
      2. If depolarization is conducted through the ventricles the QRS complex will appear normal

VIII. Ventricular tachycardia
   A. A series of four or more PVCs in sequence
IX. Ventricular fibrillation
   A. The mechanical pumping of the heart is not evident on the ECG
   B. The ECG has a bizarre baseline with prominent undulations
   C. There are no recognizable P or QRS complexes
   D. Unless controlled immediately, ventricular fibrillation will result in cardiac arrest
X. First-degree atrioventricular block
   A. The P-R interval is longer than normal
   B. This type of heart block is a result of a minor conduction defect
XI. Second-degree atrioventricular block
   A. Some atrial pulses are not conducted through the A-V node and therefore do not cause depolarization of the ventricles
   B. There are two types
      1. Type I (Mobitz Type I) or (Wenckebach A-V Block): progressive lengthening of the P-R interval on successive beats and then P waves occurring without QRS complexes
         a. P waves occurring without QRS complexes is called a "dropped beat"
      2. Type II: a constant P-R interval that is usually of normal duration with random dropped beats
XII. Third-degree atrioventricular block
   A. Also known as a complete heart block; the most severe heart block
   B. A lack of any relationship between P waves and QRS complexes; the atria beat at their own rate and the ventricles beat at their own rate
XIII. Asytole
   A. Cardiac arrest
      1. The ECG tracing will appear as a flat line

ANAL SAC EXPRESSION ▰▰▰▰▰▰▰
Definition

I. The anal sacs are located on either side of an animal's anus at approximately the four and eight o'clock positions
II. The anal sacs are filled with odorous secretions and should normally be expressed when the animal defecates
III. This procedure is commonly performed on dogs, rarely on cats

Indications

I. To decrease irritation to the animal caused by distention or inflammation
II. To instill medication in diseased anal sacs
III. Removal of material from anal sacs

Procedure

I. The dog may have to be muzzled and/or securely restrained
II. There are two methods for anal sac expression
   A. External
      1. Using rolled cotton over the dog's anus, apply pressure in a medial and slightly dorsal direction of the external anus
      2. This method does not guarantee full expression of anal sacs
   B. Internal
      1. Insert a gloved, well-lubricated index finger into the anus
      2. With cotton covering the sac, gently squeeze together index finger and thumb to milk contents of the anal sac toward the medial anus
      3. After examining the contents of secretions, roll the glove over the cotton, remove from the hand and discard
         a. Normal anal sac material should contain granular brown, malodorous material

Complications

I. Rupture of abscessed anal sac
II. Perforation of rectum

ENEMAS

Definition

I. An enema is the infusion of fluid into the lower intestinal tract through the anus
II. Enemas are used to remove fecal material from the colon

Indications

I. To prepare for radiographs with or without contrast media involvement
II. To irrigate the colon of a patient who has been poisoned
III. To relieve constipation

Procedure

I. Sedation or anesthesia may be needed in cases of severe blockage or fractious animals
II. An abdominal radiograph should be completed to rule out perforation or foreign body
III. Use an enema container with a rounded, soft, pliable piece of connected tubing
IV. Place the animal in sternal or lateral recumbency, preferably on a wash table
V. Put on examination gloves
VI. Place the enema preparation into the enema container
   A. Examples of enema preparations
      1. Mild soap and water
      2. Saline for irrigation
      3. A commercial enema preparation
   B. Hyperphosphate enema solutions should not be used in cats or small dogs
      1. These solutions may cause acute collapse associated with hypocalcemia
VII. Lubricate well the end of the flexible tubing
VIII. Insert the tip of the enema tubing to the colorectal junction
IX. Place the enema container above the animal to aid the solution to flow into the animal by gravity
X. More than one enema may be required to evacuate the animal's bowels adequately
XI. Do not continue to administer enemas if there is no sign of fecal material
XII. Do not proceed with enema if there is evidence of abdominal pain that could be associated with intestinal perforation or obstruction

Complications

I. Rupture of the colon
II. Leakage of enema fluid into peritoneal cavity through already ruptured intestinal tract
III. Hemorrhage in cases of ulcerative colitis
   A. Enemas are contraindicated in cases of ulcerative colitis, since they may increase bleeding

BANDAGING

Materials

I. Cotton roll
II. Two-inch or four-inch adhesive tape
III. Conforming gauze
IV. Elastic bandage
V. Sterile and/or unsterile gauze
VI. Cotton balls

Head and Neck

I. Reasons for bandaging
   A. Postocular surgery
   B. Repair of an aural hematoma
   C. Ear surgery
   D. To secure a jugular catheter or pharyngostomy tube

II. Precautions
  A. The bandage should be frequently checked postoperatively because edema that could be life threatening may occur
  B. Respiration and mucous membrane color must be monitored closely
    1. The bandage should be loose enough to enable two fingers to fit under the bandage
    2. If there are any changes in respirations the bandage should be loosened or changed immediately
  C. If the animal tries to remove the bandage, an Elizabethan collar can be used for restraint

Thorax

I. Reasons for bandaging
  A. To secure chest drains
  B. To protect large thoracic wounds
  C. Spinal surgery
II. Precautions
  A. If impairment of respiration occurs the bandage should be removed or cut to loosen it immediately

Abdomen

I. Reasons for bandaging
  A. To secure a gastrostomy tube
  B. After a radical mastectomy
  C. For extensive wounds or dissection of the abdominal region
II. Precautions
  A. Care must be taken when applying the bandage not to incorporate the prepuce in male dogs because this can interfere with urination
  B. Steps should be taken also to keep the bandage clean and dry from urine and feces

Limbs

I. Reasons for bandaging
  A. Immobilization of fractures
  B. Wound protection
  C. Stabilization for fluid therapy
II. Most common type: Robert Jones bandage
  A. A Robert Jones bandage can be used to temporarily stabilize fractures before surgical repair
  B. This bandage consists of several layers of rolled cotton compressed tightly with elastic gauze and elastic tape
  C. The underlying layers of cotton prevent constriction of the limb
III. Precautions
  A. When bandaging the upper portion of a limb, the entire limb should be incorporated in the bandage
  B. This allows for even distribution of pressure along the limb and maintains venous return from the paw
  C. The toes should be checked routinely for swelling, coldness, and pallor of the nail beds (where possible)
    1. If any of theses changed occur the bandage should be loosened or changed because these signs may indicate poor venous return
  D. The bandage should be loose enough to allow two fingers to slip under the bandage at all times

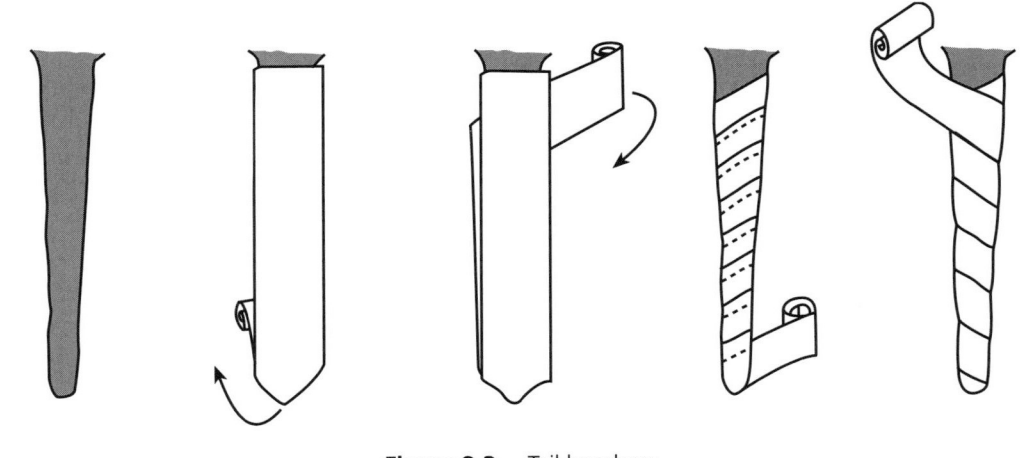

Figure 8-3   Tail bandage.

E. To keep the bandage clean and dry when walking the animal
   1. A small bag, an examination glove, or an empty fluid bag can be taped onto the proximal end of the limb and then removed after exercising

Paw

I. Reasons for bandaging
   A. Declawing of cats
   B. Dewclaw removal in dogs
   C. Repair of lacerations
II. Precautions
   A. The accessory pad should be included when bandaging the paw
   B. A piece of cotton under the pad, as well as between the digits, helps to prevent irritation or chafing

Tail (Figure 8-3)

I. Reasons for bandaging
   A. Partial tail amputation
   B. Protection of wounds
   C. Tumor removal
   D. To wrap long-haired cats or dogs with severe diarrhea to keep the area as clean as possible
II. Precautions
   A. Sedation may be needed if bleeding persists from excessive tail wagging or from hitting the remaining portion of tail on a hard surface after amputation
      1. In cases of amputation, a hard tubular object fastened to the base of the tail protecting the sight is often helpful
         a. Objects such as an empty cardboard roll can be useful
         b. Analgesics may be required for pain

Specialized Bandaging Techniques

I. Ehmer sling to support the hind limb post reduction of hip luxation
II. Velpeau sling (Figure 8-4) to support the shoulder joint after surgery
III. Hobbles can be applied to hindlimbs to prevent them from abducting excessively

Casting Materials

I. Fiberglass cast
   A. Lightweight and strong
   B. Fast-setting cast
II. Plaster of Paris
   A. Gauze roll impregnated with calcium sulphate dihydrate

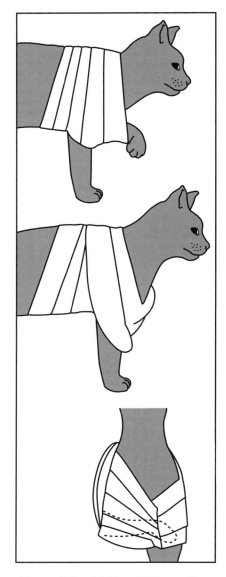

Figure 8-4 Making a Velpeau sling.

Aftercare of Bandages, Slings, and Casts

I. Close monitoring is essential
   A. Note evidence of odor, edema, discharge, or skin irritation
   B. Note warmth, color, and swelling of toes
II. Prevent the animal from chewing or licking the bandage
   A. Use discipline, sedation, an Elizabethan collar, T-shirts, or socks, or foul-tasting substances can be applied to the dressing
III. When outdoors, protect the bandage from dirt and moisture by covering it with a plastic bag
IV. Exercise should be limited

Glossary

alopecia Absence of hair from skin in areas it is normally present

anaphylaxis A manifestation of immediate hypersensitivity in which exposure of a sensitized individual to a specific antigen or hapten results in life-threatening respiratory distress, usually followed by vascular collapse and shock

anuria Complete suppression of urinary secretion from the kidneys

aseptic In a sterile manner

aspirate To apply suction and withdraw fluid out

ataxia Lack of muscle coordination

auscultate To listen to thoracic and abdominal sounds

capillary refill time (CRT) After applying pressure to the gumline to blanch them, it is the time it takes for color to return to the area, normally 1 to 2 seconds

colloid An intravenous solution containing starch or protein molecules

conjunctiva Delicate membrane lining the eyelids and surrounding the eyeball

crystalloid Isotonic electrolyte solution

distension Abnormal swelling or size

edema Abnormally large amounts of fluid in the intercellular tissue spaces of the body

extracellular Outside a cell or cells

gait Manner or style of walking

hemorrhagic shock Hypovolemic shock resulting from hemorrhage

hypoproteinemia Abnormal decrease in the amount of protein in the blood, sometimes resulting in edema and fluid accumulation in serous cavities

hypotensive Abnormally low blood pressure

hypovolemic Abnormally decreased volume of circulating fluid (plasma) in the body

hypovolemic shock Shock resulting from insufficient blood volume for the maintenance of adequate cardiac output, blood pressure, and tissue perfusion

intracellular Situated or occurring within a cell or cells

intradermal In the dermis layer of the skin

intramedullary Within the marrow cavity of the bone

intraperitoneal Within the peritoneal cavity

isotonic A solution that has equal tonicity as another solution with which it is compared

malocclusion Absence of proper alignment of teeth when the jaws are closed

myocardium Middle and thickest layer of the heart wall, composed of cardiac muscle

nystagmus Involuntary rapid horizontal or vertical movement of the eyeball

oncotic pressure Osmotic pressure due to presence of colloids in a solution; it is the force that tends to counterbalance the capillary blood pressure

palpation Using the fingers with light pressure on the surface of the body to determine consistency of the parts beneath

pancreatitis Inflammation of the pancreas

parenteral Not through the gastrointestinal tract but by another route such as intravenous

peripheral An outward structure or surface as in the limbs of the body

polyuria Production of a large volume of urine over a specific period of time

premature ventricular contraction Premature beats where the QRS complex usually has wide and bizarre complexes

pruritus Itching

purulent Containing or forming pus

pyrexic Abnormal elevation of body temperature

turgor Normal consistency of tissue or how quickly it returns to normal after being slightly pulled

urticaria A vascular reaction, usually transient, involving the upper dermis, representing localized edema caused by dilatation and increased permeability of the capillaries and marked by the development of wheals

Review Questions

1 What is a pulse deficit?
  a. Increased heart rate
  b. Pulse rate and heart rate are the same
  c. Pulse rate lower than heart rate
  d. Weak pulses

2 Where are the popliteal lymph nodes located?
  a. Cranial to the scapula
  b. On the sternum
  c. Behind the stifle
  d. Just below the hock

3 Referred sounds are generally:
  a. From the diaphragm
  b. From the trachea
  c. From the lung lobes
  d. Digestion noises

4 Oral medications would be contraindicated when:
  a. Fractured ribs are evident
  b. Pancreatitis is diagnosed
  c. Blood loss is chronic
  d. The treatment is chronic

5 A parenteral drug is administered:
  a. Topically
  b. p.o.
  c. Not via the GI tract
  d. IM only

6 What is a sign of overhydration?
  a. Decreased respiratory rate
  b. Decreased capillary refill time
  c. Increased respiratory rate
  d. Increased salivation

7 Which would be considered a colloid?
  a. Ringer's lactate
  b. 5% dextrose
  c. Plasma
  d. Saline

8 Subcutaneous fluids are contraindicated when:
   a. There is evidence of mild dehydration
   b. The patient needs dextrose
   c. The patient is very small
   d. There is evidence of chronic heart failure

9 _____ is/are recommended before performing an enema
   a. Abdominal radiographs
   b. Abdominal palpation
   c. IV fluids
   d. Large amounts of laxative

10 A canine blood donor should weigh no less than:
   a. 20 kg
   b. 25 kg
   c. 15 kg
   d. 10 kg

11 The most common vein used for blood donation is the:
   a. jugular
   b. cephalic
   c. saphenous
   d. femoral

12 What is the total amount of blood that can be collected from a feline patient at one donation?
   a. 60 mL
   b. 51.5 mL
   c. 50 mL
   d. Whatever volume is required for the recipient

13 If packed red cells are added to the anticoagulant it may cause:
   a. Contamination
   b. An incorrect ratio of blood to anticoagulant
   c. Hemolysis
   d. Crenation of the red cells

14 If a blood transfusion reaction occurs:
   a. Dilute the blood product with saline
   b. Slow down the transfusion
   c. Stop the transfusion immediately
   d. Administer drugs for the reaction and continue the transfusion

15 When an animal has sinus bradycardia, the heart rate:
   a. Is too fast
   b. Is too slow
   c. Has stopped
   d. Is normal

16 What complications can occur from a constricting bandage?
   a. Difficulty breathing
   b. Swelling or edema
   c. Coldness of the extremity
   d. All of the above

17 Anals sacs are expressed:
   a. To decrease odor caused by fecal material
   b. To decrease the chances of a ruptured anal sac
   c. Due to perforation of the rectum
   d. To instill medication in diseased anal sacs

18 The origin of electrical activity in the myocardium is:
   a. AV Node
   b. SA Node
   c. Atria
   d. Ventricle

19 What is *not* represented on an ECG tracing?
   a. Ventricular systole
   b. Atrial systole
   c. Ventricular repolarization
   d. Atrial repolarization

20 A third degree atrioventricular block is characterized by:
   a. Lack of a relationship between the P wave and QRS complex
   b. A constant long P-R interval
   c. A dropped beat
   d. A normal P-R interval with dropped beats

BIBLIOGRAPHY

Crow and Walshaw: *Manual of clinical procedures in the dog and cat,* Philadelphia, 1987, J.B. Lippincott Co.

DiBartola SP: *Fluid therapy in small animal practice,* Philadelphia, 1992, W.B. Saunders.

Dorland's Illustrated Medical Dictionary, ed 27, Philadelphia, W.B. Saunders, Harcourt Brace Jovanovich, Inc.

Edwards NJ: *ECG manual for the veterinary technician,* Philadelphia, 1993, W.B. Saunders.

Kirk RW and Bistner SI: ed 6, *Handbook of veterinary procedures and emergency treatment,* Philadelphia, 1995, W.B. Saunders.

Lane DR, Cooper B: *Veterinary nursing,* Oxford, 1994, Butterworth Heineman.

Mathews KA: *Emergency and critical care notes and protocols,* Guelph, Ontario, Canada, 1996, Lifelearn Inc, University of Guelph.

Mathews KA: *Fluid and electrolyte maintenance and replacement, Veterinary emergency and critical care manuel,* Guelph, 1996, Lifelearn.

Mathews K: *Veterinary emergency and critical care manuel,* Guelph, 1996, Lifelearn.

McCurnin D: *Clinical textbook for veterinary technicians,* ed 3, Philadelphia, 1994, W.B. Saunders.

Meltzer LE, Pinneo R, Kitchell JR: *Intensive coronary care: a manual for nurses,* ed 4, Bowie, Maryland, Robert J. Brady Co., a Prentice-Hall Publishing and Communications Company.

Muir MW, DiBartola SP: *Fluid therapy, Current Veterinary Therapy VIII,* Philadelphia, 1983, W.B. Saunders.

O'Grady MR: ECG Interpretation Workshop, Winter Conference 1995 Ontario Association of Veterinary Technicians.

Pratt PW: *Medical nursing for animal health technicians,* ed 1, Santa Barbara, 1985, America Veterinary Publication, Inc.

Pratt PW: *Medical, surgery and anesthetic nursing for veterinary technicians,* ed 2, St. Louis, 1994, Mosby.

Pratt PW: *Principles and practice of veterinary technology,* St. Louis, 1998, Mosby.

Equine Nursing and Surgery

Susan Cornwell   *Colleen Hill*

OUTLINE

Normal Values
Dental Formula and Care
   Dental Formula
   Dental Care
Gastrointestinal Ailments
   Common Clinical Signs

Rule Outs Of Gastrointestinal Ailments
Neuromuscular Disorders
   Common Clinical Signs
   Rule Outs of Neuromuscular Disorders

Respiratory Diseases
   Common Clinical Signs
   Rule Outs of Respiratory Diseases
Blood Disorder
Foot Ailments
Equine Surgery

LEARNING OUTCOMES

After reading this chapter you should be able to:

1. Recognize equine normal values.
2. Define disease, illnesses, and the technician's role.
3. Be familiar with important pre and postoperative care.

As veterinary technicians, we play a very large role in the day to day care of animals. Veterinarians rely on our instincts, knowledge, and observational skills to assist and/or alert them to the progression (or otherwise) of the animal's state of health.

NORMAL VALUES

   I. Temperature: 37° C to 38.5° C (98.6-101° F)
   II. Pulse: 28 to 45 beats/min
   III. Respiration: 8 to 20 breaths/min
   IV. Mucous membrane color: healthy pink color
   V. Capillary refill time: 1 to 2 seconds
   VI. Gastrointestinal motility (borborygmus)
     A. Bubbling

     B. Gurgling
     C. Distant thunder
   VII. Digital pulses: none to slight
   VIII. Fecal output
     A. Color varies with diet
     B. Should be well-formed moist balls that break easily when they hit the ground
     C. Frequency approximately 8 to 10 times daily
   IX. Urine
     A. Colorless to yellow
     B. Can be thick or turbid due to high mucous content

DENTAL FORMULA AND CARE
Dental Formula

   I. $2\left(I\,\dfrac{3}{3}\; C\,\dfrac{1}{1}\; P\,\dfrac{3\text{ or }4}{3}\; M\,\dfrac{3}{3} \right) = 40 \text{ or } 42$
   II. Mares usually do not have canine teeth
     A. Equine canine teeth are also called tushes
   III. Horses develop temporary and permanent teeth

Dental Care

   I. Wolf teeth or P1 are located in the upper jaw
     A. If wolf teeth (P1) do not fall out on their own, the veterinarian will have to extract them because they can interfere with the bit

II. Anatomically the horse's upper jaw is wider than the lower jaw
  A. When a horse eats it grinds food in a side to side motion
  B. This creates sharp edges on the outside of the upper teeth (buccal surface) and on the inside of the lower teeth
  C. The term *floating the teeth* is the rasping down of these sharp edges
  D. A veterinarian should check the horse's teeth at least annually to determine if teeth need floating
    1. Signs that animal's teeth need floating include:
      a. Halitosis
      b. Lacerations of oral cavity
      c. Feed dropping
      d. Head tilt
      e. Undigested food in feces

GASTROINTESTINAL AILMENTS

Common Clinical Signs

  I. Restlessness, anxiety, or agitation
  II. Pawing, pacing/stall walking
  III. Flank watching and possible biting at flank
  IV. Kicking at abdomen
  V. Sweating
  VI. Getting up and down in stall
  VII. Rolling
  VIII. Grinding teeth
  IX. Distended abdomen
  X. Increased heart rate and respiration rate
  XI. Mucous membranes can be pale, bright or brick red, or cyanotic
  XII. Toxic line (red or blue) on gums just above teeth may be present
  XIII. Increased CRT
  XIV. Gastrointestinal motility: hypermotile, hypomotile, or absent
  XV. Digital pulses bounding with increased heat in hoof wall
  XVI. Fecal output can be absent, small amounts of hard, dry balls, or cow patty to diarrhea
  XVII. Sawhorse stance (standing stretched out), or dog sitting
  XVIII. Decreased appetite
  XIX. Reflux, via nasogastric tube, is often present (can be absent or up to 15 L in an average size horse)

Rule Outs of Gastrointestinal Ailments

  I. Colic
  A. Refers to abdominal pain
    1. Most commonly seen ailment
  B. Gastrointestinal causes include
    1. Excessive gas
    2. Spasmodic colic
    3. Ileus (cessation of peristalsis)
    4. Parasitic infestations (i.e., *Ascaris* in foals and *Strongylus* in adult horses)
    5. Volvulus (torsion of small or large intestine)
    6. Intussusception
    7. Impactions
    8. Obstructions
    9. Displacement
    10. Inguinal hernias
  C. Symptoms vary with the severity of the colic and disposition of the horse
  D. All of the clinical signs listed above will not necessarily be seen in each case. Management of all ailments and diseases are at the discretion of a veterinarian
  E. Management of colics consists of:
    1. Fluid therapy
    2. Antiinflammatory drugs
    3. Mineral oil
    4. Antiflatulence medication
    5. Monitoring
  F. Monitoring includes:
    1. Vital signs
    2. Gut sounds (motility)
    3. Fecal output
    4. Hydration status (PCV and TP)
    5. Obtaining nasogastric reflux (how much, if any)
    6. Walking
    7. Gradual introduction of food to the animal
  G. In cases where surgery has been performed or toxemia occurred, digital pulses are also extremely important to monitor because laminitis is always a concern
II. Colitis
  A. An acute inflammatory process of the large colon and cecum
  B. In most cases of acute colitis a cause is unknown
  C. Several possibilities include:
    1. Dietary change
    2. *Salmonella* spp.
    3. *Clostridium perfringens* (Colitis X)
    4. Potomac Horse Fever
    5. Antibiotic therapy
    6. Overuse of NSAIDs

D. Clinically each horse tends to present the same way
  1. Inappetence
  2. Abdominal pain
  3. Diarrhea (varying from cow patty to profuse watery diarrhea)
  4. Dehydration
  5. In severe cases, shock
E. Management of colitis
  1. Fluid therapy with a balanced electrolyte solution (e.g., Lactated Ringers Solution [LRS])
F. Monitoring
  1. Vital signs
  2. PCV and TP
  3. Digital pulses and heat (signs of laminitis) in hooves
G. Usually free choice grass hay is offered but grain is withheld
H. Horses with diarrhea are kept isolated due to the possibility of *Salmonella*
I. When a horse is on intravenous fluids, it is vital that the indwelling catheter be monitored for:
  1. Heat
  2. Swelling
  3. Pain
J. This is very important because horses with colitis are prone to thrombosis of the jugular vein

III. Salmonellosis
A. A very serious problem due to zoonotic potential and high contagiousness to other horses
  1. Horses may naturally carry *Salmonella* as part of their intestinal flora
B. Causes include:
  1. Stressful situations, i.e., trailering
  2. Sudden changes in feeding
  3. Sickness
  4. Surgery
C. Clinically horses present with:
  1. Acute, profuse, watery, foul-smelling diarrhea
  2. Dehydration
  3. Depression
D. Management is extremely important
  1. The horse should be isolated
  2. Handling the animal should be kept to one person to prevent the possibility of cross contamination
  3. Anyone handling the horse should be gowned, gloved, and wear protective boot covers
  4. When leaving the isolated animal, hands should be thoroughly washed and boots should be dipped in a foot bath containing a bactericidal solution
  5. Fluid therapy with a balanced electrolyte solution is very important because hydration status is the number one concern
E. Monitor vital signs as with any other diarrhea case
F. Horse is fed hay ad libitum; grain is withheld

IV. Intestinal clostridial infections
A. An acute inflammatory process of the bowel
B. Colitis X is the most common form and is diagnosed on postmortem examination
C. Clinically horses present with:
  1. Signs similar to salmonellosis
  2. Often no initial diarrhea
  3. Severe abdominal pain
  4. Increased gut motility (hypermotile)
  5. Diarrhea within a matter of hours
D. Management is the same as for salmonellosis
E. The antibiotic bacitracin, given orally, may be effective in some cases

V. Potomac Horse Fever (PHF)
A. *Ehrlichia risticii* is the cause of PHF
B. This rickittsia-like organism is thought to be transmitted by arthropods (i.e., ticks, fleas, flies, and mosquitoes)
C. Horses can be tested for PHF by using an ELISA test and an indirect immunofluorescent antibody (IFA) test
D. Clinically horses present with the following:
  1. Depression
  2. Anorexia
  3. Pyretic symptoms
  4. Decreased gut sounds
  5. Abdominal pain and diarrhea (shown by some)
E. Management of PHF
  1. Oxytetracycline
  2. Aggressive fluid therapy with a balanced electrolyte solution
F. As in cases of *Salmonella,* the same monitoring and strict isolation procedures are applied
G. Laminitis is a major concern with PHF and should be monitored closely
H. Vaccines are available for PHF

VI. Antibiotic and NSAID therapy
   A. Overuse of antibiotics and nonsteroidal antiinflammatory drugs can cause diarrhea
   B. Clinically the horse presents with:
      1. Loss of appetite
      2. Depression
      3. Some abdominal pain
      4. Protein loss due to ulceration of the bowel or stomach
   C. Some antibiotics such as tetracycline drugs can cause diarrhea as a side effect
   D. Management
      1. Fluid therapy such as LRS and plasma
      2. Monitoring patients' vital signs
   E. Antibiotics and NSAIDs should be discontinued
   F. Gastroscopy can be performed to determine ulcerations
   G. Treatment with antiulcer medication can then be initiated if needed

VII. Anterior enteritis
   A. The cause is idiopathic; however, *Clostridium* spp. have been implicated
   B. Clinically horses present with the following:
      1. Severe colic
      2. Increased heart rate
      3. Possible pyrexia
   C. Signs are often the same as with an obstruction of the bowel
   D. Diagnosis is made by the veterinarian performing a rectal examination
   E. In the case of anterior enteritis, colic signs decrease when nasogastric reflux is obtained. With an obstruction, colic signs usually do not decrease. The horse will then become depressed
   F. Management
      1. Passage of a nasogastric tube and frequent siphoning to empty fluid buildup in the stomach
      2. Fluid therapy is important to replace fluid loss from the nasogastric reflux
   G. Monitoring is the same as with colic, although particular attention is paid to temperature because toxemia is a concern

VIII. Hyperkalemic Periodic Paralysis (HYPP)
   A. This disease originally resulted in a genetic mutation that has been traced back to a quarter horse sire
   B. Clinically horses can show any of the following:
      1. Muscle fasciculations
      2. Colic-like episodes
      3. Sweating
      4. Respiratory distress
      5. Prolapsed third eye lid
      6. Loose feces
   C. A DNA blood test has been developed and can determine:
      1. If a horse is a homozygous affected animal
      2. A heterozygous carrier
      3. Normal
   D. If the test is positive, breeding should be discouraged and owners should be made aware that riding these horses can be dangerous
   E. Management of HYPP consists of:
      1. A low potassium diet
      2. Grass or oat hay (no alfalfa hay)
      3. Plenty of fresh water
      4. Minimizing stress in these affected horses is beneficial

NEUROMUSCULAR DISORDERS ▰▰▰▰

Common Clinical Signs

   I. Ataxia
   II. Depression
   III. Circling
   IV. Head tilt
   V. Head pressing
   VI. Nystagmus
   VII. Facial paralysis, drooling
   VIII. Incoordination, limb knuckling, and toe dragging
   IX. Muscle wasting
   X. Prolapsed third eyelid
   XI. Seizure
   XII. Altered behavior

Rule Outs of Neuromuscular Disorders

   I. Tetanus (lockjaw)
   A. Caused by the bacterium *Clostridium tetani*
   B. *C. tetani* is found in the soil and infects horses through puncture wounds
   C. The bacteria produces exotoxins, which affect the horse's nervous system
   D. Symptoms
      1. Muscle stiffness (sawhorse stance)
      2. Decreased feed intake
      3. Sensitivity to light and sound
   E. Management of tetanus should begin with the infected horse receiving a booster of tetanus antitoxin. This is given because the antitoxin will bind to any circulating tetanus toxins

F. Wound treatment
1. Cleaning
2. Draining
3. Local infiltration of penicillin to the site of the wound
G. Systemically the horse should be given intravenous penicillin
H. The horse should be kept in a dark, quiet stall
I. Intravenous fluids may be needed, especially if horse is dysphagic
J. Vaccinating horses annually with tetanus toxoid to help stimulate the immune system is a preventive measure

II. Rabies
A. A virus that attacks the central nervous system
B. This virus most commonly is passed by a bite from an infected animal
C. Because the virus is found in large quantities in saliva, domestic animals, including man, can become infected through open wounds and across mucous membranes
D. Symptoms include all of the above and can also consist of:
1. Extreme aggression
2. Dysphagia
3. Hydrophobia
4. Self-inflicted wounds
E. Clinical signs are always progressive
F. Management of rabies
1. The suspected horse must be quarantined
2. Anyone handling the horse should wear protective clothing and gloves due to rabies zoonotic potential
G. Unfortunately, if rabies is highly suspected, the horse must be euthanized because of the threat to human life and because there is no cure
H. A definitive diagnoses can be made only at postmortem
I. An annual rabies vaccine should be given as a preventive measure

III. Equine Protozoal Myeloencephalitis (EPM)
A. Affects the central nervous system
B. The protozoa, *Sarcocystis falcatula,* is currently thought to be the causative agent
C. The protoza
1. Encysts in the muscle of birds
2. Opossums eat the infected birds
3. Opossum's feces contaminate the horse's feed and water supply

D. Symptoms will depend on location of lesion
E. Locations of lesions from the protozoa
1. The brain stem
2. Spinal cord
3. Peripheral nerves
F. Horses may show any of the following:
1. Ataxia
2. Facial paralysis
3. Head tilt
4. Depression
5. Blindness
6. Dysphagia
7. Circling
8. Hind end weakness and ataxia
9. Gluteal, tongue, and masticatory muscle wasting
10. Incontinence
11. In some cases recumbency
G. EPM is diagnosed by performing a cerebrospinal fluid (CSF) tap
H. The spinal fluid is then analyzed for
1. Antibodies to *Sarcocystis falcatula*
2. Protozoal DNA
I. Management of EPM consists of long-term antibiotic and antiprotozoa therapy, which usually includes trimethoprim-sulfadiazine and pyrimethamine
J. Unfortunately, affected animals often do not recover completely and post therapeutic relapses are common

IV. Equine Herpes Virus 1 (EHV-1)
A. Also known as viral rhinopneumonitis
1. It is transmitted by direct contact or aerosols
B. Clinically horses with EHV-1 can be:
1. Incoordinated
2. Incontinent
3. Ataxic in hindlimbs
4. Have loss of tail tone
5. In extreme cases horses become recumbent
C. Abortion can occur in pregnant mares
D. If affected late in gestation, abortion may not occur; however, foals are infected in utero and may be born dead or die shortly after birth
E. Management of EHV-1 depends on the severity of the disease and treatment includes:
1. Antibiotics
2. Antiinflammatories
3. Corticosteroids

F. Vaccinating horses is a preventive measure but may not be effective against abortions or neurologic diseases

V. Equine Encephalomyelitides (sleeping sickness)
   A. Three strains of this alphavirus
      1. Eastern (EEE)
      2. Western (WEE)
      3. Venezuelan (VEE)
   B. Most common to Canada and the United States: Eastern (EEE) and Western (WEE) strains
   C. Transmitted by mosquitoes
   D. Clinically horses:
      1. Can be pyretic
      2. Will head press
      3. Circle in the stall
      4. Have seizures
   E. Mortality is common
   F. Management
      1. Antiinflammatories
      2. NSAIDs
      3. Corticosteroids
      4. Anticonvulsants
      5. An emphasis on supportive nursing care
   G. Vaccinating horses against this disease is an effective preventive measure

RESPIRATORY DISEASES ▬▬▬▬

Common Clinical Signs

I. Coughing
II. Purulent or bloody nasai discharge
III. Depression
IV. Anorexia
V. Dyspnea, tachypnea
VI. Pyrexic

Rule Outs of Respiratory Diseases

I. Strangles
   A. A very contagious upper respiratory tract disease
      1. Caused by the bacterium *Streptococcus equi*
   B. It is spread by the infected animal's secretions or by fomites
   C. Another bacteria that creates similar clinical signs but is not contagious is *S. zooepidemicus*
   D. Horses develop swelling of the lymph nodes
      1. Under the mandible
      2. In the guttural pouches
      3. In the throat area

E. These abscesses can be quite painful and eventually rupture
F. Management
   1. Infected horse isolated to prevent cross contamination
   2. Abscesses hot packed (to speed maturation) or lanced to encourage proper drainage
   3. Fluids and feed slurries given if the horse is dysphagic
   4. Keep horse warm with plenty of fresh water available
   5. Possible use of antipyretics and antibiotics
G. Anything that comes into contact with the infected horse should be well disinfected or burned if possible
H. Currently available vaccines may lessen the severity of the disease but will not prevent an infection

II. Equine Herpes Virus (EHV-4)
   A. Like EHV-1, which was covered under neuromuscular disorders, this virus is also spread by direct contact or aerosols
      1. This strain of virus attacks the upper respiratory tract
   B. As well as the above clinical signs, horses will have:
      1. Increased lung sounds
      2. Possible swelling of the lymph nodes
   C. Management
      1. Isolate the infected animal to prevent cross contamination
      2. Keep the horse warm in a well ventilated stall
      3. Have plenty of fresh water available
      4. Avoid stressful situations (i.e., trailering)
   D. A vaccine is available; although it is questionable as to prevention of the disease, it does seem to lessen the severity of it

III. Equine Influenza (FLU)
   A. An extremely contagious virus that attacks the upper respiratory tract
   B. It is spread very quickly in areas of extensive horse populations as:
      1. Horse shows
      2. Race tracks
      3. Barns where horses are constantly moving in and out
   C. Like the other respiratory viruses, the influenza virus also is spread by direct contact and by aerosols

D. As well as the above clinical signs, horses may be:
    1. Lethargic
    2. Have increased lung sounds in some cases
E. Management is the same as EHV-4
F. Currently available vaccines may lessen the severity of the disease but will not prevent an infection

BLOOD DISORDER

I. Equine Infectious Anemia (EIA)
    A. Also known as swamp fever
    B. The virus is found in:
        1. The blood
        2. Semen
        3. Tissues
    C. It is transmitted by:
        1. Arthropods (most commonly biting flies)
        2. Blood transfusion
        3. Dirty needles
    D. Clinically horses will be:
        1. Pyretic
        2. Depressed
        3. Anorexic
        4. Have weight loss
        5. Anemic
    E. Diagnosis of EIA is done by taking a blood sample from the horse and having the serum analyzed for antibodies
    F. This test is known as the Coggins test; it is required for:
        1. Any horse that is traveling across borders
        2. Racehorses
        3. Show horses
        4. Horses that are being sold
    G. There is no cure or prevention for this disease
    H. Infected horses will always be carriers of this virus but may be asymptomatic
    I. Euthanasia depends on:
        1. State regulations
        2. Provincial regulations
        3. Federal regulations
    J. If horse is not euthanized, it must be isolated for the rest of its life

FOOT AILMENTS

I. Laminitis (founder)
    A. Inflammation of the sensitive laminae of the feet

1. Most commonly occurs in the front feet; however it can also occur in the hind feet
B. Caused by
    1. Grain overload
    2. Ingestion of large amounts of cold water (water founder)
    3. Endotoxemia
    4. Concussion (road founder)
    5. Hormonal influences
    6. After viral respiratory diseases
    7. After administration of drugs
    8. Overeating lush pastures, particularly in the spring
C. Clinically, horses will:
    1. Be reluctant to move
    2. Toe point
    3. Rock back on the heal to relieve the pressure on the toe
    4. Be pyrexic
    5. Be depressed
    6. Be off feed
    7. Have increased heat in the hoof wall and bounding digital pulses as a result of increased blood flow
    8. Be sensitive to hoof testers
D. In extreme cases the coffin bone rotates and can come through the sole of the foot
E. Radiographs are used to determine degree of rotation
F. Management
    1. Antiinflammatories
    2. Vasodilator (isoxsuprine hydrochloride)
    3. Acepromazine
    4. Fluids (LRS)
    5. Grass hay ad libitum, no grain
    6. Corrective hoof trimming
    7. Cold hosing and icing feet may also be done; however this treatment is controversial
II. Navicular syndrome
    A. Degeneration of the navicular bone
    B. Exact cause unknown
    C. Clinically, horses may:
        1. Stumble
        2. Have a shortened stride
        3. Be intermittently lame
    D. When pressure is applied over the sole of the foot with hoof testers, a horse with navicular disease will react by pulling the foot away in response to pain

E. To further diagnose navicular syndrome the following is performed:
1. Flexion tests
2. Nerve blocking
3. Radiographs
F. Management
1. Antiinflammatories
2. Vasodilator (isoxsuprine hydrochloride)
3. Corrective foot trimming and shoeing
4. Last resort: surgically performing a neurectomy

EQUINE SURGERY

I. Presurgical preparations
A. Take horse off feed 12 hours before surgery. Water may be left
B. TPR is performed
C. Groom horse to rid excess dirt and dander; pull shoes
D. Clip and aseptically prep jugular vein; place an intravenous catheter
E. PCV and TP, blood gas, and electrolyte analysis if available
F. Rinse out horse's mouth before induction
G. After horse is induced, the veterinarian will:
1. Direct positioning of the horse
2. Indicate the area that needs to be clipped and prepped
H. Horse's feet should be covered with gloves or plastic (i.e., rectal sleeves) to prevent contamination to the surgery suite
II. Positioning of horse
A. The following surgeries are performed in dorsal recumbency
1. All abdominal surgeries (i.e., colic, exploratory, caesarean, laryngeal ventriculectomy, umbilical and inguinal hernias)
2. Bilateral or unilateral cryptorchid
3. Carpal, hock, and stifle arthroscopies
4. Neurectomy
B. When positioning a horse in dorsal recumbency, particular attention must be paid to:
1. The padding underneath the shoulder and gluteal muscles
2. If padding is not sufficient, myositis can develop
C. The following surgeries are performed in lateral recumbency
1. Eye surgeries
2. Tooth extractions

3. Mandible fracture repair (i.e., wiring)
4. Laryngotomy
5. Laryngoplasty
6. Fetlock and shoulder arthroscopies
7. Periosteal strips
8. Castration
D. When positioning a horse in lateral recumbency:
1. Pay particular attention so that there is no pressure on the down elbow
2. The up legs should be supported with pads or leg supports
3. The down foreleg should be pulled forward to enhance circulation
E. The following can be performed when a sedated horse is standing
1. Extraction of wolf teeth (first premolar)
2. Rectovaginal tears using an epidural
3. Caslick (suturing a small portion of mare's vulva to prevent air entering the vagina, commonly known as windsucking)
4. Perianal lacerations using an epidural
5. Uncomplicated ovariectomies
6. Castrations
III. Preparation of surgical site
A. After surgical site is clipped and vacuumed, caps and masks should be worn
B. Prepping
1. Clean area with a bacteriostatic agent such as chlorhexidine or an iodine based soap
2. After site is clean, apply alcohol to defat the skin
3. Move horse inside the surgical suite, where a final germicidal prep solution of tincture of savlon or iodine is used
C. Prepping for eye surgeries
1. Clip hair around eye, including eyelashes. Take care to prevent hair getting into eyes
2. If the eye is being enucleated (removed), the eyelids are sutured closed
3. Bacteriostatic agents should be avoided because they irritate the sensitive tissue around the eye and also can damage the eyeball
4. A very dilute solution of povidone-iodine and saline can be used to clean skin around the eye
5. When flushing out the eye, saline is often used

IV. Postoperative care
   A. After the horse recovers and is stable, it can be moved back to its stall
   B. The horse should be kept warm and quiet
   C. Monitoring horse's feces is very important—ileus is always a risk with any general anesthetic
   D. Horse's vital signs, including gastrointestinal motility are monitored twice daily
   E. After horse passes feces, soft food such as a small bran mash can be introduced. A couple of hours later, a small amount of hay can be fed
   F. If horse passes more feces and vital signs are normal, horse's regular feeding schedule can be slowly introduced, beginning with gradually increasing amount of hay fed
   G. If horse does not pass any feces, a veterinarian will perform a rectal examination to determine if horse is impacted
   H. If impacted:
      1. A nasogastric tube is passed and mineral oil and warm water is introduced into the stomach to help break down the impaction
      2. Food is withheld from the horse
      3. Horse may be placed on intravenous fluids (LRS) until horse is passing feces
      4. Frequent hand walking (if surgery allows)
      5. Monitor vital signs
      6. Particular attention is paid to gastrointestinal motility (gut sounds)
      7. Horse is monitored four times daily until impaction has passed
   I. In cases of arthroscopic surgery:
      1. Bandage is monitored for any discharge
      2. Leg is monitored for any unusual heat, swelling, or pain
      3. Usually 24 hours after the surgery, hand walking for 5 minutes is introduced
   J. In cases of fracture repair:
      1. The cast is monitored for softness caused by discharge leaking from the fracture site
      2. Note any unusual smell or any unusual swelling above the cast

Glossary

arthroscopy The ability to look inside a joint through the aid of a fiberoptic scope

asymptomatic A carrier of a disease that does not show any symptoms

borborygmus Bubbling and gurgling sounds as a result of gas moving through the gastrointestinal tract

dyspnea Difficulty breathing

fasciculations Involuntary muscle contractions

ileus Cessation of intestinal motility, which leads to impactions/obstructions

in utero In the uterus

myositis Inflammation of the muscle that results when blood flow is interrupted. This results with uneven or inadequate padding. Muscles can become damaged, and it is an extremely painful condition

nasogastric Long tube placed through horse's nose into the stomach

neurectomy Cutting the digital nerves to desensitize the foot to pain

thrombosis Presence of a fibrin clot in vessels

thrombus A fibrin blood clot that remains where it is formed; can affect blood flow if it obstructs the vessels

pyrexia Presence of fever

Review Questions

1 Which of these are zoonotic?
   a. *Ehrlichia risticii* and *Clostridium* spp.
   b. *Sarcocystis falcatula* and *Streptococcus equi*
   c. *Salmonella* spp. and rabies
   d. *Ehrlichia coli* and *Klebsiella* spp.
2 Common signs of neuromuscular disease:
   a. Restlessness, anxiousness, or agitation
   b. Anorexia, pyrexia, or depression
   c. Grinding teeth and sweating
   d. Muscle wasting, head pressing, or ataxia
3 There is a vaccine available for:
   a. Equine protozoal myeloencephalitis
   b. Equine infectious anemia
   c. Sleeping sickness
   d. Hyperkalemic periodic paralysis
4 How are horses infected with equine protozoal myeloencephalitis?
   a. Fomites
   b. Opossums feces
   c. Arthropods
   d. Aerosol
5 The etiological agent for strangles is:
   a. *Streptococcus equi*
   b. *Streptococcus zooepidemicus*
   c. *Clostridium* spp.
   d. *Sarcocystis falcatula*

6 Coggins is the test for:
   a. Equine infectious anemia
   b. Equine protozoal myeloencephalitis
   c. Potomac horse fever
   d. Hyperkalemic periodic paralysis
7 What is very important when positioning a horse in dorsal recumbency for surgery?
   a. Pulling the front legs cranially
   b. Position of the head
   c. Exposure of jugular vein for intravenous access
   d. Sufficient padding for shoulders and gluteal muscles ✓
8 When prepping a surgical site, alcohol is used as what type of agent?
   a. Bacteriostatic
   b. Defatting
   c. Germicidal
   d. Bactericidal
9 Myositis is a result of:
   a. Improper padding
   b. Improper prepping
   c. Horse not taken off feed before surgery
   d. Feeding horse too soon after surgery
10 A postoperative concern for the horse is:
   a. PCV and TP
   b. Moving horse back to its stall as quickly as possible
   c. Proper grooming and shoe removal
   d. Ileus

BIBLIOGRAPHY

Anderson DM, editor: *Dorland's pocket medical dictionary,* ed 24, Philadelphia, 1989, W.B. Saunders.

Fraser CM, editor; Bergeron JA, associate editor; Mays A, associate editor; Aiello SE, assistant editor: *The Merck veterinary manual,* ed 7, Rahway, 1991, Merck & Co., Inc.

Knecht CD, Allen AR, Williams DJ, Johnson JH: *Fundamental techniques in veterinary surgery,* ed 3, Philadelphia, 1987, W.B. Saunders.

McCurnin DM: *Clinical textbook for veterinary technicians,* ed 3, Philadelphia, 1993, W.B. Saunders.

McCurnin DM: *Clinical textbook for veterinary technicians,* ed 2, Philadelphia, 1990, W.B. Saunders.

Rose RJ, Hodgson DR: *Manual of equine practice,* Philadelphia, 1993, W.B. Saunders.

Ruminant and Swine Nursing, Surgery, and Anesthesia

Sandy Agla

OUTLINE

Ruminant and Swine Nursing
  The Physical Examination
  Administering Medication and
    Sample Collection
  Venipuncture
  Intramuscular Injections
  Milk Sampling
  Diseases of Ruminants and
    Swine

Preventable Diseases
Ruminant and Swine Surgery
  Laparotomy (Bovine)
  Digit Amputation (Bovine)
  Teat Laceration Repair (Bovine
    and Caprine)
  Eye Enucleation (Bovine)
  Castration
  Dehorning

Ruminant and Swine Anesthesia
  Local and Regional Anesthesia
    (Analgesia)
  General Anesthesia

LEARNING OUTCOMES

After reading this chapter you should be able to:

1. Know techniques for administering medications and collection of samples in food animals.
2. Know some of the common diseases of cattle, small ruminants, and swine.
3. Recognize some of the preventable (by vaccination) diseases of food animals.
4. Know some of the common surgical procedures of food animals.
5. Know some of the species differences regarding surgical procedures.
6. Understand the difference between local and regional anesthesia.
7. Know the various methods of regional anesthesia in food animals.
8. Know the considerations for each species in anesthesia for food animals.
9. Know monitoring techniques for general anesthesia in food animals.

A technician in a large animal practice must be familiar with common techniques, some of the diseases, the diseases for which vaccines are available, and surgical procedures and anesthetic principles. For more in-depth information, refer to the many excellent references that are available. Some are listed at the end of this section.

RUMINANT AND SWINE NURSING
The Physical Examination

I. Observations
  A. Use all senses when performing a physical examination

B. Before entering a stall or pen, helpful information can be obtained by observation
 1. Note the animal's eyes, its stance and carriage, body condition, urine and manure output, food and water intake
 2. Know the "normals" for each type of animal. For instance, if you are used to observing beef animals, a dairy cow may look underconditioned when, in fact, her weight may be optimum for her

II. Physical examination
 A. The physical examination should proceed from nose to tail, taking note of swellings, abrasions, discharges, etc.
 B. TPRs should fall within normal ranges (see Appendix C)
 C. Rumen contractions should be noted by listening with a stethoscope at the left paralumbar fossa
 1. Normal rumen motility is 1 to 3 contractions per minute

Administering Medication and Sample Collection

I. Oral dosing
 A. Balling gun
 1. Boluses, capsules, and magnets (for dairy cattle) can be given using this device, which may be made of plastic or metal
 2. With ruminants, the animal should be secured and the head well restrained
 a. Hold the animal around the bridge of the nose, place your fingers in the interdental space, and apply pressure to the hard palate
 b. This will force the animal to open its mouth so you can introduce the balling gun at the interdigital space
 c. Position it so the medication will be deposited at the base of the tongue
 d. The head should be stabilized and held horizontally
 3. In pigs, a bar speculum can be introduced into the animal's mouth to hold the jaws open so that the balling gun can be used to deposit boluses or capsules at the base of the tongue
 B. Stomach tube
 1. For delivering large amounts of liquid medication or fluids, anthelmintics, or for transfaunation

 2. Frick speculum
 a. A hollow, stainless steel tube, used in cattle, inserted similarly to the balling gun. It is also used as a guide in introducing a stomach tube to prevent the tube from being damaged
 b. In sheep or goats, a tape roll or appropriately sized, smooth ended syringe case can be used
 3. Measure the distance from the nose to the rumen at approximately the 13th rib and insert the tube through the speculum up to the mark
 a. You may detect the odor of rumen gas to let you know you are in the correct place or have someone listen over the rumen at the paralumbar fossa with a stethoscope as you blow air into the tube
 (1) A "gurgling" sound will be heard
 b. After you verify correct placement, the liquid can be given
 c. Always kink off the tube or occlude the end before removing it to prevent the animal from aspirating any of the contents
 C. Drench
 1. Small amounts of liquid medication can be given via drench
 2. A dose-syringe or unbreakable bottle is placed in the interdental space (ruminants) or at the commissure of the mouth (swine)
 a. The head is tilted slightly so the nose is level with the eye
 b. The liquid should be given at a slow enough rate to let the animal swallow

Venipuncture

I. Cattle venipuncture
 A. Jugular is for sampling and giving large volumes of fluids
 1. Head is restrained in a head catch and drawn upward to the opposite side
 2. Injection site is cleansed with 70% alcohol and occluded
 3. A 14 or 16 gauge, 5 to 7.5 cm (2-3 inch) needle is used and pushed with one sharp motion through the skin at a 45°-90° angle
 B. Tail vein (ventral coccygeal) is for sampling and injecting small volumes
 1. Confine to an area to prevent sideways movement and bend the tail directly forward at the base

2. Cleanse with 70% alcohol
3. Use an 18 to 20 gauge, 2.5 to 3.75 cm (1-1.5 inch) needle inserted at a 90° angle on the midline between the hemal arches of the 4th to 7th coccygeal vertebrae

C. Milk vein (subcutaneous abdominal) forms hematomas easily and is under pressure. Use caution
   1. Occlusion is not necessary before entering with a 14 gauge, 5 to 7.5 cm (2-3 inch) needle
   2. Digital pressure applied for several minutes is necessary but a hematoma may still form

II. Sheep and goat venipuncture
A. Jugular is almost always used
   1. Direct a 18 or 20 gauge, 2.5-cm (1 inch) needle into the jugular furrow at about a 30°-45° angle
B. Cephalic is uncommon
C. Femoral is uncommon

III. Swine venipuncture
A. Cranial vena cava for a large volume (right side preferred because the phrenic nerve and thoracic duct are found near left external jugular vein)
   1. An 18 or 20 gauge, 7.5 to 10 cm (3-4 inch) needle is used for adult pigs
   2. The jugular fossa near the manubrium sterni, a bony projection on the ventral midline cranial to the forelegs, is used as a guideline
   3. The needle is inserted perpendicular to the plane of the neck and toward the left shoulder
B. Caudal auricular (ear) for small volumes
   1. An 18 or 22 gauge, 2.5 to 3.75 cm (1-1.5 inch) needle is usually used with slight negative pressure maintained on the syringe
   2. A 19 or 21 gauge butterfly is commonly used for IV administration

Intramuscular Injections

I. Cattle
A. Locations used are gluteal, semimembranosis, semitendinosis, and occasionally lateral cervical muscles
B. Needle commonly used for adults is 16, 18, or 20 gauge, 3.75 to 5 cm (1.5-2 inch) with a 15 to 20 mL maximum volume of medication per site

C. Smaller gauge used for calves and up to 10 to 15 mL, depending on muscle mass
D. When giving intramuscular injections to cattle it is customary to place the needle before attaching the syringe
   1. A couple of slaps with the flat part of the fist before inserting the needle tends to desensitize the area and allows the animal to steady itself before the needle goes in

II. Sheep and goats
A. Best given in the semimembranosis or semitendinosis but sometimes gluteals are used
B. Use an 18 to 20 gauge, 3.75 cm (1.5 inch) for adults and a 20 to 22 gauge needle for young animals
C. The average volume for adults is 5 to 10 mL with a maximum of 15 mL

III. Swine
A. Dorsolateral neck muscles are best for swine destined for meat (gluteals can be used)
B. For adult pigs use an 18 to 20 gauge, 3.75 cm (1.5 inch) needle
C. Depending on the site, a maximum of 1 to 15 mL should be given

Milk Sampling

I. An important aspect of dairy herd health is early detection and treatment of mastitis. Because of rising laboratory costs, milk sampling (for culture) is often done on a herd basis
A. Quarters are sampled into one tube and individual quarter sampling done on only those animals that showed positive on the herd testing
B. Sampling should be done before routine milking or at least 6 hours after
C. Each teat should be washed, wiped with an alcohol swab, and allowed to dry
   1. Clean in the order of far to near
D. The first part of the stream should be discarded into a strip cup and a midstream sample taken horizontally is directed into the sample vial, which is held horizontally out from under the near side of the animal
E. Sampling is done from the nearest side first

II. Determination of subclinical mastitis and a rough estimate of somatic cell count can be done using an on-site procedure called the California Mastitis Test (CMT)
A. The test consists of a paddle with four shallow cups and a reagent containing a pH indicator

B. A small amount of milk is mixed with an equal amount of CMT reagent
C. The paddle is gently rotated and an interpretation made based on the amount of precipitation
D. The amount of precipitate formed is given a 0 to 4 rating

Diseases of Ruminants and Swine

I. Hypocalcemic parturient paresis (milk fever)
  A. Incidence
    1. The incidence of milk fever in cattle increases in high-performing animals at 5 to 9 years of age. It is greater in Channel Island breeds (Jersey). It usually occurs at 48 to 72 hours postpartum
    2. Milk fever in sheep is most common in late pregnancy but can occur in early lactation
    3. The condition is rare in sows but may occur within a few hours of farrowing
  B. Serum calcium level is decreased, serum magnesium may be increased (flaccid paralysis) or decreased (tetany)
    1. Low serum phosphorus may be a contributing factor
  C. Clinical signs initially include muscle tremors, weakness, and staggering gait
    1. Classical signs include sternal recumbency, head turned into flank, anorexia, dry muzzle, atonic rumen, increased heart rate (with decreased intensity of heart sound), mydriasis, myositis, and nerve damage if down too long
    2. If left untreated, depression of the circulatory system and bloat as a result of lateral recumbency will be fatal
  D. Characteristically, a quick positive response is obtained with treatment of intravenous calcium borogluconate
    1. Careful attention must be paid to the heart during infusion because calcium salts affect the heart muscle
  E. Animals should be fed a ration high in phosphorus and low in calcium during the later stages of pregnancy
II. Ketosis (acetonemia in cattle; pregnancy toxemia in ewes)
  A. Ketosis is a metabolic disease
    1. Can occur in the period from just after calving until peak lactation in the cow (2-6 weeks after calving)
    2. Generally occurs in the last trimester of pregnancy in ewes

B. As a result of increased demand for glucose for the production of milk in high-producing cows and the demands of the developing fetus (or fetuses), the dam is in a negative energy balance
    1. Body fat is mobilized to provide energy
    2. Ketone bodies are produced in excess of tissue needs and clinical ketosis results
  C. Ketosis may be secondary to any underlying disease that causes inappetance
  D. There is a characteristic acetone odor to the breath, milk, and urine
  E. Two forms of the disease may manifest: the wasting and the nervous forms
    1. Wasting form: more common
      a. The cow may begin by being off grain alone, then silage, but may continue to eat hay
      b. Weight loss exceeds what one might expect from loss of appetite alone
      c. Milk production declines
    2. Nervous form: presents acutely with head pressing, delirium, teeth grinding, and staggering
      a. In ewes and does, signs of the disease are more like the nervous form, and ketones may be detected on the breath
  F. Treatment
    1. Intravenous infusion of glucose (dextrose) is usually successful in cows, although it often needs to be repeated
    2. Oral doses of propylene glycol and hormonal therapy may be useful
    3. The same treatment in ewes is less satisfactory
    4. Lambs may have to be removed by C-section to save the ewe
  G. Most incidences of ketosis can be prevented by adhering to a careful management and ration plan
III. Displaced abomasum
  A. Left displaced abomasum (LDA)
    1. Occurs when the abomasum is displaced from its normal position on the abdominal floor to the left side of the abdomen between the rumen and the abdominal wall
    2. Occurs most commonly in large, high-producing, mature dairy cows immediately after calving
    3. Clinical signs are decreased appetite, lower milk production, decreased rumen

motility, intermittent diarrhea, secondary ketosis, and the presence of an auscultable "ping" in the left flank caused by the entrapment of gas

B. Right displaced abomasum (RDA)
   1. Occurs within a few weeks of calving and may be complicated by abomasal torsion
   2. Less common than LDA but clinical signs are similar
   3. Abomasal torsion will present with acute, severe abdominal pain
   4. Surgical correction is done using any of left flank, right flank, or ventral paramedian laparotomy and abomasopexy (and/or omentopexy)
   5. There is an increased incidence of displaced abomasum in cows fed a high grain diet (zero grazing) in conjunction with confined housing

IV. Vagus indigestion
   A. Vagus indigestion is a common disease in cattle; uncommon in sheep
      1. Characterized by anorexia, decreased movement of ingesta through the stomachs, and distention
   B. Most common cause: hardware disease (traumatic reticuloperitonitis)
      1. Hardware disease usually results from perforation of the reticulum and sometimes the rumen by an ingested foreign object
      2. Clinical signs are a sudden decrease in milk, anorexia, "hunching," and groaning
      3. Often the cow will grunt if pressure is applied over the xyphoid ("grunt test")
      4. Rumen becomes atonic, fecal output is decreased, and ketosis often occurs
      5. Treatment includes antibiotics and placing a magnet into the reticulum
      6. If unsuccessful, a rumenotomy may be performed
      7. Because dairy cattle are most often affected, most cases can be prevented by the administration of a bar magnet to all heifers at 6 months of age and careful adherence to debris-free forage
   C. *Actinobacillosis* of the rumen also can cause vagal indigestion in cattle
   D. In sheep the cause may be peritonitis due to *Sarcosporidia*

V. Rumenal tympany (bloat)
   A. Bloat is an acute overdistention of the rumen in the form of free gas or froth mixed with ingesta
      1. Frothy bloat occurs in cattle on legume pasture and on high-level grain diets
         a. The froth produced prevents the escape of normal gases during eructation
      2. Gas bloat is caused by a physical obstruction of the gases and a failure of eructation
   B. If the bloat is not life threatening, the passage of a large bore tube into the rumen to allow the escape of gas may be sufficient
   C. If the bloat is severe, the distention causes compression of the diaphragm and the animal is unable to breathe
      1. An emergency rumenotomy may be necessary to save the animal
      2. The left paralumbar fossa can be incised using a sharp knife or a trocar and cannula
      3. Antifermentive and antifrothing agents are usually administered
   D. Frothy bloat can be controlled to some degree by careful pasture and feed management

VI. Rumen acidosis (grain overload)
   A. Grain overload is an accumulation of excessive quantities of highly fermentive carbohydrates that produce lactic acid in the rumen
      1. As lactic acid increases, rumen pH may drop below 5.0 and metabolic acidosis occurs
      2. Cattle and sheep are affected
      3. Usually occurs due to accidental access to large quantities of grain
   B. Clinical signs include severe toxemia, weakness, dehydration, fluid-filled static rumen, incoordination, and recumbency, leading to death
   C. Principles of treatment include decreasing fermentation and acid production in the rumen using antimicrobials, neutralizing metabolic acidosis, and rehydrating the animal using intravenous fluids with sodium bicarbonate

VII. Neonatal diarrhea
   A. An important disease of farm animals with multiple infectious and noninfectious causes
      1. Stresses such as cold weather, changes in diet or housing, weaning, and failure

of passive transfer of gamma globulins from colostrum predispose the neonate to infection

   2. Absorption of IgG occurs optimally in calves within the first 6 to 8 hours of life but may occur up to 24 hours; in goats up to 4 days; in lambs, maximally to 15 hours but up to 24 to 48 hours; in piglets up to 12 to 24 hours

   3. Dietary diarrhea also can be due to ingestion of increased quantities of milk or inferior milk replacers

   B. Neonatal diarrhea is characterized by profuse, watery, yellow diarrhea, dehydration, metabolic acidosis, shock, and death

   C. Successful treatment of diarrhea depends on cause and duration

   1. Replacing fluid and electrolytes lost and correcting metabolic acidosis should be the main objectives

   D. Infectious causes of neonatal diarrhea can be controlled with a vaccination regime and provision of good quality colostrum (see Preventable Diseases)

VIII. Mastitis

   A. An inflammation of the mammary gland that can occur in all species, although it assumes economic importance only in species used for milk

   B. A large proportion of cases are subclinical and can be detected only by screening tests based on the leucocyte count

   C. Clinical mastitis is characterized by heat, pain, and swelling of the gland and marked changes in the milk such as discolorization and clots

   D. A few of the major bacteria involved are: *Staphylococcus aureus, Streptococcus agalactiae,* and some of the coliform bacteria

   E. Treatment must include removal of infection from the quarter and returning the milk to its normal composition

   F. Several treatments are available and depend on the severity of infection; they include frequent milking out of the infected quarter (stripping), udder infusions, systemic antibiotics, and perhaps drying off of the infected quarter (i.e., not milking it)

   G. Prevention of mastitis through a prophylactic routine of regular screening, proper milking technique, maintenance of milking equipment, and early recognition and treatment of subclinical cases is the best course

IX. Porcine reproductive and respiratory syndrome (PRRS or mystery swine disease)

   A. A new disease in North America, making its appearance in the 1980s

   B. Characterized by reproductive failure and increased mortality in farrowing and nursery room pigs

   1. Reproductive problems include return to estrus, abortion, and delivery of mummified, stillborn or poorly viable piglets

   2. Increased mortality in piglets is associated with a "thumping" respiration with severe interstitial pneumonia and several secondary infectious diseases such as diarrhea and septicemia

   C. PRRS appears to be spread by movement of pigs between farms and by airborne dispersion over distances of less than 3 kilometers

   D. Recent development of a vaccine has proved encouraging

Preventable Diseases

A comprehensive herd health program should encompass a vaccination regime suited to the particulars of the geographic area and specific herd requirements. The following is a list of diseases that may be controlled through vaccination.

I. Bovine

   A. Bovine Respiratory Disease Complex, including:

   1. Infectious Bovine Rinotracheitis (IBR) (viral)

   2. Bovine Viral Diarrhea (BVD)

   3. Parainfluenza III (PI3) (viral)

   4. Bovine Respiratory Syncytial Virus (BSRV)

   5. *Haemophilus somnus* and *Pasteurella haemolytica*

   B. Clostridial diseases

   1. Blackleg—*Clostridium chauvoei*

   2. Malignant edema—*Clostridium septicum* and *Clostridium sordellii*

   3. Infectious necrotic hepatitis—*Clostridium novyi* Type B

   4. Bacillary hemoglobinuria—*Clostridium haemolyticum*

   5. Pulpy kidney—*Clostridium perfringens* Type D

   6. Hemmorhagic enterotoxemia—*Clostridium perfringens*

   7. Tetanus—*Clostridium tetani*

C. Others
  1. Vibriosis—*Campylobacter fetus*
  2. Brucellosis—*Brucella abortus*
  3. Leptospirosis—*Leptospira pomona*
  4. Anthrax—*Bacillus anthracis*
  5. Anaplasmosis—*Anaplasma marginale*
  6. Listeriosis—*Listeria monocytogenes*
  7. *Escherichia coli* diarrhea in calves
  8. White muscle disease
    a. To prevent, give injection of vitamin E and selenium

II. Sheep and goats
  A. Clostridial diseases: See Bovine
  B. Brucellosis—*Brucella ovis*
  C. Vibriosis—*Vibrio fetus*
  D. Listeriosis—*Listeria monocytogenes*
  E. Foot Rot—*Bacteroides nodosus*
  F. Others
    1. Contagious ecthyma (soremouth, orf) (viral)
    2. Bluetongue (viral)
    3. Enzootic Abortion in Ewes (EAE)—*Chlamydia psittaci*
    4. White muscle disease—injection of vitamin E and selenium

III. Swine
  A. Leptospirosis—*Leptospira pomona*
  B. Neonatal porcine colibacillosis—*Escherichia coli*
  C. Atrophic rhinitis—*Bordetella bronchiseptica, Pasteurella multocida, Haemophilus pleuropneumoniae*
  D. Erysipilas—*Erysipelothrix rhusiopathiae*
  E. Meningitis—*Streptococcus suis*
  F. Porcine parvovirus
  G. Transmissible Gastroenteritis (TGE)—porcine rotavirus
  H. Porcine Reproductive and Respiratory Syndrome (PRRS)—(viral)
  I. Enteric disease in piglets—*Clostridium perfringens* Type C
  J. Swine dysentery—*Treponema hyodysenteriae*
  K. Pseudorabies—(viral)

RUMINANT AND SWINE SURGERY
Laparotomy (Bovine)

I. A laparotomy for diagnostic purposes or for surgical intervention of a condition such as LDA or RDA or for Caesarean section or rumenotomy is routinely performed with the animal standing in a chute or stocks using local anesthetic (information is found in the next section)

II. The incision is made in the paralumbar fossa and the area to be prepped includes a wide margin surrounding the incision site

III. The hair is clipped, any gross debris is removed, and a surgical prep is performed over the entire area

IV. The tail should be tied to the animal's hindleg or attached by rope to her halter, on the same side as the incision. Never tie a cow's tail to a post or rail because she can easily amputate her tail

V. Sutures should be removed 2 to 3 weeks post-op

VI. On occasion the surgeon may elect to perform a paramedian or ventral midline celiotomy for an RDA or caesarean. In this instance the cow is cast with ropes and placed in dorsal recumbency

Digit Amputation (Bovine)

I. The cow is placed in lateral recumbency with the affected claw up

II. The claw and interdigital space are thoroughly cleaned of manure and debris

III. The area is clipped from mid-metacarpus to the hoof and prepped in a routine manner

IV. Anesthesia is achieved with a ring block or intravenous local using rubber tubing as a tourniquet distal to the carpus or hock

V. Obstetrical or gigli wire is used to amputate the claw

VI. After surgery, the foot is bandaged for 2 to 3 weeks (unless complicated by infection) and may need to be changed frequently

Teat Laceration Repair (Bovine and Caprine)

I. This surgery may be performed with the cow standing or in dorsal recumbency

II. A ring block is used on the affected teat and a complete surgical prep performed
  A. Rubber tubing used as a tourniquet will control bleeding and milk leakage
  B. A teat prosthesis may be inserted at the time of repair

III. Postoperatively, the insert will allow the affected teat to drain while the other quarters are being milked

IV. Hand milking should not be done because it may interfere with the suture line

V. Sutures are removed in about 2 weeks

VI. Similar surgical technique is used on the doe

Eye Enucleation (Bovine)

I. The cow will have to be restrained in a chute while a halter secures its head to one side

II. Regional anesthesia is done with a Peterson Eye Block or a four-point retrobulbar block

III. Usually the eyelids are sewn together, then the area is clipped and surgically prepped

IV. Typically, the prep is complicated by necrotic and contaminated tissue

V. Post-op care will include antibiotics and perhaps a wound spray on the surgical site

Castration

I. Bovine

    A. Calves are usually castrated at from 1 to 4 weeks of age

    B. No anesthesia or surgical prep is generally used, for financial reasons

    C. For "open" castration, an incision is made in the scrotum and an emasculator is used to sever and crush the spermatic cord

    D. Calves should be vaccinated for clostridial infections before or at the time of castration

    E. An emasculatome is used for "closed" castration

        1. This device crushes and severs the spermatic cord without having to incise the skin of the scrotum

    F. Calves are sometimes castrated using an elastrator, or elastic band, around the testicles

        1. This procedure is best done within 2 to 3 days of age

II. Small ruminants

    A. Lambs (if used for wool) are castrated within the first 1 to 2 weeks of life using an elastrator and are tail-docked at the same time, also using an elastic or rubber band

    B. Sometimes an "open" or closed method of castration is used, as described for calves above

    C. Lambs destined for meat are usually only tail docked and are often not castrated because they reach market weight before sexual maturity

    D. Kids are castrated within the first 1 to 3 weeks of life using methods as described above

    E. Other procedures performed at this time include vaccination against clostridial infection and injection of vitamin E and selenium

III. Swine

    A. Pigs are usually castrated at 1 to 2 weeks of age using an open technique

    B. Other procedures performed before or at this time are iron dextran injection to prevent anemia, tail docking to prevent cannibalism in confined housing, and clipping of milk or needle teeth (canines and third incissors) to prevent injury to the sow

    C. Frequently, inguinal hernias are discovered in the piglet at the time of castration

        1. The skin of the inguinal area should be prepped with an antiseptic solution before repair

        2. Piglets should be placed in a clean, warm pen until recovered

Dehorning

I. Calves: dehorning in cattle is done to prevent injury from fighting

    A. It is preferable to disbud calves at 1 to 2 weeks of age using an electric dehorner

        1. Caustic pastes should be avoided

    B. If the horn buds are 1 to 2 (0.5 to 1 inch) cm in length, a gouge-type dehorner (Barnes) can be used

    C. Mature horns can be removed with a Keystone dehorner, a hardback saw, or a wire saw

    D. Local analgesia for dehorning can be achieved with a cornual nerve block or ring block

    E. Considerations are control of pain and hemorrhage and protection against fly strike in the dehorn wound

II. Goats

    A. Goats should be dehorned using an electric dehorner as soon as the horn buds are palpable

    B. Goats are very susceptible to pain and can die of shock and fright so analgesia is often administered

    C. Brain tissue is superficial in young goats and may be damaged if the iron is left on too long

RUMINANT AND SWINE ANESTHESIA ▬▬▬

Local and Regional Anesthesia (Analgesia)

Local and regional anesthetics are commonly used in large animal practice because they are often safer and more convenient than general anesthetics. Local anesthesia is the desensitization of the tissues of the surgical site by infiltration of an anesthetic agent. Regional anesthesia is desensitization of the surgical site by blocking the nerves to the region.

    I. Cattle

    Regional anesthesia in cattle is commonly done for standing laparotomy. The following techniques (or a variation) are frequently used. In every case, the animal is adequately restrained, the area is clipped and prepped, and attention is paid to aseptic technique.

A. Inverted L block
1. Nerves supplying the paralumbar fossa travel in a ventral-caudal direction from the spine
2. Local anesthetic is infiltrated in a horizontal line just ventral to the transverse processes of the lumbar vertebrae and a vertical line just caudal to the last rib
   a. In this way the nerves supplying the incision site are blocked
3. A variation of this technique is used for regional analgesia for a ventral midline approach

B. Paralumbar block (Cornell block)
1. Local anesthetic is injected below the lateral edges of the transverse processes of the first four lumbar vertebrae
   a. The needle is placed horizontally below each process directed toward the midline
   b. Twenty to twenty-five mL of local anesthetic is injected at each site, using an 18 g × 1.5 inch needle
2. In this way the branches of T13, L1, L2 (and L3), which supply the surgical site, are blocked

C. Paravertebral block
1. The nerves are blocked as they come off the spinal column (T13, L1, L2, and L3)
   a. At a position about 4 cm (1.5 inch) off the midline, using a long (4-6 inch) needle, local anesthetic is injected at the caudal edges of L1, L2, and L3
2. Heat and muscle relaxation and desensitization of the skin and deeper tissues will result if the block is successful

D. Epidural block
1. Indications for use:
   a. To stop straining for obstetrical manipulations
   b. To facilitate the reduction of rectal and vaginal prolapses
   c. Perineal surgery, udder surgery
   d. To stop straining during laparotomies and caesareans
   e. Urethrostomies
2. It is achieved by injecting a small quantity of anesthetic agent in the epidural space between the first and second coccygeal vertebrae (cranial epidural) or the sacrococcygeal junction (caudal epidural). The area blocked includes the anus, vulva, perineum, and caudal aspects of the thighs
3. If a larger quantity of local is used (high epidural) it may provide 2 to 4 hours of analgesia for laparotomy, limb surgery, teat surgery, etc.
4. The animal will not remain standing in the latter case

E. Cornual nerve block: used to provide anesthesia for dehorning
1. The cornual nerve runs along the frontal crest from the lateral canthus of the eye to the horn
2. The head must be firmly secured and the area clipped and prepped
3. Five to ten mL of local is injected about halfway along the nerve at the lateral border of the frontal crest

F. Peterson eye block: employs a specialized, curved needle
1. First a skin bleb is made at the point where the supraorbital process meets the zygomatic arch
   a. The needle is inserted through the bleb and 15 to 20 mL of local are deposited in the area of the optic nerve
2. Second, local is injected subcutaneously lateral to the zygomatic arch
   a. This technique will desensitize the globe and surrounding tissues of the eye for enucleation

G. Retrobulbar (four point) block: local anesthetic is injected into the dorsal and ventral eyelids and at the medial and lateral canthi
1. Then approximately 30 to 40 mL of local anesthetic is directed to the nerves at the apex of the orbit with a curved needle
2. Both block techniques can be used for enucleation or extirpation of the eye

H. Ring block
1. Local anesthetic agent is deposited subcutaneously and deep into the tissues completely around the surgical site, as in teat surgery, dehorning, claw amputation, etc.

II. Sheep and goats
A. Regional anesthesia such as paravertebrals and epidurals can be used in sheep and goats

B. Goats have a low pain threshold and require sedation

C. A technique similar to the above described cornual nerve block can be used to dehorn mature goats

D. Some texts recommend using dilute solutions of lidocaine in sheep and goats because of an apparent toxicity potential

III. Swine

A. A line block, inverted L block, or an epidural can be used for ceasarean section in the sow (high epidural)

1. The injection site for epidural in the sow is the lumbosacral space

General Anesthesia

I. Cattle

A. Bloat and regurgitation of rumen contents are problems associated with general anesthesia in cattle

1. Feed should be withheld from bovine patients before general anesthesia, if possible

2. Withhold roughage for 48 hours, grain and concentrates for 24 hours, and water for 12 hours

B. Tranquilizers are not usually administered as a preanesthetic because they do not work well to calm fractious cattle and violent recoveries are not a problem in bovine

C. Anesthesia can be induced with a number of drugs, including, but not limited to, the following:

1. Chloral hydrate given slowly as a 7% solution to effect

2. Thiamylal sodium

3. Thiopental sodium

a. Induction is not as prolonged as with thiamylal sodium and may cause transient apnea

4. Guaifenesin with 2 g of a thiobarbiturate

5. Ketamine and xylazine intramuscularly

6. A mixture of 5% guaifenesin containing 1 mg/mL ketamine and 0.1 mg/mL of xylazine

D. In a recumbent cow, bloat and aspiration of regurgitated rumen contents are a concern

1. If possible, position so that the animal is in right lateral recumbency, which keeps the rumen up

a. Elevate the neck so head is downward

b. Position so upper front and hindlimbs are parallel to the table surface

2. Position in sternal recumbency as soon as possible

3. It is suggested to extubate with the cuff inflated

E. An endotracheal tube with inflated cuff should be placed even if inhalants are not used. Also use a stomach tube for the escape of rumen gases

1. On induction, a mouth speculum is inserted to aid in the introduction of the endotracheal tube

F. The surgical table should be covered with protective padding to prevent postanesthetic complications due to nerve paralysis

G. Halothane is usually employed when inhalation anesthesia is chosen. At surgical plane, the bovine will have slow, regular breathing, a slight palpebral reflex, and anal reflex. The pupil is centered between the upper and lower lids

1. If light or deep, the eye is rotated ventrally and the pupil is rotated medially below the lower lid

2. Oxygen should be continued 5 to 10 minutes postanesthetic delivery

H. The technician should monitor heart rate, pulse strength, muscle relaxation, respiratory rate, mucous membranes, CRT, and blood pressure

II. Sheep and goats

A. Injectable anesthesia regimes and the use of halothane for general anesthesia are similar to that outlined for bovine

B. Withhold feed for 24 hours and water for 12 hours

C. Small ruminants should be intubated to prevent aspiration from regurgitation

D. Eye position as a measurement of anesthetic depth is not as accurate in small ruminants as in cattle

III. Swine

A. Some concerns when anesthetizing swine

1. A higher incidence of malignant hyperthermia

2. Fewer accessible superficial veins and arteries

3. Tracheal intubation is difficult in adult pigs because the larynx is long and mobile

a. Laryngeal spasm is common

B. Induction can be achieved using:

1. Thiamylal or thiopental sodium

a. These can be used alone for short procedures

2. Ketamine can be used with thiobarbiturates or halothane
3. A mixture of guaifensen (5% solution), ketamine (1 mg/mL) and xylazine (1 mg/mL) can be used in adult pigs
4. Halothane by face mask
5. Droperidol and fentanyl (Innovar-Vet) intramuscularly
6. Stresnil (azaparone)

C. Eye reflexes and position are unreliable for monitoring pigs
D. Heart rate, respiratory rate, muscle relaxation, and pulse strength (if possible) should be monitored
E. As with ruminants, continue oxygen 5 to 10 minutes postinhalation and position the animal in sternal recumbency as soon as possible
F. Unless there is evidence of regurgitation, extubate with the cuff deflated

Glossary

abomasopexy The abomasum is fixed to the abdominal wall using a permanent suture. The technique is used to correct a displacement of the abomasum

enucleation Surgical removal of the globe of the eye

extirpation Surgical removal of everything within the orbit of the eye, including globe, muscles, adipose tissue, and lacrimal gland

omentopexy The omentum is anchored to the abdominal wall similarly to abomasopexy. It is usually used in the case of right torsed abomasum

paralumbar fossa Area in the flank bordered dorsally by the spinous processes of the lumbar vertebrae, cranially by the last rib, and caudally by the tuber coxae. It provides a flank approach to the abdomen for laparotomy

rumenotomy A surgical procedure for the evacuation of the rumen. A left flank approach is used. A rumenotomy is indicated in the following conditions: removal of metallic foreign bodies (traumatic reticuloperitonitis), rumen overload, obstructing foreign bodies, and rumen impaction

semimembranosus, semitendinosus Hamstring muscles of the hindlimb

tetany A condition in which localized spasmodic contraction of the muscle takes place. It results from a decreased level of blood calcium

transfaunation Reconstitution of the rumen flora through the use of cud transfer

Review Questions

1 The most dangerous defence strategy of cattle is:
   a. Herding
   b. Charging
   c. Biting
   d. Kicking
2 Which is *not* a common site for IM injection in cattle?
   a. Gluteals
   b. Semimembranosus
   c. Brachiocephalicus
   d. Pectorals
3 To auscult the rumen place the stethoscope over the:
   a. Right paralumbar fossa
   b. Left paralumbar fossa
   c. Animal's left side just below the point of the elbow
   d. Animal's right side just below the point of the elbow
4 Screening for subclinical mastitis can be done by:
   a. Monitoring milk output
   b. CMT
   c. Observation
   d. Palpating the udder for heat and pain
5 Parturient paresis is commonly known as:
   a. Milk fever
   b. Hardware disease
   c. Pizzle rot
   d. Mastitis
6 A common clinical sign in LDA is:
   a. Toxemia
   b. Auscultable ping
   c. Hunching
   d. Head pressing
7 Gas bloat is caused by:
   a. Increased amounts of lactic acid in the rumen
   b. Ingestion of too much grain
   c. A physical obstruction to eructation
   d. A negative energy balance
8 Blackleg is a disease of ruminants caused by:
   a. *Pasteurella haemolytica*
   b. *E. coli*
   c. Anthrax
   d. *Clostridium chauvoei*
9 Which of the following veins should be used with caution when taking a blood sample from a cow?
   a. Jugular vein
   b. Lateral thoracic vein
   c. Milk vein
   d. Coccygeal vein
10 Which of the following is *not* a part of Bovine Respiratory Disease Complex?
   a. Leptospirosis
   b. *Haemophilus somnus*
   c. Bovine viral diarrhea
   d. IBR

11 A "closed castration":
a. Uses an emasculator
b. Eliminates the possibility of fly strike
c. Is performed on pigs at 1 to 2 weeks of age
d. Employs a local nerve block

12 Disbudding in kid goats generally employs:
a. Keystone dehorners
b. Barnes dehorner
c. Hot iron
d. Gigli wire saw

13 Which of the following is not an indication for laparotomy in ruminants?
a. RDA
b. Uterine prolapse
c. Rumenotomy
d. Exploratory

14 Claw amputation in the cow is accomplished:
a. With the cow in lateral recumbency
b. Using a low epidural block
c. With the cow in a standing stock and the head well restrained
d. With the cow in dorsal recumbency

15 Which of the following is *not* a feature of swine anesthesia?
a. Laryngospasm
b. High incidence of malignant hyperthermia
c. High incidence of toxicity from local anesthetics
d. Difficulty in monitoring pulse strength

16 Which of the following is *not* used for a standing laparotomy in the bovine?
a. Peterson block
b. Paralumbar block
c. Inverted L block
d. Paravertebral block

17 Goats require sedation in addition to local anesthetic for most procedures because:
a. They have a low pain threshold
b. They have a high pain threshold
c. Most goat farms do not have proper chutes
d. They are difficult to restrain

18 Which of the following statements is true?
a. Aseptic technique is unnecessary in food animals
b. Cows have tough hide and therefore do not require analgesics
c. Due to the disposition of cattle, most surgical procedures can be done with local anesthetic and restraint
d. Cattle often experience violent recoveries from general anesthesia

19 The paralumbar block is also known as:
a. Cornell
b. Peterson
c. Tufts
d. Cornual

20 The paravertebral block inhibits the following nerves:
a. L1, L2, and L3
b. Orbital apex
c. L7, S1, and S2
d. T13, L1, L2, and L3

BIBLIOGRAPHY

Blood DC, Henderson JA, Radostits OM: *Veterinary medicine: a textbook of the diseases of cattle, sheep, pigs and horses,* ed 5, London, 1979, Bailliere Tindall.

McCurnin DM: *Clinical textbook for veterinary technicians,* ed 3, Philadelphia, 1994, W.B. Saunders.

Pratt P: *Medical, surgical and anesthetic nursing for veterinary technicians,* ed 2, Goleta, 1994, American Veterinary Publications, Inc.

Reibold TW, Goble DO, Geiser DR: *Large animal anaesthesia: principles and techniques,* Ames, 1982, Iowa State University Press.

The Merck veterinary manual, ed 6, New Jersey, 1986, Merck and Co. Inc.

Turner AS, McIllwraith CW: *Techniques in large animal surgery,* ed 2, Philadelphia, 1989, London, Lea & Febiger.

CHAPTER 11

Veterinary Dentistry

Barbara Donaldson

OUTLINE

Occlusion

Oral Lesions

Dental Problems

Anatomy of the Tooth

Dentition

Tooth Surfaces

Tooth Roots

Tooth Function

Numbering Teeth

Dental Instruments

Dental Prophy

Safety

Gum Disease

Dental Radiography

Home Care

LEARNING OUTCOMES

After reading this chapter you should be able to:

1. Recognize normal and abnormal dental structures, conditions, and lesions.
2. Identify teeth by means of the Anatomical and Triadan Numbering Systems.
3. Use dental terminology to chart dental morphology accurately.
4. Recognize and correctly use, care for, and sharpen dental hand instruments.
5. List the steps to perform a complete dental prophylaxis.
6. Describe the causes and stages of gingivitis and periodontitis.
7. Perform dental radiography.
8. Recommend a dental home care program.

I t is estimated that 85% of all dogs and cats over the age of 2 years have periodontal disease. Periodontal disease is a progressive condition that affects the supporting tissues of the teeth. Bacterial plaque is the initial cause of periodontitis. It can lead to tooth loss and infections of the heart, liver, and kidney. Proper dental consideration is a vital part of the veterinary care necessary to ensure a healthy and happy pet.

OCCLUSION

   I. Normal bite
     A. Scissor bite
     B. The upper incisors close just in front of the lower incisors
     C. The lower canines lie between the upper incisors and canines without touching either
     D. The lower first premolars are the most rostral with the upper arcade fitting into the spaces between the lower premolars forming a zigzag pattern
     E. The upper fourth premolars overlap the lower first molars, forming the carnassial teeth in dogs
     F. In cats the upper third and fourth premolars tightly overlap the lower fourth premolars, as well as the first molars. The upper fourth premolars and lower molars are the feline carnassial teeth
  II. Malocclusions
     A. Prognathism
       1. Undershot jaw
       2. Mandible longer than maxilla
       3. Normal for brachycephalic breeds
       4. Often associated with anterior crossbite

B. Brachygnathism
  1. Overshot jaw or parrot mouth
  2. Maxilla longer than mandible
C. Level bite
  1. End to end bite of the incisors
  2. Genetically a degree of prognathism
D. Wry mouth
  1. One half of the head is longer than the other half
  2. Genetically only affects one side of the head
E. Posterior crossbite
  1. Mandible is wider than the maxilla in the area of the premolars
  2. Occurs occasionally in boxers and long nosed breeds
F. Oligodontia
  1. Fewer teeth than normal
G. Anodontia
  1. Missing teeth
H. Polydontia
  1. More teeth than normal
I. Dental interlock
  1. Deciduous teeth that erupt in an abnormal pattern
  2. The upper deciduous canine teeth are pushed rostral to the lower canine teeth, which prevents the forward growth of the mandible
J. Retained deciduous teeth
  1. Permanent teeth erupt lingually to the deciduous teeth (except the upper canine teeth)
  2. Common in toy breed dogs

ORAL LESIONS

I. Malignant tumors
A. Melanoma
  1. Most common in dogs; rare in cats
  2. Spreads slowly, invades bone
B. Squamous cell carcinoma
  1. Second most common tumor in dogs; most common in cats
  2. Spreads slowly, invades bone
C. Fibrosarcoma
  1. Third most common tumor in dogs
  2. Guarded prognosis
II. Nonmalignant tumors
A. Epulis (an oral mass—osseous or fibromatous lesion)
  1. Requires biopsy to differentiate
  2. Three classifications: fibromatous, ossifying, acanthomatous

  3. Involves the periodontal ligament
  4. Can be locally invasive to bone
III. Gingival hyperplasia
A. Thickening of gingiva as a result of chronic inflammation
IV. Stomatitis
A. Inflammation of soft tissue of the oral cavity
B. Can be caused by foreign bodies, chemical or electrical burns, or can be immune related
V. Contact ulcers
A. Lesions caused when a tooth contacts the mucosa
VI. Eosinophilic ulcers
A. Rodent ulcers that occur on the lip of cats, benign
VII. Cervical line lesions
A. External Odontoclastic Resorptions: EORs
B. Occur at the neck of the tooth in cats
C. Unknown cause
D. Odontoclasts actively resorb the dentin and enamel
E. Graded from Class I to Class V (the most advanced)

DENTAL PROBLEMS

I. Gemini
A. One root with two crowns
II. Fusion
A. Two tooth buds grow together to form one larger tooth
III. Enamel hypoplasia
A. Known as "distemper teeth" where sections of enamel are reduced or missing
IV. Misdirected teeth
A. Teeth that erupt in an abnormal direction
V. Retained deciduous
A. Retained primary teeth
VI. Tetracycline staining
A. Yellow stain due to the administration of tetracycline to a pregnant dog or to young pups
VII. Impaction
A. The inability of the tooth to erupt through the gum
VIII. Abscessed teeth
A. Advanced periodontal disease may result in root abscesses
B. Most commonly seen abscessed tooth in dogs is the upper fourth premolar
IX. Oronasal fistula
A. Caused by an abscess of the maxillary canine and can show clinical signs of nasal discharge and/or swelling over the root

X. Caries
   A. True coronal caries not a common problem in carnivores as compared with humans
   B. If present are often multiple advanced lesions affecting several teeth
   C. Upper first and second molars and lower first molar are most commonly affected
XI. Worn teeth
   A. Exhibit a brown center but do not allow access by an explorer
XII. Neck lesion
   A. Resorptive lesion that destroys the crown
XIII. Trauma
   A. Caused by chewing hard objects or by blows to the head

ANATOMY OF THE TOOTH

I. Tooth structure (see Figure 11-1)
   A. Enamel
      1. Outer covering of the crown composed of hydroxyapatite
      2. In hypsodont teeth (long crown) of herbivores such as horses, the enamel is also invaginated into longitudinal grooves and infundibula (cups) of the teeth
   B. Dentin
      1. Comprises the bulk of the tooth
      2. Formed by odontoblasts in a tubular fashion
      3. Capable of repair by producing secondary dentin
   C. Pulp
      1. Occupies the interior cavity
      2. In the root it is called the root canal
      3. Rich with blood vessels, nerves, and lymphatics
   D. Cementum
      1. A type of bone that covers the root of the tooth
      2. Attached by the periodontal ligament fibers
   E. Cementoenamel junction
      1. Junction between crown and root (CEJ)
II. Tooth supporting structure
   A. Periodontal ligament
      1. Holds the tooth in the alveolus (socket)
      2. Comprised of collagen and elastic fibers
   B. Alveolar bone
   C. Gingiva
      1. Soft tissue providing epithelial attachment

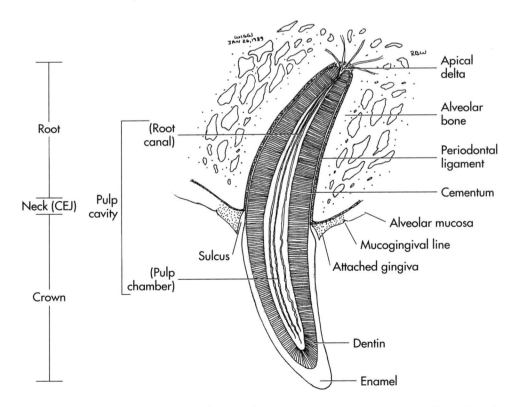

Figure 11-1 Anatomy of a tooth and supporting structures. (From Pratt PW: *Principles and Practice of Veterinary Technology,* St Louis, 1998, Mosby.)

D. Gingival sulcus
  1. Space between the gingiva and the tooth
  2. Normal depth in dogs is 1-3 mm; in cats, 0.5-1 mm
E. Crevicular fluid
  1. Secreted from the gingiva
  2. Flushes the sulcus
  3. Rich in immunoglobulins and other antimicrobial properties

DENTITION

I. Dogs
  A. Deciduous teeth: 28
  B. Permanent teeth: 42
    1. Formula $= 2\times \left(I\dfrac{3}{3}\ C\dfrac{1}{1}\ P\dfrac{4}{4}\ M\dfrac{2}{3} \right)$
II. Cats
  A. Deciduous teeth: 26
  B. Permanent teeth: 30
    1. Formula $= 2\times \left(I\dfrac{3}{3}\ C\dfrac{1}{1}\ P\dfrac{3}{2}\ M\dfrac{1}{1} \right)$
    2. The three upper premolars are numbered 2, 3, 4 and the lower premolars are numbered 3 and 4
      a. Anatomists conclude that the first upper premolar and the lower first and second premolars are missing
III. Horse
  A. Deciduous teeth: 24
  B. Permanent teeth: 40 to 42 (stallion); 30 to 36 (mare)
    1. Formula $= 2\times \left(I\dfrac{3}{3}\ C\dfrac{1}{1}\ P\dfrac{3-4}{3}\ M\dfrac{3}{3} \right)$
      a. Mares often do not have the canine teeth
IV. Swine
  A. Deciduous teeth: 32
  B. Permanent teeth: 44
    1. Formula $= 2\times \left(I\dfrac{3}{3}\ C\dfrac{1}{1}\ P\dfrac{4}{4}\ M\dfrac{3}{3} \right)$
V. Ruminants (e.g., sheep, cattle)
  A. Deciduous teeth: 20
  B. Permanent teeth: 32
    1. Formula $= 2\times \left(I\dfrac{0}{4}\ C\dfrac{0}{0}\ P\dfrac{3}{3}\ M\dfrac{3}{3} \right)$
VI. Hamsters, gerbils, mice, and rats
  A. Permanent teeth: 16
    1. Formula $= 2\times \left(I\dfrac{1}{1}\ C\dfrac{0}{0}\ P\dfrac{0}{0}\ M\dfrac{3}{3} \right)$
VII. Guinea pigs
  A. Permanent teeth: 20
    1. Formula $= 2\times \left(I\dfrac{1}{1}\ C\dfrac{0}{0}\ P\dfrac{1}{1}\ M\dfrac{3}{3} \right)$
VIII. Rabbits
  A. Permanent teeth: 28
    1. Formula $= 2\times \left(I\dfrac{2}{1}\ C\dfrac{0}{0}\ P\dfrac{3}{2}\ M\dfrac{3}{3} \right)$

TOOTH SURFACES

I. Crown
  A. Above the gum line
II. Root
  A. Below the gum line
III. Buccal
  A. Surface toward the cheek
IV. Lingual
  A. Surface toward the tongue
V. Labial
  A. Surface toward the lips
VI. Palatal
  A. Surface toward the soft palate
VII. Mesial
  A. Surface toward the rostral end, or front, of the mouth
  B. Incisor is the edge closest to the midline
VIII. Distal
  A. Surface toward the back of the tooth
IX. Occlusal
  A. Chewing surface
X. Furcation
  A. The space between two roots where they meet the crown

TOOTH ROOTS

I. Dogs
  A. One root: incisors, canines, first premolars, third molar of lower jaw
  B. Two roots: second and third premolars, fourth premolars of lower jaw, first and second molars of lower jaw, possibly third molars of lower jaw
  C. Three roots: fourth premolars of upper jaw, first and second molar of upper jaw
II. Cats
  A. One root: incisors, canines, first premolars of upper jaw, first molars of upper jaw
  B. Two roots: second premolars upper jaw, two premolars of lower jaw, and lower molars
  C. Three roots: third premolars upper jaw

TOOTH FUNCTION

I. Incisors
  A. Cutting, nibbling
II. Canines
  A. Holding, tearing

III. Premolars
    A. Cutting, shearing, holding
IV. Molars
    A. Grinding
V. Carnassial teeth
    A. Largest cutting teeth
    B. Dogs: upper fourth premolars and lower first molars
    C. Cats: upper fourth premolars and lower molars

NUMBERING TEETH

I. Anatomical system
    A. Upper case letters: permanent teeth
    B. Lower case letters: deciduous teeth (primary)
    C. Superscript right: upper right teeth
    D. Subscript right: lower right teeth
    E. Examples
        1. I_2: second permanent incisor, lower right
        2. ^1c: primary canine, upper left
        3. Sp^1: supernumerary first primary premolar, upper right
II. Triadan system
    A. Uses quadrants with three-digit numbers
    B. First number indicates the quadrant the tooth is found in and the type of tooth
    C. Permanent teeth begin with the numbers 1, 2, 3, 4
    D. Deciduous (primary) teeth begin with the numbers 5, 6, 7, 8

Upper right quadrant	Upper left quadrant
1 if permanent tooth	2 if permanent tooth
5 if deciduous tooth	6 if deciduous tooth
Lower right quadrant	**Lower left**
4 if permanent tooth	3 if permanent tooth
8 if deciduous tooth	7 if deciduous tooth

    E. The second and third numbers refer to the specific tooth in each quadrant, always beginning from the midline of the mouth
    F. EXAMPLES
        1. 103: upper right third permanent incisor
        2. 308: lower left last permanent premolar
    G. Cats are missing teeth 105, 205, 305, 306, 405, 406
    H. Cats

(101-103)	104	(106-108)	109	Upper right
I	C	P	M	
(401-403)	404	(407-408)	409	Lower right

I. Dogs

(101-103)	104	(105-108)	(109-110)	Upper right
I	C	P	M	
(401-403)	404	(405-408)	(409-411)	Lower right

DENTAL INSTRUMENTS

I. Hand instruments
    A. Three parts: handle, shank, and working end
    B. Instruments are held in a modified pen grasp
    C. Sickle scaler
        1. Has a sharp pointed tip with two sharp sides
        2. Used for supragingival calculus
    D. Curet scaler
        1. Has a U-shaped tip with one sharp side
        2. Used for subgingival calculus and root planing
    E. Periodontal probe
        1. Has no sharp sides
        2. Used to measure the depth of the gingival sulcus
        3. Measured in millimeters
    F. Shepherds hook or explorer
        1. Has a sharp tip only
        2. Used to detect subgingival calculus and tooth mobility
        3. Used to detect feline neck lesions (EORs)
        4. Used to detect cavities and broken teeth
II. Mechanical scalers
    A. Ultrasonic scaler
        1. Magnetostrictive: tip vibrates in an elliptical motion
        2. Piezoelectric: tip vibrates in a linear motion
        3. Sonic: tip vibrates in an elliptical motion
        4. Used for gross calculus above the gum line
        5. Used lightly on the teeth to avoid heat buildup and pitting of the enamel with possible pulpal damage
        6. Maximum of 20 seconds per tooth
    B. Roto-pro burs
        1. Spins at 300,000 to 400,000 rpm
        2. Used to remove tartar and calculus
        3. Can easily damage the enamel, dentin, and soft tissue
III. Sharpening hand instruments
    A. Sharpen after each use before sterilizing
    B. Use an acrylic stick to test for sharpness
    C. If light reflects from the cutting edge, the instrument is dull
    D. Sharpening stones vary from coarse to fine
        1. Ruby stone: coarse; water lubricant
        2. Arkansas stone: fine; oil lubricant

3. India stone: fine or medium; oil lubricant

4. Carborundum stone: coarse; water lubricant

5. Ceramic stone: fine or medium; water or dry lubricant

DENTAL PROPHY

I. Examine the patient, beginning with the history
   A. Look for symmetry of the head and face
   B. Look for nasal, ocular discharges, or swellings
   C. Examine lips, mouth, and tongue
   D. Examine teeth and gums
   E. Measure gingival sulcus
      1. May be measured after the prophy
   F. Scale the teeth above and below the gum line
      1. Use proper method and equipment as discussed previously
   G. Polish to remove microscopic grooves left by the scaling process and to remove plaque
      1. Keep prophy cup moving to avoid heating of the tooth
      2. Use plenty of paste
      3. Wet teeth with water to cool them
      4. Use a light touch but enough pressure to flare the cup
      5. Polish the enamel in the sulcus
      6. Use a medium or fine paste
      7. Set the polisher below 3000 rpm
   H. Flush the gingival sulcus with 0.12% chlorhexidine
   I. Wipe and air dry the teeth
   J. Can use a disclosing solution to reveal any remaining plaque (solution may stain hair or clothing)
   K. Apply fluoride and leave on 1 to 4 minutes
      1. Serves as an antibacterial agent
      2. Desensitizes the teeth
      3. Strengthens the enamel
      4. May not be necessary if fluoride is found in the prophy paste but many think the teeth must be dry for fluoride to be effective
   L. Wipe off the fluoride

SAFETY

I. Animal
   A. Use sterile and well-maintained instruments and equipment
   B. Use an appropriately sized mouth gag to avoid problems in the temporomandibular joints
   C. Use a cuffed endotracheal tube
   D. Place gauze sponges in the back of the throat as a protection against excessive water and debris
   E. Keep the patient's head downward
   F. Cover the patient's eyes
   G. Roll the patient with the sternum under, especially in large breed dogs

II. Human
   A. Wear a surgical mask, glasses, and gloves
   B. May help to spray the patient's mouth with 0.12% chlorhexidine to reduce the bacterial load
   C. Work comfortably seated on a stool at a proper height
   D. Support the working hand on a surface in the same quadrant you are working

GUM DISEASE

I. Gingivitis
   A. Inflammation of the gingiva
II. Periodontal disease
   A. Inflammation of the supporting structures of the teeth
III. Causes
   A. Lack of daily dental care
   B. Accumulation of plaque, which is composed of bacteria
   C. Formation of calculus, which is mineralized plaque
   D. Plaque can form within 6 hours
   E. Plaque can mineralize within 24 to 48 hours
IV. Classification of gum disease
   A. Healthy
      1. Sharp gingival margin
      2. Shrimp color
      3. No odor
   B. Grade I
      1. Marginal gingivitis
      2. Slight redness, not swollen, mild odor
      3. Gram-positive aerobic cocci and rods
   C. Grade II
      1. Moderate gingivitis
      2. Swelling begins, ruby red, plaque
      3. Bleeding on probing
   D. Grade III
      1. Severe gingivitis, early periodontitis
      2. Red and purple margins, beginning of pocket formation with swelling and bleeding on probing
      3. No tooth mobility
      To this point conditions are reversible

E. Grade IV
   1. Moderate periodontitis
   2. Severe inflammation and swelling with deep pockets
   3. Slight tooth mobility
F. Grade V
   1. Severe periodontitis
   2. Tooth mobility and loss
   3. Lots of pus, 50% bone loss
   4. Anaerobic gram-negative rods
V. Treatment
   A. Depends on disease classification and discretion of the veterinarian
      1. Complete prophy
      2. Root planing
      3. Antibiotics
      4. Possible gum surgery
      5. Possible tooth extraction
      6. Home care
      7. Dry food
      8. Chew toys

DENTAL RADIOGRAPHY

I. Purpose
   A. Ascertain condition of teeth and gingival sulcus
   B. Identify cavities and resorptive lesions
   C. Identify retained roots
   D. Identify bone and root system of the teeth
   E. Help evaluate intraoral neoplasia
   F. Identify number of teeth in the mouth
   G. Identify periapical abscesses
II. Recommendations
   A. Conduct routine dental x-rays in young animals to identify the permanent dentition
   B. In the treatment of periodontal disease, perform x-rays every 12 to 24 months

C. Use x-rays before extractions to determine condition of the roots and number of teeth and roots involved
D. X-ray during endodontic procedures to confirm the procedure
E. Perform x-rays as follow up to root canal procedure to check the file depth
III. Equipment
   A. Intraoral film for detail
   B. Chair side darkroom to free up the main dark room
   C. Rapid processing solutions
   D. Dental x-ray machine with a lead lined cone to achieve greater detail and versatility
   E. Protective shielding, film holding devices, finger-ring dosimeter badges
IV. Positioning
   A. Routine dental survey of 6 films

		Technique
Each mandible	2 films	parallel lateral oblique
Each maxilla	2 films	bisecting angle
Mandibular canines and incisors	1 film	bisecting angle
Maxillary canine and incisors	1 film	bisecting angle

V. Techniques
   A. Parallel (Figure 11-2)
      1. Place the dental film parallel to the end of the x-ray tube and the long axis of the tooth

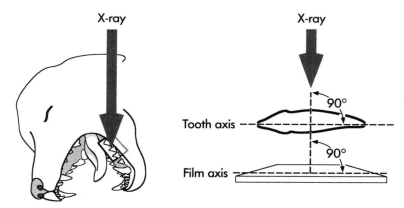

Figure 11-2 Parallel position technique for dental radiographs of the mandibular premolar teeth. (From Harvey CE, Emily PE: *Small Animal Dentistry,* St Louis, 1993, Mosby.)

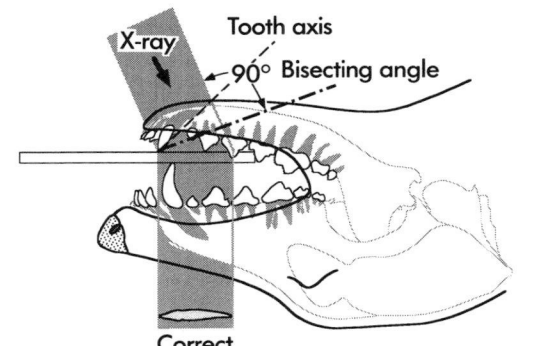

Figure 11-3 Bisecting angle technique for dental radiographs. **A,** Lower canine tooth. **B,** Carnassial tooth. (From Harvey CE, Emily PE: *Small Animal Dentistry,* St Louis, 1993, Mosby.)

2. The central ray will be perpendicular to the teeth and the film
3. Place folded gauze between the top edge of the film and the occlusal surfaces of the teeth to securely push the film down into the bottom of the mouth
   B. Bisecting angle (Figure 11-3)
1. Place the film inside the animal's mouth behind the affected tooth
2. Direct the central ray perpendicular to the line that bisects the angle formed by the film and the long axis of the tooth
3. This technique will reduce the artifact of foreshortening or elongation
4. Can be used for intraoral and extraoral films

HOME CARE

I. Goal: to control plaque and tartar buildup
II. Daily brushing with veterinary products
III. May involve use of antibacterial and fluoride products
IV. Feed hard food that does not stick to the teeth as well as other products
V. Use chew toys to provide an abrasive action, to strengthen the periodontal ligaments, and to increase crevicular flushing
VI. Do not feed dried hooves, which may cause slab fractures

Glossary

alveolar bone Cancellous bone adjacent to tooth roots
anodontia Absence of teeth
apex Bottom of the root
apical Toward the apex
attached gingiva Gingiva from the free gingival groove to the mucogingival line
brachygnathism Overshot jaw
buccal Tooth surface nearest the cheek
calculus Mineralized plaque
canine tooth Large single rooted tooth used to grasp and tear
caries Cavities
carnassial tooth Upper fourth premolar and lower first molar used to shear
cementoenamel junction Where the enamel meets the cementum
cementum Bony tissue covering the dentin of the root
coronal Toward the crown
crevicular fluid Secreted from the gingiva
crown Portion of the tooth covered by enamel
cusp Tip of the crown
deciduous teeth Baby or primary teeth
dental quadrant Half of an arch when divided by the midline
dentin Bulk of the tooth covered by cementum in the root and enamel in the crown
distal Away from the midline
enamel The hydroxyapatite covering of the crown
epulis Fibrous tumor of the gum
erosion Loss of tooth structure by chemical means not involving bacteria
free gingiva Portion of gingiva not attached to the tooth
free gingival margin Free edge of the gingiva on the tooth
furcation Space between two roots where they join the crown
gingiva Soft tissue surrounding the teeth
gingival hyperplasia An increase in the amount of gingival tissue
gingival sulcus Space between the free gingiva and the tooth
incisal Biting surface of the anterior teeth
interdental Area between the proximal surfaces of adjacent teeth in the same arch
labial Surface of the incisors nearest the lips
lingual Surface of the mandibular teeth nearest the tongue
malocclusion Deviation from the normal bite
mandible Bone of the lower jaw
maxilla Bone of the upper jaw
mesial Toward the midline of the dental arch; can also be the surface or edge of the tooth closest to the rostral end (front of the mouth)
molar Large multicusped tooth used for grinding

mucogingival Line where the gingiva meets the alveolar mucosa

neck Cementoenamel junction

occlusal Chewing surface of the posterior teeth

odontoblast Cell in the pulp that produces dentin

oligodontia Fewer teeth than normal

oronasal fistula Abnormal opening between the nasal and oral cavities

palatal Surface of the maxillary teeth nearest the palate

palate Structure separating the oral and nasal cavities

periapical abscess Abscess at the apex of the tooth

periodontal ligament Network of fibers connecting the tooth to the bone

periodontium Supporting structures of the teeth

plaque Thin film covering the teeth composed of bacteria, saliva, food, and epithelial cells

premolars Teeth between the canines and the molars used for shearing

primary teeth The first teeth to erupt

prognathism Undershot jaw

proximal Surface of the tooth adjacent to another tooth

pulp Soft tissue inside the tooth composed of blood vessels, nerves, lymphatics, and connective tissue

resorption Loss of substance by a physiological or pathological process

root Part of the tooth covered by cementum

root canal Part of the tooth containing the pulp

root planing Scaling of the tooth root

saliva Secretions from the salivary glands, containing enzymes

subgingival curettage Removal of plaque and calculus from the gingiva below the gum line

Review Questions

1 The percentage of dogs and cats over the age of 2 years with some form of periodontal disease has been estimated to be:
   a. 50
   b. 65
   c. 75
   d. 85

2 The normal bite of a dog is best described as:
   a. An anterior crossbite
   b. A scissor bite
   c. A level bite
   d. A posterior bite

3 Retained deciduous teeth:
   a. Present no problems for the pet
   b. Affect larger breeds more often
   c. Occur commonly in a Wry Bite
   d. Cause malocclusions and gingivitis

4 The most common oral tumor in dogs is a(an):
   a. Melanoma
   b. Squamous cell carcinoma
   c. Fibrosarcoma
   d. Eosinophilic ulcer

5 The lesion that occurs at the neck of the tooth in cats is called:
   a. An epulis lesion
   b. A crevicular lesion
   c. A root cavity
   d. An external odontoclastic resorption (EOR)

6 The bulk of the tooth is comprised of:
   a. Enamel
   b. Dentin
   c. Cementum
   d. Pulp

7 The lower left fourth premolar is tooth number:
   a. 108
   b. 208
   c. 308
   d. 408

8 The surface of the incisor tooth facing the roof of the mouth is:
   a. Lingual
   b. Buccal
   c. Palatal
   d. Labial

9 The number of permanent teeth in cats is:
   a. 26
   b. 30
   c. 35
   d. 42

10 The instrument used to scale the root of the tooth is a:
   a. Sickle
   b. Explorer
   c. Probe
   d. Curet

11 The normal depth of the gingival sulcus in a dog is:
   a. 0.5 to 1 mm
   b. 1 to 2 mm
   c. 1 to 3 mm
   d. 4 to 6 mm

12 Severe inflammation and swelling with deep gingival pockets and slight tooth mobility occur in periodontal disease at stage:
   a. II
   b. III
   c. IV
   d. V

BIBLIOGRAPHY

Antony J: Pacific dental services, lecture notes, Vancouver, British Columbia, November 1991.

Bellows J: *Home study course,* American Society of Veterinary Dental Technicians, 1995.

Eisner ER: Problems associated with veterinary dental radiography; *Prob Vet Med* 2(1):46-61, 1990.

Emily P, Penman S: *Handbook of small animal dentistry,* 1990, Pergamon Press, Canada Ltd.

Emily P: Intraoral radiography, *Veterinary clinics of North America, small animal practice* 16:801, 1986.

Frost P: *Canine dentistry,* ed 5, J.H. Day Communications Inc., 1995.

Hale F: Veterinary dental services, lecture notes, Fergus, Ontario, September 1994.

Harvey C: Periodontal disease in dogs and cats, *Veterinary Technician Magazine,* June 1991.

Harvey CE, Flax BM: Feline oral dental radiographic examination and interpretation, *Vet Clin North Am Small Anim Pract* 22:1279-1295, 1992.

Hawkins J: Applied dentistry for veterinary technicians: lesson one, *Veterinary Technician Magazine,* January/February 1991.

Hawkins J: Waltham applied dentistry for veterinary hospital staff, Veterinary Learning Systems Co., Inc., 1993.

Miller B, Harvey C: Sharpening of dental instruments, *Veterinary Technician Magazine,* January 1994.

Piasentin W: Techniques of veterinary dental radiography, *Veterinary Technician Magazine,* June 1996.

Radiography

Marg Brown

OUTLINE

X-ray Production
X-ray Tube
X-ray Machine
Image Receptors
Darkroom and Processing Tech-
  niques
  Darkroom Considerations
  Manual Film Processing Pointers
  Automatic Film Processing
Radiographic Quality
  Definition

Radiographic Density
Contrast
Radiographic Detail or Definition
Technical Errors and Artifacts
Developing a Technique Chart
Radiation Safety
  Responsibilities
  Hazards of Ionizing Radiation
  Radiation Measurement
  Maximum Permissible Dose
    (MPD)

Safety Practices
Positioning Techniques
  Basic Principles
  Basic Criteria and Principles of
    Positioning and Restraint
Contrast Radiography
  Basic Concepts
  Media
  Patient Preparation
  Specific Studies

LEARNING OUTCOMES

After reading this chapter you should be able to:

1. Understand some of the basic principles involved with x-rays and their production.
2. Describe the anatomy of the x-ray tube.
3. Briefly explain the components of the x-ray machine.
4. Understand the principles of accessory x-ray equipment and image receptors used in veterinary practice so that diagnostic radiographs are consistently produced.
5. Properly process radiographs based on your understanding of darkroom principles.
6. Explain what is meant by radiographic quality, including density, contrast, and detail and the factors influencing these.
7. Identify common technical errors and artifacts and know how to prevent or correct them.
8. Understand the concepts involved with setting up a technique chart.
9. Describe the effects that could occur if proper radiation safety is not practised.
10. State the units of radiation and the MPD allowed.
11. List practical methods that can be employed to reduce radiation exposure.
12. List and define proper directional terminology used in radiography.
13. List basic guidelines for veterinary radiographic positioning and restraint.
14. Explain what is meant by contrast media, giving examples.

Radiography is an important diagnostic tool available to veterinary practice. To arrive at a proper diagnosis, high quality images must be produced. This chapter discusses basic but essential information needed to produce diagnostic radiographs. Radiation physics, positioning and restraint, technique charts, and specialized procedures are discussed briefly and can be further investigated by consulting the excellent texts listed under Bibliography.

X-RAY PRODUCTION ▰▰▰▰▰▰

I. Definition of radiation: propagation of energy through space and matter
II. Three types of radiation
    A. Particulate radiation
        1. "Particles" of the atom
            a. EXAMPLES: neutrons, protons, electrons, alpha particles, beta particles
            b. Some particles may have a positive, a negative, or a neutral charge
        2. Cannot reach the speed of light
        3. Process that occurs in the x-ray machine is an example
    B. Electromagnetic radiation
        1. Definition: transport of energy through space without matter
        2. EXAMPLES: radiowaves, television waves, microwaves, x-rays, gamma rays
        3. Has wavelength: defined as the distance from one crest of a wave to the next
        4. Has frequency: the number of crests passing a particular point per unit of time. It is measured in hertz (Hz)
        5. Energy associated with electromagnetic radiation is the ability to do work and is measured in electron volts (eV)
        6. Electromagnetic radiation is measured in frequency, energy, and wavelength
            a. Wavelength and frequency are inversely related
                (1) The shorter the wavelength, the greater the energy
            b. The greater the energy, the greater the ability to penetrate
        7. When matter and electromagnetic radiation interact, wave and particle behavior can be described
        8. X-rays have similar physical properties as other forms of electromagnetic radiation
    C. Ionizing radiation
        1. Definition: particulate and electromagnetic radiation with sufficient energy to cause ionization
        2. Radiation must have greater energy than the electron binding energy
        3. Ionization causes damage to tissues
III. Definition of X-rays
    A. X-rays are a form of radiation that result when the energy of the electrons is converted to electromagnetic radiation
    B. X-ray beam is composed of bundles of energy or quanta referred to as photons that travel in a wave
    C. Photons have no mass or electrical charge
IV. Production of x-rays
    A. X-rays are produced when the fast moving electrons or particulate radiation collide with matter
    B. This is best achieved in an x-ray tube. The tube consists of a negative electrode known as the cathode and a positive anode
    C. A cloud of electrons (negative particulate radiation) forms at the cathode and accelerates across the tube where the electrons interact with the target material at the positive anode
    D. This interaction forces the high speed electrons to lose their energy, resulting in the production of 1% x-radiation and 99% heat
    E. The electrons that travel across the tube have different energies, measured in kilovoltage (kVp)
    F. A setting on the x-ray machine determines the kVp of the electrons and thus the x-ray penetrating power
    G. Thus to produce x-rays, one needs a source of electrons, a method of accelerating electrons, a directed path, a target, and an envelope to provide vacuum, all of which are provided in the x-ray tube
V. Discovery of x-rays
    A. Wilhelm Conrad Roentgen on November 8, 1895
    B. Used a cathode ray tube (Crookes), which was an evacuated glass tube with two electrodes through which an electrical current was passed
    C. X-rays were used almost immediately for medical and surgical diagnosis
    D. Changes in skin color, similar to sunburn, due to radiation exposure were reported as early as April 1896

X-RAY TUBE ▰▰▰▰▰▰▰▰▰▰

I. Cathode (electrically negative portion of the x-ray tube, Figure 12-1)
    A. Provides the source of electrons and a directed path
    B. The filament is a coiled wire that emits electrons when heated up
        1. When heated, electrons are held less tightly by the nucleus of the atom. After the binding energy of the electrons is exceeded, an electron cloud available for travel is formed

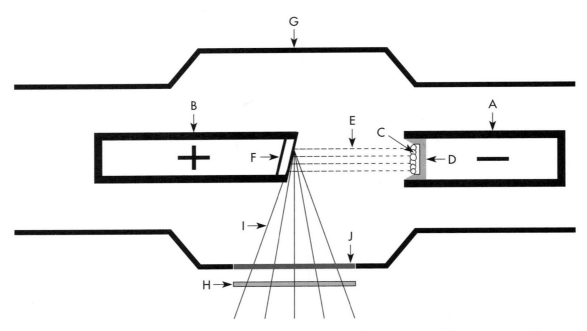

Figure 12-1 Anatomy of an x-ray tube. *A*, Cathode. *B*, Anode. *C*, Tungsten filament. *D*, Focusing cup. *E*, Accelerating electrons. *F*, Tungsten target. *G*, Glass envelope. *H*, Aluminum filter. *I*, Generated x-rays. *J*, Beryllium window. (From Pratt PW: *Principles and Practice of Veterinary Technology*, St Louis, 1998, Mosby.)

2. The flow of current to the filament is controlled by the step-down transformer, which is regulated by the milliamperage (mA) control
3. Filament is constructed of tungsten, which has a high melting point and atomic number
4. Most machines contain a small and a large filament

C. The focusing cup is a cavity in which the filaments sit
   1. It is maintained at the same negative potential as the heated filament
   2. Because like charges repel, the electron beam is directed to a small area on the anode

D. Acceleration of the electrons is controlled by the kVp

II. Anode (electrically positive portion of the x-ray tube)
   A. Provides the target for the interaction of the electrons
   B. Composed of the target and a copper stem
   C. Tungsten is used also for the target material to dissipate the high temperatures while the copper stem conducts the heat away from the target
   D. The actual area on the target that the electrons hit is the focal spot

1. Size of the spot affects the x-ray image
2. Size is determined by the filament size chosen
   a. The smaller the focal spot the sharper the image but there is less heat dissipation
3. Because of the target angle, more x-rays leave the cathode side of the x-ray tube than from the anode side, resulting in an uneven distribution of x-rays on the image (this is known as the heel effect)
   a. Most noticeable when using largest film size and low kVp techniques
   b. May be advantageous to place the thickest part of the animal toward the cathode side

E. Two types of anodes: stationary anode and rotating anode
   1. Stationary anodes are found in dental and small portable units used in large animals
      a. These units have a small capacity for x-ray production and are unable to withstand a lot of heat
      b. Consists of a beveled target angled toward the window embedded on a cylinder of copper

2. Rotating anode
   a. An approximate 3 inch disk shaped anode rotates on an axis through the center of the tube
   b. Filament from the cathode directs electron stream against the beveled edge of this tungsten disk mounted on a molybdenum spindle
   c. Position of the focal spot remains fixed while this circular ring rotates rapidly (3350 times per minute), using a larger target area for the electrons to dissipate their heat
   d. Can use higher tube currents, shorter exposure time, and smaller filament

III. Tube envelope
   A. Traditionally made of Pyrex glass that has been evacuated to form the vacuum necessary for x-ray production
   B. Window is the thin segment of the glass that allows maximum emission of x-rays and minimum absorption by the glass (also called aperture)

IV. Tube or machine housing
   A. Metallic structure that covers and protects the x-ray tube or in the case of portable units, the entire machine
   B. Lined internally with lead and contains insulating oil

V. Causes of x-ray tube failure
   A. More than 95% is due to operator error
   B. Most damage is related to heat accumulation in the tube, which may lead to filament evaporation, broken filaments, cracked anodes, anode melting or pitting, and burned out or frozen bearings

VI. Tube rating chart
   A. Provided by all manufacturers of x-ray tubes
   B. A composite graph that shows the maximum combination of kVp, mA, and exposure time that can be used safely in a single exposure to avoid injury to the x-ray tube from excessive heat production

X-RAY MACHINE

I. Electrical circuits for x-ray tube control
   A. High voltage circuit
      1. Purpose is to provide high electrical potential needed to accelerate the electrons from the cathode to the anode
      2. High potential (kVp peak or potential) generated by a step-up transformer
         a. Incoming wall voltage (110 or 220 V) must be changed to kilovolts (1000 × greater)
         b. Most machines have a range of 40 to 120 kVp
      3. kVp selection switch controlled by autotransformer
      4. Line voltage compensator also associated with circuit
   B. Low-voltage (filament) circuit
      1. Purpose is to provide electricity (amperage) needed to heat the filament
      2. Tungsten filament needs minimal energy so a step-down transformer needed to reduce incoming voltage
      3. Connected to the milliamperage (mA) control
   C. Timer switch
      1. Purpose is to control the length of exposure time during which high voltage is applied across the tube
      2. Best to have exposure times of less than one thirtieth of a second (0.03 second) to minimize potential of patient movement
   D. Rectification circuit
      1. Purpose is to change the alternating current coming into the tube into direct current to ensure that there are no negative deflections of the wave when no electrons are generated
      2. Various possibilities exist, depending on the type of x-ray machine

II. Technique selection or control panel
   A. Quality (energy, penetrating ability) of x-rays produced, controlled by kVp potential, while milliamperage (mA) and time (sec) control the quantity (intensity)
   B. Product of mA and time is milliampere seconds (mA × sec = mAs)
   C. Methods available for technique selection depends on machine
      1. Three factor: operator can control kVp, mA, and sec
      2. Two factor: kVp and product of mAs only
      3. One factor: kVp selection only

III. Tube stand
   A. Apparatus that supports x-ray tube

IV. Accessory x-ray equipment
   A. Filtration
      1. Total filtration is result of inherent (filtering by glass envelope) and added (aluminum disk placed over window) filtration

2. Purpose is to selectively remove less energetic, less penetrating (nondiagnostic) x-rays from primary beam
3. Filtered primary x-ray beam decreases the amount of undesirable patient exposure by increasing the mean beam energy but decreasing the overall beam intensity. This necessitates increasing the exposure time or mA

B. Collimation
   1. Beam restricting device that limits the primary beam
   2. Purpose is to prevent unnecessary patient exposure and to decrease production of scatter (secondary) radiation, thereby resulting in greater patient safety, increased operator safety, and an improved quality radiograph
   3. Beam restricting devices include lead aperture diaphragm, lead cone, lead cylinder, adjustable lead aperture shutter
   4. Most regulatory agencies require some evidence of collimation on the films

C. Grids (Figure 12-2)
   1. Series of thin linear strips of alternating radiodense (lead) and radiolucent (plastic or aluminum) materials encased in an aluminum protective cover
   2. Placed between patient and film
   3. Generally used when area radiographed is greater than 9, 10, or 11 cm, depending on the reference source. This author uses 10 cm
   4. Purpose is to prevent scatter radiation from reaching the film. This improves quality of the radiograph
   5. Part of the primary beam is also absorbed so exposure needs to be increased (usually mA or sec)
   6. Characteristics
      a. Grid ratio: relationship of the height of the lead strips to the distance between them (e.g., if the lead strips are eight times as high as the space between them, the ratio is 8:1)
         (1) The greater the ratio, the better the absorption of scatter radiation, but the disadvantages of a higher ratio are: greater exposure needed, more perfect centering required, narrower focusing range permitted
      b. Grid pattern: determined by orientation of lead strips

         (1) Linear grid: lead strips in one direction (most common)
         (2) Crossed grid (crosshatch): two linear grids sandwiched together so that the strips are at right angles to each other
      c. Types of grids
         (1) Parallel grid: strips perpendicular to face of grid and parallel to each other

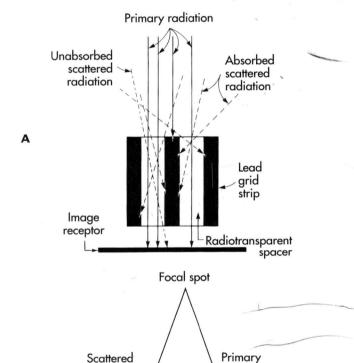

Figure 12-2 Cross-section of a grid. **A,** Diagram of a small section of a grid showing how a large proportion of the scattered radiation is absorbed and image-forming primary radiation passes through to the image detector. **B,** Diagram of focused Potter-Bucky diaphragm being moved toward the right. (From Eastman Kodak Co.: *The Fundamentals of Radiography,* ed 12, Rochester, NY, 1980, Eastman Kodak Co., Radiographic Markets Division.)

(2) Focused grid: strips placed parallel to the primary x-ray beam. Angle begins at 90° to the surface at the center of the grid and progresses to greater angles toward both edges of the film. Most common

 d. Lines per cm or inch (grid frequency)

  (1) As the number of lead strips per cm or inch increase, they become narrower, which means the lines will be less objectionable on the radiograph

  (2) The increased frequency also means less absorption of scatter, increased exposure factors, and increased cost

 e. Mode of movement

  (1) Stationary grid: the grid does not move, which means that the grid lines are identifiable on the radiograph

  (2) Moving grid (Potter-Bucky diaphragm): through a mechanical device the grid lines are blurred, resulting in a clearer radiograph

IMAGE RECEPTORS

 I. Definition

  A. Mechanisms involved with transferring the invisible ionizing radiation into a visible image

 II. Cassette

  A. Rigid film holder designed to keep the intensifying screen and the film in close contact

  B. The front, which is made of plastic, light metal, or carbon fiber, must face the x-ray tube

  C. The back is made of heavy steel to sustain the weight of the patient if necessary

  D. Do not drop the cassette, and keep it clean

 III. Intensifying screens

  A. Layers of tiny luminescent phosphor crystals bound together on a plastic base and covered with a protective coating

  B. X-ray film is sandwiched between the two intensifying screens that are positioned on the inner surfaces of the cassette

  C. When the phosphor crystals in the screen are struck by x-radiation, they fluoresce and emit light

   1. This visible light exposes the light sensitive emulsion of the x-ray film

   2. Over 95% of exposure to film is due to this light emitted from the intensifying screens (indirect imaging)

  D. The primary purpose is to reduce the amount of exposure required to produce a diagnostic image

  E. Screen construction

   1. Base material for support

   2. Reflective layer to redirect light toward the film to increase efficiency of film

   3. Phosphor layer composed of calcium tungstate or rare earth crystals to convert the energy of the remnant x-ray beam into visible light

    a. These phosphorescent crystals:

     (1) Have a high atomic number

     (2) Have a high level of x-ray absorption

     (3) Must have high x-ray-to-light conversion with suitable energy and color

     (4) Should stop emitting light when the x-ray exposure ceases

   4. Protective coating applied to phosphor to prevent abrasion and allow transmission of light

  F. Care of intensifying screens

   1. Important to clean regularly (monthly) with a cleaner that is recommended (best) or 70% alcohol

   2. Make sure surface is dry before loading films

   3. Any debris on screen surface will cause artifacts

   4. Avoid "digs and scratches" on the screen surface when loading and unloading film

  G. Phosphor types

   1. Calcium tungstate phosphor

    a. Emits blue light

    b. Has good x-ray absorption ability but lacks in light conversion efficiency

    c. Traditionally used in phosphor layer

   2. Rare earth phosphors

    a. Primarily emit in the green light spectrum

    b. Greater x-ray-to-light conversion, resulting in decreased exposure required

  H. Screen speed (Figure 12-3)

   1. Relative term referring to the measure of exposure necessary to produce a diagnostic film

   2. Screen speed ratings

    a. Slow (high definition, ultra-fine, fine grain): designed for optimal detail

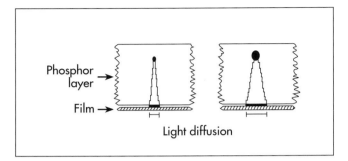

Figure 12-3 Increasing the size of the phosphor crystals increases the speed of the screen. However, the image appears more grainy.

with minimal concern for exposure time

b. Medium (regular, midspeed, normal, par speed): good resolution with relatively low exposures

c. Fast (high speed) used when reduced exposure time or increased patient penetration required

3. Fast screens

a. Require less radiation exposure than slower speed screens to produce the same degree of blackness on the film

b. Generally have larger crystals to increase the x-ray absorption and light conversion

c. Usually have a thicker phosphor layer

d. The larger crystals and thicker layer mean more blurriness (high grain) and less detail

e. Because of greater absorption and conversion, rare earth screens can produce the same (or better) degree of radiographic detail as calcium tungstate with less radiation exposure

4. Quantum mottle resulting in a spotty or mottled radiograph is a disadvantage of increased film speed

IV. X-ray film

A. Purpose is to provide a permanent diagnostic record

B. Film composition

1. Transparent polyester base

2. Adhesive to attach emulsion to base

3. Emulsion that consists of gelatin and silver halide crystals (that appear as tiny grains under the microscope—billions per mL)

4. Protective coating to protect emulsion from scratching

C. Latent image

1. Definition: an invisible image on the x-ray film after it has been exposed by ionizing radiation or visible light before the film has been processed

2. On a screen-type film, the grain of silver halide absorbs the emitted light photon and begins to split apart

3. The partially split crystals will convert to metallic silver and turn black after the film is developed

4. The greater the number of converted silver halide crystals, the blacker the film

5. Unexposed crystals will be cleared away by the fixer

D. Film types

1. Screen film

a. Silver crystals are more sensitive to wavelengths of light emitted from the intensifying screens than from direct ionizing radiation

b. Less exposure needed to produce a diagnostic radiograph

c. Must be sensitive to the light emitted by the intensifying screens

2. Nonscreen film

a. Designed to be more sensitive to direct ionizing radiation

b. Greater exposure factors required because there is no intensification of the x-ray beam

c. Packaged in a light-tight heavy envelope

d. Useful in bone or dental radiography where greater detail is required

(1) Dental film speed that is available is usually designated as D or E (range for dental film is A to F, with A being the slowest)

E. Film speeds (see Table 12-1)

1. Depend on size of the crystal

2. Generally the smaller the crystal, the wider the latitude or exposure factors that can be used without significantly changing the film density, and the greater the resolution

3. Medium film represents a compromise between fine grain and speed; it is mostly used in veterinary radiography

Table 12-1 Comparison of film speed

Characteristic	Fast film (ultraspeed)	Slow film (high detail)
Crystal size	Larger crystals	Smaller crystals
Exposure required	Lower needed	More needed
Film latitude	Less latitude	Greater latitude
Image	Grainier image	Less grainy image
Definition	Less resolution	Greater resolution

F. Film care
1. Store film boxes on end so film is in a vertical position
2. Store in a cool (10°-15° C; 50°-59°) room with low relative humidity (40%-60%)
3. Store away from ionizing radiation, and vapors such as formalin, hydrogen peroxide, or ammonia
4. Use before expiration date to prevent radiographic fogging
5. Film can be placed in a plastic bag and stored in a refrigerator or freezer to prolong usefulness

V. Film-screen systems
A. Combined speed determines exposure requirements
B. Must determine most desirable system for your clinic based on image detail and speed requirement
C. A numeric value is assigned to each film and screen combination
D. The numerical value differs for each company so that proper comparisons can be made only for that particular company
E. As a rule 300-400 speed is medium speed and considered most versatile
F. The speed of the system is inversely related to the mAs setting—as you increase the speed (higher number) you decrease the mAs
G. Values are similar to ISO (ASA) of photographic film

VI. Legal records and identification
A. Must be properly identified (in film emulsion) to be legal
B. Identification should include:
1. Patient identification
2. Owner identification
3. Date of examination
4. Name of hospital

C. A numeric system employing a patient case number or file number facilitates record keeping
D. Methods of labeling a radiograph include:
1. Lead markers
2. Lead-impregnated tape
3. Photoimprinting label system
4. Miscellaneous markers
a. Right (Rt) or Left (Le) is essential
b. Labeling of front (F) or hind (H) limbs and medial (M) or lateral (L) in equine radiography
c. Time sequence labels for special procedures
d. Position markers
e. Technician identification markers

VII. Film filing
A. Must be properly labeled and filed for future referral or follow-up examinations
B. Because these are legal records, province and state associations require a minimum file and retrieval period before they are allowed to be discarded

DARKROOM AND PROCESSING TECHNIQUES ■■

Radiography begins and ends in the darkroom, where films are loaded into cassettes and returned for processing into finished radiographs. Most mistakes made in radiography of animals are related to the processing of radiographs.

Darkroom Considerations

I. Cleanliness is absolutely essential
II. Good ventilation and temperature control
III. Light-proofed so that film fogging does not result
IV. Darkroom safelight
A. Filter must match sensitivity of film used
1. Amber for blue sensitive
2. Dark red (e.g., Kodak GBX) can be used for blue and green
B. Correct wattage (usually 6½ to 15 watts)
C. At least 4 feet from working area
D. Work as quickly as possible
V. Fogging due to light leaking or improper safelight illumination can be evaluated as follows
A. Place an unradiographed film on the counter
B. Cover three fourths of it with a piece of cardboard for 1 minute
C. Move the cardboard covering one half of the film for 1 additional minute
D. Shift the cardboard so that only one fourth of the film is covered for 1 additional minute

E. Remove the cardboard and expose the entire film for 1 additional minute (4 minutes in total)

F. Process normally

G. Darkened areas are indicative of fogging

VI. Organize into a wet and dry area to minimize processing artifacts

VII. State, provincial, or federal regulations require proper use of gloves, protective eye wear, eye wash bottle (WHMIS/OSHA)

Manual Film Processing Pointers

I. Basic steps include developing, rinsing or stop bath, fixing, washing, and drying

II. Chemical solutions are usually required by manufacturer to be diluted—follow steps carefully

III. Keep all solutions at required temperature

A. Optimum temperature is 20° C or 68° F

B. Less activity occurs at lower temperatures; greater activity occurs at higher temperatures

IV. Make sure chemicals are well mixed before using

V. Carefully follow manufacturer's suggestion for time-temperature development

VI. Agitate film intermittently in solutions to prevent air bubbles

VII. Avoid letting film drain back into chemical solutions when removing from the tanks

VIII. Keep lids on the solution tanks whenever possible

IX. Developer: primary function is to reduce or convert the exposed silver halide crystals of the film to black metallic silver

A. Developer consists of developing agents, accelerators, preservatives, restrainers, and a solvent

B. pH is alkaline in a range of 9.8 to 11.4

C. Solution needs replacing when it turns a brown to green color or when the processed radiographs do not have the expected density or contrast

D. Maintain level of solution with fresh replenisher

X. Rinse bath: purpose is to stop developing process and prevent contamination of the fixer

A. Rinse in circulating water for about 30 seconds

XI. Fixer: primary functions are to remove and clear away the unexposed, undeveloped silver halide crystals, as well as hardening the film to make the film a permanent record

A. Fixer consists of clearing or fixing agents, preservative, hardeners, acidifiers, buffers, and a solvent

B. pH is acidic

C. Film can be briefly viewed after it is cleared (about 1 minute but it is safer to wait at least 2 minutes) but must be returned and fixed in total for about double the development time

D. Change fixer when time required for the film to change from cloudy to clear exceeds 2 to 3 minutes

E. Replenish when solution is low as evidenced by film artifact (see Table 12-5)

XII. Wash bath: purpose is to remove processing chemicals from the film, thereby preventing film discoloration and fading over time

A. Wash in clean, circulating water about 15 to 20 minutes

XIII. Drying

A. Place hanger in drier or hang on rack

B. Avoid dusty areas

XIV. Maintenance and replenishing

A. For optimum chemical efficiency, it is suggested to daily remove 8 oz (250 mL) of developer and fixer, and replenish same amount

B. Solutions should be changed at least every three months or when 15 gallons (60 L) of working replenisher have been used

Automatic Film Processing

I. Mechanized film processing is a more accurate term

II. Films carried from solution to solution and through the dryer by a roller assembly

III. Processing times vary from 90 seconds to 8 minutes depending on temperature (77°-96° F [20°-35° C]) with temperature inversely related to length of processing times

IV. Chemicals are more concentrated with similar properties and procedures to the manual processing but there are a few exceptions

A. A hardener is included in the developer

B. No rinsing occurs between developing and fixing

V. Keep processor clean at all times—especially rollers, roller racks, and cross over rollers

VI. Change chemicals as required

VII. As cost of units decrease, automatic processing will become more popular in veterinary clinics

RADIOGRAPHIC QUALITY
Definition

I. That "feature of a diagnostic radiograph that describes to what degree the shadows identified on the film clearly depict the anatomical features under investigation" (Morgan)

II. A film of good diagnostic quality should have optimal density, correct scale of contrast, and excellent detail with minimal magnification and distortion
   A. See Table 12-2 for technical errors related to density

Radiographic Density

I. Definition: the degree of darkness or blackness on the film

II. Determined by the number of photons that have affected the film—the greater the number, the darker the film

III. Influenced by several factors, including:
   A. Total number of x-rays that reach the film (mAs) (Figure 12-4)
      1. mAs (milliampere-seconds) is a quantity factor that controls the number of x-rays produced (beam intensity)
      2. If more x-rays are produced the film will be darker
   B. Penetrating power of the x-rays (kVp)
      1. Kilovoltage potential (kVp) is a quality factor that affects the energy of the x-rays
      2. At higher kVp settings, more x-rays with more energy are produced, there is a better penetration through the tissue, and as a result the film density increases
   C. Developing time and temperature
   D. Forms of beam attenuation such as filters or grids
   E. Tissue density and patient thickness (Figure 12-5)
      1. Tissue and film density are inversely proportional
      2. In order of increasing film density (white to black) and decreasing tissue density (most dense to least) we have metal, bone, water (organs), fat, gas
   F. Other physical factors are film and screen speed, use of contrast agents, source image distance (formerly called focal film distance)

IV. Can be measured by a densitometer

Contrast

I. See Table 12-3 for technical errors related to contrast

II. Definition: refers to the visible difference between two adjacent radiographic densities
   A. Can be divided into radiographic contrast and subject contrast

III. Radiographic contrast

Table 12-2 Technical errors affecting film density

	Decreased film density	Increased film density
Machine factors	Underexposure: too low kVp, mAs Drop in incoming line voltage Equipment malfunction	Overexposure: too high kVp, mAs Surge in incoming line voltage Equipment malfunction
Physical factors	Undermeasurement of anatomical part Increased subject density Source image distance (SID) too great Grid used and not accounted for Positive contrast media used Slow speed screen/film used No exposure	Overmeasurement of anatomical part Decreased subject density SID too short No grid used and not accounted for Negative contrast media used Fast speed screen/film used Double exposure
Processing factors Wet-tank	Underdevelopment Developer time short Developer temperature too cold Exhausted developer Contaminated developer Diluted developer Developer improperly mixed Defective thermometer	Overdevelopment Developer time too long Developer temperature too high Inaccurate thermometer Solutions too concentrated Bromide missing from developer
Automatic processors	Under-replenishment Developer temperature too low Exhausted developer Developer improperly mixed	Over-replenishment Developer temperature high Light leak from cover or in darkroom Rollers malfunctioning

A. Refers to the various shades of black, gray, and white on a radiographic film and the differences between them
B. High contrast film means a very black and white film with few grays

1. Referred to as having a short latitude or scale of contrast—fewer, but bigger steps
2. Preferred for spine and extremity films

C. Long latitude or scale films have a larger number of shades of gray but little differ-

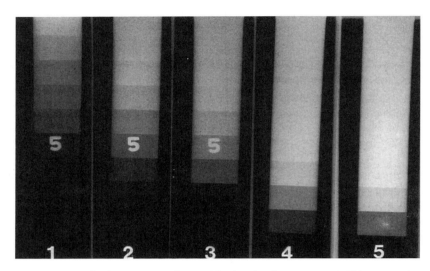

Figure 12-4   Image 1 displays more radiographic density than Image 5. This means Image 1 was exposed with a higher mAs. (From Han CM, Hurd CD: *Practical Guide to Diagnostic Imaging; Radiography and Ultrasonography*, St Louis, 1994, Mosby.)

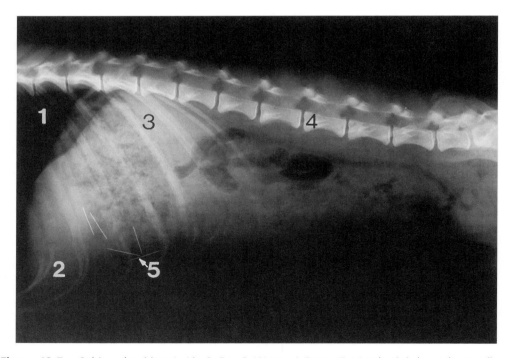

Figure 12-5   Subject densities: *1*, Air. *2*, Fat. *3*, Water. *4*, Bone. *5*, Metal. Air is least dense, allowing x-rays to penetrate and expose the film. Metal is the most dense, absorbing most of the x-rays and allowing only a few to penetrate, exposing the film. (From Pratt PW: *Principles and Practice of Veterinary Technology*, St Louis, 1998, Mosby.)

Table 12-3 Technical factors affecting radiographic contrast

Low contrast	
Machine factors	Over-penetration from too high kVp
Physical factors	Slower speed screens, film, or those manufactured with lower levels
	Fog due to:
	• Light leak such as safelight or while in cassette or during loading or unloading
	• Scatter radiation if not using a grid for thick parts
	• Direct or scatter radiation:
	If left lying near machine during other exposures
	If film bin exposed
	• Film stored in too hot or too humid place
	• Outdated film
	Beam not collimated
	Over-filtration
	Negative contrast used
	Low subject contrast
	Excessive pressure on emulsions of unprocessed films
Processing factors	
Wet-tank	Prolonged development
	Developer temperature too high
	Solutions contaminated or exhausted
	Fixed for too short of time or turning on light too soon
	Luminous clocks and watch faces
Automatic processors	Prolonged development
	Developer temperature too high
	Exhausted or contaminated solutions

ences or contrast between them—more but smaller steps

    1. Preferred for soft tissue

  D. Kilovoltage has the greatest influence on radiographic contrast

    1. X-ray beam is polychromatic, which means that it contains a spectrum of energies (average energy is one half to one third the peak energy)

    2. At lower kVp there are more lower energy photons and a greater difference in energy levels

    3. As kVp increases, the difference between the energy levels lessen, allowing for greater penetration of the x-ray beam through the tissue

    4. The absorption of the x-ray beam by the various tissues at higher kVp is more uniform, resulting in lower radiographic contrast

  E. Scatter radiation (that nonimage forming radiation that is scattered in all directions resulting from objects in the path of the beam) adds a grayness to the film

    1. Inappropriate areas of the film are being exposed, thus decreasing contrast

  F. Processing factors and other physical factors (beam attenuation, fogging) affect radiographic contrast

  G. mAs does not affect contrast if sufficient quantity is used because an increase or decrease in mAs affects the number of x-rays evenly

  IV. Subject contrast is defined as the difference in density and mass between two adjacent anatomic structures

  A. Subject contrast depends on the thickness and density of the anatomic part

  B. Subject contrast affects radiographic contrast

    1. High subject density means high tissue density

    2. The greater the subject density (e.g., bone) the greater the difference between the blacks and whites on the radiograph

    3. High subject contrast then increases radiographic contrast

Radiographic Detail or Definition (See Table 12-4 for Technical Errors Related to Detail and Figure 12-6 to 12-8)

  I. Refers to definition of the edge of an anatomic structure

  II. Image sharpness, clarity, distinctness, and perceptibility are synonymous

  III. Lack of detail or penumbra may be due to many factors

TECHNICAL ERRORS AND ARTIFACTS ▬▬▬

Several errors in handling x-ray film, manipulating exposure factors, or setting up a procedure could result. See Table 12-5 for artifacts and other errors.

DEVELOPING A TECHNIQUE CHART ▬▬▬

A technique chart is a table with predetermined X-ray machine settings that enables one to select the correct machine settings based on the thickness of the tissue and the anatomical portion to be radiographed.

  I. Each machine requires its own technique chart

  II. Several charts may be needed (screen/nonscreen, grid/no grid, species specific, anatomy specific, various film/screen combinations)

  III. Can use variable kVp chart, variable mAs chart, or a combination of both

IV. Whatever method is used certain concepts should be kept in mind
   A. Standardize as many factors as possible (speed of screens, age of screens, speed of film, source-image distance, beam filtration, temperature, and age and time of processing, type of grid)
   B. Keep in mind that mAs is directly proportional to film density but does not appreciably alter film contrast if the density is correct
   C. Kilovoltage is directly proportional to film density and inversely proportional to film contrast—low kVp means a high scale of contrast
   D. Source-image density (SID) squared is inversely proportional to film distance
      1. Change in SID means a change in film density
      2. SID does not alter film contrast if film density is correct
      3. Also referred to as focal-film distance (FFD)
   E. Change in thickness requires a change in kVp setting. For each additional thickness in patient cm add:
      1. 2 kVp if under 80 kVp
      2. 3 kVp if in 80 to 100 kVp range
      3. 4 kVp if over 100 kVp
   F. A general relationship exists between mAs and kVp

Table 12-4 Common errors relating to lack of radiographic detail or definition (penumbra)

Machine factors	Too large a focal spot used Focal spot damaged
Physical factors	Motion unsharpness 　　Motion of patient, cassette, machine 　　Too slow time used Geometric unsharpness 　　Poor contact of intensifying screen and film 　　Increased object film distance 　　Decreased source image distance 　　Patient too thick 　　Rounded area of interest Geometric distortion and magnification 　　Patient/part not parallel to the film 　　Patient/part not perpendicular to the beam 　　Primary beam not centered over the area of interest 　　Area of interest not close to the film Radiographic noise 　　Film graininess (film speed too fast) 　　Structure mottle (intensifying screen speed too fast) 　　Quantum mottle (too few photons producing an image)

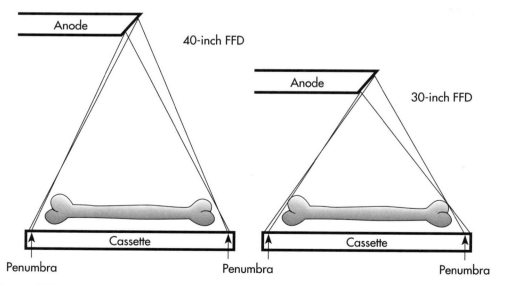

Figure 12-6 Increasing the focal-film distance (FFD) decreases the amount of penumbra, increasing the radiographic detail. (From Pratt PW: *Principles and Practice of Veterinary Technology,* St Louis, 1998, Mosby.)

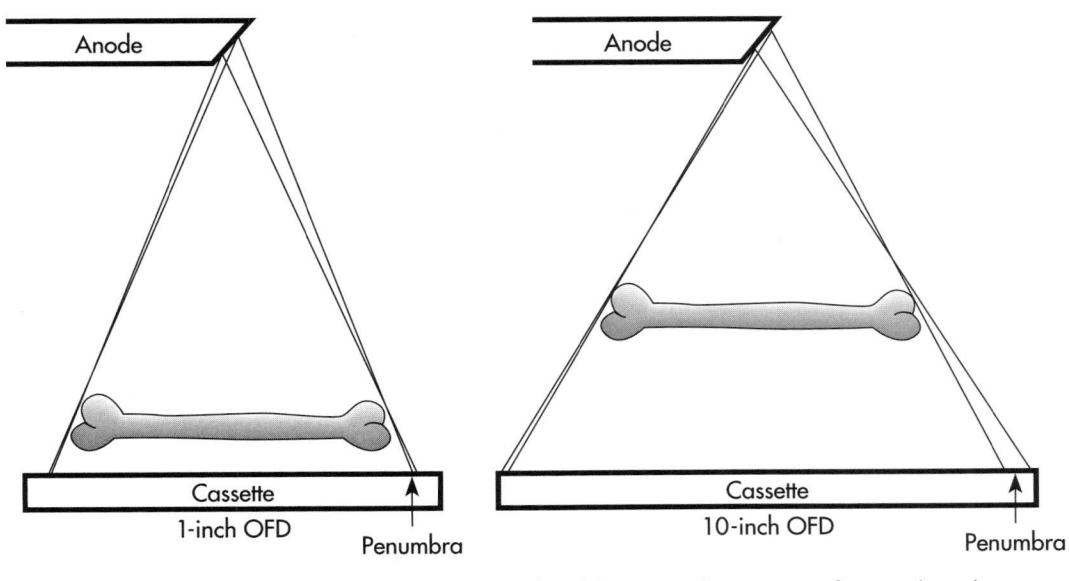

Figure 12-7   Increasing the obect-film distance (OFD) increases the amount of penumbra, decreasing the radiographic detail. (From Pratt PW: *Principles and Practice of Veterinary Technology,* St Louis, 1998, Mosby.)

Table 12-5   Artifacts and other technical areas

Black marks
Film scratches usually after exposure but before processing
Crescent marks: rough handling, finger-nail
Light leak: defective cassettes, storage in bin
Static electricity: linear dots or tree pattern from too low humidity or improper handling
Developer drops before processing
Film stuck together while in fixer
Linear lines due to grid cutoff
Roller lines of automatic processor—film jammed

Yellow radiograph
Exhausted fixer solution
Fixing time too short
Inadequate rinsing
Film sticking together during processing

Slow drying
Waterlogged films due to prolonged washing, water too warm, or improper hardening by the fixer
Air too humid or cool
Automatic processor—
  Thermostat malfunction
  Too low dryer temperatures
  Improper hardening
  Inadequate air venting

White marks or clear areas
Film emulsion scratched off usually before exposure or during processing
Debris on surface of film
Defective screens (pitted, scratched)
Smudges of fixer on fingers before developing
Grit due to remnant fixer not washed
Increased atomic number of object (e.g., positioning device, lead contrast media on cassette)
Air bubble on film during developing procedure
Developing solution low
Film touching side of tanks during manual developing
Reticulation due to improper stirring of solutions
Blank film: unexposed or fixed before developed
Evidence of collimation

Brittleness of finished radiograph
Excessive drying temperature, time
Excessive hardening in fixer

Green areas or films
Processing solutions low
  Two films stuck together during processing

1. If film density is too dark, to correct the error:
   a. Have mAs setting or subtract 10 kVp (in 70-90 range) (Morgan)
   b. Decrease mAs 30% to 50% or kVp 10% to 15% (Lavin)

2. If film density is too light, to correct error:
   a. Double mAs setting or add 10 kVp (in 70-90 kVp range) (Morgan)
   b. Increase mAs 30% to 50% or kVp 10% to 15% (Lavin)

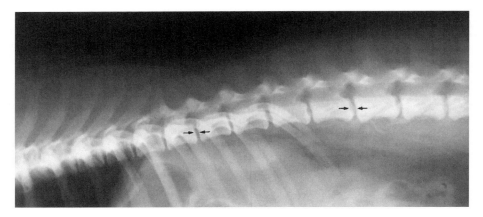

Figure 12-8 The intervertebral spaces appear narrow toward the edges of the radiograph *(arrows)* as compared with the spaces in the center of the radiograph. (From Pratt PW: *Principles and Practice of Veterinary Technology,* St Louis, 1998, Mosby.)

G. Exposure factors must also be increased for conditions such as:
   1. Pleural fluid/cardiomegaly
   2. Ascites
   3. Obesity
   4. Plaster cast
   5. Special positive radiographic procedures
H. To determine if kVp or mAs should be changed
   1. If film is too dark but contrast has not significantly been altered (i.e., soft tissue is dark but bones are relatively white) mAs should be decreased
   2. If film is too dark and bones are gray the problem is overpenetration or too much kVp
   3. If film is too light and anatomical parts, especially in cranial abdomen, are not clearly visible, an increase of kVp will improve density and contrast

RADIATION SAFETY

The major objective of a veterinary practice that uses ionizing radiation should be to obtain the maximum amount of information with the minimal exposure to all concerned. "Radiation should be respected . . . . not feared." (Lavin)

Responsibilities

I. It is the practice owner's responsibility to:
   A. Ensure that proper radiation safety measures are observed
   B. Meet state or provincial requirements: dosimetry devices, proper protection devices, registration, room design, etc. Usually regulated by the Department of Health
   C. Instruct personnel in proper radiation safety and use

Hazards of Ionizing Radiation

I. All tissues are sensitive to ionizing radiation
   A. Ionizing radiation refers to the excitation of orbital electrons in an atom so that the atoms are separated into charged particles
      1. The molecule may break or alter
      2. Charged molecules may function improperly or not at all
   B. The interaction between x-rays and tissues occurs at the atomic level but it is theorized that visible injury results from molecular derangements of macromolecules and water
   C. Injury to cells, tissues, and organs occurs at the time of exposure but may require hours, days, or generations to show damage
II. Types of cellular damage in the body
   A. Genetic damage occurs to DNA (genes) of reproductive cells
      1. Manifestation not detectable until future generations
   B. Somatic cell damage occurs in all other cells and becomes evident at some point in the individual's life, although it may never become obvious due to tissue repair
   C. Nucleus of proliferating somatic and genetic cells is considered to be the most sensitive area of the cell to the ionizing effects
   D. Greater sensitivity occurs with:
      1. Younger tissues and organs

Table 12-6 Maximum permissible dose

WHOLE BODY DOSE FOR OCCUPATIONALLY EXPOSED OVER 18 YEARS OF AGE		
Weekly	0.001 Sv	(0.1 rem)
Quarterly	0.03 Sv	(3 rem)
Calendar year	0.05 Sv	(5 rem)
Accumulated over lifetime	0.05 (N-18) Sv	(5[N-18]rem)

N = age in years.

2. Higher metabolic activity
3. Greater proliferation rate of cells and growth rate of tissues
E. Organ tissues considered critical because of their sensitivity are dermis, thyroid, eye, lymphatics, blood forming tissues, bone, and germinal epithelium or gonads

Radiation Measurement

I. Absorbed dose is the unit of ionizing radiation that measures the energy transferred by this radiation to a body part.
  A. SI unit is Grey (Gy)
  B. Previous unit was rad (1 Gy = 100 rad)
II. Dose equivalent makes allowances for the fact that ionizing radiation affects all tissues differently
  A. SI unit is Sievert (Sv)
  B. Previous unit was rem (1 Sv = 100 rem)

Maximum Permissible Dose (MPD)

I. See Table 12-6 for specific MPD
II. Definition: maximum dose of radiation that a person may receive in a given period
III. Set by the National Committee on Radiation Protection and Measurement (NCRP)
IV. NCRP and most provincial and state regulations allow occupationally exposed persons to restrain and position animals when *absolutely necessary* but other states or provinces prohibit any manual restraint
V. Various dosimeters or personal exposure monitoring devices are available but these and MPD are meaningless unless:
  A. Each individual involved in taking radiographs properly wears the dosimeter every time he or she takes radiographs
  B. Dosimeters are routinely sent to a federally approved lab for evaluation
VI. For more information contact Radiation Protection Service of the Department of Health of your state or province

Safety Practices

I. Exposure and damage to tissue can occur from:
  A. Primary beam: *Never* allow any part of the body to be in the primary beam even if properly protected
    1. Primary beam will penetrate through lead aprons and gloves
  B. Secondary or scatter radiation that is produced when the primary beam interacts with objects in its path
    1. Amount and direction of scatter depends on kVp level, volume of tissue irradiated, field size, and composition of tissue
  C. X-ray machine leakage
II. Important safety practices
  A. Never permit anyone under 18 years of age or pregnant women in the room during exposure
  B. Remove unnecessary personnel and rotate personnel during procedures
  C. Use nonmanual restraint such as chemical restraint, sandbags, sponges, tape, and restraining devices whenever possible. A little patience and creativity will go a long way
  D. Always wear protective gloves, thyroid protector, and aprons
    1. Minimum 0.5 mm lead equivalent
    2. Routinely inspect and radiograph for any damage
  E. Never permit any part of the body, even if it is shielded, to be in the primary beam
  F. Consider use of protective goggles (0.25 mm lead equivalent) and larger shielding devices
  G. Collimate so there is at least an unexposed border on each film proving that the primary beam is limited and scatter radiation reduced
  H. Wear dosimeter outside of apron near the collar
  I. Never hand hold an x-ray machine
  J. Do not direct the x-ray beam at any individual or occupied adjacent room
  K. Use 2.5 mm aluminum filter to remove the lower energy portion of the x-ray beam
  L. Regularly have the machine calibrated and checked
  M. Use fastest film-screen systems compatible with obtaining diagnostic radiographs
  N. Plan each procedure carefully to avoid retakes
  O. Keep an exposure log identifying the patient, study, and exposures

P. Follow state and provincial radiation safety codes

III. Remember the big three methods of radiation safety (McCurnin)
- A. Time: avoid retakes, do it correctly the first time
- B. Distance: keep as far as possible from patient and x-ray beam
- C. Shielding: always wear protective apparel

POSITIONING TECHNIQUES

Proper positioning is essential to obtain diagnostic radiographic examinations. Refer to texts that thoroughly explain specific procedures for various species

Basic Principles

I. Common terms and abbreviations used (based on American Committee of Veterinary Radiologists and Anatomists) (Figure 12-9)
- A. Left (Le)
  Right (Rt)
- B. Refers to limbs
  1. Medial (M)
  2. Lateral (L)
- C. Cranial (Cr)
  1. Toward head
  2. For limbs proximal to carpus/tarsus
- D. Cd (caudal), toward tail
- E. Dorsal (D)
  1. Toward back
  2. Also cranial portion of limb distal to carpus/tarsus

F. Ventral (V)
  1. Toward abdomen
G. Palmar (Pa)
  1. Caudal portion of pectoral limb from carpus distally
H. Plantar (P1)
  1. Caudal portion of pelvic limb from tarsus distally
I. Oblique (O)
  1. Less than 90° to axis
J. Rostral (R)
  1. Used for head—toward the nares

II. Beam direction
- A. Lateral: the side closest to the film is marked (i.e., side it is lying on)
  1. EXAMPLE: Rt L = lying on right side
- B. Abbreviated term indicates direction of beam: first letter is where the x-rays enter the body, second letter is where x-rays leave the body, (part that lies against the film)
  1. EXAMPLE: VD (ventrodorsal)—the animal would be lying in dorsal recumbency or on its back
- C. Oblique views are usually in reference to limbs
  1. The first two letters indicate where the beam enters the body, the next two letters indicate where it exits (the body part that is specifically against the film)
  2. First letter in each pair describes front or back; second letter of each pair describes the side of the limb

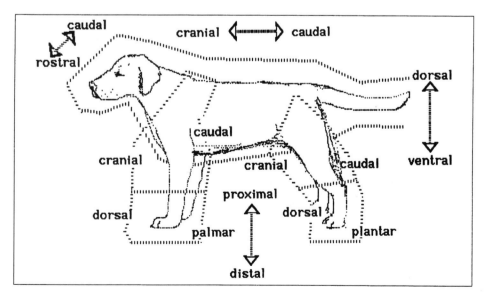

Figure 12-9 Veterinary anatomic terminology. (From Han CM, Hurd CD: *Practical Guide to Diagnostic Imaging; Radiography and Ultrasonography,* St Louis, 1994, Mosby.)

3. EXAMPLE: Dorsomedial-palmarolateral oblique (DMPaLO) of the carpus
   a. Carpus is rotated (O) so that the x-ray beam is aimed at the front of the limb (D) toward the medial side (M). This faces you
   b. This means that the beam exits from the back of the limb (Pa) so that the opposite side (L) faces or is against the film

Basic Criteria and Principles of Positioning and Restraint

I. Keep comfort and welfare of patient in mind
   A. Be prepared before patient positioning
   B. Use steady, slow, gentle movements
   C. Use minimum restraint through chemical and/or mechanical assistance
II. Minimize exposure to radiation of assistants by using nonmanual restraint whenever possible
III. Measure with callipers the area of interest in centimeters
IV. Have two views at right angles to each other except
   A. Thoracic views, contrast studies, and equine radiography often require more views
   B. Injury may allow only a lateral view
V. Have the area of interest as close to the film as possible
VI. Center the beam to area of interest and include specific anatomy for each anatomic area
VII. Keep the area of interest parallel to the film and perpendicular to the x-ray beam
VIII. Collimate using the smallest field size possible to accommodate essential anatomy
IX. When radiographing extremities, include the proximal and distal joints of the long bone being radiographed
   A. If radiographing a joint, include at least one third of the long bones distal and proximal to that joint
X. Make sure patient is adequately prepared
XI. When using positioning aids, minimize placing radiolucent and radiopaque devices over the area of interest
XII. Plan your procedure carefully to avoid retakes

CONTRAST RADIOGRAPHY ▬▬▬▬

Basic Concepts

I. Used to enhance the visualization of individual organs and structures that are not adequately visible on the survey radiographs
II. Contrast means density difference

Media

I. Two classes of contrast media
   A. Positive contrast (radiopaque) such as barium, iodine
      1. Absorb more x-rays than bone so appear even whiter on a radiograph
      2. May be classified as
         a. Insoluble: barium, which is used mainly for gastrointestinal studies. Never give barium parenterally
         b. Soluble: all other positive contrast media; contains iodine that can be used for renal, articular, vascular, myelographic, and gastrointestinal studies
         c. Soluble iodinated contrast agents are hyperosmotic and though rare may also cause toxic reactions
   B. Negative contrast (radiolucent) such as air, carbon dioxide
      1. No x-rays are absorbed so the media appears black on the radiograph
   C. Double contrast studies incorporate positive and negative contrast medium

Patient Preparation

I. Depending on the procedure, the patient may have to:
   A. Have food withheld 12 to 24 hours
   B. Be given an enema or cathartic 4 to 12 hours before the procedure
II. Have a survey radiograph completed before the procedure

Specific Studies

Please refer to the excellent references available for actual studies

Glossary

absorbed dose The amount of energy that tissue receives when it is bombarded by ionizing radiation, measured as Grey (Gy) or rads

actual focal spot The area of the focal spot when viewed from 90° to the target

amperage Term used to describe the flow of electrons through a current

anode Positive electrode in the x-ray tube that contains the target

artifact That which decreases the diagnostic quality of a radiograph

binding energy Energy that must be surpassed before an electron can be removed from its orbit

calipers Measuring device to determine patient thickness

cathode Negative electrode in the x-ray tube that supplies the electrons

caudocranial (CdCr) Directional term indicating that the x-ray beam enters from toward the tail and exits toward the head. Opposite is CrCd. Usually in reference to limbs, proximal to the carpal and tarsal joints

detail Part of film quality indicating clear resolution and definition of the shadows on the radiographic image

distal Further away from the point of origin. Opposite is proximal

dorsopalmar (DPa) Directional term that refers to limbs distal to and including the carpus. The beam enters from the front of the limb and exits at the back of the limb. PaD is opposite

dorsoplantar (DPl) Directional term that refers to limbs below, including the tarsus (see above)

dorsoventral (DV) Directional term that indicates that the x-ray beam enters from the back of the animal and exits out its belly. The animal would be lying in ventral recumbency (on its abdomen). Opposite term is VD

dosimeter A device used to measure the radiation exposure that personnel receive

effective focal spot Area of the focal spot as seen through the x-ray tube window and directed on the film

electromagnetic radiation Propagation of ionizing energy through space in the form of photons

electron Negatively charged particle of the atom that circles around the nucleus

electron beam Beam of electrons that is accelerated from the cathode to the anode by a high electrical potential in the x-ray tube

filament Coiled wire of the cathode that emits the electron beam

film contrast A characteristic of the film that influences radiographic contrast. Often film contrast and latitude are inversely related

film graininess Loss of detail caused by the size of the individual silver halide crystals; usually more pronounced in faster speed film; also referred to as radiographic mottle

film latitude Exposure range that will produce acceptable density on the film

focal range Distance from the grid to the x-ray tube that will minimize grid cutoff

fogging An overall grayness that does not contribute to the diagnostic quality of the film; may be caused from chemicals as well as undesirable radiation

geometric unsharpness Loss of detail due to geometric distortion, also referred to as penumbra

grid cutoff When a grid is not used correctly and the primary beam is more than normally absorbed

grid ratio Ratio of the height of the lead strips as compared to the space between them (r = h/d)

heel effect Due to the angle of the target, a greater intensity of x-rays are emitted from the cathode side, rather than from the anode side

ionization A process of transferring enough energy to an atom so that the outer electron is removed; the atom is positively charged

kilovoltage peak (kVp) Maximum energy of the x-ray beam that determines the quality or penetrating power of the beam

latent image Invisible image produced on the x-ray film after exposure and before processing

maximum permissible dose (MPD) Maximum amount of radiation that an individual is allowed over a given time period

milliampere-seconds (mAs) Amount of current flowing through the tube times the exposure time in seconds; milliampere = one one thousandth ampere

object film distance Space between the film and the part being radiographed

penumbra Loss of detail due to geometric unsharpness

photon A bundle of radiation energy, also known as quanta

polychromatic beam An x-ray beam that has a broad spectrum of energies; depends on the kVp—the lower the kVp the more polychromatic the beam

quality Term referring to the average energy of the x-ray beam or its penetrating ability (kVp)

quantity Term that refers to the total number of x-ray photons (controlled by mA)

quantum mottle Loss of radiographic detail that occurs in faster screens because of the uneven distribution of the phosphor crystals within the screen

radiodense or radiopaque An object or tissue that absorbs radiation so that the image on the film is lighter

radiographic contrast Variation in degree of darkness between two adjacent areas on the film

radiographic density Degree of darkness found on the radiograph

radiographic quality How well the shadows on the radiograph are clearly identified

radiography The making of radiographs

radiology The use of radiant energy in the diagnosis and treatment of disease

radiolucent A tissue or device that allows most of the x-ray beams to pass through unaffected

rectification The process of changing alternating current to current flowing in one direction only (direct current)

remnant beam Primary radiation emitted from the x-ray tube

scatter radiation or secondary radiation Caused by interaction of the primary beam with tissue or matter in its path

source image distance (SID) Formerly called focal film distance, it is the distance from the focal spot or source of the x-rays to the image receptor or film

speed The exposure required to produce a diagnostic film density

structure mottle A loss of radiographic detail that occurs because of phosphor variations found in intensifying screens; more noticeable with fast speed screens

subject contrast Contrast resulting from the difference in density, mass, and atomic number of adjacent tissue structures

thermionic emission Heating of the filament so that the energy produced forces the electrons to be released from their atomic orbits

thermoluminescent dosimeter A form of personnel radiation dosage monitor

x-ray A short wavelength, high energy form of electromagnetic radiation

Review Questions

1 What is the maximum permissible dose (MPD) or radiation that the whole body is allowed in a year?
  a. 5 SV   (5.00 mRem)
  b. 0.05 (N-18) SV   (5[N-18]rem)
  c. 0.05 SV   (5 rem)
  d. 0.03 SV   (3 rem)

2 Which factor does not appreciably affect contrast?
  a. kVp
  b. mAs
  c. Film speed
  d. Processing

3 For a diagnostic radiograph, what will a "high plus" speed film need in comparison to a par speed film?
  a. Use of a grid
  b. Longer processing time
  c. More mAs or kVp
  d. Less mAs or kVp

4 The main purpose of the developer is to:
  a. Remove unexposed, undeveloped silver halide crystals
  b. Reduce exposed silver halide crystals to black metallic silver
  c. Change the calcium tungstate crystals to black calcium
  d. Create a latent image

5 Density is decreased on a film by:
  a. Increasing the kVp
  b. Decreasing the tissue density
  c. Decreasing the mAs
  d. Increasing the processing chemical temperatures

6 A higher grid ratio means that:
  a. The lead plate is thicker
  b. Less scatter radiation is absorbed
  c. More scatter radiation is absorbed
  d. Less primary radiation is absorbed

7 X-rays:
  a. Are a type of electromagnetic radiation
  b. Have less energy than radio waves
  c. Have longer wavelengths than radio waves
  d. Are measured in meters

8 There will be more scattered radiation noticed on the film with:
  a. Use of a grid
  b. Increased kVp
  c. Decreased kVp
  d. Decreased patient thickness

9 A radiograph using 70 kVp and 10 mAs is too dark. Which technique would be most reasonable for the repeat?
  a. 80 kVp and 5 mAs
  b. 85 kVp and 10 mAs
  c. 60 kVp and 20 mAs
  d. 70 kVp and 5 mAs

10 If an animal had its right side against the film this view is known as a:
  a. Right lateral
  b. Side view

  c. Ventrodorsal
  d. Left lateral

11 The purpose of an aluminum filter in an x-ray machine is to:
  a. Limit the size of the x-ray beam
  b. Focus the x-ray beam to the focal spot
  c. Remove the long wavelength x-rays from the x-ray beam
  d. Remove short wavelength x-rays from the beam

12 The degree of overall blackness on a radiograph is termed:
  a. Density
  b. Contrast
  c. Radiolucent
  d. Radiopaque

13 An example of positive contrast media that may be injected intravascularly is:
  a. Nonsoluble barium
  b. Water soluble barium
  c. Water soluble iodine
  d. b and c

14 To increase the radiographic detail or definition
  a. Increase the object film distance
  b. Decrease the source image distance
  c. Increase the source image distance
  d. Increase the focal spot size

15 There is approximately a 1 cm, or 0.5 inch, clear band along one of the narrow film edges of the processed radiograph. This occurred because the:
  a. Developer is too low
  b. Fixer is too low
  c. Field size was collimated in too far
  d. Film edge was exposed to light

BIBLIOGRAPHY

Curry TS, Dowdy JE, Murray RC: *Christensen's physics of diagnostic radiology,* ed 4, Philadelphia, 1990, Lea & Febiger.

Darby ML, editor: *Mosby's comprehensive review of dental hygiene,* ed 3, St. Louis, 1994, Mosby-Year Book, Inc.

Douglas SW, Herrtage ME, Williamson HD: *Principles of veterinary radiography,* ed 4, Philadelphia, 1987, Bailliere Tindall.

Eastman-Kodak Company: Kodak: *The fundamentals of radiography,* ed 12, Rochester, New York, 1980.

Kleine LJ, Warren RG: *Small animal radiography,* St. Louis, 1982, CV Mosby.

Lavin L: *Radiography in veterinary technology,* Philadelphia, Pennsylvania, 1993, W.B. Saunders.

McCurnin D: *Clinical textbook for veterinary technicians,* ed 3, Philadelphia, Pennsylvania, 1994, W.B. Saunders.

Morgan JP: *Techniques of veterinary radiography,* ed 5, Ames, 1993, Iowa State University Press.

NCRP: *Radiation protection in veterinary medicine,* #36, Bethesda, Maryland, 1970.

NCRP: *Structural shielding design and evaluation or medical use of x-rays and gamma rays of energies up to 10 meV,* #49, Bethesda, Maryland, 1970.

Owens JM: *Radiographic interpretation for the small animal clinician,* St. Louis, 1982, Ralston Purina Company.

Rendano VT, Ryan G, Bassano: Radiation safety—transparent leaded-plastic panels: a product evaluation, *J Am An Hosp Assoc* 23:141-4, 1987.

Rendano VT, Ryan G: Technician assistance in radiology, Part II. Basic consideration and radiation safety, *Comp Contin Ed* 9:547-51, 1988.

Ryan GD: *Radiographic positioning of small animals* Philadelphia, 1981, Lea & Febiger.

Smallwood JE et al: A standardized nomenclature for radiographic projections used in veterinary medicine, *Vet Radiol J* 26:2-9, 1985.

Ticer JW: *Radiographic technique in veterinary practice,* ed 2, Philadelphia, Pennsylvania, 1984, W.B. Saunders.

CHAPTER 13

Ultrasonography

Pierry Kuskis

OUTLINE

Basic Physics of Ultrasound
  Image Production
  Sound Waves
  Attenuation
  Acoustic Impedance
Ultrasound Machine
  Transducers
  Transducer Crystals
  Piezoelectric Effect
  Bandwidth
  Types of Transducers
  Equipment Controls
Equipment Controls
  Brightness and Contrast
  Gain and Power
  Time-Gain Compensation

Image Physics
  Resolution
  Sound Beam Zones
  Focusing
The Display
  Display Format
Final Image
  Image Characteristics
  Organ Appearance
  Scanning Planes
Artifacts
  Propagation Artifacts
  Attenuation Artifacts
  Other Artifacts
Examination
  Preparing the Patient

Sonographic Appearance of Organs
  Spleen
  Liver
  Gallbladder
  Kidneys
  Bladder
  Prostate
  Uterus
  Stomach and Bowel
  Pancreas
  Adrenal Glands
Lesions
  Appearance
  Classification of Lesions

LEARNING OUTCOMES

After reading this chapter you should be able to:

1. Have a better understanding of the basic physics of ultrasound.
2. Be familiar with the basic functioning of the ultrasound machine.
3. Understand the concepts of image physics.
4. Have an understanding of the concepts of the final image and artifacts.
5. Differentiate between the sonographic appearance of anatomical features and artifacts.
6. Properly prepare a patient for routine ultrasonography.
7. Explain the equipment controls responsible for the images.

Ultrasound is a diagnostic modality used to image various organs in the living body. By noninvasive means, the veterinary technologist may use ultrasound to determine and compare the location, size, and echogenicity of certain structures. Imaging can be done easily to most animals without tranquilization so that even the most critically ill patient can tolerate the examination. It is important to understand the basic fundamentals of physics concerning ultrasound. Without this knowledge, it would be difficult to understand the applications and limitations of ultrasound. In this chapter, the ultrasound machine, organ characteristics, artifacts, and patient preparation will be discussed.

BASIC PHYSICS OF ULTRASOUND

Definition: waves of sound that are of a frequency beyond the range of human hearing

Image Production

I. Waves travel through media, transferring energy from one location to another

II. Sound waves are reflected back to the transducer, analyzed by a computer, and displayed on a screen

Sound Waves (Figure 13-1)

I. Wavelength (λ)

A. Definition: the distance that a wave must travel in one cycle

B. Ultrasound has a shorter wavelength than that of audible sound

C. Wavelength is determined by the characteristics of the transducer

II. Frequency (f)

A. Definition: the number of cycles per unit of time (seconds)

B. As frequency increases, the wavelength decreases

C. Ultrasound waves are in the 2 to 10 MHz range compared to human hearing, which is around 20,000 Hz

III. Velocity (v)

A. Definition: the speed at which sound travels through an object = frequency × wavelength

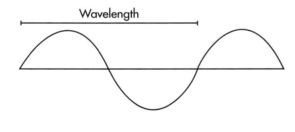

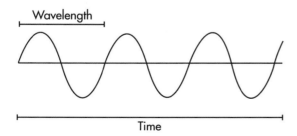

Figure 13-1 Frequency and wavelength are inversely related. As the wavelength increases, the frequency decreases. (From Han CM, Hurd CD: *Practical Guide to Diagnostic Imaging; Radiography and Ultrasonography,* St Louis, 1994, Mosby.)

B. When the sound wave returns, the computer records the time

C. The computer will use the time taken for the echo to return to calculate the depth at which the sound was reflected

IV. Amplitude: intensity or loudness of a wave

V. Period (T): time needed to produce one cycle

Attenuation

I. Definition: the loss of intensity of the ultrasound beam as it travels through tissue due to:

A. Absorption: production of heat as sound passes through soft tissue, causing loss of energy

B. Scattering: sound is reflected in different directions from dissimilar tissue interfaces

C. Reflection: the return of a part of the ultrasound beam toward the transducer

Acoustic Impedance

I. Definition: the ability of tissue to resist or allow the transmission of sound

II. Impedance depends on the density of certain tissue

III. Air and bone have a high acoustic impedance, hindering the passage of the ultrasound wave, whereas tissue, with a low acoustic impedance, is favorable

ULTRASOUND MACHINE

Transducers

I. Definition: the part of the ultrasound machine used to scan a patient

A. Devices that convert one form of energy to another

B. Send out a series of sound pulses and collect the returning echoes

II. Pulsed wave transducers

A. A short burst of sound is emitted from this transducer. It waits until the echo comes back before sending another one

B. Most common

C. One transducer alternately transmits and receives

III. Continuous wave

A. Contains two transducers: one transducer constantly sends sound waves while the other one listens

Transducer Crystals

I. Definition: the active element required to promote the conversion of electrical energy to ultrasound

A. Natural crystals: quartz, tourmaline, rochelle salt

B. Synthetics: most common; lead zirconate titonate, barium titanate, and lithium sulfate
C. The crystal produces sound by vibrations through the piezoelectric effect
D. After pulses are sent, the crystals are dampened to stop vibrations
E. Struck by the echoes returning, they start to vibrate again
F. Crystals convert echoes into electrical energy

Piezoelectric Effect

I. Definition: the conversion of electrical energy to pressure energy (ultrasound or acoustic)
II. Piezoelectric means pressure electricity

Bandwidth

I. Definition: the entire range of frequency
II. A transducer can produce more than one frequency above or below its center frequency

Types of Transducers

I. Mechanical sector
A. Consists of one or more crystals mechanically steered to produce a 'pie-shaped' image
II. Linear array
A. Consists of a small row of crystals sequentially pulsed
B. Produces parallel lines and allows the image to be rectangular
C. Ideal for transrectals and equine tendons
III. Phased array sector scanner
A. Contains about 20 crystals, which are electronically steered through a sector
B. Commonly used in echocardiography
C. Usually small and expensive

EQUIPMENT CONTROLS

The ultrasound machine has many controls for adjusting the image. Improper use may decrease quality of the image and possibly produce lesions that, in fact, don't exist.

Brightness and Contrast

I. Display monitor controls should be adjusted so that black, white, and all different shades of gray can be seen

Gain and Power

I. Affects brightness of the image
II. The higher the overall gain or power, the brighter the image
III. Increasing the power increases the intensity of the sound leaving the transducer and the waves returning to it, since gain amplifies the returning echoes

Time-Gain Compensation (TGC)

I. TGC adds increasing amounts of electronic gain to the more distant echoes
II. It enables the returning echoes from different depths to have the same brightness on the monitor
III. TGC consists of near-field, far-field, gain, and delay controls

IMAGE PHYSICS

Resolution

I. Definition: the ability to separately identify small structures on the ultrasound image
A. The frequency of the transducer dictates the resolution of the image
B. The higher the frequency (i.e., 7.5 MHz) the shorter the wavelength and thus the better the resolution
II. Lateral resolution
A. The ability of the ultrasound beam to separate two structures lying perpendicular to the beam; depends on the beam diameter (width)
B. The distance between two interfaces must be greater than the beam width for each interface to be identified separately
III. Axial resolution
A. Depends on the wavelength of the sound frequency used
B. Ability of the ultrasound beam to separate two structures lying along the path of the beam
C. By using the narrowest beam width possible, one can achieve the best resolution

Sound Beam Zones

Sound beam zones are determined by the dimensions and design of the transducer.
I. Near field
A. The portion of the sound beam where the beam width narrows as the distance increases until it reaches the narrowest portion
B. The area of the beam closest to the crystal
II. Focal point
A. Where the beam reaches its narrowest point
III. Far field
A. The area of the beam in which the boundaries diverge

Focusing

I. Definition: the method of moving the focal point closer to the image, to narrow the width and improve resolution

II. Transducers are focused by shaping the crystal, addition of a lens, or combining both concepts

THE DISPLAY
Display Format

I. Definition: how the returning echo, or the image, appears on the screen
   A. Can be rectangular or sector
II. A mode: (amplitude mode) (Figure 13-2)
   A. One-dimensional graphic display
   B. Returning echoes are viewed as a series of peaks on a graph
   C. The greater the intensity, the higher the peak

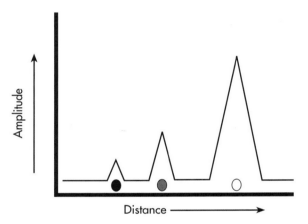

Figure 13-2 Where A-mode uses peaks on a graph to depict the strength of the returning echoes, B-mode uses bright pixels, or dots, on a monitor. The brighter the pixel, the stronger the returning echo. (From Han CM, Hurd CD: *Practical Guide to Diagnostic Imaging; Radiography and Ultrasonography,* St Louis, 1994, Mosby.)

III. B mode (brightness mode) (see Figure 13-2)
   A. Depicts dots on a screen as a two-dimensional image
   B. Brightness of the dot depends on the intensity of the returning echo
   C. The position of the dot on the base line depends on the depth of the reflecting structure
IV. M mode (motion mode) (Figure 13-3)
   A. A two-dimensional display of a reflector over time
   B. The position of a reflector is displayed on the vertical axis and time is displayed on the horizontal axis
   C. Stationary objects result in straight lines while moving ones will be wavy
   D. Mainly used in cardiology to assess cardiac valves, walls, and chamber size

FINAL IMAGE
Image Characteristics (Figure 13-4)

The format used for ultrasound display is a black background on which echo information appears in white. Size, shape, and margins of the organs should be known so that any deviation from the normal can be documented.

I. Echogenic (echoic)
   A. Tissue that produces enough echoes to return to the transducer to be displayed
   B. Appears white on the screen
   C. The greater the difference between two adjacent organs, the greater the echo reflection between them
II. Sonolucent
   A. Majority of the sound is penetrating deeper into the tissue with only a few echoes being reflected back

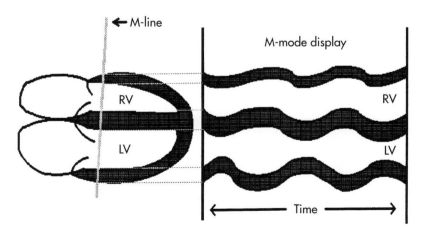

Figure 13-3 M-mode displays the motion of a thin slice of an organ over time. (From Han CM, Hurd CD: *Practical Guide to Diagnostic Imaging; Radiography and Ultrasonography,* St Louis, 1994, Mosby.)

III. Anechoic
 A. Describes tissue that transmits all the sound to deeper tissue
 B. Appears black on the screen and is usually fluid filled
IV. Hyperechoic
 A. Appears brighter than surrounding tissue and thus more echogenic
 B. Tissue that reflects more sound back to the transducer than the area around it
 V. Hypoechoic
 A. Area appears darker than surrounding tissue
 B. Reflects less sound back than the area of tissue around it
VI. Isoechoic
 A. Tissue equal in appearance to that of surrounding tissue

Organ Appearance

 I. Contour
 A. Is the organ outline smooth, rough, or irregular?
 II. Texture
 A. Is the organ parenchyma homogeneous?
III. Shape
 A. Does the organ have its proper shape?
IV. Size
 A. Specific organs should be measured to determine whether or not they are within normal parameters

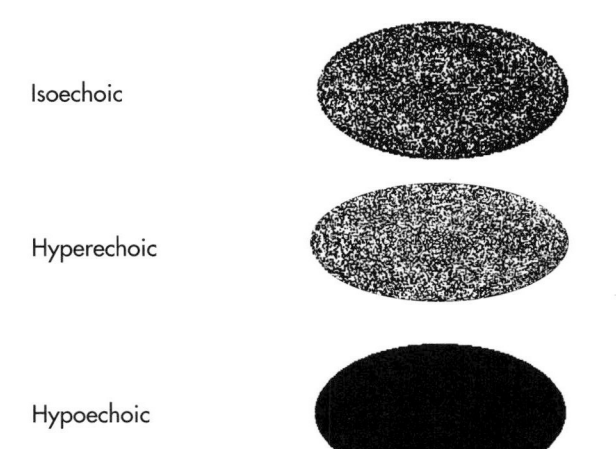

Isoechoic

Hyperechoic

Hypoechoic

Figure 13-4 An area within an organ or the whole organ that is brighter or whiter than surrounding tissue is described as hyperechoic. Areas that are darker than surrounding tissue are descibed as hypoechoic. Areas that are the same as surrounding tissue are described as isoechoic. (From Han CM, Hurd CD: *Practical Guide to Diagnostic Imaging; Radiography and Ultrasonography,* St Louis, 1994, Mosby.)

Scanning Planes

The animal should be scanned laterally or in dorsal recumbency and the organs should be scanned in two planes.
 I. Sagittal (longitudinal) or long axis
 A. Transducer marker should be constantly held to the cranial or caudal end of the animal
 II. Transverse (short axis)
 A. Transducer marker should be 90° to the longitudinal plane

ARTIFACTS

Definition: refers to something seen on an ultrasound image that anatomically, does not exist
 I. Artifacts occur during imaging
 II. Some are a direct benefit; others are not
III. It is important to distinguish between artifacts and real structures

Propagation Artifacts

 I. Reverberations
 A. Appear as many linear echoes
 B. Occur when sound is reflected constantly between a strong reflector (i.e., bone or air and the transducer surface)
 II. Refraction
 A. Occurs when the sound beam changes direction as it passes from one medium to another
 B. Allows the organ to appear in different positions
III. Mirror image
 A. Appears when an organ lies next to a reflector; on the image, the organ appears to be present on both sides of the reflector
 B. Often occurs in the region of the diaphragm and liver

Attenuation Artifacts

 I. Acoustic shadowing
 A. Occurs when sound is totally reflected or absorbed by an object
 B. Prevents sound from traveling to a greater depth
 C. Calculi, bowel gas, etc. can cause this posterior shadowing
 II. Enhancement
 A. Echoes beside a fluid-filled structure will not be as strong as the ones behind it
 B. Enhancement occurs because sound transmitted through fluid is less attenuated than the tissue beside it
 C. This artifact can determine if the lesion is a hypoechoic mass or a cyst

Other Artifacts

I. Ring down
   A. Similar to reverberation
   B. Produces many parallel echoes
   C. Associated with gas bubbles
II. Comet tail
   A. Similar to reverberation
   B. Caused by a strong reflector
   C. Consists of thin lines with close echoes

EXAMINATION

Preparing the Patient

I. Shaving
   A. Essential, because the ultrasound beam would otherwise pass and reflect through air-filled haircoat before penetrating the skin
   B. For abdominal ultrasounds, the abdomen should be shaved, using a #40 clipper blade, from the xyphoid process to the pubis, then, laterally, from the rib cage to the flanks
   C. For cardiac ultrasounds, the cardiac region is shaved using a #40 blade
   D. Alcohol can be used to wipe away residual dirt and hair
II. Positioning
   A. Small animals should be placed in dorsal recumbency in a padded V-shaped trough for abdominal ultrasounds
   B. Cardiac small animal patients are placed in sternal or lateral recumbency with the shaved cardiac region situated over a hole in the table so that the transducer may be passed through it
   C. Ultrasound is usually performed with large animals in a standing position.
III. Acoustic coupling gel should be used so that no air is present between the transducer and the skin surface
IV. Physical and/or chemical restraint should be used as needed
V. Each ultrasound examination, should be done in the same systematic order so as not to miss anything
VI. Small dogs and cats can be scanned using a 7.5 MHz transducer. It provides better detail and greater attenuation but less depth penetration. Larger dogs can be scanned with a 5 MHz transducer. The lower frequency increases the depth of penetration but results in less detail and attenuation

SONOGRAPHIC APPEARANCE OF ORGANS

Spleen

I. Most hyperechoic
II. Uniform, granular appearance
III. Surrounded by a bright capsule
IV. Seen best on left side of the patient
V. Lies close to the surface

Liver

I. Less echogenic than the spleen
II. Contains many vessels and bile channels
III. Overtexture is coarse
IV. Contains gallbladder

Gallbladder

I. Anechoic with a bright wall
II. Sometimes contains sludge
III. Can be large in an animal that has fasted

Kidneys

I. Ovoid shape
II. Surrounded by a bright capsule
III. Cortex is hypoechoic
IV. Medulla is anechoic
V. Bright central area is pelvic fat
VI. A saggital view should be measured to assess size

Bladder

I. Anechoic with a hyperechoic wall
II. Debris often seen

Prostate

I. Can be visualized by following the urethra into the pelvic inlet
II. Surrounds urethra and is bilobed with a bright appearance

Uterus

I. If enlarged, can be seen adjacent to the bladder
II. Wall is hypoechoic

Stomach and Bowel

I. Difficult to image due to gas
II. Walls seen as white or dark gray
III. Rugal folds can be visualized in the stomach

Pancreas

I. Adjacent to duodenum and between stomach and spleen

Adrenal Gland

I. Hypoechoic
II. Uniform gray color
III. Found medial and cranial to, or beside, the cranial pole of the kidneys
IV. Caudal pole of the adrenal is next to the renal artery as it joins the aorta

LESIONS

Disease can appear as an alteration in echo texture in an organ.

Appearance of Lesions

I. Focal changes
   A. Readily identified
   B. Can be in one specific area of the organ
II. Diffuse
   A. Can be subtle changes
   B. Can affect the whole organ, thus texture needs to be assessed by comparisons with other organs

Classification of Lesions

I. Cystic
   A. Well-defined borders
   B. No internal echoes
   C. Shows posterior enhancement
II. Solid
   A. Contains many echoes, which can be spread throughout
   B. No posterior enhancement
III. Mixed
   A. Contains cystic and solid lesions
   B. Borders may be irregular

Glossary

A mode Demonstrates returning ultrasound beam as peaks on a graph; the more intensified the beam, the higher the peak

acoustic impedance Ability of tissue to hinder the transmission of sound

amplitude Intensity or loudness of an ultrasound wave

anechoic Waves are transmitted to deeper tissue; none are reflected back

attenuation Loss of intensity of the ultrasound beam as it travels through tissue, caused by absorption or scatter

axial resolution Ability of the ultrasound beam to identify separate structures

B mode Uses bright dots or pixels on the screen to identify the intensity of ultrasound echoes; the position of the dot depicts the depth of the reflecting structure

cystic lesion Has a well-defined border with no internal echoes and shows posterior enhancement

diffuse Subtle chances that can affect an entire organ

echoic Tissue that produces enough echoes when it is returned to the transducer and displayed

focal changes Readily identified lesions found in a specific area of an organ

frequency The number of cycles per unit of time

hyperechoic Tissue that reflects more sound back to the transducer than the surrounding tissues; appears bright

hypoechoic Tissue that reflects less sound back to the transducer than the surrounding tissue; appears dark

isoechoic Tissue that has the same ultrasonic appearance as that of the surrounding tissue

lateral resolution The ability of the ultrasound beam to identify separate structures that lie in a plane perpendicular to the sound beam

linear scanner A scanner that produces a rectangular image

M mode A mode of ultrasound that displays a two-dimensional image over a timed baseline

mixed lesion Borders are irregular and contain cystic and solid areas

piezoelectric effect The conversion of electrical energy to ultrasound

saggital Transducer marker is held to the cranial or caudal end of the animal; provides a scan of the long axis of an organ

sector scanner Scanner that produces a "pie-shaped" image with a narrow near field and a wide far field

solid Contains many echoes spread throughout

transducer The part of the machine that actually scans the patient, emits pulses of sound, and receives the returning echoes

transverse Transducer marker held 90° to the longitudinal plane; provides short axis view of organs

ultrasound The method of sending high frequency sound waves into tissues and receiving the returning echoes as an image; a noninvasive diagnostic procedure

velocity The speed at which sound travels through an object

wavelength The length that a wave must travel in one cycle

Review Questions

1 When the sonographer chooses a higher frequency transducer, it must be kept in mind that there is:
   a. Less resolution but greater depth penetration
   b. Better resolution but less depth penetration
   c. Less resolution and less depth penetration
   d. Better resolution and better depth penetration

2 A hyperechoic lesion appears:
   a. Brighter than surrounding tissue
   b. Darker than surrounding tissue
   c. Dark with posterior enhancement
   d. Same as surrounding tissue

3 At which area does the ultrasound beam reach its narrowest point?
   a. Focal point
   b. Near field
   c. Far field
   d. Reverberation point

4 The purpose of the Time-Gain Compensation is to:
   a. Adjust brightness of the image
   b. Make tissues look alike
   c. Decrease contrast of the image
   d. Increase speed of the returning image

5 The transducer needs crystals that can transform electrical energy into sound, etc. The effect exhibited by these crystals is:
a. Electromagnetic
b. Impedance
c. Piezoelectric
d. Attenuation

6 The artifact that is exhibited posterior to a bladder stone is:
a. Mirror image
b. Reverberation
c. Refraction
d. Shadowing

7 Ultrasound uses sound that is in what range of human hearing?
a. Within
b. Below
c. Above
d. Equal to

8 A Mechanical Sector Scanner consists of one or more crystals mechanically moved to produce what type of image?
a. Rectangular
b. Square
c. Pie-shaped
d. Linear

9 A structure that contains cystic and solid lesions is:
a. Hypoechoic
b. Anechoic
c. Complex
d. Sonolcent

10 Lateral resolution depends on beam:
a. Bandwidth
b. Frequency
c. Wavelength
d. Width

11 Which organ is the most echogenic?
a. Bladder
b. Liver
c. Kidney
d. Spleen

12 Hertz refers to:
a. Velocity
b. Density
c. Cycles per second
d. Wavelength

BIBLIOGRAPHY

Han C, Herd C, Kerklis L: *Practical guide to diagnostic imaging: radiography and ultrasonography,* Goleta, California, 1994, American Veterinary Publications Inc.

McCurnin, DM, editor: *Clinical textbook for veterinary technicians,* ed 3, Philadelphia, 1994, W.B. Saunders.

Odwin C, Dubinsky T, Fleischer A: *Appleton and Lange's review for the ultrasonography examination,* ed 2, Norwalk, Connecticut, 1993, Appleton and Lange.

CHAPTER 14

Sanitation, Sterilization, and Disinfection

Pat Cutler

OUTLINE

Levels of Microbial Resistance
Degrees of Microbial Control
How Microbial Control Methods
  Work
  Mode of Action
  Efficacy of Microbial Control
Methods of Microbial Control
  Physical Methods
  Chemical Methods

Autoclave
  Advantages
  Disadvantages
  Function
  Types
  Operation

Quality Control For Sterilization and
  Disinfection
  Sterilization
  Disinfection

LEARNING OUTCOMES

After reading this chapter you should be able to:

1. List the classes of pathogenic organisms in order of their resistance to destruction.
2. State the percentages of microorganisms destroyed by sanitation, disinfection, and sterilization.
3. List the different ways that microbial control methods destroy or inhibit pathogenic organisms.
4. List the five categories of physical methods of microbial control.
5. Name and describe the twelve physical methods of microbial control.
6. Identify the level of microbial control achieved with each of the twelve physical methods.
7. State an example of the application of each of the twelve physical methods of microbial control.
8. List the properties of the "ideal chemical agent" for microbial control.
9. Name and describe the ten classes of microbial control chemicals.
10. Identify the level of microbial control achieved by the ten chemical classes.
11. State an example of each of the ten chemical classes of microbial control.
12. List three advantages and two disadvantages of the autoclave in animal care facilities.
13. Explain the function of the autoclave.
14. Compare the gravity displacement autoclave and the prevacuum autoclave.
15. Describe the preparation of each of the following for processing in the autoclave:
    Linen packs
    Pouch packs
    Hard goods
    Liquids
    Contaminated objects
16. List the guidelines for loading the autoclave chamber.
17. Compare the three different autoclave cycles.
18. List and define the five methods of quality control for sterilization.
19. List and define the two methods of quality control for disinfection.

The objective in sanitation, sterilization, and disinfection is to **control microorganisms,** or **pathogens,** in the environment, thus protecting patients and staff from contamination and disease and thereby promoting optimum healing and wellness.

LEVELS OF MICROBIAL RESISTANCE

    I. Pathogens are microorganisms that cause disease. As shown in Figure 14-1, all microorganisms are not equal; some are easily destroyed and some are much more resistant

    II. Microbial control is achieved by using methods of sanitation, disinfection, and sterilization to a degree that is practical, efficient, and cost effective. Sterility is used only when necessary; in many situations sanitation and disinfection create acceptable levels of microbial control

DEGREES OF MICROBIAL CONTROL

    I. Sterilization is the elimination of all life from an object, or complete microbial control. Disinfection, sanitization, and cleaning remove most microorganisms but not all (Figure 14-2).

HOW MICROBIAL CONTROL METHODS WORK
Mode of Action

Different physical and chemical methods destroy or inhibit microorganisms in several ways:

    I. Damage cell walls or membranes

    II. Interfere with cell enzyme activity

    III. Destroy microbial cell contents by oxidation, hydrolysis, reduction, coagulation, denaturation, or the formation of salts

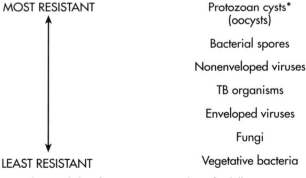

MOST RESISTANT

Protozoan cysts*
(oocysts)

Bacterial spores

Nonenveloped viruses

TB organisms

Enveloped viruses

Fungi

LEAST RESISTANT

Vegetative bacteria

*No chemical disinfectant carries a claim for killing oocysts; the best method for eliminating them is to use heat and agitation (or the autoclave).

Figure 14-1 Ranking of microorganisms according to resistance to destruction by chemical methods. (Courtesy McLaughlin S.)

Efficacy of Microbial Control

The effectiveness of all microbial control methods depends on the following factors:

    I. Time: most methods have minimum effective exposure times

    II. Temperature: most methods are more effective as temperature increases

    III. Concentration and preparation: chemical methods require appropriate concentrations of agent; disinfectants may be adversely affected by mixing with other chemicals

    IV. Organisms: type, number, and stage of growth of target organisms

    V. Surface: physical and chemical properties of the surface to be treated may interfere with the method's activity; some surfaces are damaged by certain methods

    VI. Organic debris or other soils: if present, will dilute, render ineffective, or interfere with many control methods

    VII. Method of application: items may be sprayed, swabbed, or immersed in disinfectants; cotton and some synthetic materials used to apply or store chemicals may reduce their activity

METHODS OF MICROBIAL CONTROL
Physical Methods

    I. Dry Heat (mode of action: oxidation)

       A. Incineration (efficacy: complete sterilization)

          1. Material or object is exposed to a hot fire

          2. Object must become red hot as in 'loops' for microbiology

          3. Used to dispose of tissue or carcasses; must be burned to ashes

       B. Hot air oven (efficacy: complete sterilization)

          1. Sterility requires 1 hour of exposure to 170° C (340° F)

          2. Useful for powders and nonaqueous liquids such as paraffin or vaseline

          3. Used in some animal care facilities

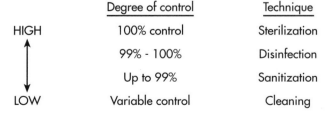

	Degree of control	Technique
HIGH	100% control	Sterilization
	99% - 100%	Disinfection
	Up to 99%	Sanitization
LOW	Variable control	Cleaning

Figure 14-2 Degree of microbial control by various techniques. (Adapted from Minshall DK: *CALAS Training Manual.*)

4. Useful for domestic applications (e.g., the kitchen oven)
C. Drying (efficacy: incomplete sterilization)
   1. Most organisms require humidity to survive and grow
   2. A clothes drier is best but any exposure to dry circulating air greatly reduces organism numbers

II. Moist heat (mode of action: denatures microbial protein)
   A. Hot Water (efficacy: incomplete sterilization)
      1. Used to clean and sanitize surfaces
      2. Addition of detergents increases efficacy by emulsifying oils and suspending soil so they are rinsed away
   B. Boiling (efficacy: may be complete sterilization)
      1. Requires 3 hours of boiling to achieve sterility
      2. Boiling for 10 minutes will destroy vegetative bacteria and viruses but not spores
      3. Addition of 2% calcium carbonate or sodium carbonate will inhibit rust and increase efficacy
      4. Useful for "field work"
   C. Steam (efficacy: incomplete sterilization)
      1. Similar to boiling because the temperature is the same
      2. Exposure to steam for 90 minutes kills vegetative bacteria but not spores
   D. Steam under pressure (efficacy: complete sterilization)
      1. Autoclave: most efficient and inexpensive method of sterilization for routine use in animal facilities

III. Radiation (mode of action: damages cell enzyme systems and DNA)
   A. Ultraviolet (UV) (efficacy: may be complete sterilization)
      1. Low energy ultraviolet radiation is a sterilant when items are placed at close range; UV has no penetrating ability
      2. Used to sterilize rooms
      3. Very irritating to eyes
   B. Gamma radiation (efficacy: complete sterilization)
      1. Ionizing radiation produced from Cobalt-60 source
      2. Good penetrating ability in solids and liquids
      3. Used extensively in commercial preparation of pharmaceuticals, biological products, and disposable plastics

IV. Filtration (mode of action: physically traps organisms that are too large to pass through the filter)
   A. Fluid filtration (efficacy: can be complete sterilization)
      1. Fluid, by means of positive or negative pressure, is forced through a fiber filter or more commonly a screen filter
      2. Used to sterilize culture media, buffers, and pharmaceuticals
      3. Pore size of 0.45 microns removes most bacteria but microplasmas and viruses require 0.01 to 0.1 micron pore size
      4. May be used in conjunction with a prefilter to remove larger particles
   B. Air filtration (efficacy: can be complete sterilization)
      1. Used extensively in animal care facilities in surgical masks, laboratory animal cage tops, and air duct filters
      2. Fibrous filters made of various paper products are effective for removing particles from air
      3. Efficacy is influenced by air velocity, relative humidity, and electrostatic charge
      4. HEPA: high efficiency particle absorption; filters are 99.97% to 99.997% effective in removing particles over 0.3 microns in size
      5. Surgical masks are designed to protect the patient from the wearer and *not* the wearer from the patient; special masks are available for protecting personnel from pathogens in animals
      6. Masks must fit snugly on the face, stay dry, and be changed at least every 4 hours to be effective

V. Ultrasonic vibration (mode of action: coagulates proteins and disrupts cell walls)
   A. Cavitation (efficacy: incomplete sterility)
   B. High frequency sound waves passed through a solution create thousands of cavitation "bubbles"
   C. Bubbles contain a vacuum—as they implode or collapse, debris is physically pulled from objects
   D. Effective as an instrument cleaner

Chemical Methods

Many chemicals are available to sterilize, disinfect, or sanitize but none are the "ideal" agent. Chemicals penetrate organism cell walls and react with cell components in various ways to destroy or inhibit growth. Many chemicals are disinfectants with varying levels of activity (see Table 14-1); a few are sterilants

I. Ideal chemical agent
   A. Effective against all pathogenic organisms
   B. Effective in a short time
   C. Safe for all surfaces and tissues
   D. Inexpensive and easy to store and use
   E. Not affected by organic debris or other soil
   F. Effective at any temperature
   G. Nontoxic, nonpyrogenic, nonantigenic
   H. Residual and cummulative action
II. Chemicals
   A. Soaps
      1. An anionic cleaning agent made from natural oils
      2. Ineffective in hard water
      3. Does not mix well with quaternary ammonium compounds and diminishes the effectiveness of halogens
      4. Minimal disinfectant capability and is not antimicrobial
   B. Detergents
      1. Synthetic soaps
      2. Anionic, cationic, or nonionic; anionic combined with cationic will neutralize both
      3. Anionic and nonionic soaps are good cleansers; cationic soaps are better disinfectants
      4. Most are basic; a few are acidic
      5. Emulsify grease and suspend particles in solution
      6. May contain wetting agents
III. Quaternary ammonium compounds (Quats)
EXAMPLES: Centrimide, benzalkonium chloride (Zephiran, Quatsyl-D, Germiphene)
   A. Active against
      1. G$^+$ bacteria
      2. Some G$^-$ bacteria
      3. Some fungi
      4. Some viruses—new formulations
   B. Organically substituted ammonium compounds
   C. Inactivated by organic material, soap, hard water, cellulose fibers
   D. Bacteria not destroyed may clump together; those inside are protected
   E. More effective in basic pH
   F. A cationic detergent
   G. Deodorizes
   H. Dissolve lipids in cell walls and cell membranes
IV. Phenols
EXAMPLES: phenol, carbolic acid, coal tar phenols, cresol
   A. Active against
      1. G$^+$ bacteria
      2. G$^-$ bacteria
      3. Lipophilic viruses
      4. Some fungi
   B. Developed from phenol or carbolic acid
   C. Synthetic phenols are prepared in soap solutions that are nontoxic and nonirritating
   D. Standard by which other disinfectants are measured
   E. Toxic to cats, since they lack inherent enzymes to detoxify
   F. May be toxic to rabbits and rodents
   G. Activity decreased by Quats
   H. Not inactivated by organic matter, soap, or hard water
   I. Toxic to skin and mucous membranes (except synthetic phenols)
V. Aldehydes
EXAMPLES: gluteraldehyde, formaldehyde
   A. Active against
      1. G$^+$ bacteria
      2. G$^-$ bacteria
      3. Most acid-fast bacteria

Table 14-1 Levels of disinfection

Some manufacturers refer to low, medium, and high level disinfectants. Higher level products are effective against a greater variety of organisms. They must kill hydrophilic and lipophilic viruses. They must also kill spores. Medium level disinfectants must be tuberculocidal. Low level products kill vegetative bacteria.

	Bacteria			Viruses		
LEVEL	VEGETATIVE	ACID-FAST	SPORES	LIPOPHILIC	HYDROPHILIC	EXAMPLE
HIGH	+	+	+	+	+	aldehydes, VPHP, chlorine-dioxide
MEDIUM	+	+	0	+	+/−	alcohols, phenols, 7th gen. Quats
LOW	+	0	0	+/−	0	Quats

Courtesy McLaughlin S.

     4. Bacterial spores

     5. Most viruses

     6. Fungi

     7. Considered to be a *sterilant* but may require 12 hours of contact

  B. Gluteraldehyde (Cidex)

     1. Noncorrosive

     2. Supplied as an acid, activated by adding sodium bicarbonate

     3. Good for plastics, rubber, lenses in "cold sterilization"

     4. Inactivated by organic material

     5. Irritating to respiratory tract and skin

  C. Formaldehyde (Formicide)

     1. Aqueous solution 37%-40% w/v formaldehyde

     2. May be diluted with water or alcohol

     3. Irritating to tissue and respiratory tract; toxic

     4. A vapor phase surface disinfectant that slowly yields formaldehyde

VI. Biguanide

EXAMPLES: chlorhexidine gluconate (Hibitane, Precyde)

  A. Active against

     1. G^+ bacteria

     2. Most G^- bacteria

     3. Some lipophilic viruses

     4. Fungi

  B. Efficient disinfectant, used mostly as an antiseptic

  C. Inactivated by organic material and hard water

  D. Has immediate, cummulative, and residual activity

  E. Used as a surgical scrub and handwash

  F. Low toxicity

VII. Chlorine and chlorine releasing compounds

EXAMPLES: chlorine gas, chlorine dioxide

  A. Active against

     1. G^+ bacteria

     2. G^- bacteria

     3. Most acid-fast bacteria

     4. Bacterial spores

     5. Lipophilic and hydrophilic viruses

     6. Fungi

     7. Considered to be a sterilant

  B. Commonly available as sodium hypochlorite (household bleach)

  C. Cheapest and most effective chemical disinfectant

  D. Available chlorine equals oxidizing ability

  E. Bleaches fabrics, corrosive to metals

  F. Inactivated by organic debris

VIII. Halogens

EXAMPLES: chlorine, iodine, flourine, and bromine

  A. Active against

     1. G^+ bacteria

     2. G^- bacteria

     3. Acid-fast bacteria

     4. Lipophilic and hydrophilic bacteria

     5. Fungi

  B. Iodine most common; used in solution with water or alcohol

  C. Iodophors: iodine and detergent, nonstaining and nonirritating; used as a surgical scrub (Betadine)

  D. Inactivated by organic material

  E. The darker the color the greater the activity

  F. Aqueous forms are staining and irritating

IX. Alcohols

EXAMPLES: ethyl alcohol, isopropyl alcohol, methyl alcohol

  A. Active against

     1. G^+ bacteria

     2. G^- bacteria

     3. Acid-fast bacteria

     4. Lipophilic bacteria

     5. Hydrophilic bacteria (ethanol only)

  B. Most effective when diluted to 60%-70% (isopropyl), 70%-80% (ethyl)

  C. Used as a solvent for other disinfectants and antiseptics

  D. Low toxicity

  E. Irritating to tissues

  F. Fogs lenses, hardens plastics, dissolves some cements

  G. Inactivated by organic debris

  H. Ineffective after evaporation

  I. Defatting agent

X. Peroxygen compounds

EXAMPLES: peracetic acid

  A. Active against

     1. G^+ bacteria

     2. G^- bacteria

     3. Acid-fast bacteria

     4. Lipophylic and hydrophylic bacteria

     5. Fungi

     6. Classed as a sterilent; may not kill pinworm eggs

  B. Applied as a 2% solution for 30 minutes at 80% humidity

  C. Explosive

  D. Damages iron, steel, rubber

XI. Ethylene oxide (EO)

EO is a colorless, nearly odorless gas that diffuses and penetrates rapidly. It is flammable, explosive, toxic, carcinogenic, and irritating to tissue.

A. Active against
   1. G$^+$ bacteria
   2. G$^-$ bacteria
   3. Acid-fast bacteria
   4. Lipophilic and hydrophilic viruses
   5. Fungi
   6. Bacterial spores
   7. Classified as a sterilent
B. Effective sterilant for heat labile objects
C. Used in a chamber with a vacuum
D. May be mixed with CO_2, ether, or freon
E. Used at temperatures of 21° to 60° C (70°-140° F) (works more quickly at higher temperatures); exposure times of 1 to 18 hours
F. Requires minimum relative humidity of 30% (40% is optimum)
G. Items must be clean and dry and may be wrapped in muslin, polyethylene, polypropylene, or polyvinyl
H. Sterilized items *must* be ventilated in a designated area for 24 to 48 hours to remove residual EO
XII. Figure 14-3 ranks chemicals in order of their ability to destroy microorganisms.

AUTOCLAVE

Advantages

I. Consistently achieves complete sterility
II. Inexpensive and easy to operate
III. Safe for most surgical instruments and equipment, drapes and gowns, suture materials, sponges, some plastics and rubbers
IV. Safe for patients and personnel

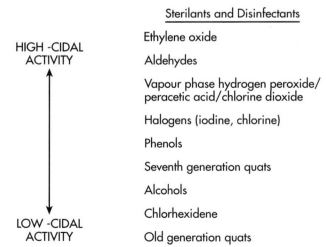

Sterilants and Disinfectants

HIGH -CIDAL ACTIVITY

Ethylene oxide

Aldehydes

Vapour phase hydrogen peroxide/peracetic acid/chlorine dioxide

Halogens (iodine, chlorine)

Phenols

Seventh generation quats

Alcohols

Chlorhexidene

LOW -CIDAL ACTIVITY

Old generation quats

Figure 14-3 Ranking of chemicals according to -cidal activity. (Courtesy McLaughlin S.)

V. Established protocols and quality control indicators are easy to access

Disadvantages

I. Staff may overestimate the ability of the autoclave—sterility depends on saturated steam of the appropriate temperature having contact with all objects within the autoclave for a sufficient length of time
II. Requires a thorough understanding of techniques to insure that the above occurs

Function

I. Heat is the killing agent in the autoclave
II. Steam is the vector that supplies the heat and promotes penetration of the heat
III. Pressure is the means to create adequately heated steam
IV. Complete sterilization is achieved after 9 to 15 minutes of exposure to 121° C (250° F)
V. The temperature of steam at sea level is 100° C (212° F); an increase in pressure results in an increase in the temperature of the steam
VI. The minimum effective pressure of the autoclave is 15 psi, which provides steam at 121° C (250° F)
VII. Many autoclaves attain pressures of 35 psi, which creates a steam temperature of 135° C (275° F) (Table 14-2)
VIII. Exposure times must allow penetration and exposure of all surfaces to 121° C (250° F) steam
IX. Exposure time is decreased by increasing pressure, which increases steam temperature

Types

I. Gravity displacement autoclave
   A. Simple autoclave that heats water in a chamber; the continued application of heat by an electric element creates pressure within the chamber, this pressure raises the boiling point of the water, and thus the ultimate temperature of the steam

Table 14-2 Steam sterilization temperature/pressure chart

Pressure (psi)	Temperature °C	°F	Time (minutes)
0	100	212	360
15	121	250	9-15
20	125	257	6.5
25	130	266	2.5
35	133	272	1

Adapted from Minshall D: *CALAS training manual,* 1995.

B. Known as gravity displacement autoclave because the steam gradually displaces the air contained within the chamber—the air is forced out through a vent

C. Timing of the cycle begins when the temperature in the chamber reaches at least 121° C (250° F)

D. After sufficient exposure time, the steam is exhausted through a vent into a reservoir

E. Air that has been sterilized within the jacket and then filtered is admitted into the chamber to replace the exhausting steam

F. If the chamber is improperly loaded or there is insufficient steam there will be air pockets remaining in the chamber that will interfere with steam penetration and result in nonsterile areas

G. Load must be dried within the autoclave

II. Prevacuum autoclave

A. Usually a much larger and more costly machine; equipped with a boiler to generate steam and a vacuum system

B. Air is forced out of the loaded chamber by means of the vacuum pump

C. Steam at 121° C (250° F) or more is introduced into the chamber; the steam immediately fills the chamber to eliminate the vacuum

D. Exposure time starts immediately

E. At completion of exposure cycle the steam is vacuumed from the chamber and replaced by hot, sterile, filtered air, which dries the contents

F. Airpockets are eliminated and processing times are reduced due to use of vacuum

G. Often equipped with readout and/or printout of chamber temperatures and pressures

Operation

I. Preparation of load

A. Linen packs

1. All instruments in packs are scrupulously cleaned and rinsed in deionized water

2. Instruments are disassembled and ratchets are open

3. Solid bottom trays or kidney dishes are not included

4. Appropriate linens are in good repair and freshly laundered

5. Disposable linens (drapes, wrappers, etc.) are *not* reused

6. An indicator is included in every pack

7. The pack is wrapped using correct technique with at least two layers of material

8. Pack is sealed with autoclave tape and labeled with date, contents, and operator

9. Pack should not exceed 30 × 30 × 50 cm (12 × 12 × 20 inches) in size

10. Pack should not exceed 5.5 kg (12 lb) in weight

11. Pack should not exceed 115.3 kg/m^3 in density

B. Pouch packs

1. Used for single instruments, sponges, etc.

2. Above guidelines apply (see Linen packs)

3. Pouches are heat sealed or ends are rolled three times and securely taped with autoclave tape

4. Labeled as above

C. Hard goods

1. Stainless steel or other hard instruments, trays, bowls, laboratory cages, and other equipment may be autoclaved without wrapping

2. Must be physically clean and rinsed in deionized water

3. Syringes are separated before autoclaving

D. Liquids

1. Contained in pyrex flask three times larger than contents require

2. Cover with *loosely* applied lid or place a needle through stopper to allow air exchange (the sterility of liquids processed in the autoclave is in question; removing liquids from the chamber is hazardous to personnel)

E. Contaminated objects

1. Used before disposal to decontaminate syringes, culture plates, etc., that contain biohazard waste

2. Place objects in appropriate container for disposal—special autoclavable biohazard bags are available

II. Loading the chamber

A. Must allow free circulation of steam; use perforated or wire mesh shelves

B. Linen packs have 2.5 to 7.5 cm (1-3 inch) space between; place multiple packs on edge instead of stacking

C. Paper/plastic pouches are placed in specially designed baskets that support them on edge with paper side of each package facing the plastic side of the adjacent package

D. Solid bowls or basins are placed upside down or on edge

E. Mixed loads (hard goods and wrapped goods) have wrapped goods on upper shelf

III. Autoclave cycles

A. Wrapped goods

1. Has "dry" cycle that allows wrapped packs to dry
2. Used for most surgical packs

B. Hard goods

1. Has no dry cycle; used for trays, bowls, cages, etc. that will not be maintained in a sterile condition
2. Also used for "flash autoclave" to quickly sterilize instruments that are needed immediately

C. Liquids

1. Exhausts steam more slowly than other cycles
2. Used for liquids that would be forced from containers during a faster exhaust

QUALITY CONTROL FOR STERILIZATION AND DISINFECTION

The effectiveness of any method of microbial control must be monitored regularly.

Sterilization

I. Recording thermometer

A. Displays temperature of autoclave chamber—operator observes for correct temperature during cycle

B. Some autoclaves are equipped with printed tape of chamber temperatures and pressures

II. Thermocouple

A. Used in steam, dry heat, and chemical sterilization chambers

B. Temperature sensors are placed in the part of a test pack that is most inaccessible to steam penetration

III. Chemical indicator

A. Definition: paper strips impregnated with sensitive chemicals that change color when conditions of sterility are met

B. Used with autoclaves and ethylene oxide systems

IV. Biological indicator

A. Bacterial spores are exposed to autoclave or ethylene oxide and then cultured

V. Bowie Dick Test

A. Tests prevacuumed autoclaves for complete removal of air and uniform steam penetration

B. Uses a pack made to specific dimensions with a cross of autoclave tape in the center

Disinfection

I. Surface sampling

A. Surface to be tested is swabbed with a sterile applicator and transferred to a suitable media plate for growth

B. Surface or item may be rinsed with sterile solution, which is examined for contaminants

C. "Contact plate" of media is touched to surface and incubated

II. Serology

A. The presence of viruses in the environment is monitored by serological testing of animals to determine the presence of antibodies

Glossary

antiseptic A chemical antimicrobial that is applied to the skin or mucous membranes

bacteriostat An agent that stops or prevents the growth of bacteria but does not necessarily kill the bacteria

cide, cidal To kill or destroy; used as a suffix after bacteria, virus, spore, etc. to denote "death to"

cleaning Physical removal of organic and inorganic soils and many microbial contaminants

disinfectant An agent, usually chemical, that is applied to inanimate objects to destroy or inhibit microorganisms

hydrophilic Affinity for water

lipophilic Affinity for fat

microorganism Microbe, especially pathogenic bacterium

pathogen Any disease-producing microorganism

sanitize The process of removing infectious material and reducing numbers of pathogens in an environment to promote health; the application of a detergent combined with a disinfectant

sterilize To eliminate all forms of life, including viruses and spores

Review Questions

1 The following microorganisms are listed from *most* to *least* resistant:

a. Fungi, spores, protozoan cysts, vegetative bacteria
b. Spores, protozoan cysts, lipophylic viruses, vegetative bacteria
c. Protozoan cysts, TB organisms, fungi, lipophylic viruses
d. Spores, protozoan cysts, lipophylic viruses, hydrophylic viruses

2 Disinfection controls (kills) _____ of the microorganisms on an object.

a. 90%

b. 99%

c. 98%

d. 95%

3 An agent that stops or prevents the growth of microorganisms but does not necessarily kill them contains the suffix:

a. –cidal

b. Pathogen

c. –stat

d. –biotic

4 A chemical antimicrobial that is applied to the skin or mucous membranes is a/an:

a. Antiseptic

b. Disinfectant

c. Antibiotic

d. Germicide

5 Factors that affect the efficacy of any method of microbial control include:

a. Temperature

b. Size of object

c. Surface of the object

d. a & c

6 Incineration and hot air ovens destroy microorganisms by what mode of action:

a. Oxidation

b. Disruption of cell membranes

c. Hydrolyzation

d. None of the above

7 The efficacy of boiling as a method of microbial control is increased by adding ——————— to the water.

a. Sodium chloride

b. Calcium chloride

c. Sodium bicarbonate

d. Sodium carbonate

8 HEPA filters are:

a. High efficiency particle absorption filters

b. Able to remove particles over 0.3 mm in size

c. The same as surgical face masks

d. Able to filter all viruses

9 Hibitane is an example of which class of disinfectant?

a. Phenols

b. Quaternary ammonium compounds

c. Biguanides

d. Halogens

10 The following chemicals are classed as sterilants:

a. Ethylene oxide, peroxygen compounds, alcohols

b. Ethylene oxide, aldehydes, quaternary ammonium compounds

c. Aldehydes, peroxygen compounds, halogens

d. Aldehydes, peroxygen compounds, ethylene oxide

11 The killing agent in the autoclave is:

a. Steam

b. Heat

c. Pressure

d. Time

12 All the following techniques promote adequate steam penetration within the autoclave *except:*

a. Unratcheting surgical instruments

b. Including basins and kidney bowls in instrument packs

c. Leaving at least 2.5 cm (1 inch) of space between packs in autoclave

d. Using freshly laundered wraps on all packs

13 The following methods of quality control use biological tests to determine the presence or absence of microorganisms on an object:

a. Serology

b. Bowie Dick test

c. "Contact" plates

d. a & c

e. None of the above

14 The minimum effective pressure in an autoclave is ——————— .

a. 5 psi

b. 20 psi

c. 25 psi

d. 15 psi

15 At 135° C (275° F) microorganisms are destroyed in ——————— minutes.

a. 3

b. 2

c. 1

d. 5

BIBLIOGRAPHY

Duggins T, Kelly B, editors: *Effective sterilization in hospitals by the steam process,* Rexdale, Ontario, 1991, Canadian Standards Association.

Duggins T, Kelly B, editors: *Recommended standard practices for emergency (flash) sterilization,* Rexdale, Ontario, 1992, Canadian Standards Association.

Kagan KG: Care and sterilization of surgical equipment, *Veterinary Technician* Vol. 13, No. 1, 1992.

Knecht CD, Allen AR, Williams DJ, Johnson JH: *Fundamental techniques in veterinary surgery,* ed 3, Philadelphia, 1987, W.B. Saunders.

McCurnin DM, editor: *Clinical textbook for veterinary technicians,* ed 3, Philadelphia, 1995, W.B. Saunders.

Minshall DK, English DRA: *Chemical disinfection of animal facilities,* parts 1 & 2, CALAS Continuing Education Compendium, pp 33-50, May, 1992.

National standards and recommended practices of sterilization, Arlington, 1988, Association for the Advancement of Medical Instrumentation.

Olfert ED, editor: *CALAS training manual,* revised 1995.

Tracy DL: *Small animal surgical nursing,* ed 2, St. Louis, 1994 Mosby.

CHAPTER 15

Surgical Preparation and Instrument Care

Melanie Harris

OUTLINE

Surgical Instruments
    Scissors
    Forceps
    Needle Holders
    Retractors
    Common Orthopedic Instruments

Miscellaneous Instruments
    Needles and Suture Material
Instrument Care and Pack Preparation
    Instrument Care
    Preparing Instrument Packs

Patient Preparation
Surgeon and Sterile Assistant Surgical Scrub
Operating Room

LEARNING OUTCOMES

After reading this chapter you should be able to:

1. Recognize common surgical instruments and define their intended use.
2. Identify types of surgical needles.
3. Identify suture material.
4. Understand the sizing of suture material.
5. Describe proper instrument care.
6. Describe pack preparation for sterilization.
7. Understand the principles of sterilization monitors.
8. Describe aseptic technique while performing a patient surgical preparation and patient positioning.
9. Describe how to maintain asepsis in a surgical suite.
10. Describe correct surgical scrubbing and conduct in the operating room.
11. List possible duties of a sterile surgical assistant.

This chapter contains basic information on identification of instruments, instrument care, and sterile technique. The chapter also includes a summary of aseptic patient preparation, pack preparation, and preparation of the surgical suite.

Acting as sterile assistant to a surgeon or as a circulating nurse during surgery are important aspects of the veterinary technician's role in a veterinary hospital. These concepts are not only learned and memorized but by experience become second nature.

SURGICAL INSTRUMENTS

The veterinary technician should be familiar with basic surgical instruments and their intended use (Figure 15-1). The following are some common instruments used in veterinary surgery.

Scissors

I. General purpose scissors can be described in three ways
   A. Type of point (e.g., blunt/blunt, sharp/blunt, or sharp/sharp)
   B. Shape of the blade (e.g., straight or curved)
   C. Cutting edge (e.g., plain or serrated)
II. Operating scissors are designed for use on specific types of tissue
   A. Mayo scissors work well for cutting and dissecting dense tissue (Figure 15-2).
   B. Metzenbaum scissors have fine tips and long handles for cutting and dissecting more delicate tissue

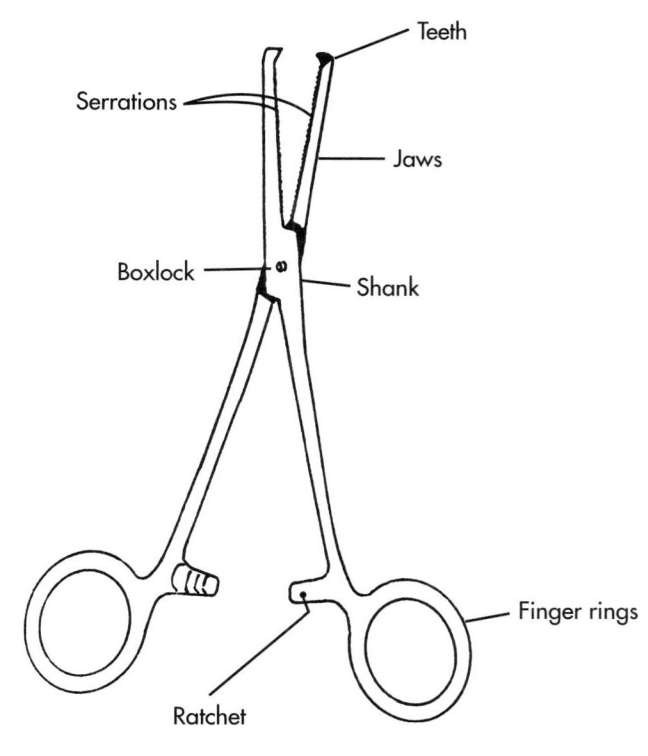

Figure 15-1 Parts of surgical instruments. (Courtesy The Ohio State University. In Tracy DL: *Small animal surgical nursing,* ed. 2, St. Louis, 1994, Mosby.

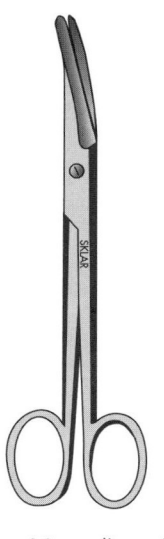

Figure 15-2 Mayo dissecting scissors.

III. Wire cutting scissors have short, thick jaws with serrated edges for cutting wire suture material
IV. Littauer and Spencer suture removal scissors are used to cut and remove sutures postoperatively
    A. Blunt tips with one blade terminating into a thin curved hook
    B. Spencer scissors are smaller than Littauer scissors
V. Lister bandage scissors are used to cut under a bandage without puncturing the patient's skin (Figure 15-3)
    A. One blade has a flat, thick edge and a blunt tip
    B. Available in various sizes

Forceps

I. Thumb forceps are hand held in a pencil grip for holding tissue
    A. Adson tissue forceps provide good tissue grip with minimal damage to tissue due to tiny rat tooth tips
    B. Brown-Adson tissue forceps have multiple fine intermeshing teeth on edges of the tips

(Figure 15-4). The sides of the blades are wider for ease of handling
    C. Dressing forceps have serrations but no teeth on the jaws; useful for handling dressing material
    D. Russian tissue forceps have rounded tips and are used for holding hollow viscera
II. Self-retaining forceps use a ratchet-locking device to grasp and retract tissue
    A. Allis tissue forceps have intermeshing teeth that ensure a secure grip
    B. Babcock tissue forceps are similar to the Allis forceps but have no gripping teeth
    C. Sponge forceps have a hole in the center of circular tips
    D. Backhaus towel clamps are considered forceps and are used to secure drapes to the patient's skin (Figure 15-5)
III. Hemostatic forceps can be straight or curved and are used for ligating vessels and tissues
    A. Halsted mosquito forceps control capillary bleeders (Figure 15-6)
        1. Length up to 10 cm (4 inches)
        2. Serrations transverse the entire jaw length
    B. Kelly and Crile forceps are for grasping intermediate size vessels
        1. Standard lengths are 12.5 cm (4.5 inches)
        2. Kelly forceps have distal transverse grooves
        3. Crile forceps have complete transverse grooves

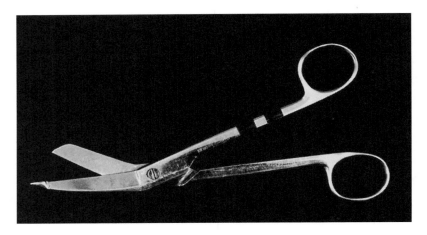

Figure 15-3　Lister bandage scissors. (In Tracy DL: *Small animal surgical nursing,* ed. 2, St. Louis, 1994, Mosby.)

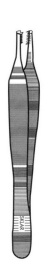

Figure 15-4　Brown-Adson tissue forceps.

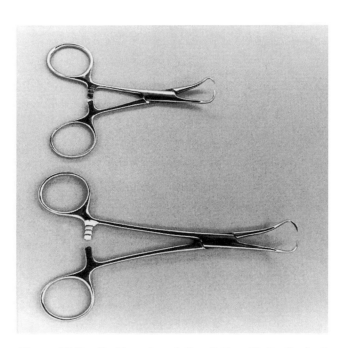

Figure 15-5　Backhaus towel clips. (In Tracy DL: *Small animal surgical nursing,* ed. 2, St. Louis, 1994, Mosby.)

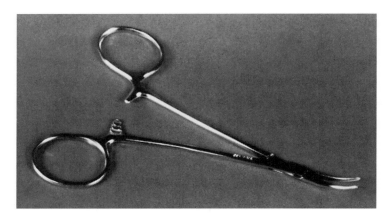

Figure 15-6　Halsted mosquito forcepts, curved. (Courtesy The Ohio State University. In Tracy DL: *Small animal surgical nursing,* ed. 2, St. Louis, 1994, Mosby.)

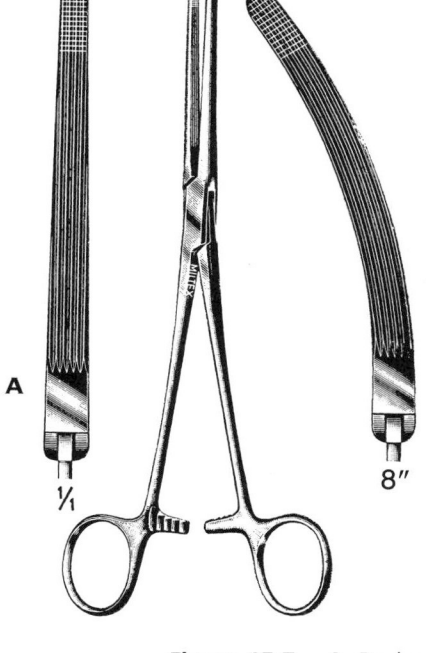

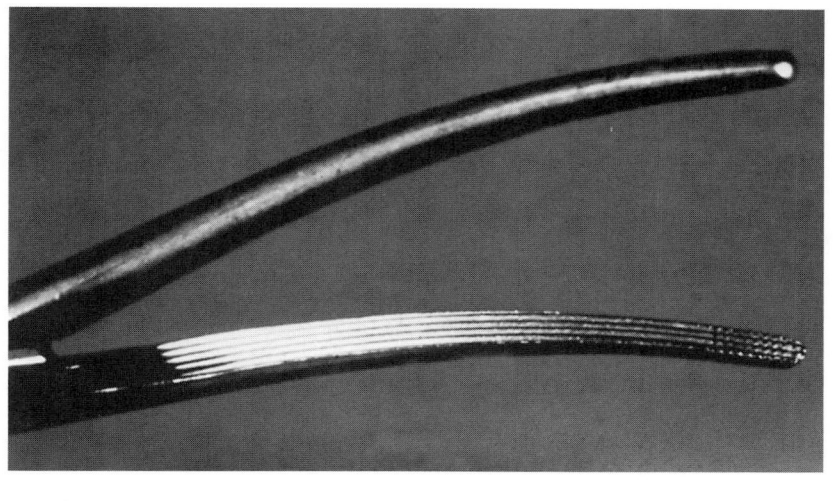

Figure 15-7 **A,** Rochester-Carmalt forceps. **B,** Rochester-Carmalt forceps have longitudinal serrations and cross-hatched pattern at tips of each jaw. (Courtesy Miltex and The Ohio State University. In Tracy DL: *Small animal surgical nursing,* ed. 2, St. Louis, 1994, Mosby.)

C. Rochester-Pean and Rochester-Carmalt forceps are commonly used in stump and pedicle ligation (Figure 15-7)
   1. Generally are 20 cm (7-9 inches) in length
   2. Carmalts have longitudinal grooves and distal transverse grooves
   3. Peans have transverse grooves
D. Rochester-Oshner forceps are similar to Rochester-Pean but also have 1:2 teeth at the tips

Needle Holders

I. Type of forceps used for holding curved needles and aid in tying sutures
II. Surgical preference determines the type of needle holder used
III. Mayo-Hegar (Figure 15-8) and Olsen-Hegar are commonly used in veterinary surgery
   A. Olsen-Hegar combine a needle holder with scissors to cut suture without using a separate scissor
   B. Mayo-Hegar can be used only as a needle holder (no scissor)

C. Crisscross grooves assist in grasping the needle
IV. Mathieu needle holders do not have rings for the fingers and spring open and closed by finger pressure

Retractors

I. Senn retractors are for skin and superficial muscle retraction
II. Meyerding, Hohmann, and U.S. Army are handheld retractors for larger muscle masses (Figure 15-9)
III. Self-retaining retractors have a locking mechanism
   A. Gelpi retractors have a single tip that extends outward to retract muscles
   B. Weitlanders are similar but have multiple prongs at the tips
   C. Balfour retractors are useful in abdominal surgery and several sizes are available
   D. Finochetto retractors are for thoracic surgery
IV. Ovariohysterectomy hook or spay hook is a type of retractor (Figure 15-10)
   A. Snook has a broad flat handle and a flat curved tip

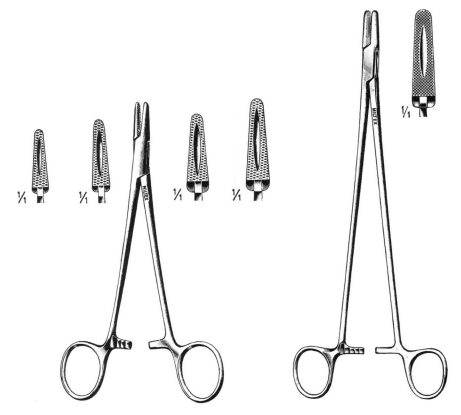

Figure 15-8 Mayo-Hegar needle holder. (Courtesy Miltex. In Tracy DL: *Small animal surgical nursing,* ed. 2, St. Louis, 1994, Mosby.)

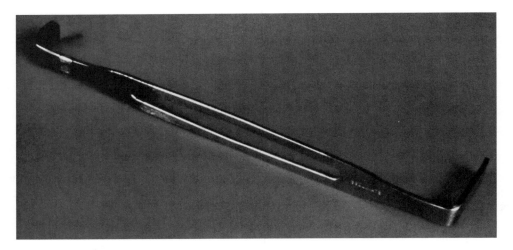

Figure 15-9 U.S. Army retractor. (Courtesy The Ohio State University. In Tracy DL: *Small animal surgical nursing,* ed. 2, St. Louis, 1994, Mosby.)

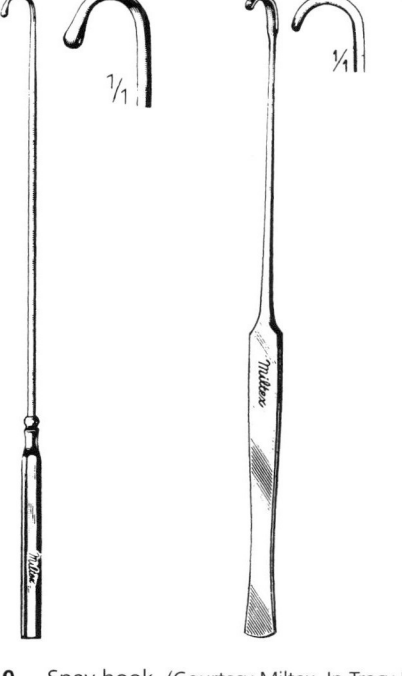

Figure 15-10   Spay hook. (Courtesy Miltex. In Tracy DL: *Small animal surgical nursing,* ed. 2, St. Louis, 1994, Mosby.)

B. Covault has an octagonal handle and a buttoned tip

Common Orthopedic Instruments

I. Kern and Richards forceps have strong gripping teeth; some have a ratchet to manipulate bone fractures to reduction

II. Verbrugge and reduction forceps can hold bone fragments in reduction while inserting fixators

III. Wire twisters look like a larger needle holder

IV. Jacobs chucks are used to advance pin placement

V. Rongeurs, such as the Lempert, are used to break up and remove bone

VI. Periosteal elevators, such as the Freer and Langbeck, are used to remove muscle from bone by releasing the periosteum

Miscellaneous Instruments

I. Suction tip chosen depends on its intended use
A. Poole tips work well to remove abdominal fluid without being plugged by omentum
B. Frazier-Ferguson tips allow variable suction strength for removing blood
C. Yankauer tips are best for removing fluid but not blood

II. Bard-Parker scalpel handle is used with a detachable blade
A. Use a needle holder to attach and remove the blade
B. A size #3 handle with a #10, #11, #12, or #15 blade are most commonly used in small animal surgery
C. A size #4 handle and a #20 blade can also be used

III. Groove directors are sometimes used to assist in making an incision

Needles and Suture Material

I. Surgical needles are available in several sizes and forms
A. Can be straight, curved, half curved, or half circle
1. Curved needles are most commonly used
2. Curved needles are described by their circle size (i.e., ¼, ⅜, ½, ⅝ circle)
3. One half curved needles are straight except for a curved tip
B. Needle points are cutting or tapered (noncutting)
1. Type of cutting points can be reverse, triangular, or side cutting for skin, cartilage, or tendons
2. Taper point needles are round or oval with reverse cutting points for tissues that may tear easily
C. Needles can be eyeless (swaged) or with an eye (round, square)
1. Needles "swaged on" to the suture are less traumatic, since needle size is relative to suture size
2. Using a separate needle and suture can cause tissue damage if used improperly
a. Needle and suture should be close to the same size
b. Thread suture through curved needles from the inside without tension

II. Commonly used absorbable suture material
A. Surgical gut is the most common nonsynthetic material
B. Examples of synthetic suture material
1. Polyglycolic acid (Dexon, Davis-Geck): synthetic polyester from hydroxyacetic acid
2. Polygalactin acid (Vicryl, Eithicon): copolymer of lactic and glycolic acids
3. Polydioxanone (P.D.S., Ethicon) and polyglyconate (Maxon, Davis-Geck): synthetic polyester

III. Nonabsorbable suture material can also be natural or synthetic
- A. Examples of natural fibers for suture material
  1. Silk is considered nonabsorbable even though its tensile strength is usually lost after 6 months
  2. Cottons and linens have been used for suture material
  3. Stainless steel is used in veterinary surgery but can be difficult to work with due to decreased flexibility
- B. Examples of synthetic nonabsorbable suture material
  1. Polypropylene (Prolene, Ethicon): synthetic plastic
  2. Polyamide/nylon (Ethilon, Ethicon): polymerized plastic
  3. Polymerized caprolactrum (Vetafil, B. Braun, Melsungen AG): coated synthetic fiber commonly used for skin closure

IV. USP (Pharmacopeia) sizing is generally used when asking for suture material
- A. EXAMPLE: 4-0, 3-0, 2-0, 0, 1, 2 . . . (pronounced 4 ought)
- B. As the number increases to the right after 0, the diameter of the suture becomes heavier; thus the size increases (i.e., size 3 suture is larger than size 2 suture)
- C. As the number increases to the left of 0, the diameter of the suture is thinner; thus the size decreases (i.e., size 2-0 is larger than size 3-0)
- D. Wire suture is also sized by gauge, which varies from 18 to 40 gauge
  1. The lower the gauge number, the thicker the diameter of the wire suture

V. Suture material and needle size used are based on many factors determined by the surgeon

INSTRUMENT CARE AND PACK PREPARATION ■

Stainless steel instruments are in general expensive and high quality. If maintained well, stainless steel instruments will last a life time.

Instrument Care

I. Clean instruments in warm water and a neutral pH detergent with a hard-bristled nylon brush
II. Use an ultrasonic cleaner to clean instrument joints that are difficult to clean manually
- A. Instruments should be placed in cleaner with boxlocks and ratchets open
- B. Follow manufacturer recommendations for use
III. Use hot water to rinse the instruments

IV. Place instruments in a surgical milk solution
- A. The surgical milk solution is an excellent lubricant and rust inhibitor
- B. In general, surgical milk must be used on all instruments cleaned by ultrasound, since all traces of lubricants are lost in cleaning
- C. After immersion in instrument milk the instruments should be put on a clean paper or cloth towel to drain
V. Instruments should be examined before being packed for resterilization
- A. Check that all surfaces are clean and free of foreign material
- B. Make certain that boxlocks work smoothly and are not loose
- C. Instrument tips should close tightly and evenly, especially on all forceps and needle holders
- D. Scissors should be sharp along the entire edge of the blade

Preparing Instrument Packs

I. The packing of instruments, drapes, and gowns should be consistent and allow the greatest amount of steam sterilization
- A. Leave boxlocks and ratchets in the open position or locked no more than one click
- B. Place heavier instruments on the bottom of the packs and place first used items such as towel clamps on top
- C. Fold gowns and drapes accordion style
- D. Surgical gowns should be wrapped inside out with all ties folded inside neatly and sleeves on top of the gown
  1. The gown pack can also include a towel for drying hands after a surgical scrub
- E. Laporatomy sheets, drapes, skin towels, should be folded using the accordian pleat method (accordian pleat drape and fold in three).
  1. Some surgeons prefer to have one corner of the drape folded over for easier grasping of the drape
- F. Double linen wrappers should be used for the outside wrapper or two linen/paper wrappers can be used
- G. Packs must fit the size of the autoclave and leave ample room for steam movement
II. The wrapping of instrument packs, drapes, and gowns should be consistent for proper sterile handling technique when opened
- A. Place a minimum of two appropriate sized wrapping materials in front of you in a diamond shape

B. Place the instrument pack or linen in the center of the first or inner wrapper

C. Begin with the corner nearest you and fold over the top of the pack

D. Take a small part of that corner and fold it back toward you to leave a tab

E. Do the same with one of the side corners, then the opposite side

F. The side furthest away from you should always be folded over last

G. Tuck this last corner inside the two sides, leaving a tab that can be pulled to open

H. Repeat the same folding technique with the second or outer wrapper

III. Tape should be used on the outside of every pack and linen

A. The tape keeps the packs sealed tighter and prevents corners from unfolding

B. Useful for labeling information

1. Contents of item (i.e., large gown, general pack, etc.)

2. Complete date item was sterilized (i.e., 96-01-05)

3. Name of the technician who prepared and sterilized the pack

IV. Types of sterilization monitors

NOTE: More than one sterilization monitor should be used to ensure optimum sterility of the pack.

A. Indicator tape indicates only that an item has been exposed to steam

1. Lines on the tape will change color

2. The color change does *not* indicate that temperature has been met and maintained for a certain period of time

3. Indicator tape on the outside of the pack means only the outside of the pack has been exposed to steam

B. Chemical indicator strips change color when exposed to steam for a certain period of time

1. Place in the center in the least accessible place for steam: between folds of drapes or gown. Do not place the indicator directly on instruments

2. Must remember to check the strip as soon as pack is open

C. Biological indicators are excellent monitors of sterility

1. Tests for the most heat resistant bacteria

2. However, it does not give an immediate answer

D. Visual monitoring of sterilization should always occur to insure that adequate time and temperature has been achieved

PATIENT PREPARATION

The goal of patient preparation is to achieve asepsis or a preparation site free of germs that could cause disease or decay.

I. Hair removal should produce minimal skin trauma

A. Bathing should be done the day before surgery if possible (elective surgery)

B. Surgical hair removal should be completed with electric clippers and a #40 blade

1. Blades should be well lubricated and have no missing teeth that may tear the skin

2. Coolants prevent clipper blades from overheating

II. Start clipping at the proposed incision and work laterally against the direction of hair growth

A. Thick-coated animals sometimes require clipping with the direction of hair first, perhaps using a #10 blade initially

B. Try not to allow clipped areas to touch unclipped areas

C. In general, clip more hair rather than too little hair

D. By consulting the surgeon and the patient file, determine the proper site and the size of the site before clipping

III. Technicians should be familiar with common general surgical clips and animal placements for surgery

A. Most laparotomies such as the ovariohysterectomy and splenectomy have a standard preparation site

1. Begin by expressing the bladder before clipping

a. The bladder must be empty to increase the space in the abdominal cavity and to prevent the animal from eliminating on the surgery table while under anesthetic

2. Animals are placed in dorsal recumbency

3. Hair is removed cranially to the xiphoid process and caudally to the pubis

4. Hair is removed laterally

a. For cats, approximately one clipper blade width past the nipple line

b. For large dogs at least 4 inches of hair either side of the midline should be removed

B. Canine castrations require hair removal from the scrotum and prepuce extending into the inguinal area

1. Some surgeons prefer that the tip of the prepuce remain unshaven to reduce irritation

C. Feline castrations require less hair removal and can be done by plucking the hair from the testes and around the scrotum

D. Puppy dewclaw removal and tail docking, as well as feline declawing, do not require hair removal before surgical scrub

E. For perineal urethrostomies, rectal fistulas, and anal sac surgeries the animal is in ventral recumbency with its hindlegs hanging down over the edge of the table. The tail is tied or clipped to the top or side of the body
  1. Surgical table can be tilted upward for surgeon comfort
  2. Hair removal should be outward from the rectum and extended up the base of the tail and down both legs

F. Orthopedic surgeries require a larger surgical area prepared to enable the surgeon to manipulate the limb (e.g., lateral and medial hindlimb for a femoral intramedullary pinning)

IV. After clipping, a dust buster or central vacuum is useful to remove all loose hair from the surgery site and the surrounding area of the preparation table

V. If performing a limb surgery, the unclipped area of hair on the foot should be wrapped
  A. Plastic bags or examination gloves secured with tape work well
  B. Wrapping after the hair is clipped prevents loose hair from sticking to the tape

VI. Recommended scrub solutions are chlorohexidine or povidone-iodophor products

VII. Scrubbing process should be done with sterile gloves, gauze, and scrub bowl
  A. Begin at the incision and work outward in a circular motion
  B. Never return to the incision area without getting a new gauze square
  C. Produce a good lather but do not scrub too hard
  D. Scrubbing process should be completed a minimum of three times
    1. Gauze squares should appear clean after the final scrub
    2. Ask yourself if the skin is aseptic for surgery before continuing to the next step
  E. Apply isopropyl alcohol, chlorhexidine, or iodine as an antiseptic
  F. Final preparation should be completed in a manner such that the area of the incision is the most aseptic

  1. There are several methods to accomplish the final aseptic application
    a. Method #1: Using a nonsterile gauze square with antiseptic, make the first stroke medially down the incision line. Each subsequent stroke of antiseptic is to the right or left of the incision site, ending at the outermost border
    b. Method #2: Begin similar to Method #1, complete one side, use a new sponge soaked with antiseptic to complete the opposite side in the same manner
    c. The objective is that no stroke of antiseptic is repeated, thereby maintaining asepsis
    d. Many practices use antiseptic spray as the final prep in the operating room

VIII. Surgical preparation should be performed outside of the operating room, then carefully move the patient into surgery, trying not to contaminate the surgical scrub
  A. Reapply antiseptic after patient is positioned, using one of the above methods
  B. Repeat entire preparation if contamination occurs

IX. The patient should be tied to the table in the appropriate position
  A. The knot should be a half hitch on the limb to facilitate easy release in case of an emergency
    1. Apply ties with two contact points per limb to reduce pressure problems
    2. Do not secure too tightly, since this may cause muscle problems

SURGEON AND STERILE ASSISTANT SURGICAL SCRUB

I. Purpose: remove dirt, grease, and decrease bacterial flora from the hands and arms

II. Before scrubbing set out sterile scrub brush, any packs and surgical equipment that may be needed. Put on cap and mask, remove jewelry, ensure nails are fingertip length and that fingernails are free of nail polish
  A. There are many variations of a surgical scrub. All variations are based on timed or stroke methods of scrubbing the surface of the hands and arms. For the purposes of this text, a stroke method will be used as an example
    1. Turn on water, checking for comfortable water temperature; thoroughly wash both hands and arms; clean nails

2. Begin with a sterile scrub brush or prepackaged soap/brushes; wet the brush and/or apply antiseptic soap to it

3. Begin with one hand, scrubbing fingertips, using 12 strokes. Proceed in a methodical fashion from the baby finger to thumb, scrubbing each plane of each finger 12 times

4. Progress to the palm, then back of hand and lateral hand

5. Move to wrist area, scrubbing all four planes

6. Scrub the remaining portion of the arm, ending 2 inches proximal to the elbow

7. Rinse the brush, apply more antiseptic to the brush and begin the same procedure on the opposite hand and arm

8. After right and left arms have been scrubbed, rinse hands and arms from the fingertips to the elbows, continuing to hold hands upward

9. Drying of hands and arms: hold sterile towel away from the body. Using one side of the sterile towel, dry one hand first, followed by the arm. Use the other side of the towel for the opposite hand and arm

III. Gowning and gloving should be completed immediately after drying hands

A. Gowning

1. Hold gown by inside shoulder seams, carefully pick the gown up and away from the counter

2. The gown will unfold open

3. Slide one arm into the sleeve and then the opposite arm into the remaining sleeve

4. Allow unsterile personnel to tie the gown

B. Gloves should fit snugly but not so tightly as to cut off circulation of the hands.

C. There are two standard methods of gloving: open and closed

1. Open gloving

a. With left hand, grasp inside cuff of the right glove; pull glove over the right hand and cuff of the gown

b. The left glove can now be handled with the gloved right hand by placing the fingertips on the inside of the folded back cuff of the glove and pulling it on the left hand and over the cuff of the gown

2. Closed gloving

a. With fingertips of the right hand covered by the cuff of the gown, pick up the glove and place it on the covered left hand with fingertips of the glove facing the shoulder

b. The thumb of the glove is on top of the left hand thumb

c. Pull the glove over the cuff and push the hand into it while pushing out of the gown cuff

d. The same procedure is used for the right hand glove

e. After both gloves are in place, the gloves can be repositioned for comfort

3. After gloving is completed the hands should be held above the waist and in front of the body

OPERATING ROOM

All operating rooms have the same strict rules that must be followed. Knowing and understanding aseptic technique will help any technician adapt to any operating room.

I. Aseptic conditions must be applied to the surgical suite and the patient

A. Patients and surgery staff prep in another room

B. Only surgery related equipment belongs in the operating room

C. Always clean from ceiling to floor. Every item in the operating room must be removed and cleaned regularly with disinfectants

D. Clean daily before surgeries begin and between cases

II. Proper surgical attire is a must

A. Scrubs are specially designed for operating rooms

1. Street clothes should never be worn

2. Smocks should be worn over scrubs while clipping hair and when outside the surgical area

B. Everyone entering the surgical area must wear a cap and mask

C. Foot covers or surgery shoes must be worn

III. Talking in the operating room should be minimal

A. Talking can distract a surgeon's concentration

B. Saliva weakens the filtration of the surgical mask

IV. Movement within the operating room should be limited, since the increased air movement can increase the risk of contamination

A. Prepare any equipment that may be used before the surgery begins

B. An organized surgery suite layout will prevent movement in the room to retrieve needed equipment and material

C. The surgery suite should be located in an isolated area of the hospital with decreased traffic volume

V. An imaginary line should be drawn around the sterile field of the surgeon, operating table, and instrument tray

A. When passing sterile equipment, do not cross that line but stand near it

B. Stand to the right or to the left, so the surgeon does not have to turn his/her back to the patient

C. Hold a sterilized packaged item away from your body when opening

D. When opening items wrapped as described earlier:

1. Open the side furthest away from you using the tab

2. Proceed to do one side then the other without allowing your arms to pass overtop of the item

3. Then pull the last tab (one closest to your body) toward you, exposing the item or second sterile wrap

4. Only outer pack wrappers should be opened by unsterile personnel before surgery: keeping the inner wrap closed ensures sterility of the contents

E. How to open items in sterilization pouches

1. Determine which end is marked to be opened

2. Hold both hands in fists with thumbs on top of your index finger

3. Grab each side of the pouch, holding it between your thumb and index finger

4. Separate the seal by rolling your fists outward

5. Lower part of your fist can apply pressure to the item in the pouch to prevent it from sliding out

F. Always allow the surgeon to approach you to retrieve a sterile item or place the item in a sterile manner on the pack

VI. Surgical gowns should be considered sterile only on the front side above the waist to the shoulder and down the arms

A. Keep hands clasped in front, close to the body, and above the waist or above the surgery table

B. If trading places, pass back to back with hands folded, never turn your back toward the patient

VII. A sterile surgical assistant can perform the following functions:

A. Receive sterile equipment

1. Lift items up and out

2. Do not reach over a patient or sterile field

B. Keep the surgical table organized

C. Anticipate and pass needed equipment and instruments

1. Hand in the correct position for immediate use

2. Tap the surgeon's palm with the instrument to insure proper contact

D. Maintain hemostasis for the surgeon

1. Place suction tip near tissue not directly on the tissue

2. Dab area with gauze square, do not wipe

3. Keep count of the gauze squares used and discarded

E. Provide retraction of muscles and tissues with minimal trauma and good surgical exposure

F. Cut suture material after suture placement

VIII. If a sterile item touches an unsterile item, it immediately becomes unsterile and is discarded

A. Any item that is dropped, punctured, or wet is unsterile

B. The patient's skin is aseptic, not sterile, avoid contact

C. If in doubt, it is not sterile

Glossary

asepsis In surgery, referring to the destruction of organisms before they enter the body

fistulas Any abnormal passage within body tissue; generally a passage leading from two internal organs or an internal organ to the body surface

intramedullary Within the marrow cavity of a bone

laparotomies An incision into the abdominal wall; exploratory laparotomy often used to physically examine the abdominal organs (also referred to as celiotomy)

ligating Application of a ligature or material such as wire or suture material to tie off blood vessels to prevent bleeding or constrict tissue

ovariohysterectomy Surgical excision of the ovaries and uterus; commonly called a "spay"

pedicle A stem or stemlike structure

perineal Situated on the perineum

perineum External region between the vulva and the anus in the female or between the scrotum and anus in the male

ratchet A step-locking device on surgical instruments. The ratchet consists of a notched bar on each handle of an instrument, the notches are facing and overriding when the handles are closed and locked

serrations Having a sawlike edge or border

splenectomy Excision of the spleen

swaged-on A type of suture material that is fused to the end of the needle

transverse Extending from side to side or at right angles to the long axis

urethrostomies Creation of a permanent hole for the urethra in the perineum

viscera Internal organs enclosed within a cavity

Review Questions

1 Scissors with long handles used for cutting delicate tissue are:
   a. Littauer
   b. Metzenbaum
   c. Mayo
   d. Lister

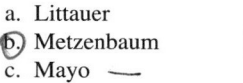

2 20 cm (7-9 inch) forceps with longitudinal grooves are:
   a. Rochester-Pean
   b. Rochester-Carmalt
   c. Kelly
   d. Crile

3 A needle holder combined with a scissor is called:
   a. Mathieu
   b. Rochester-Pean
   c. Mayo-Hegar
   d. Olsen-Hegar

4 Self-retaining tissue forceps with multiple fine intermeshing teeth at the tips are called
   a. Allis
   b. Babcock
   c. Adson
   d. Brown-Adson

5 Which of the following is *not* a type of needle point?
   a. Reverse cutting
   b. Taper
   c. Side cutting
   d. Swaged

6 An example of a nonsynthetic absorbable suture material is:
   a. Surgical gut
   b. P.D.S.
   c. Silk
   d. Nylon

7 What is the scientific name for Vetafil?
   a. Polyglycolic acid
   b. Polypropylene
   c. Caprolactrum
   d. Polydioxanone

8 What type of detergent should be used to clean instruments?
   a. Slightly acid pH
   b. Neutral pH
   c. Slightly alkaline pH
   d. Does not matter

9 The minimum number of surgical scrubs on a surgical site that should be completed is:
   a. One
   b. Two
   c. Three
   d. Four

10 Which of the following is not a recommended antiseptic for patient preparation?
   a. Chlorohexidine
   b. Alcohol
   c. Roccal
   d. Iodine

BIBLIOGRAPHY

Berg J: Sterilization. In Slatter: *Textbook of small animal surgery,* ed 2, vol 1, Philadelphia, 1993, W.B. Saunders.

Egger EL: Surgical assistance and suture material. In McCurnin DM: *Clinical textbook for veterinary technicians,* ed 3. Philadelphia, 1994, W.B. Saunders.

Fries CL: Assessment and preparation of the surgical patient. In Slatter: *Textbook of small animal surgery,* ed 2, vol 1. Philadelphia, 1993, W.B. Saunders.

Hobson HP: Surgical facilities and equipment. In Slatter: *Textbook of small animal surgery,* ed 2, vol 1. Philadelphia, 1993, W.B. Saunders.

Knecht CD et al: Operating room conduct. In *Fundamental techniques in veterinary surgery,* ed 3. Philadelphia, 1987, W.B. Saunders.

Knecht CD et al: Selected small animal surgical procedures. In *Fundamental techniques in veterinary surgery,* ed 3. Philadelphia, 1987, W.B. Saunders.

Knecht CD et al: Surgical instrumentation. In *Fundamental techniques in veterinary surgery,* ed 3. Philadelphia, 1987, W.B. Saunders.

Knecht CD et al: Suture material. In *Fundamental techniques in veterinary surgery,* ed 3. Philadelphia, 1987, W.B. Saunders.

McCurnin DM, Jones RL: Principle of surgical asepsis. In Slatter: *Textbook of small animal surgery,* ed 2, vol 1. Philadelphia, 1993, W.B. Saunders.

Miltex surgical instruments, Lake Success, New York, 1986, Miltex Instrument Co., Inc.

Nieves MA, Merkley DF, Wagner SD: Surgical instruments. In Slatter: *Textbook of small animal surgery,* ed 2, vol 1. Philadelphia, 1993, W.B. Saunders.

Oakes AB, Oakes MG, Seim III, HB: Small animal surgical nursing and dentistry. In McCurnin DM: *Clinical textbook for veterinary technicians,* ed 3. Philadelphia, 1994, W.B. Saunders.

Schwarz P, Blass C: Instrumentation and principles of aseptic technique. In McCurnin DM: *Clinical textbook for veterinary technicians,* ed 3. Philadelphia, 1994, W.B. Saunders.

Tracy DL: *Small animal surgical nursing,* ed. 2 St. Louis, 1994 Mosby.

Anesthesia

Cynthia Stoate

OUTLINE

Preanesthetic Medication
  Advantages
  Disadvantages
  Examples
Injectable Anesthetics
  Barbiturates
  Propofol
  Neuroleptanalgesics
  Ketamine
Inhalation Anesthetics
  Advantages
  Examples
Nitrous Oxide
  Advantages
  Disadvantages
  Method of use

Breathing Systems
  Rebreathing System
  Nonrebreathing System
  Partial rebreathing System
Breathing Circuits
  Circle System
  Universal F-circuit
  Bain System
Vaporizers
  Classification
  Location
Parts of an Anesthetic Machine
Stages of Anesthesia (depths)
Monitoring
  Eye
  Pedal Reflex (pain response)

Jaw Tone
Cardiovascular System
Respiratory System
Capillary Refill Time (CRT)
Mucous Membrane Color
Temperature
Analgesia
Muscle Relaxants
Ventilation
Fluid Therapy
  Fluid Characteristics
  Fluid Calculation
Blood Loss
Acid-Base Balance
Oxygenation Problems

LEARNING OUTCOMES

After reading this chapter you should be able to:

1. Understand the indications, advantages, disadvantages, effects on the body, and the associated adverse side effects of the commonly used preanesthetics.
2. Explain the rationale, effects on the body, advantages and disadvantages of the commonly used IV, IM, and inhalation anesthetic agents.
3. Identify or describe the components of general anesthesia, including the various stages and planes.
4. Know the rationale for and the various parameters that should be monitored during anesthesia.
5. Understand the differences between advantages and disadvantages of rebreathing and nonrebreathing systems.

6. Be familiar with the various parts of the anesthetic machine.
7. Differentiate between a precision and nonprecision vaporizer and recognize the advantages and disadvantages of each.
8. Understand the important concepts of analgesics and muscle relaxants.
9. Understand the techniques of assisted and controlled ventilation.
10. Know the principles involved with providing proper fluid therapy and for maintaining the acid-base balance.
11. Identify oxygenation problems that might occur.

Anesthesia is a broad subject and could involve extensive reading. This chapter condenses the information by dealing with commonly used anesthetic agents, equipment, and procedures. Although much of this chapter could pertain to any species, the emphasis is on domestic dogs and cats.

PREANESTHETIC MEDICATION

Advantages

I. Advantages will vary with different drugs but may include:
  A. Reduced stress of animal
  B. Smoother induction and recovery
  C. Decreased amount of induction and possibly maintenance agent required
  D. Analgesia intra and postoperatively
  E. Reduced secretions
  F. Reduced autonomic reflexes
  G. Handler safety

Disadvantages

I. Disadvantages are minimal
  A. Cost can be balanced by the possible reduction of induction and maintenance cost
  B. Time delay can be avoided, if necessary, by giving certain preanesthetic medications IV that will work almost immediately
  C. Some (e.g., xylazine, acetylpromazine, opioids, and diazepam) have been associated with temporary behavior and personality changes

Examples

I. Anticholinergics (parasympatholytics): for example, atropine, glycopyrrolate
  A. Indications
    1. To prevent or treat bradycardia by suppressing stimulation of the vagal nerve
    2. To reduce salivary secretions (antisialogogic) and tear secretions
    3. Dilate pupils (mydriatic)
    4. Promotes bronchodilation
    5. In combination with opioids
  B. Contraindications
    1. Tachycardiac patients
    2. Possibly with geriatrics or with other conditions such as congestive heart failure that could not handle a potential tachycardia
    3. Conditions such as constipation or ileus, which would further reduce peristaltic action of the intestine

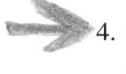

    4. Glycopyrrolate and atropine produce basically the same effect but glycopyrrolate has a slower onset of action and generally has less potential for producing a tachycardia or cardiac dysrhythmia
      a. Salivation is also more effectively suppressed with glycopyrrolate

II. Phenothiazines (tranquilizers): for example, acepromazine, chlorpromazine
  A. Indications
    1. Good sedation for healthy, elective procedures
    2. Antiemetic
  B. Contraindications
    1. Convulsing/epileptic patients, seizure history, head trauma
      a. Acepromazine may reduce the seizure threshold of the animal
    2. Shock (hypovolemic) and hypothermia due to peripheral vasodilation that can lead to hypotension
    3. Depressed
    4. Caution with geriatrics and pediatrics, use a lower dose
    5. Liver or kidney diseases
    6. Allergy testing due to antihistamine effect
  C. Other effects
    1. Antidysrhythmic effect
    2. May cause excitement rather than sedation
    3. Personality changes that usually subside within 48 hours

III. Benzodiazepines (tranquilizers): for example, diazepam (Valium), zolazepam, midazolam (Versed), and lorazepam (Ativan)
  A. Indications
    1. Convulsing/epileptic patients, seizure history, CSF tap and/or myelogram
    2. Minimal cardiovascular or respiratory depression so useful in geriatric and pediatric animals
    3. Works better in older, depressed, or anxious patients
  B. Contraindications
    1. Normal, excitable, healthy animal (may cause excitement in some dogs, cats, and horses)
      a. Doesn't sedate or tranquilize animals but has antianxiety and calming effects that may make animal more difficult to control when inhibitions and anxieties are removed
    2. Neonatal animals and animals with poor hepatic dysfunction because of poor metabolism

C. Rarely used alone and usually given intravenously because the carrier, propylene glycol, causes pain when given intramuscularly
   1. May precipitate if administered in the same syringe as other agents

IV. Alpha-2 agonists (thiazine derivative): for example, xylazine (Rompun, Anased) romifidine, detomidine (Dormosedan), and medetomidine (Domitor)
   A. Indications
      1. Potential side effects limit use to sedation only, not for preanesthetic medication
      2. Can use to sedate a vicious animal before euthanasia
      3. Have some short (16-20 minutes) analgesic effect
      4. Will cause vomiting in up to 50% of dogs and 90% of cats
      5. Xylazine and detomidine are used most frequently in horses
      6. Xylazine is used in ruminants also
         a. Use low doses in small and large ruminants
   B. Contraindications
      1. Considerable potential for adverse side effects, especially when given intravenously
      2. Whenever concerned about bradycardia, hypotension, arrhythmias, heart block, respiratory depression, hepatic and renal function, and if prone to gastric dilation and torsion
   C. Yohimbine (Yobine) can reverse the effects of xylazine
      1. Tolazoline and 4-aminopyridine can reverse the effects also
   D. Xylazine can be absorbed through skin abrasions or mucous membranes: wash any drug spilled on human or animal skin immediately

V. Opioid: for example, butorphanol (Torbugsic, Torbutrol), meperidine (Demerol, Pethidine), morphine, oxymorphone (Numorphan)
   A. Can be used for preanesthetic, for induction, or for analgesia and sedation
      1. Commonly used as preanesthetic mixture, along with an anticholinergic and a tranquilizer
      2. Also used as neuroleptanalgesia in combination with tranquilizer (fentanyl-droperidol; Innovar-Vet)
   B. Various levels of respiratory and cardiovascular depression and gastrointestinal effects,

depending on patient condition, drug, and dose
      1. Other side effects include cough suppression, miosis in dogs and mydriasis in cats, increased responsiveness to noise, excessive salivation, physical dependence
   C. Reversible by use of agent such as naloxone
   D. Some opioids may cause bizarre behavior in cats and horses
   E. Indications
      1. For good analgesia, especially acute postoperative pain
         a. More pronounced effect if given before pain perception
      2. Moderate sedation
   F. Contraindications
      1. Previous history of opioid excitement
      2. Morphine has a higher incidence of producing vomiting (depending on the dose), avoid with cases of G.I. obstruction, diaphragmatic hernia
      3. Do not give meperidine IV as it produces histamine release when given by this route
   G. Classified as narcotic in Canada and schedule II in the US with strict regulations

VI. Phencyclidines (cyclohexamine): for example, ketamine (Ketaset, Ketalean, Vetalar) and tiletamine hydrochloride (in combination with zolazepam [Telazol])
   A. Produces cardiovascular stimulation
   B. Increases muscular rigidity
   C. Causes salivation
   D. Indications
      1. Immobilization of patient
      2. Mucous membrane application via the mouth is effective
   E. Contraindications
      1. Never use alone except in cats
      2. Avoid as a preanesthetic medication in dogs
      3. Avoid in animals with seizure history
         a. Can cause convulsions with high doses
            (1) More likely to occur with dogs
            (2) Can be minimized by combining with a tranquilizer
      4. Produces poor visceral analgesia
      5. Caution with cats with chronic or acute renal failure or blocked urethra (renal excretion of ketamine in cats)
      6. Prolonged, unreliable recoveries

VII. Neuroloptanalgesics
  A. Any combination of an analgesic and a tranquilizer (e.g., Innovar Vet [fentanyl and droperidol], oxymorphone and acepromazine)
  B. Indications
    1. Heavier sedation (depending on dose) for short procedures (i.e., wound suturing, porcupine quill removal)
    2. Cardiac or shock cases
  C. Contraindications
    1. Animal will become hyperactive to auditory stimulus
    2. May defecate or vomit
    3. May pant
    4. May cause bradycardia

INJECTABLE ANESTHETICS
Barbiturates

I. Classified as:
  A. Oxybarbiturates: e.g., phenobarbital (considered as an anticonvulsant, not an anesthetic) and pentobarbital (Nembutal or Somnotol)
  B. Thiobarbiturates: for example, thiopental (Pentothal) and thiamylal (Surital, Bio-Tal)
  C. Methylated oxybarbiturates: methohexital (Brevital)
II. Also classified by speed of onset of action
  A. Long acting (e.g., phenobarbital)
  B. Short acting (e.g., pentobarbital)
  C. Ultra short acting (e.g., thiopental and methohexital)
III. Barbiturates in general can be used for sedation, anticonvulsants, and general anesthesia
  A. Commonly used as induction agents to allow endotracheal intubation followed by maintenance with an inhalant anesthetic such as halothane or isoflurane
IV. Causes unconsciousness at an adequate dose
V. Depresses respiration and cardiovascular system to a variable extent
  A. Give to effect (amount necessary to induce anesthesia)
  B. Give as a bolus (usually one third to one half of the calculated dose given rapidly)
VI. Nonreversible
VII. Protein binding
  A. Level of plasma protein can alter rate and amount of absorption of the barbiturates
  B. Barbiturates will bind to protein
    1. The amount of barbiturate free in the circulation and not bound to protein will increase if the patient is hypoproteinemic

    2. More barbiturate will thus be available to penetrate the CNS and cause unconsciousness
VIII. Lipid solubility increases in the barbiturates from the long acting to the ultrashort acting
  A. There is quicker onset of action with the shorter acting barbiturates because they cross the blood-brain barrier faster
  B. This also accounts for the quicker recovery of the shorter acting barbiturate
  C. Recovery from these drugs depends on a combination of redistribution (to muscle and fat) and hepatic metabolism
  D. If a drug has a low lipid solubility there is little or no redistribution and recovery depends mostly on metabolism (a slow process)
  E. If a drug has a high lipid solubility it is readily redistributed from the blood to the muscle and fat tissue where it is not available to act on the brain
    1. Recovery from a highly lipid soluble drug is thus faster
  F. As the blood levels decline due to metabolism, small quantities of the redistributed drug reenter the circulatory system from muscle and fat and are also metabolized
    1. These low levels that arise from the muscle and fat stores are not enough to clinically alter the level of consciousness
IX. Examples of barbiturates
  A. Phenobarbital
    1. Used mostly as a sedative for excitable dogs or as an anticonvulsant for epileptic type seizures
    2. Sedation can last up to 24 hours, depending on the dose
  B. Pentobarbital
    1. Once used commonly for anesthetic inductions, it now has been replaced mostly by the ultrashort acting barbiturates
    2. It can also be used to control seizures (although EEG seizure activity may persist)
    3. It can be administered intramuscularly for sedation, without tissue reaction
    4. With IV induction there is significant effect at 1 minute postinjection; maximum effect is in 5 minutes
    5. Recovery by metabolism is slow and rough in all animals except in sheep where recovery is smoother and faster

C. Methohexital
1. Highly lipid soluble and rapidly metabolized; therefore it has the quickest onset, shortest duration, and quickest recovery (even if used for long-term maintenance)
2. Best choice of barbiturates for sight hounds or other patients of excessive lean body
   a. These patients seem to be extremely sensitive to barbiturates (due to poor ability to metabolize and a lack of fat storage) and they have prolonged recoveries
3. Good choice for brachycephalics to obtain quick and smooth intubation and rapid recoveries without "hang over" effects
4. Induction effect is noted 15 seconds postinjection
5. Induction and/or recoveries may be accompanied by convulsions or recoveries may simply be rough but this effect is less likely if good sedation is given
D. Thiopental
1. Has a high lipid solubility
   a. It is redistributed to muscle and fat tissue and metabolized very slowly
   b. Initial recovery is by redistribution; therefore it is fairly quick
2. Problems with recovery will occur if subsequent doses have been given for maintenance of anesthesia and if the muscle and fat tissues are saturated
   a. Recovery will be slow and possibly rough
   b. Best to use for induction only or a maximum maintenance of one half hour
3. Significant effect is noted 15 to 30 seconds postinjection
4. There is an arrhythmogenic potential with this drug

Propofol (Diprivan, Rapinovet)

I. Used for sedation, induction, and/or anesthesia maintenance by repeated bolus injections or continuous infusion
II. Rapid acting with smooth, excitement free induction
III. Rapid smooth recovery due to redistribution and rapid metabolism
   A. Vomiting may occur with recovery in some patients

IV. Ideal for induction of sight hounds and other lean body patients
V. Ideal for injectable maintenance of anesthesia, since there is no accumulation
VI. Minimal cardiovascular and respiratory effects
   A. May have tachycardia or bradycardia
   B. Transient apnea has been reported after rapid IV injection
VII. Good anticonvulsant
VIII. Nonirritating with incidental perivascular injection
IX. Some muscle relaxation occurs but analgesia is poor

Neuroleptanalgesics

I. Examples are Innovar Vet (fentanyl and droperidol) or any other combination of an analgesic and a tranquilizer such as oxymorphone and diazepam
II. Minimal cardiovascular depression
III. Produces CNS depression
IV. Partially reversible
V. Disadvantages
   A. Patients are hyper-responsive to sound
   B. Opioid analgesics may produce respiratory depression, making transfer to inhalation anesthesia difficult
   C. Patient may also defecate, urinate, and possibly vomit

Ketamine

I. Produces catalepsy, amnesia, and questionable analgesia
II. Pharyngeal-laryngeal reflexes are partially intact
III. Excessive skeletal muscle tone
IV. Mild cardiac stimulation and some respiratory depression
V. Small percentage of cats will show convulsive behavior
   A. Other side effects: tissue irritation, increased salivation, increase in cerebral spinal fluid (CSF) pressure, open eyes with central dilated pupil, nystagmus (repetitive side-to-side motion of the eyeball), an increase in intraocular pressure, temporary personality changes, and excited recoveries
VI. Dogs are more likely to seizure and therefore ketamine should be combined with a tranquilizer (i.e., acepromazine or diazepam when used with dogs)
VII. Metabolized by the liver and also excreted somewhat in an unchanged form through kidneys in dogs

VIII. Excreted primarily by the kidneys in cats
IX. Use with caution in seizure disorders or those undergoing neurological system procedures

INHALATION ANESTHESIA

Advantages

I. Advantages over injectable anesthesia
   A. Easier to control and change depths of anesthesia
   B. Excreted mainly by respiration; therefore recovery is fairly rapid and there is little metabolism
   C. Requires administration of oxygen (O_2) to the patient, which provides a patent airway if an endotracheal tube is used
   D. Respiratory and cardiovascular depression are minimal at safe concentrations
   E. Provides some analgesia and muscle relaxation
   F. Less accumulation, and recoveries are rapid

Examples

I. Examples of inhalation agents
   A. Methoxyflurane: MAC 0.23% (minimal alveolar concentration)
      1. Advantages
         a. Good analgesia and muscle relaxation
         b. Minimal arrhythmogenicity
         c. Low vapor pressure: can use with a precision or nonprecision vaporizer
         d. Slow plane changes reduces chance of sudden overdose
      2. Disadvantages
         a. Increased solubility leads to slow induction and slow recovery
         b. Possible renal toxicity (environmental pollution concerns)
         c. Respiration depression at deep surgical planes
         d. Slow response to changes in concentration, which may be a concern if surgical bleeding occurs
         e. Not suitable for mask induction
   B. Halothane: MAC 0.8%
      1. Advantages
         a. Less respiratory depression
         b. Lower solubility than methoxyflurane and therefore faster induction and recoveries and faster response to changes in concentration
         c. Not nephrotoxic
         d. Can mask induce
      2. Disadvantages
         a. Higher vapor pressure requires an out-of-circle precision vaporizer for maximum safety
         b. Arrhythmogenic potentials
         c. Cardiac depression resulting in hypotension (dose related)
         d. Little analgesia
         e. Hepatotoxic
   C. Isoflurane: MAC 1.2% in dogs; 1.6% in cats
      1. Advantages
         a. Cardiovascularly safer with reduced arrhythmogenicity and better cardiac output
         b. Minimal liver metabolism
         c. Lower solubility and therefore faster induction and recoveries and a faster response to changes in concentration (faster than halothane)
      2. Disadvantages
         a. Respiratory depression
         b. Occasional stormy recoveries
         c. More expensive
         d. Similar higher vapor pressure as halothane, therefore requires an out-of-circle precision vaporizer
         e. Vasodilation results in similar blood pressure as with halothane (dose related)

NITROUS OXIDE (N_2O)

Advantages

I. Can be used to speed inhalation induction by the second gas effect
   A. N_2O initially passes from the alveoli into the blood in large volumes
   B. The inhalant agent and O_2 are at a lower percentage
   C. This difference effectively increases the concentration of the inhalant agent and O_2 in the alveoli
      1. Advantages
         a. Availability to the blood is affected
II. Provides additional analgesia (species variable)
   A. When used during anesthesia maintenance it reduces the amount of other anesthetic agents required (i.e., reduces the percent of halothane or isoflurane)
III. Minimal cardiovascular and respiratory effects
IV. Rapid effects
V. No metabolism

Disadvantages

I. Cannot be used alone (MAC >100%)
II. Danger of hypoxia if not used properly

III. Since use of N_2O reduces inspired O_2 levels to 33% there is a danger of hypoxia if used with patients with respiratory problems
   A. These problems include pneumonia, lung tumors, pulmonary edema, diaphragmatic hernia, or other conditions compromising the patient's ability to oxygenate
IV. Cannot be used with animals with gas-occupying cavities (i.e., GDV, intestinal obstruction, pneumothorax)
   A. N_2O has an increased partial pressure and low solubility in blood
   B. Therefore nitrous oxide will diffuse into gas-occupying cavities faster than the rate at which resident gases leave
   C. This causes an increased pressure in these cavities

Method of Use

I. For mask induction
   A. Initially use 100% O_2 with gradual increases in percentage of inhalant anesthetic agent
   B. When high levels of inhalant agent are reached, turn on N_2O at a $N_2O:O_2$ ratio of 2:1 to continue induction
      1. This provides 66% N_2O and 33% O_2
II. If you plan to use N_2O as part of your anesthetic maintenance, continue with the 2:1 ratio
III. To ensure adequate oxygenation of the patient
   A. Never have O_2 levels below 500 mL/min (flow meters may not be accurate below this)
   B. Never have O_2 levels below 30 mL/kg/min (three times metabolic requirements) to ensure adequate oxygenation of the patient
   C. When using N_2O with a partial rebreathing or nonrebreathing system (i.e., Bain) make sure total fresh gas flow (N_2O and O_2 combined) are at least 130 mL/kg/min, of which 33% should be O_2 (see section on breathing systems)
IV. If the patient's O_2 saturation or mucous membrane color deteriorates (gray, cyanotic) at any time through the procedure it is best to discontinue N_2O use in case hypoxia is impending
V. When the procedure is complete
   A. Turn off the N_2O at the same time as the inhalant anesthetic
      1. If N_2O is turned off too soon you may be withdrawing a necessary analgesic source and therefore will have to increase the inhalant anesthetic agent to continue the procedure
   B. Increase the O_2 flow rate to 100 mL/kg/min with a rebreathing system or 300 mL/kg/min with a nonrebreathing system
   C. Keep patient on this increased O_2 flow rate for at least 5 minutes to prevent diffusion hypoxia
      1. When N_2O is turned off there is a flood of N_2O from the blood back into the alveoli
         a. This displaces the O_2 in the lower respiratory tract and limits the O_2 available to the patient
   D. Observe the patient for at least 5 minutes after O_2 source is removed to ensure that the patient is oxygenating well on room air
      1. Supplemental O_2 by a face mask should be used if needed

BREATHING SYSTEMS

Rebreathing System

I. Rebreathing systems (e.g., To-and-Fro- or Circle systems)
   A. Rebreathing refers to breathing a mixture of expired gases and fresh gases
   B. The amount of carbon dioxide (CO_2) in rebreathed gases depends on:
      1. If the breathing system has a CO_2 absorber
      2. The flow rate of fresh gases (the higher the fresh gas flow rate the more expired gas pushed out the scavenger and not rebreathed)
   C. Depending on the flow rate of fresh gas the system is classified as a closed system (total rebreathing of expired gases) or a semiclosed system (partial rebreathing of expired gases)
   D. Closed system
      1. With closed systems the fresh gas flow rate does not exceed patient's metabolic O_2 consumption of 5-10 mL/kg/min
         a. The system may be used with a closed pop-off and a fresh gas flow of 5-10 mL/kg/min
         b. Expired gases are recirculated (after CO_2 removed) with incoming fresh gases
      2. It is economical and there is minimal pollution
      3. It takes longer to change planes of anesthesia
      4. N_2O build up is common so don't use N_2O with this system

5. This system requires constant monitoring to ensure pressures do not build up in the system if the O_2 flow delivered exceeds the metabolic requirement

6. It is the author's belief that unless uninterrupted observation of this system is permitted, it can be dangerous to run a rebreathing system with the pop-off valve closed, if the pop-off valve has no safety release at high pressures

   a. It is recommended to leave the pop-off slightly open to prevent increases in pressure in the system and adjust the O_2 flow rate accordingly to prevent the rebreathing bag from collapsing

      (1) If the bag does not collapse you can be confident you are delivering enough O_2 to meet the patient's metabolic requirement

E. Semiclosed system

   1. With semiclosed systems the fresh gas is delivered in excess of metabolic consumption at 40-50 mL/kg/min (suggested economical flow)

   2. The gas escapes through the pop-off to the scavenger or after having the CO_2 removed it recirculates with the fresh gases

      a. Higher flows can be used and less rebreathing then will occur

   3. N_2O buildup is not a concern with this system

Nonrebreathing System

I. There is no mixing of inhaled and exhaled gases and no rebreathing of expired gases; all expired gas goes to the scavenger

II. Fresh gas flow rates required at 200-300 mL/kg/min

III. CO_2 absorber not required

Partial Rebreathing System (With No CO_2 Absorber)

I. Some exhaled gases, including CO_2, are rebreathed back into patient

II. Maintenance of a normal CO_2 level depends on increased respiratory effort or the assumption that the rebreathed gas fills only the dead space of the breathing system (a small amount)

III. Fresh gas flow rate of 130 mL/kg/min with the Bain system

BREATHING CIRCUITS

There are many kinds of breathing circuits available. The most common in veterinary medicine are circle systems, universal F-circuits, and Bain systems.

Circle System

I. Consist of a CO_2 absorber (i.e., soda lime) with inspiratory and expiratory unidirectional valves, two breathing hoses connected with a 'Y' piece to the patient, rebreathing bag, and pop-off valve

II. Can be used as a nonrebreathing system (200 mL/kg/min), partial rebreathing system (40-50 mL/kg/min), or total rebreathing system (5-10 mL/kg/min)

III. An advantage is the mixture of expired gases with incoming gases, which humidifies and warms the incoming gases

IV. The main disadvantages of the circle system are with smaller patients:

   A. Excess weight and bulk of the hoses
   B. Excess dead space
   C. The resistance to breathing through unidirectional valves

Universal F-Circuit

I. Basically a modified circle system where the inspiratory hose is placed within the expiratory hose

II. Still requires a CO_2 absorber, rebreathing bag, unidirectional valves and pop-off valve

III. Incoming fresh gas is warmed also by expired gases

IV. The advantage is lighter weight and less bulk

V. A disadvantage is that if the circuit is stretched when in use, the end of the inspiratory hose pulls away from the end of the expiratory hose

   A. This is considered a safety feature to prevent breakage of hoses but it increases the amount of dead space
   B. When not stretched the dead space is at least comparable to the circle system

Bain System

I. Consists of one tube inside another tube

   A. The fresh gases flow through the inner tube and the unused fresh gases and exhaled gases flow through the outer tube
   B. There is also a rebreathing bag with a pop-off valve but no CO_2 absorber

II. Between breaths the fresh gases flow through the inner tube toward the patient then back through the outer tube toward the pop-off valve

III. When the patient inspires, the gases are drawn from the inner tube, which will be 100% fresh gases or a mixture of fresh gases and expired gases, depending on the fresh gas flow rate
IV. This system can be used as a nonrebreathing system with a fresh gas flow rate of 200-300 mL/kg/min
    A. The high flow rate pushes exhaled gases away down the outer tube so there is no rebreathing of exhaled gases
V. This system can be used also as a partial rebreathing system with a flow rate of 130-200 mL/kg/min
    A. The flow rate pushes most of the exhaled gases away but there is partial rebreathing of some exhaled gases
VI. The Bain system is ideal for small patients
    A. It is light weight
    B. Has minimal dead space
    C. There is little resistance to breathing
VII. This system is good for all small animals in general but is not economical when patient is over 10 kg
VIII. Limiting factors to size of patient
    A. The O_2 flow meter must provide flow rates required for a partial or nonrebreathing system (130-300 mL/kg/min)
    B. The total volume of the Bain hose must be greater than the tidal volume of respiration of the patient to effectively prevent rebreathing
IX. Good for procedures involving the head (less tubing in the way)
X. Good for procedures with a lot of manipulation (i.e., radiography, since there is less weight pulling on the animal)
XI. Warming and humidification is minimal with partial rebreathing
XII. Requires a precision vaporizer

VAPORIZERS

Vapor pressure is characterized by the amount of vapor related to its liquid in a closed container; the pressure exerted by the gas is called the vapor pressure and will increase with increases in temperature. Since most anesthetics vaporize at a concentration higher than necessary for clinical anesthesia we use a vaporizer to deliver diluted anesthetics to patients

Classification

I. Accuracy
    A. Precision vaporizer
        1. Enables delivery of controlled concentrations of anesthetic vapor independent of time, temperature, and fresh gas flow rate
            a. The temperature and flow rate are compensated for by the vaporizer or manually by the anesthetist
        2. Percentage of anesthetic is determined by dial, chart, or mathematical calculation
        3. Because of internal resistance, precision vaporizers must always be placed out-of-circle because the patient cannot physically draw gases through them
        4. A disadvantage is that they are more complex and therefore more expensive and require more servicing
    B. Nonprecision vaporizer
        1. Do not deliver a constant percentage due to changes in temperature, fresh gas flow rates, ventilation changes, liquid and wick surfaces, and the amount of liquid anesthetic in vaporizer
        2. Percentage of anesthetic delivered cannot be calculated
        3. Little internal resistance, therefore can be used in-the-circle
        4. Although they can be used out-of-circle, the nonlinear concentrations delivered make anesthesia depth hard to control
        5. Vaporizers are simple, less expensive, and require less servicing

Location

I. Location of vaporizer in-the-circle
    A. VOC (vaporizer out-of-circle)
        1. Vaporizer is added to the system between the O_2 flow meter and the circle (circle consisting of inspiratory and expiratory valves, breathing hoses, CO_2 absorber, pop-off, and rebreathing bag)
    B. VIC (vaporizer in-the-circle)
        1. Vaporizer is placed inside the breathing system, usually between the inspiratory valve and the patient
        2. VICs are always nonprecision
        3. The carrier gas (i.e., O_2) passes over the surface of the anesthetic liquid or past a wick
        4. Incoming gases mix with warmed exhaled gases in the system
        5. Better vaporization of liquid is obtained when low fresh gas flows are used
            a. High flows cool liquid and reduce vaporization

6. These vaporizers are also safest when used with agents with low vapor pressure (e.g., methoxyflurane)

PARTS OF AN ANESTHETIC MACHINE ▰▰▰

I. Pressure reducing valve (or regulator): reduces the pressure of the oxygen or nitrous oxide leaving the tank to 50 psi

II. Flowmeter
   A. Measures oxygen or nitrous oxide in L/min
   B. Allows the anesthetist to set the oxygen or nitrous oxide flow rates that will be delivered to the animal
   C. Newer machines have a low flow (less than 1 L) and a high flow meter (0-5 L) for oxygen

III. Inhalation/exhalation flutter valves or check valves
   A. Ensures a unidirectional flow of gas to and from the animal when delivering via a circle system

IV. Y-connector
   A. Connects the endotracheal tube to the inspiratory and expiratory tubes of a circle system

V. Rebreathing bag or reservoir bag
   A. Allows the animal to breathe easier from a reservoir of gas
   B. The reservoir bag can also be used to deliver oxygen (with or without anesthetic gas) and manually assist respirations, which is commonly called bagging

VI. Carbon dioxide absorber/soda lime canister
   A. Used in rebreathing systems as a filter of any gases not leaving the system through the exhaust valve
   B. Exhaust gases enter a canister containing soda lime or barium hydroxide lime that absorbs carbon dioxide and water vapor in the circuit
   C. When the soda lime or barium hydroxide granules turn color or become hard instead of crumbly, they are exhausted
   D. When in use granules will produce heat and condensation inside the canister
   E. The spent granules should be thrown out and replaced with new granules

VII. Exhaust valve
   A. Also called "pop-off" valve or pressure relief valve
   B. Exhaust gases leave the system via this valve
   C. The valve can be open or partially open when a patient is on the machine
   D. The valve is closed for leak tests or when filling the reservoir bag for assisted respirations

VIII. Manometer
   A. Measures the pressure in the system in mm of Hg or cm of H_2O
   B. The pressure should be at 0

IX. Oxygen flush valve
   A. O_2 bypasses vaporizer, delivering 100% O_2 to breathing system
   B. Enables the anesthetist to flush the system with pure oxygen
   C. It can be used to fill the reservoir bag and system for leak tests
   D. It can be used to flush anesthetic gases out of the circuit and replace gases with 100% O_2
   E. Never use O_2 flush with Bain system attached to a small animal because it produces too much pressure

X. Scavenger system
   A. Attached to the exhaust valve
   B. A basic scavenger system consists of tubing that collects waste gases and directs them outside of the building or to a charcoal canister that absorbs waste anesthetic gases
   C. Scavengers can be active systems (e.g., vacuum pump or a fan) or passive systems (e.g., tubing to a hole in an exterior wall of the building)

XI. Negative pressure relief valve
   A. Some newer machines have this safety valve
   B. If negative pressure is created in the system the valve will open and allow room air into the circuit
   C. Negative pressure could be due to an active scavenger system or a low to nil oxygen supply

STAGES OF ANESTHESIA (DEPTHS) ▰▰▰

I. Stage 1
   A. Induction stage, stage of analgesia, and altered consciousness
   B. From beginning to loss of consciousness
   C. Sensations become dull
   D. Loss of pain
   E. Pupils are normal in size, then begin to dilate when entering stage 2
   F. Blood pressure may be elevated
   G. Respiration rate is generally increased, may be irregular
   H. Vomiting, retching, and coughing may occur

II. Stage 2
   A. Stage of delirium or excitement
   B. Excitement and involuntary muscular movement
   C. Eyes closed, jaw set

D. Pupils dilated, light reflex still present

E. Respiration irregular

F. Vomiting may occur

III. Stage 3

A. Stage of surgical anesthesia

B. Respiration full and regular

C. Pupils begin to constrict

D. Palpebral blink is absent (or minimal with methoxyflurane)

E. Four subplanes

1. Subplane I

a. Eyeball begins to rove, pupil is light responsive, and medial palpebral still present

b. Muscle tone still present

c. Pain reaction still present

d. Respiration is one half thoracic and one half abdominal

e. Blood pressure and heart rate are normal

2. Subplane II

a. Regular respiration

b. Fixed eyeball

3. Subplane III

a. Increased abdominal respiration, delayed thoracic inspiratory effect (intercostal paralysis)

b. Eyeballs fixed and converged

c. Pupils begin to dilate

d. Pulse fast and feeble

e. Blood pressure decreased

4. Subplane IV

a. Progressive respiratory paralysis

b. Tidal volume decreased

c. Palpebral and corneal reflexes absent

d. Pupils dilated and not light responsive

e. Heart rate decreased

f. Apnea

IV. Stage 4

A. Stage of medullary paralysis

B. Apnea

C. Cardiac arrest

MONITORING

The signs you receive from monitoring may differ depending on the species and the anesthetic agents being used. The following signs are general for domestic small animals (i.e., cats and dogs).

Eye

I. Position

A. The eye will rotate ventral-medially during a good plane of anesthesia

B. The eye will return to central when the patient is too light or too deep

II. Palpebral reflex (blink)

A. Stimulated by lightly touching the medial or lateral canthus of the eyelids

B. The lateral palpebral reflex is eliminated before the medial palpebral reflex as the patient becomes deeper

C. The reflex will become slow, weak, then absent in a good surgical plane with most inhalant agents

D. If a good analgesic has been given, or injectable anesthesia alone or methoxyflurane is used, then a mild medial palpebral reflex is acceptable

III. Corneal reflex

A. Stimulated by lightly touching the cornea of the eye

B. This reflex should be present under anesthesia

C. Absence of this reflex indicates anesthesia overdose

D. Considering the potential damage that can be inflicted on the cornea and the wide range of other monitoring options available this reflex should not be tested unless necessary

IV. Pupil size

A. Generally dilated when in a light, nonsurgical plane

B. Constricted in a light surgical plane

C. Dilated in a deep plane

D. Note that sympathetic responses such as pain or certain drugs (e.g., Atropine) will dilate the pupils

Pedal Reflex (Pain Response)

I. Stimulated by pinching the skin between the toes

II. Normal response is to withdraw the leg

III. This response should become slower and weaker to absent as the anesthetic plane becomes deeper, being completely eliminated by a light surgical plane

Jaw Tone (Muscle Tone)

I. Stimulated by attempting to spread the jaws apart two to three times

II. Normal response is to resist

III. This response should become weaker as the anesthetic plane becomes deeper and should be absent in a light surgical plane

IV. If a good analgesic or methoxyflurane has been used then mild jaw tone can remain if all other monitoring signs indicate an appropriate plane of anesthesia

V. Some breeds will appear to have increased jaw tone due to increased muscle mass in this area (e.g., Rottweiller)

Cardiovascular System

I. Heart rate
  A. Most accurately measured by stethoscope
  B. Can also be measured by digital readout of mechanical monitoring equipment
  C. Normal rates are 70-140 for dogs and 110-140 for cats
  D. Heart rate may decrease with deepening anesthetic plane but may also stay constant or increase with a dangerously deep plane and/or with hypotension
  E. Bradycardia (decreased heart rate) is not always a sign of deep anesthesia. Heart rate may decrease with:
    1. Certain drugs prone to producing bradycardia
    2. End stage hypoxia (e.g., due to respiratory obstruction)
    3. Vagal nerve stimulation (e.g., pressure on the eyes; manipulation of abdominal contents)

II. Pulse rate
  A. Measure by palpation of an artery
  B. Pulse deficits (difference between heart rate and pulse rate) should be noted

III. Rhythm
  A. Arrhythmias can be monitored by arterial palpation but are more accurately monitored with an electrocardiogram

IV. Blood pressure
  A. Palpation of a peripheral pulse can indicate drastic increases or decreases in blood pressure but not actual values
  B. Blood pressure is more accurately measured by an indirect or direct arterial blood pressure monitoring system
  C. Normal blood pressures
    1. Systolic: 100-160 mmHg
    2. Mean: 80-120 mmHg
    3. Diastolic: 60-100 mmHg
  D. Generally blood pressure will decrease as the anesthetic plane deepens
  E. Hypovolemia will reduce blood pressure
  F. Hypercapnia will increase blood pressure

Respiratory System

I. Monitor rate and depth (character) of the ventilation

II. Normal rate is 8-20 breaths per minute and normal tidal volume is 10-15 mL/kg

III. In a very light plane of anesthesia the ventilation will be irregular in depth and rate in response to stimulation

IV. In a surgical plane the rate and depth are generally regular

V. In a deep plane of anesthesia, breathing may become shallow and rapid or both the rate and depth may decrease

VI. As the plane gets deeper there will be some thoracic muscle paralysis producing paradoxical breathing (abdomen rises and chest falls during an inspiration)

VII. Blood gas levels can also be monitored
  A. O_2 levels will define the patients oxygenating ability
  B. CO_2 levels will define the ventilation status
  C. Hypoventilation is indicated by increased CO_2 levels (respiratory acidosis)
  D. Hyperventilation is indicated by decreased CO_2 levels (respiratory alkalosis)

Capillary Refill Time (CRT)

I. Acquired by digital compression on any unpigmented mucous membrane and timing between release of pressure and return of blood flow to the area

II. A normal CRT is 1-2 seconds

III. Good indication of how well cardiac output is affecting peripheral perfusion

IV. The time will generally become longer with deepening anesthetic planes and hypovolemia

Mucous Membrane Color

I. Generally pink in unpigmented areas

II. Mucous membranes may change color to a grey tinge or blue with decreased O_2 levels in the blood; however, this change may be delayed and is not considered a good forewarning sign

III. High CO_2 due to hypoventilation may produce a very bright pink, vasodilated, mucous membrane color

IV. Pale mucous membranes may occur with anemia, hypothermia, or with light planes of anesthesia when pain is occurring

Temperature

I. Decreases in body temperature and slow metabolism can reduce the amount of anesthetic agent required

II. It is important to monitor and support body temperature from the time of sedation through recovery

III. Monitor rectal or axilla peripheral temperature with a digital thermometer, or monitor core temperature with an esophageal temperature probe

IV. Hypothermic patients should be actively rewarmed to 37.5° C (99° F), after which heat sources should be removed to prevent hyperthermia

V. To prevent burning of the patient any heat source used (e.g., hot water circulating blanket, heat lamp, warm water bottles or oat bags) should not produce heat over 42.0° C (107.6° F)

VI. To prevent burning, physical sources of heat (e.g., warm water bottle or oat bags) should be wrapped in a towel before placing against the patient

ANALGESIA

I. Depending on the individual patient and the procedure, consider:
   A. Which agent to use
   B. Timing (pre, intra, or post procedure) of administration
   C. The length of analgesia required
   D. The choice of route of administration (e.g., systemic [SQ, IM, IV], local, regional, or epidural)

II. If the patient is in pain, analgesics should be provided in the preanesthetic medication to help alleviate pain and anxiety and provide for a smoother induction

III. Administration of analgesics pre and intra operatively will allow reduction of induction and/or maintenance anesthetic agent required by the patient and maintain a level plane of anesthesia with proper analgesia

IV. Analgesics should be provided during and/or after any surgical or otherwise painful procedure before recovery from anesthesia
   A. Application of analgesia before conscious awareness of pain will have a positive influence on the effect of the analgesia

V. By decreasing pain on recovery, stress of the patient is decreased and therefore a quicker, more successful recovery is promoted

VI. Some examples of choices of analgesic agents
   A. (NSAIDs) Nonsteroidal antiinflammatory drugs, for systemic use
   B. Opioids for systemic and epidural use
   C. Local anesthetics for systemic, local, regional, or epidural use

MUSCLE RELAXANTS

I. Neuromuscular blocking agents are used to:
   A. Relax skeletal muscles for better manipulation of joints and bones
   B. Obtain better surgical exposure
   C. Control ventilation
   D. Assist tracheal intubation
   E. Immobilize the eyes for ocular surgery
   F. To reduce amount of anesthetic agent used when deep anesthesia will not be tolerated by the patient

II. Requires ventilation of the animal at all times

III. Requires some form of additional analgesia

IV. Requires close monitoring for depth of anesthesia because several monitoring signs will be eliminated (i.e., jaw tone, eye position, palpebral blink, spontaneous breathing)

V. Nerve stimulators are an asset
   A. Aid in the assessment of effect of the neuromuscular block
   B. Indicate time to give subsequent doses
   C. Indicate when to reverse

VI. Some examples of neuromuscular blocking agents: succinylcholine, gallamine, pancuronium, atracurium, and vecuronium
   A. Doses, length of effect, side effects, and reversal agents differ

VENTILATION

I. Assisted (occasional sigh or additional breaths) or controlled (intermittent positive pressure ventilation—IPPV)

II. Manual or mechanical

III. Goal is to maintain near normal acid-base status and oxygenation and to counteract CO_2 retention

IV. In some cases only assistance is needed (e.g., obese patient, patient in head down recumbency, hypothermia, pulmonary disease)
   A. Occasional 'sighing' or 'bagging' the patient (e.g., once or twice a minute) may achieve the above goals

V. In many cases it is necessary to control the ventilation (IPPV) (i.e., when using neuromuscular blocking agents, thoracic surgery, diaphragmatic hernia, gastric torsion, any patient obviously hypoventilating)

VI. Observed guidelines and reassess results continually
   A. Rate 8 to 12 breaths/minute
   B. Inspiration to expiration ratio of 1:2
   C. Tidal volume of 12 to 20 mL/kg (30 mL/kg for open chest)
      1. 12 mL/kg >40 kg
      2. 20 mL/kg <10 kg
   D. Inspiratory pressure of 15 to 20 cm H_2O (30 cm H_2O with open chest)

VII. The goal of using these parameters is to decrease CO_2 levels slightly below normal, thereby eliminating spontaneous breathing and allowing control of ventilation
   A. Therefore in most cases it is not necessary to use a neuromuscular blocking agent to perform IPPV
VIII. Double check all ventilation with visualization for "normal" chest movement; reassess other parameters of the patient (mucous membrane color, capillary refill time, heart rate, pulse strength, and blood gases when available)
   IX. Concerns
   A. Generally decrease percentage of inhalant anesthetic delivered to the patient because you will be ventilating better for the patient than if it were spontaneous; therefore more anesthetic will be delivered
   B. If the patient breathes spontaneously while IPPV is performed it is an indication of:
      1. Underventilation
         a. An indication for you to increase the minute volume by increasing the rate and/or volume of breaths
      2. Patient is in pain
   C. If you are ventilating adequately the patient will not attempt to breath spontaneously
   D. Overventilation
      1. Overventilation has potential to damage an animal's lungs
         a. Rupture of alveoli, leading to pneumothorax or mediastinal emphysema
      2. Decreased cardiac output and venus return
      3. Excessive CO_2, leading to respiratory alkalosis
   E. With pneumothorax, ventilate with caution and be prepared for the possibility of a tension pneumothorax
      1. When the chest is closed and there is a hole in the lungs, gases will escape from the lungs to the thoracic cavity as you ventilate—where they build up pressure around the lungs to the point where the lungs can no longer expand
      2. You will notice difficulty squeezing the rebreathing bag or an increased pressure will register on the pressure gauge of the ventilator or anesthetic machine with chest expansion
   F. When removing the patient from the ventilator, continue to ventilate for several minutes after discontinuing inhalant anesthetic; this will help eliminate the inhalant from the patient's system and speed recovery
      1. Decrease the minute volume (rate and/or volume) to allow CO_2 levels to increase slightly in the patient's system to stimulate the patient to breath spontaneously

FLUID THERAPY

If time allows, the patient should be stabilized for fluid imbalances, electrolyte imbalances, anemia, and hypoproteinemia before proceeding with an anesthesia.

Fluid Characteristics

I. Most stable anesthetic cases are maintained on an intravenous replacement crystalloid such as Normosol R or Plasmalyte 148 as opposed to a maintenance crystalloid such as Normosol M or Plasmalyte 56
II. Replacement crystalloids should have high sodium and chloride levels and a low potassium level, similar to plasma
III. Replacement crystalloids are administered at 5 to 10 mL/kg/hr for routine, healthy anesthesia or surgery
IV. Having the patient on intravenous fluids allows you to:
   A. Replace fluid loss due to preoperative water and/or food restriction, evaporation from open body cavities, and/or breathing dry gases
   B. Maintain hydration, tissue perfusion, and organ function (especially, renal)
   C. Replace some blood loss
   D. Maintain a patent intravenous access in the case of an emergency

Fluid Calculation

I. For dehydrated patients, if time does not allow hydration status to be fully stabilized before anesthesia, 50% of the fluid deficit can be replaced IV over the 20 to 30 minutes required for effective premedication
II. Total volume to treat dehydration is calculated as:

$$\frac{\% \text{ dehydration}}{100} \times \text{weight (kg)} \times 1000 = \text{mL to give 100}$$

A. EXAMPLE: 20 kg dog that is 7% dehydrated

$$\frac{7}{100} \times 20 \times 1000 = 1400 \text{ mL}$$

III. Give 700 mL in 20 to 30 minutes before anesthesia induction
   A. Recognizing that instability may persist until the entire deficit is replaced, continue at an increased fluid administration rate of 20 to 90 mL/kg/hr during the remainder of anesthesia or until the deficit is replaced to maintain good blood pressure
IV. A maximum fluid rate of 60 (cats and older dogs) to 90 (other dogs) mL/kg/hr to replace the calculated fluid loss is a safe rapid administration rate in awake and anesthetized patients
V. Other abnormal losses such as surgical bleeding are replaced in addition to this deficit and surgical maintenance fluids

BLOOD LOSS

I. Anemia from acute blood loss is more critical
II. Patients with chronic anemia will tend to compensate and may tolerate a lower PCV
   A. If PCV is <25% in dogs or <20% in cats, whole blood or packed red cells (colloids) should replace the surgical fluids and be started before anesthesia if possible
   B. If PCV is normal but TP is <3.5 gm/dl plasma, dextrans or starch should replace surgical fluids (artificial colloids)
III. The total volume to improve PCV or TP is calculated as follows:

$$\frac{\text{desired PCV(TP)} - \text{recipient PCV (TP)}}{\text{donor PCV(TP)}} \times \text{wt (kg)} \times 50 = \text{mL (vol)}$$

IV. When blood or plasma is used to correct anemia or hypoproteinemia during surgery the rate of administration is 3 to 10 mL/kg/hr
   A. The blood should be given slowly for the first 5 to 10 minutes to observe for transfusion reactions
   B. Observe for reaction signs: hypotension, tachypnea, tachycardia, poor CRT, vomiting (if awake), pallor, and urticaria
V. When blood, plasma, or artificial colloids are given to treat chronic anemia the rate of administration should not exceed 20 (cats and older dogs) to 30 (other dogs) mL/kg/hr
VI. For acute intraoperative blood loss, 10% to 15% of the total body blood volume can be replaced with replacement crystalloid fluids, provided the PCV and TP were normal to begin with
   A. To calculate the volume lost, consider that the total body blood volume is approximately 100 mL/kg in dogs and 75 mL/kg in cats, for example:

   1. For a 10 kg dog:
      10 kg dog × 100 mL/kg = 1000 mL total blood volume
      10% blood loss = 100 mL
   B. When replacing a 10% to 15% blood loss with crystalloids, replace at 2 to 3 times the volume lost (in addition to the surgical fluid rate)
      1. Only one third of the crystalloid volume will stay in the vascular compartment
      2. The remainder two thirds of the crystalloid volume will move into the interstitial space (e.g., for the same 10 kg dog with a 10% blood loss, a total of 100 mL blood lost, replace this with 200 to 300 mL of crystalloids)
   C. If >15% blood loss is replaced with crystalloids there is a risk of hemodilution
      1. Any blood loss over 15% of the total body blood volume may require replacement with whole blood or packed red cells
      2. Unlike crystalloids, the whole volume of colloids administered will remain in the vascular compartment; therefore the volume of colloid administered will be equal to the volume of blood lost
      3. If the condition of the patient allows, begin with an initial slow drip rate for 5 minutes to watch for transfusion reaction, then continue administration of the remainder of the colloid as fast as the loss occurs
   D. In an emergency situation the slow initial administration may not be possible, the need for fast administration of blood may outweigh the risk of a transfusion reaction

ACID-BASE BALANCE

Defined by pH, which is the result of processes in the body tending toward acidosis or alkalosis.
I. Mechanisms that regulate pH are respiratory or metabolic in nature and are maintained by three systems
   A. Chemical buffers
      1. Bicarbonate (carbonic acid)
      2. Phosphate (RBCs, kidneys)
      3. Hemoglobin
   B. Respiratory
      1. By breathing and alteration of CO_2 the lungs can regulate the concentration of carbonic acid
   C. Kidney
      1. Elimination of excess acid or bases: carbonic acid—carbon dioxide equilibrium

$$CO_2 + H_2O <=> H_2CO_3 <=> H^+ + HCO_3^-$$
(respiratory)   (metabolic)

II. Disturbances in acid-base balance can be found in one of four categories
   A. Respiratory acidosis
      1. CO_2 production is greater than CO_2 excretion
      2. Indicated on blood gas analysis by an increase in CO_2 levels
      3. Caused by anything that depresses ventilation (hypoventilation) and impairs excretion of CO_2 (i.e., deep anesthesia, pulmonary disease, respiratory obstruction)
      4. May also be caused by increased CO_2 production with malignant hyperthermia
      5. Increase in CO_2 causes a gain in acids and therefore the pH decreases
      6. Other signs: increased cardiac output (hypertension), vasodilation, ventricular arrhythmias
      7. Natural compensation of the body with time through the kidneys (though chronic hypercapnia is rare)
      8. Respiratory acidosis can be treated by
         a. Ventilating the patient with a higher minute volume (increase the tidal volume and/or respiration rate) than what the patient was breathing spontaneously to help remove some of the CO_2
         b. Treatment of the underlying disease (i.e., pneumonia)
   B. Respiratory alkalosis
      1. CO_2 excretion is greater than CO_2 production
      2. Indicated on blood gas analysis by a decrease in CO_2 levels
      3. Caused by excessive controlled ventilation (IPPV) or anything that stimulates spontaneous hyperventilation and therefore removal of CO_2 such as pain, excitement
      4. Causes excess loss of H^+ and gain in bases
      5. Other signs: may produce tachycardia and ECG changes
      6. Natural compensation of the body with time through the kidneys, though chronic hypocapnea is rare; therefore compensation is seldom seen
      7. Respiratory alkalosis can be treated by
         a. Decreasing the minute volume if the patient is being ventilated
         b. If the patient is breathing spontaneously and hyperventilating, assess and treat the cause of hyperventilation such as light anesthesia, pain
   C. Metabolic acidosis
      1. Indicated on blood gas analysis by low adjusted base excess (ABE) or low HCO_3^-
      2. Common causes are lactic acid gain (commonly caused by decreased tissue perfusion), renal failure, body secretions rich in HCO_3^- that are lost and not reabsorbed (i.e., diarrhea)
      3. Causes loss of HCO_3^-, which means a H^+ gain
      4. Natural compensation by rapid response of respiratory system by hyperventilating
      5. Metabolic acidosis can be treated
         a. For a mild imbalance give an alkalinizing IV solution (containing lactate, gluconate, acetate)
         b. For more severe imbalances treat with sodium bicarbonate
            (1) Dose is calculated as follows: one half of ABE × wt (kg) × 0.3 = mEq of sodium bicarbonate
            (2) This volume should be given *slowly* IV (over 15 to 30 minutes)
            (3) Deaths have occurred during fast administration of sodium bicarbonate in dehydrated animals
               (a) HCO_3^- combines with H^+ to produce CO_2 and H_2O
               (b) The CO_2 will rapidly enter the brain; the HCO_3^- will take longer to enter cells
               (c) Excess CO_2 in the brain will drop the pH of the CNS farther, resulting in coma and death: paradoxical CNS acidosis
   D. Metabolic alkalosis
      1. Indicated on blood gas analysis by high adjusted base excess (ABE) or high HCO_3^-
      2. Caused by stomach vomiting (loss of H^+), hypochloremia (increased renal absorption of HCO_3^-)

3. Natural compensation through the respiratory system by hypoventilation resulting in a mild respiratory acidosis
4. Metabolic alkalosis can be treated, if severe, by replacing the lacking element
   a. Potassium may be necessary if hypokalemic
   b. Chloride may be necessary in the vomiting patient

III. Interpretation of blood gas results
   A. Normal values
      pH   7.35 to 7.45
      pO_2 400 to 500 mm Hg
              (arterial, 100% inspired O_2)
              150 to 250 mm Hg
              (arterial, $N_2O:O_2$ mix inspired)
              90 to 100 mm Hg
              (arterial, room air inspired)
              50 to 200 mm Hg
              (venous, 100% inspired O_2)
              30 to 60 mm Hg
              (venous, room air inspired)
      pCO_2 35 to 45 mm Hg
              (arterial, will increase by 6 mm Hg with venous sample)
      HCO_3^- −20 to 24 mEq
      ABE   −4 to +4
   B. When interpreting values of blood gas there may be two disorders: a primary disorder and a secondary (compensating) disorder
      1. First look at the pH
         a. pH <7.35 = acidosis
         b. pH >7.45 = alkalosis
      2. Then look at the pCO_2 and ABE to determine respiratory and metabolic conditions respectively
      3. Generally the pH will vary in the direction of the primary disorder
      4. Generally the component with the greatest change is the primary disorder
         a. Natural compensation is usually not 100% and seldom will there be an over-compensation
         b. pCO_2 >45 = Respiratory acidosis
            pCO_2 <35 = Respiratory alkalosis
            ABE <−4 = Metabolic acidosis
            ABE >+4 = Metabolic alkalosis
      5. ABE (adjusted base excess) considers any alteration of pCO_2 and adjusts, so even if the CO_2 is abnormal the ABE can be relied on to determine the metabolic state

6. HCO_3^- can be used as an indication of metabolic state if the CO_2 is normal
   a. HCO_3^- <20 = Metabolic acidosis
   b. HCO_3^- >26 = Metabolic alkalosis

OXYGENATION PROBLEMS

I. If patient seems to be poorly oxygenating it may be due to something as simple as a mechanical problem such as a detached endotracheal tube, disconnected or leaking rebreathing bag, or a kinked or blocked breathing hose or endotracheal tube
   A. The correction for such problems is obvious once the problem is isolated
II. Other problems may be clinical problems such as pneumonia, lung pathology, diaphragmatic hernia, pulmonary edema, etc.
   A. These cases may best be handled anesthetically with a neuroleptanalgesic, in which case supplemental O_2 is required, either through a nasal catheter or face mask
   B. If a general anesthetic is used on these cases, oxygenation may be improved by assisting or controlling the ventilation

Glossary

acidosis Increase in acid pH in blood and body tissue
adjusted base excess Measures the change in HCO_3^- when the effects of CO_2 are eliminated
alkalosis Increase in base pH in blood and body tissue
analgesia Relief of pain
anemia Decrease in erythrocytes
apnea Cessation of breathing
arrhythmia Any variation from the normal rhythm of the heartbeat
brachycephalic Breeds with short, wide heads
bradycardia Decreased heart rate
catalepsy Rigidity of muscles
hypercapnia Excess of carbon dioxide in the blood
hypertension Increased arterial blood pressure
hyperventilation Increased rate and/or depth of ventilation leading to a decreased carbon dioxide level
hypotension Decreased blood pressure
hypoventilation Decreased rate and/or depth of ventilation leading to an increased carbon dioxide level
hypovolemia Decreased volume of plasma in the body
hypoxia Low oxygen levels in the blood
IPPV Intermittent positive pressure ventilation
minimal alveolar concentration The concentration that prevents 50% of patients from responding to painful stimulus
tachycardia Increased heart rate

tachypnea Increased respiration, usually shallow and rapid
urticaria Vascular reaction in the skin resulting in red, slightly
  raised patches
vasodilation Dilation of a vessel

Review Questions

1 Which of the following is an indication to include an anti-
  cholinergic in preanesthetic medication?
  a. To produce analgesia
  b. To produce sedation
  c. To prevent bradycardia
  d. To treat tachypnea
2 Which opioid preanesthetic agent has a higher incidence of
  producing vomiting and should be avoided with cases such
  as GI obstruction or diaphragmatic hernia?
  a. Butorphanol
  b. Meperidine
  c. Morphine
  d. Oxymorphone
3 Which inhalation anesthetic agent has the quickest induction and recovery?
  a. Halothane
  b. Isoflurane
  c. Methoxyflurane
  d. Pentobarbital
4 How do you prevent diffusion hypoxia after discontinua-
  tion of N_2O use in general anesthesia?
  a. Increase the O_2 flow rate for at least 5 minutes
  b. Provide intermittent positive pressure ventilation
  c. Increase the intravenous fluid rate
  d. Turn off inhalant anesthetic agent
5 To reduce the amount of rebreathing during the use of a rebreathing system, which of the following would you do?
  a. Increase the total fresh gas flow rate
  b. Decrease the total fresh gas flow rate
  c. Increase % of inhalant anesthetic gas
  d. Decrease % of inhalant anesthetic gas
6 During a surgical plane of anesthesia the eye position will
  be where?
  a. Ventral-medial
  b. Dorsal-medial
  c. Lateral
  d. Central

7 Paradoxical breathing is characterized as which of the following?
  a. Holding of breath on inspiration
  b. Increased respiration rate
  c. Abdomen rising and chest falling during an inspiration
  d. Increased tidal volume
8 Which of the following is an indication of hypoventilation?
  a. Respiratory acidosis
  b. Respiratory alkalosis
  c. Metabolic acidosis
  d. Metabolic alkalosis
9 Replacement crystalloids during anesthesia are administered at which of the following rates?
  a. Up to 5 ml/kg/hr
  b. 5-10 ml/kg/hr
  c. 10-15 ml/kg/hr
  d. 15-20 ml/kg/hr
10 If the patient's total protein is <3.5 gm/dL, which of the
  following is not considered a suitable choice for intravenous fluids during anesthesia?
  a. Plasma
  b. Crystalloids
  c. Dextran
  d. Starch

BIBLIOGRAPHY

Catcott EJ: *Animal health technology,* ed 2, Santa Barbara,
  1977, American Veterinary Publications, Inc.
Kirk RW, Bistner SI: *Handbook of veterinary procedures and
  emergency treatment,* ed 6, Philadelphia, 1995, W.B. Saun-
  ders.
Lumb and Jones: *Veterinary Anesthesia,* ed 3, Baltimore, 1996,
  Williams and Wilkins.
McCurnin D: *Clinical textbook for veterinary technicians,* ed.
  3, Philadelphia, 1994, W. B. Saunders.
McKelvey D, Hollingshead KW: *Small animal anesthesia,* St.
  Louis, 1994, Mosby–Year Book, Inc.
Muir WW, Hubbell JAE: *Handbook of veterinary anesthesia,*
  St. Louis, 1989, C.V. Mosby.
Sawyer DC et al: *Anesthetic principles and techniques,* ed 6,
  East Lansing, 1981, Michigan State University Press.
Short CE: *Principles and practice of veterinary anesthesia,*
  Baltimore, 1987, Williams and Wilkins.

CHAPTER 17

Parasitology

Mary Lake

OUTLINE

Procedures
    Feces Examination

Commercial Flotation Kits
Blood Parasite Examination

Tables: External and Internal
Parasite Identification

LEARNING OUTCOMES

After reading this chapter you should be able to:

1. List scientific and common names of parasites.
2. Define and describe life cycles of various parasites.
3. Describe clinical signs associated with each parasite.
4. Describe how to identify a parasite infestation.
5. Define treatment and control of parasite infestations.
6. Define various basic laboratory techniques for identification of parasites.

The parasite/host relationship is unique. A parasite is an organism that in its natural habitat feeds and lives on or in another organism. The parasite may cause clinical signs in the host but its goal is to use the host to live and reproduce without causing death. However, a parasite infection in large enough numbers can overwhelm the host and subsequently cause death. Familiarity with life cycles helps us to control parasites. For example, heartworm in dogs can be controlled with preventives. In other cases such as flea infestation the environment and the host need to be treated. Proper identification of para-

This chapter is based on original material published by Michelle Metz, RVT.

sites or ova allows the veterinarian to determine which treatment regimen is appropriate. This chapter describes common parasites by host, beginning with domestic dog and cat and moving on to horses, food animals, and some common lab animals (Tables 17-1 to 17-5).

PROCEDURES

Feces Examination

Gross Examination of Feces

  I. Gross characteristics of feces should be recorded and reported to the veterinarian

  II. Characteristics noted include consistency, color, presence of blood, mucus or adult parasites, including tapeworm segments

Standard Vial Gravitation Flotation Technique

  I. Based on specific gravity of parasitic material and fecal debris

    A. Specific gravity of most parasite eggs is between 1.100-1.200 g/mL

    B. Specific gravity of water is 1.000

    C. The flotation solution must have a higher specific gravity than that of the parasitic material to facilitate flotation of parasite eggs, oocysts, etc.

  II. A simple, inexpensive technique but of poor efficiency

    A. Materials

      1. Vial (approximately 2″ deep by 1″ in diameter)

2. Two paper cups
3. Wire strainer, cheese cloth, or gauze square
4. Tongue depressor
5. Glass slide and coverslip
6. Solution of sodium nitrate with specific gravity of 1.340 g/mL
    a. Other common flotation solutions
        (1) Sugar solution: inexpensive, does not crystallize or distort eggs, specific gravity of 1.330 g/mL
        (2) Zinc sulfate solution: for protozoal organisms, specific gravity of 1.180 g/mL
        (3) Saturated sodium chloride solution, specific gravity 1.200 g/mL
B. Fill a paper cup with approximately 60 mL of sodium nitrate solution
C. Using a tongue depressor, add approximately 2-4 g (0.5-1 teaspoon) of feces
D. Mix feces well with sodium nitrate solution
E. Strain, using wire strainer, into a second cup. Remove as much fluid as possible from the fecal material in the strainer
F. Discard feces on the strainer and wash strainer with hot water for reuse
G. Swirl strained fecal suspension in the cup to randomly disperse eggs and pour mixture into vial until fluid projects above rim of the vial, creating a positive meniscus
H. Place a coverslip on top of the fluid and allow eggs to float upward
I. After 15 to 20 minutes, remove coverslip horizontally, trying not to tilt fluid back into vial, and place it on a glass slide
J. Using 10X objective, systematically examine *entire* area under the coverslip, noting type and number of parasites seen
K. Although the procedure cannot be classified as quantitative, results are reported as follows:
    1. 1-100 eggs seen: graded as one plus (+)
    2. 101-300 eggs seen: graded as two plus (++)
    3. 301-greater seen: graded as three plus (+++)

Commercial Flotation Kits

I. Common examples
    A. Ovassay (Synbiotics, San Diego, CA)
    B. Fecalyzer (EVSCO Pharmaceuticals, Buena, NJ)
    C. Ovatector (BGS Medical Products, Venice, FL)
II. Kits are easy to use but expensive
III. A kit generally comes with a vial, which may or may not have a cap, an insert (or funnel or filter) to collect or pick up feces, and possibly flotation solution
IV. Instructions
    A. Remove insert and push into stool sample
    B. Replace insert containing fecal material into vial
    C. Fill vial with flotation solution (sodium nitrate)
    D. Mix solution and fecal material by gently rotating the insert back and forth in vial
    E. Push insert funnel firmly into place in vial
    F. With additional flotation solution, fill vial completely to form a positive meniscus
    G. Float coverslip on meniscus for 15 to 20 minutes
    H. Place coverslip on slide and examine
    I. Close cap and dispose of vial

Direct Smear

I. A direct smear is used to
    A. Detect protozoa in feces
    B. Quickly estimate the number of parasites
II. Materials
    A. Microscope slides and coverslip
    B. Applicator sticks or tongue depressors
    C. Lugol's iodine or new methylene blue stain (optional)
III. Procedure
    A. Place a drop of saline or water on a slide with an equal amount of feces. A drop of stain may be added at this time
    B. Mix feces and saline with applicator stick
    C. Make a very thin smear on the slide
    D. Remove large pieces of feces on slide for easier viewing
    E. Examine smear using 10X objective for parasite eggs and larvae and 40X objective for protozoal organisms

Blood Parasite Examination (*Dirofilaria immitis* and *Dipetalonema reconditum*)
Modified Knott's Technique

I. Materials
    A. 15 mL centrifuge tube and centrifuge
    B. 2% formalin
    C. Methylene blue stain
    D. Pasteur pipettes and bulbs
    E. Slides and coverslips

Text continued on p. 203

Table 17-1 Common parasites of dogs and cats

Scientific name	Common name	Life cycle	Final site of adult parasite	Clinical signs	Treatment/control	Diagnosis	Misc.
NEMATODES							
Toxocara canis/cati *Toxascaris leonina*	Ascarid, roundworm	1. Ingestion of infective egg directly 2. Via transport host 3. Transplacentally followed by liver-lung migration, then tracheal migration	Free in lumen of small intestine, stomach; feed on intestinal contents	Poor growth, emaciation, intestinal blockage, vomiting, diarrhea, death	Oral anthelmintics	I/D of eggs on flotation *T. canis*: dense cytoplasm, spherical thick pitted shell 90 μ *T. leonina*: spherical thick colorless smooth shell, transparent cytoplasm, 90 μ	Zoonotic Visceral larval migrans Worms in adult dogs tend to somatic migration Eggs hard to remove from the environment
Ancylostoma caninum/ tubaeforme *Uncinaria stenocephala*	Hookworm	1. Transmammary infection 2. Ingestion of larvae 3. Cutaneous penetration by larvae followed by tracheal migration	Attach to intestinal mucosa + suck blood	Microcytic hypochromic anemia, emaciation, weakness, melena, death	Oral anthelmintics	I/D of elliptical, morulated eggs *Ancylostoma* <70 × 35 μ *Uncinaria* >70 × 35 μ	Zoonotic Cutaneous larval migrans
Trichuris vulpis	Whipworm	Direct ingestion of infective eggs	Threaded in mucosa of cecum + large intestine + suck blood	Watery diarrhea with overt blood, emaciation, death possible	Anthelmintics, though resistant to many	I/D of double operculate egg Approx 70 μ Differentiate from *Capillaria* spp.	Prepatent period 74-87 days—therefore clinical signs may appear before eggs shed
Dioctophyma renale	Giant kidney worm	Intermediate host: #1: mudworm #2: fish ingested by final host	(usually right) kidney	Vague abdominal pain after kidney rupture	Surgical removal	I/D of eggs in urine Lemon shaped, double operculate, thick lumpy brown shell, 75 μ	Common in mink

COMPARISON OF MICROFILARIAE

	Dirofilaria immitis	Dipetalonema reconditum
Motility	Coils and uncoils in one spot	Undulates with progressive movement
Anterior end	Tapered	"Broomstick handle," parallel sided
Length	270–325 μm	240–290 μm
Width	6.7–7.3 μm	3.5–6.5 μm

Organism						
Dirofilaria immitis	Heartworm (HW)	Int. host: mosquito 6.5 month prepatent period	Right ventricle, pulmonary artery	Panting, fainting, lethargy, right-sided cardiac enlargement, immiticide kidney + liver changes	1. Kill adults in heart with caparsolate, immiticide 2. Kill circulating microfilaria with ivermectin, levamisole 3. Preventative medication examples: Filaribits, Heartgard, Interceptor	I/D of (1) microfilariae in blood using direct blood smear, Modified Knott's Test or (2) ELISA or Filter Test antigen tests	Must differentiate from *Dipetalonema reconditum*; microfilariae HW seen in other hosts (i.e., coyotes, foxes, cats)

CESTODES

Organism						
Dipylidium caninum	Tapeworm	Int. host: flea larva ingests eggs; dog swallows adult flea	Attach to intestinal wall with suckers and absorb intestinal contents	Usually none, loss of condition, dry coat possible	Oral anthelmintic effective against tapeworms; treat animal and environment for fleas	Identification of egg packets in fecal flotation in crushed proglottid, 125 μ	Zoonotic (need to eat a flea containing a cysticeroid stage — caution crawling children)
Taenia pisiformis	Tapeworm	Int. host: rabbit	Attach to intestinal wall with suckers and absorb intestinal contents	Usually none, loss of condition, dry coat possible	Oral anthelmintics effective against tapeworms Control dog's hunting if possible	I/D of spherical radially striated egg on flotation or in crushed proglottid —40 μ, hexacath larvae	Eggs indistinguishable from other *Taenia* spp. and *Echinococcus granulosus*; Egg is immediately infective to intermediate host only

Continued

Table 17-1 Common parasites of dogs and cats—cont'd

Scientific name	Common name	Life cycle	Final site of adult parasite	Clinical signs	Treatment/ control	Diagnosis	Misc.
				CESTODES—cont'd			
Taenia hydatigena	Tapeworm	Int. host: sheep	Attach to intestinal wall with suckers and absorb intestinal contents	Usually none, loss of condition, dry coat possible	Oral anthelmintic effective against tapeworms; treat animal and environment for fleas	I/D of spherical radially striated egg on flotation or in crushed proglottid —40 μ, hexacath larvae	Eggs indistinguishable from other *Taenia* spp. and *Echinococcus granulosus* Egg is immediately infective to intermediate host only
Echinococcus granulosus	Tapeworm	Int. host: sheep, deer, moose Hydatid cyst grows in liver or lung	Attach to intestinal wall with suckers and absorb intestinal contents	Usually none, loss of condition, dry coat possible	Oral anthelmintic effective against tapeworms; treat animal and environment for fleas	Adult consists of 3-5 proglottids only I/D of egg as for *Taenia* spp.	Zoonotic Man and domestic animals involved when grazing livestock or man ingests food or vegetables contaminated with dog feces
				TREMATODES			
Paragonimus kellicotti	Lung fluke	Int. host: #1: snail #2: crayfish, ingested by dog	Air passages of lungs	Moist, cough, hemoptysis, bronchopneumonia	Limit dog's access to marshland, raw crayfish	I/D of operculated eggs on flotation 95 μ amber color cytoplasm Egg collapses by osmosis on fecal flotation media	Not host specific, can affect a variety of final hosts, including cats

PROTOZOA

Organism		Life cycle	Pathology	Signs	Treatment	Diagnosis	Notes
Isospora spp. Sarcocystis spp.	Coccidia	1. Direct ingestion of sporulated oocyst 2. Sporocysts invade intestinal epithelial cells, produce schizonts (meronts), which invade further cells 3. Macrogamete and microgametocyte produce new oocysts shed in feces	Inside epithelial cells of intestinal lining, break down lining	Persistent diarrhea, dehydration, death (especially pups)	Sulfadimethoxine for 14-21 days	I/D of oocysts of fecal flotation Thin shelled, single celled if fresh Sporulated 2 sporocysts by 4 sporozoites Size range 10-50 μ	Sarcocystis spp. oocysts shed sporulated Isospora spp. shed unsporulated
Giardia spp.		Trophozoites develop to cyst stage in small intestine	Transmission: cyst passed in feces and ingested by dog or cat Final site: lumen of small intestine	Persistent diarrhea, may lead to dehydration, and death (carrier state—no clinical signs)	Prevent fecal contamination of feed and water supply. Disinfect environment with chlorine bleach 1% Treat with metronidazole	I/D of cysts in routine fecal exam—10 μ, elliptical with 4 nuclei Make saline wet mount of fresh warm feces to look for trophozoites under high dry power—10-15 μ, spear shaped, monkey face with 2 nuclei and long flagellae from anterior end	Man potentially infected from all animals and vice versa

Continued

Table 17-1 Common parasites of dogs and cats—cont'd

Scientific name	Common name	Life cycle	Transmission	Clinical signs	Treatment/ control	Diagnosis	Misc.
				ECTOPARASITES			
Ctenocephalides canis or felis	Fleas	Egg→larvae→ pupae→adult	1. Adult fleas hop on host and suck blood 2. Female lays white eggs, which mature to larvae in the environment 3. Larvae feed on organic matter (including *Diplydium caninum*) 4. Pupate and adult emerge when disturbed or detect a host nearby	Irritation, itching, anemia with heavy infestation; flea allergy dermatitis	Anti-flea products (sprays, powders, mousses, dips, growth regulators, monthly preventions) for use on animal and environment	Adults visible to the naked eye, seen in haircoat Eggs often seen as tiny white round pearls Flea dirt seen in haircoat as black, often curly flecks that turn red when wet	Fleas generally not species specific May bite cats, dogs, rodents, birds, humans, though generally not cattle, sheep, horses, goats
Order: Anoplura (sucking) Mallophaga (chewing or biting)	Lice	Eggs→nymph→ adult Adults have 6 legs Cause pediculosis Generally host specific Whole life cycle is spent on the animal Adult lives on skin surface Eggs (nits) are attached to hairs 6-legged nymphs emerge from eggs and develop to adults	Transmitted by direct contact Lice are host specific	**Sucking lice** Barely move Feed on blood Cause anemia, weakness, death Not itchy **Biting lice** Very active on animal Feed on skin debris Cause itchiness, irritation Not deadly Smaller than sucking lice	Various topical treatments Some systemic anthelmintics (ivermectin)	**Sucking lice:** head *narrower* than thorax **Biting lice:** head *wider* than thorax	Swine and man have sucking lice only Birds and cats have biting lice only Other animals have *both* biting and sucking lice

Ticks Families: Argasid (soft ticks) Ixodid (hard ticks)	Eggs→Larva→ nymph→adult Picked up from wooded areas Feed on blood Visible to the naked eye Often carry disease causing organisms (e.g., Q-fever, Rocky Mountain spotted fever, Lyme disease) Can be one host, 2- host, or 3-host ticks Causes acariasis	1. Adults climb on- to host from grasses; female engorges with blood and drops off, lays eggs, which hatch in- to larvae 2. Larva has 6 legs; wait to grab on- to a passing warm blooded host, feeds and moults to nymph 3. Nymph has 8 legs and feeds on host blood then moults to adult	Anemia, weakness, death if infesta- tion is heavy	Mitaban, ether, chloroform applied to tick to facilitate removal of whole tick; If the parasite is on the skin of the animal, is grossly visible, and has 8 legs it is probably a tick	Specialized— usually sent to a lab for iden- tification do not leave mouthparts of tick in animal's skin to abscess
Mites	Eggs→Larva (6 legs), →nymph (8 legs), → adult (8 legs)	Transmitted by dir- ect contact	Cause mange, usually involving hair loss, scabs, thickening of skin	Usually treat with topical miti- cides or iver- mectin	Diagnosis with skin scraping All stages can be found on the skin
Demodex sp.		Causes demodi- cosis	May show no lesions or they clear up with no treatment In some dogs, pro- duces general- ized hair loss; not usually itchy; problem appears to be immune- deficiency, per- haps genetically transmitted "red mange"	Cigar shaped mite with 8 stumpy legs May see mites and eggs on fecal floats due to licking lesions	Can affect cattle and goats, cause hard nodules on skin

Continued

Table 17-1 Common parasites of dogs and cats—cont'd

Scientific name	Common name	Life cycle	Transmission	Clinical signs	Treatment/control	Diagnosis	Misc.
				ECTOPARASITES—cont'd			
Sarcoptes sp.		Deep skin mite, bores into skin, therefore difficult to diagnose; often need repeated scrapings		Causes 'scabies'; characterized by hair loss, intense itching, scabs, rapid spread throughout body		Round mite with short stubby legs, unjointed pedicles, and dorsal spines	Fairly common in dogs; seen occasionally in cattle and pigs
Cheyletiella sp.				Causes 'walking dandruff' characterized by tiny moving white spots on skin surface with itching, signs of self-inflicted trauma, occasionally weakness, dehydration, and death		Identified by examining dandruff and skin debris Microscopic mite with upside-down pear-shaped body with comb on end of feet	Common in rabbits; occasionally seen in dogs and cats
Otodectes sp.	Ear mites			Mites live in ear canal, cause itching, increased wax production, otitis externa, self inflicted trauma, aural hematomas, possibly from head shaking		Mite identified from ear swab in mineral oil Mite has tulip-like suckers on 4 front feet	Common in cats; uncommon in dogs
Notoedres sp.				Causes 'head mange' in cats Characteristic dry grey crusty lesions on head and face		May be confused with Sarcoptes sp. but it has no dorsal spines	
Chorioptes sp.				Causes crusty lesions		Pear shaped mite with long legs and tulip suckers on front legs	Common mange of cattle Seen around fetlocks of horses

II. Procedure
   A. Place 1 mL of uncoagulated blood in a 15 mL conical centrifuge tube
   B. Add 9 mL of 2% formalin
   C. Mix by inversion and shake to lyse the RBC
   D. Centrifuge for 5 minutes at 1000 rpm *or* let stand for one hour
   E. Decant supernatant by inverting tube once and let drain
   F. Add 2 drops of methylene blue stain to the sediment and mix with a pipette by gently aspirating the mixture
   G. Place a drop of the mixture on a slide, add coverslip, and examine under 10× objective
   H. Examine entire slide for microfilariae

Commercial Filter Technique

   I. Common examples of commercial kits
   A. Di-Fil (EVASCO, Buena, NJ)
   B. Filarassay*F Heartworm Diagnostic Test Kit (Pitman-Moore, Mundelein, IL)
   II. These kits come with filters, lysing solution, stain, and directions
   III. Most kits require 1 mL of whole blood to test for heartworms
   IV. Mix blood with 10 to 12 mL of lysing solution
   V. Place a new filter in the filter holder, inject the fluid into the filter holder, rinse with 10 mL of water
   VI. Place the filter on a slide, add a drop of stain
   VII. Add a coverslip to the slide and examine slide

Buffy Coat Method

   I. A concentration method using a small amount of blood
   II. Quick and can be performed after evaluation of a PCV and before total protein evaluation
   III. Materials
   A. Microhematocrit tubes and sealer
   B. Centrifuge
   C. Microscope slides and coverslips
   D. Saline
   E. Methylene blue stain
   F. Small file or glass cutter
   IV. Procedure
   A. Centrifuge blood-filled microhematocrit tube for 3 minutes
   B. Read PCV
   C. Examine surface of buffy coat (WBC) layer of the blood under microscope
      1. When centrifuging a blood-filled microhematocrit tube, the blood seperates into three layers
         a. Plasma
         b. WBC layer (buffy coat)
         c. RBC layer
   D. Use a file to scratch tube at level of the buffy coat. Snap tube and gently tap tube to place buffy coat on slide
   E. Add a drop of saline and a drop of stain to the buffy coat. Add coverslip and examine for microfilariae
   F. Use remaining plasma from the PCV to evaluate total protein

Enzyme-linked Immunosorbent Assay (ELISA Test)

   I. ELISA kits do not detect microfilariae. Only the host's response to parasites or antigens present in the blood are detected
   II. This type of test can be used to identify
   A. Occult heartworm
   B. *Dirofilaria immitis*
   C. *Dipetalonema* infection
   III. Common examples
   A. Dirocheck (Synbiotics, San Diego, CA)
   B. CITE Heartworm Test Kit (IDEXX, Portland, ME)
   C. Snap Whole Blood Heartworm Antigen Test (IDEXX, Portland, ME)
   IV. ELISA antigen detection system
   A. Monoclonal antibody is bound to the walls of a well in a test tray, to a membrane, or to a plastic wand
   B. If the specific antigen is present in the sample it will bind to this antibody and to the second enzyme-labeled antibody that is added
   C. When a color-producing agent is added to the mixture, the agent reacts to develop a specific color that indicates presence of the antigen in the sample
   D. If the sample contains no antigen, the second antibody is washed away during a rinsing process and no other color reactions take place
   V. ELISA tests are easy to perform when following manufacturer directions and take approximately 15 to 20 minutes to complete

External Parasite Identification
Skin Scraping

   I. Materials
   A. #10 scalpel blade
   B. Mineral oil in a dropper bottle
   C. Microscope slides
   D. Microscope

Text continued on p. 218

Table 17-2 Common parasites in horses

Scientific name	Common name	Life cycle	Transmission	Clinical signs	Treatment/control	Diagnosis	Misc.
				NEMATODES			
Parascaris equorum	Ascarid	1. Direct ingestion of infective egg 2. Larva hatches, follows liver-lung cycle and tracheal migration	Feed on intestinal contents in lumen of small intestine	Especially in foal with heavy infection, weakness, lethargy, loss of condition colic possible	Oral anthelmintics Limit foals' access to stale manure	I/D of subspherical eggs with pitted amber shell or smooth clear shell, 95 μ	Extremely hardy eggs, can survive in the environment for many years
Strongylus vulgaris	Bloodworm, large strongyle	Direct ingestion of infective larvae in soil, which then migrate along wall of small arteries to wall of anterior mesenteric artery + develop, break into lumen of artery + repenetrate lumen of large intestine	Attach to lining of large intestine and suck blood	1. Verminous arteritis from larvae growing in artery wall: inflamed enlarged wall with reduced blood flow to gut 2. Gut stasis from decreased circulation, thrombus formation, and death 3. Effect of adults as below	Oral anthelmintics	I/D of elliptical, morulated egg on fecal flotation, approx. 70-100 μ	Eggs not distinguishable from other large and small strongyles. Prepatent period of all large strongyles >7 months, therefore strongyle eggs in foals <7 months old are from small strongyles
Strongylus equinus *Strongylus edentatus*	Bloodworm, strongyle	Ingestion of infective larvae in soil, which then migrate to liver + other viscera, eventually breaking out in lumen of large intestine	Attach to lining of large intestine and suck blood	Larvae not too pathogenic, may cause colic when penetrating gut wall if in large numbers Adults may cause anemia, loss of condition	Oral anthelmintics	I/D of elliptical, morulated egg on fecal flotation, approx. 70-100 μ	Eggs not distinguishable from other large and small strongyles. Prepatent period of all large strongyles >7 months, therefore strongyle eggs in foals <7 months old are from small strongyles

The Cyathostomes	Small strongyles	Direct ingestion of infective larvae in soil, which penetrate and develop in gut wall, then reenter lumen	Free in lumen of large intestine	Poor growth, loss of condition	Oral anthelmintics	I/D of elliptical, morulated egg on fecal flotation approx. 70-100 μ. Eggs not distinguishable from other large and small strongyles. Prepatent period of all large strongyles >7 months, therefore strongyle eggs in foals <7 months old are from small strongyles
Oxyuris equi	Pinworm	1. Direct ingestion of infective egg 2. Larva hatches and penetrates colon wall to develop, returns to lumen 3. Female lays eggs on skin around anus	Lumen of rectum	Intense anal itching, rubbing of hind end on stalls, fence posts, etc.	Scrub stalls with soap and water to remove eggs, prevent reinfection	1. I/D on flotation of operculate, oval, larvated egg, often flattened on 1 side 90 μ. 2. I/D of egg mass in the perianal region (looks like whip cream) 3. I/D of adult worms passed in feces
Strongyloides westeri	Threadworm	Infective larvae penetrate skin or are transmitted transmammarily or by direct ingestion	Small intestine	Usually none, occasionally diarrhea in foals	Oral anthelmintics	I/D of larvated egg on flotation, approx. 40 μ. Seen for a short period of time in foals
Setaria equina		Int. host: mosquito picks up microfilariae, which develop to infective stage and are injected into horse	Free in abdominal or thoracic cavity	Usually none, occasionally microfilariae in eyes cause clouding of vision	Usually none necessary	Adult worms found during abdominal surgery or necropsy microfilariae seen in blood

Continued

Table 17-2 Common parasites in horses—cont'd

Scientific name	Common name	Life cycle	Transmission	Clinical signs	Treatment/control	Diagnosis	Misc.
			NEMATODES—cont'd				
Habronema muscae *H. microstoma* *Draschia megastoma*		1. Eggs + larvae laid in feces ingested by flies + develop inside 2. Horse ingests flies (e.g., in water bucket or flies feed on open skin wounds) 3. Infective larvae leave fly and remain in wound	Adults in stomach, larvae in open wound	Larvae in skin cause Summer sore: itchy, red-brown weepy sores that don't heal very rapidly		Usually only at necropsy Eggs not recovered in feces	
Dictyocaulus arnfeldi	Lungworm	Larvated egg coughed up and swallowed, larva passed in stool, reingested from pasture, migrate to lungs via lymphatics	Adults in bronchi and bronchioles	Rare, coughing	Anthelmintics	Larvae with brown granules recovered by Water Baermann technique	

CESTODE							
Anoplocephala magna A. perfoliata	Tapeworm	Ingestion of intermediate host: pasture mite containing cysticercoid	Attached in small intestine	Usually none, occasionally diarrhea, colic from gut irritation	Most anthelmintics not effective	I/D of squarish eggs with hexacanth larvae and pyriform apparatus, approx. 70 μ. Segments not usually seen in feces	May be hard to recover on routine fecal float nitrate sodium nitrate fecal float usually seen in feces
PROTOZOA							
Eimeria leukarti	Coccidia	Most of life cycle unclear	Cells of small intestine	None	Not indicated	I/D of dark brown thick-shelled large oocyst on flotation, 65 μ	Rare—only shed for a few weeks during lifetime
ARTHROPODS							
Gasterophilus spp.	Stomach bot	1. Adult female flies lay eggs attached to hairs 2. Horse licks, larvae enter gums and tongue, mature for 3-4 weeks, re-emerge and are swallowed, attach to stomach mucosa—9-10 months pass in feces, pupate in soil	See life cycle	Adult flies annoying to horse Bots in tongue cause ulcers, possibly pain and decreased desire to feed Bots in stomach may depress, occ. cause perforation	Treat in fall with anthelmintics effective against bots	I/D of eggs on hair, bots in tongue	G. nasalis: eggs on the face G. intestinalis: eggs on legs, withers, neck, and mane Bot identified by double rows of spines

Table 17-3 Common parasites in cows and sheep

Scientific name	Common name	Life cycle	Final site	Clinical signs	Treatment/control	Diagnosis	Misc.
GASTROINTESTINAL NEMATODES							
Haemonchus placei in cattle *Haemonchus contortus* in sheep	GIN, large stomach worm, barberpole worm	Direct ingestion of infective larvae in pasture	Suck blood in abomasum	Anemia, poor growth, bottle-jaw occasionally, death esp. pathogenic in sheep	Oral anthelmintics	I/D of GIN eggs on flotation Eggs of different GIN species indistinguishable from one another Elliptical, morulated egg with a size range of 60-90 μ	Perform fecal egg count mid-summer to determine extent of pasture contamination
Ostertagia ostertagi in cattle *Ostertagia circumcinta* in sheep	GIN, medium stomach worm	Direct ingestion of infective larvae in pasture	Suck blood in abomasum	Esp. pathogenic in cattle	Oral anthelmintics	I/D of GIN eggs on flotation Eggs of different GIN species indistinguishable from one another Elliptical, morulated egg with a size range of 60-90 μ	Perform fecal egg count mid-summer to determine extent of pasture contamination
Trichostrongylus axei in cattle *T. colubriformis* in sheep	GIN, small stomach worm	Direct ingestion of infective larvae in pasture	Feed on contents of abomasum	Scours, loss of condition, decreased milk production	Oral anthelmintics	I/D of GIN eggs on flotation Eggs of different GIN species indistinguishable from one another Elliptical, morulated egg with a size range of 60-90 μ	Perform fecal egg count mid-summer to determine extent of pasture contamination
Cooperia spp.	GIN, small intestinal worms	Direct ingestion of infective larvae in pasture	Small intestine	Scours, loss of condition, decreased milk production	Oral anthelmintics	I/D of GIN eggs on flotation Eggs of different GIN species indistinguishable from one another Elliptical, morulated egg with a size range of 60-90 μ	Perform fecal egg count mid-summer to determine extent of pasture contamination

Strongyloides spp.	GIN, small intestinal worms	Direct ingestion of infective larvae in pasture	Small intestine	Scours, loss of condition, decreased milk production	Oral anthelmintics	Larvated egg laid	Perform fecal egg count mid-summer to determine extent of pasture contamination
Nematodirus spp.	GIN, small intestinal worms	Direct ingestion of infective larvae in pasture	Small intestine	Scours, loss of condition, decreased milk production	Oral anthelmintics	Egg very large but otherwise similar to all other GIN eggs, more pointed ends; 125-150 μ	Perform fecal egg count mid-summer to determine extent of pasture contamination
Bunostomum phlebotomum in cattle *B. trigonocephalum* in sheep	Hookworm	Direct ingestion or bore through skin, follow tracheal migration	Attach to mucosa of small intestine and suck blood	Anemia	Oral anthelmintics	I/D of GIN-type egg. Adult worm reddish in color	Perform fecal egg count mid-summer to determine extent of pasture contamination
Oesophagostomum radiatum in cattle *O. columbianum* and *O. venulosum* in sheep	Nodular worm	Direct ingestion of infective larvae on pasture	Coil up in submucosa and form nodules	Diarrhea, weight loss	Oral anthelmintics	I/D of GIN-type egg	Organs are condemned at meat inspection if nodules seen
Trichuris spp.	Whipworm	Direct ingestion of infective eggs from pasture	As in dogs	Usually low worm burdens	Difficult to treat	I/D of lemon-shaped egg with bipolar plugs on flotation, 70 μ	Not transmissible to dogs
Dictyocaulus viviparus	Lungworm	1. Direct ingestion of infective larvae from pasture, which then travel in bloodstream, break out into air passages of lungs 2. Larvated eggs coughed up into mouth, swallowed and passed in feces	Lung Trachea/bronchi	Mucus and froth production, difficult breathing, coughing, loss of condition	Oral anthelmintics	Larvated eggs in saliva, or hatched larvae recovered from feces Larvae with dark staining granules	

Continued

Table 17-3 Common parasites in cows and sheep—cont'd

Scientific name	Common name	Life cycle	Final site	Clinical signs	Treatment/control	Diagnosis	Misc.
				CESTODE			
Moniezia benedeni in cattle *M. expansa* in sheep	Tapeworm	Intermediate host: pasture mite, swallowed while cattle, sheep graze	Attach to small intestine with suckers	Not very pathogenic, decreased weight gain possible	Oral anthelmintic effective against tapeworms	I/D of squarish crystal-like eggs on flotation Proglottids seen, pyriform apparatus with hexacanth larvae visible, approx. 60 µ	
				TREMATODE			
Fasciola hepatica	Liver fluke	Int. host: miracidium encysts on snail, develops through 3 stages; then metacercariae develop on grass and are swallowed during grazing	Bile ducts of liver	Liver changes, weight loss		I/D of operculate egg on flotation Granular cytoplasm Approx. 130-150 × 63-90 µ	
				PROTOZOA			
Eimeria spp.	Coccidia	See general Coccidia life cycle	As for dogs	None, or scours; especially in young	Oral amprolium	I/D of oocyst on flotation, many sizes and shapes Unsporulated in fresh feces	Sporulated oocysts contain 4 sporocysts containing 2 sporozoites each

ECTOPARASITES

		Life cycle		Effects / signs	Control / treatment	Diagnosis / notes
Melophagus ovinus	Sheep ked	1. Adult female releases larvae 2. Pupa forms attaches to wool, hatches in 3-5 weeks	Adults live entire life on host, feed on blood	Heavy infection may cause anemia, weakness, irritation, itching, and damage to wool	Die when off host (e.g., when wool shorn off)	I/D of adults in wool; motile, hairy, 6-legged wingless fly
Oestrus ovis	Nose bot in sheep	Adult fly strikes at sheep and injects maggot in nostril, which grows through winter Pupates in soil	Maggot in nostril	Sheep bothered by adult flies Maggots cause nasal irritation, mucus production, sneezing	Control of flies	In spring, I/D of fully developed larva with brown stripes on underside
Hypoderma bovis *Hypoderma lineatum*	Warble grubs in cattle	1. Adult flies lay eggs on hairs (*H. bovis* 1 egg per hair, *H. lineatum* 5-15 eggs per hair) 2. Larvae hatch and migrate (*H. bovis* to spinal canal, *H. Lineatum* to esophagus/ trachea area) 3. Both then migrate to back cut breathing hole, drop to ground, and pupate	See life cycle	Adults cause stress, decreased milk production, decreased weight gain, damage to leather, decreased value of meat	1. Control adult flies in environment 2. Treat in early fall with insecticides 3. Dangerous and potentially life-threatening to treat during larval migration in body	I/D of eggs on hairs, especially lower leg, of larvae on back Check milk/meat drug withdrawal times after treatment

Table 17-4 Common parasites in pigs

Scientific name	Common name	Life cycle	Final site	Clinical signs	Treatment/control	Diagnosis	Misc.
NEMATODES							
Hyostrongylus rubidus	Red stomach worm	Ingestion of infective larvae	Suck blood in stomach	Decreased weight gain	Oral anthelmintics Housing on cement or grating instead of dirt	I/D of oval eggs on flotation GIN type egg approx. 75 μ	Eggs indistinguishable from *Oesophagostomum dentatum* Need to culture eggs and Baermann to differentiate larvae
Oesophagostomum dentatum	Nodular worm	Direct ingestion of infective larvae	Penetrate mucosa of small and large intestine and form nodules	Decreased weight gain	Oral anthelmintics Housing on cement or grating instead of dirt	I/D of oval eggs on flotation GIN type egg approx. 75 μ	
Ascaris suum	Ascarid	Ingestion of infective eggs, migrate in bloodstream to liver and lungs; follow tracheal migration	Lumen of small intestine	Dyspnea during migration in nursing piglets Decreased weight gain in growing pigs	Oral anthelmintics Housing on cement or grating instead of dirt	I/D of subspherical eggs with lumpy or smooth shell, approx. 65 μ	Zoonotic
Trichuris suis	Whipworm	Direct ingestion of infective eggs	Threaded in mucosa of cecum	Heavy infections may cause diarrhea with overt blood	Oral anthelmintics Housing on cement or grating instead of dirt	I/D of lemon shaped egg with bipolar plugs on flotation, approx. 55 μ	
Trichinella spiralis		Female adult releases larvae, which migrate in bloodstream and encyst all over body When meat containing cysts eaten, larvae released and mature	Adults in mucosa of small intestine/ larvae coiled up in microscopic cysts in body tissues	None in pigs	Avoid feeding raw pork or pork products to pigs	No routine testing currently done in Canada of meet inspection	Zoonotic Infection by ingestion of viable larvae in meat

Metastrongylus apri	Lungworm	Intermediate host: earthworm, eaten by rooting pig	Migrate in bloodstream to lungs and break out into air passages	Coughing and predisposition to bacterial and viral respiratory infections	Oral anthelmintics	I/D of larvated egg with finely scalloped shell on flotation, approx. 50 μ
CESTODE						
Taenia solium	Tapeworm of humans	Pig is int. host, picks up infective eggs from human feces, cyst forms in muscle	Human ingests cysts from undercooked pork, attach to small intestine	None in pig	Humans should avoid undercooked pork products	Proglottids, eggs recovered from human feces
ACANTHOCEPHALAN						
Macracanthorhynchus hirundinaceus	Spiny-headed worm	Int. host: grub	Attaches to intestinal wall and absorbs nutrients	Few		I/D of oval dark brown eggs on flotation
PROTOZOA						
Eimeria spp. *Isospora* spp.	Coccidia	See general *Coccidia* life cycle as for dogs		*Eimeria* not considered pathogenic; *Isospora* causes diarrhea, dehydration, death in nursing piglets	Usually not treated	Allow feces to become stale—2-3 days, oocysts to sporulate, can then tell *Isospora* (with 2 sporocysts) versus *Eimeria* (with 4 sporocysts)

Table 17-5 Common parasites in laboratory animals

Parasite	Etiology	Transmission	Clinical signs	Treatment/control	Diagnosis	Misc.
			MICE/RATS			
Oxyuriasis (pinworm)	*Syphacia obvelata:* common parasite of mice Direct lifecycle of 11-15 days *Aspicularis teraptera* is similar but has a life cycle of 21-27 days, parasite does not live in the cecum Eggs are rounded, not deposited around the perianal region and adult morphology is different Young mice, certain species, and males may be more susceptible	Generally contamination of environment	Often not seen but heavily infected animals may suffer fron intussusception, rectal prolapse, enteritis, fecal impactions, and poor weight gains	Piperazine in drinking water for 1 week Use a detergent wash to remove ova from perineum and environment	Oxyurid eggs from perineum, fecal flotations, or with clear tapes Presence of adult worms in large intestine or cecum	*Syphacia* reported in humans
Dwarf tapeworm	Hymenolepsis nana —*Taenia taeniaforms* as larval form (*Cysticercus fasciolaris*)	*H. nana* has 3 cycle variations, prepatent period is 15-30 days	May be none or mild to moderate enteritis, constipation, catarrhal, diarrhea, weight loss, and death	*H. nana* Yomesan; thiabendzole; praziquantel in feed for 1 week	Oval ovum of *H. nana* with embryo and 3 pairs of hooks in proglottids shed in feces	*H. nana* is pathogenic for man and may cause enteric disease

Dwarf tapeworm —con't	Predisposing factors Mice in 5-7 week old range are most often infected Debility and lack of previous exposure Susceptibility and reaction varies		*H. diminuta* is less pathogenic and host specific to mice *H. nana* may stay in environment and keeps autoinfection potential Prevent by eliminating vermin and vectors Keep food and bedding clean Prevent by placing clean stock into clean premises	Animals compromised by long periods of therapy *Taenia taeniaforms*—on necropsy, larvae are detected in liver Adults seen on necropsy found in small intestine
Acariasis—in mice the usual fur mite species: *Myobiomusculi* *Mycoptes muscalinis* *Notoedres muris* Arachnids Adults have 8 legs Live on skin surface with eggs attached to hair shafts Cycles average 10-21 days, eggs hatch in 8 days Predisposing factors include young, old, or compromised; black strains are more susceptible	Spread by direct contact Adult female may live a week or more off the host Commonly infect rabbits and rodents Species are usually host specific	Generally only cause scratching but may be more of a problem in susceptible mice —follicular mite (*Psorergates simplex*) inhabit hair follicles and sebaceous glands and may be seen as white nodules, which are often noticed at necropsy	Once infection established treatment will control rather than eliminate Dusting of adult fur with permethrin dust on host and bedding weekly Some sources suggest lindane or other dips Vapona strip hung at appropriate levels (48 hour periods at several weekly intervals but be careful!)	Can impress cellophane tape against the hair and examine microscopically Can also diagnose on necropsy

Continued

Table 17-5 Common parasites in laboratory animals—cont'd

Parasite	Etiology	Transmission	Clinical signs	Treatment/control	Diagnosis	Misc.
RABBITS						
Oxyurids (pinworm)	*Passalurus ambiguus*	Ingestion of feces			Ova in feces *Passalurus* sp. does not deposit ova in the perianal area	
Cestodes	*Taenia pisiformis* Generally subclinical signs *Multiceps serialis* Larval stage		Cyst formation under the skin or in other tissues, including muscles and brain			
Coccidia	*Eimeria* sp. A healthy adult rabbit will normally have oocysts in feces	Introduction into young or old Clinical signs vary	Weight loss, soft to watery feces, mild to severe dehydration, intense thirst Feces may have mucus or blood, foul odor Mortality may be high or low, depending on *Eimeria* sp., immune status, degree of infection		I/D of oocysts on flotation	
Hepatic coccidiosis— protozoal disease of rabbits and wild lagomorphs	*Eimeria stiedae* prepatent period of 15-18 days Sporulated oocysts excyst in duodenum and pass via lymph and blood to liver and other organs Schizogony and gametogony→ biliary epithelium→unsporulated oocysts→ bile ducts to intestine	Ingestion of sporulated oocysts in feces (need 2 or more days outside of the host to sporulate); thus coprophagy not likely route of infection Long lasting immunity after initial exposure Extremely resistant —may be infectious several months	Subclinical —can see: anorexia, failure to gain or weight loss, enlarged abdomen icterus, diarrhea and death Young susceptible rabbits with large number oocysts—up to 50% mortality Alteration of liver tests Adults usually show no signs	Appear to be sensitive to penicillins, especially ampicillin Get disturbance of normal intestinal microflora and produce diarrhea Sanitation: Regularly examine all rabbits and purchase from reputable, single source Important to isolate sick animals	Oocysts in feces but hard to determine if due to incidental low grade infection or associated with primary disease Intestinal scrapings Microscopic examination Lesions in intestine, on necropsy, yellow-white foci-raised, fuzzy edged and ooze yellow-green fluid when cut Bile ducts, gallbladder, hepatomegaly	

Acarids	*Psoroptes cuniculi* Life cycle 21 days (ear mite)		Accumulation of serum and brown crusts with skin beneath hairless, moist and raw, may be scratching and head shaking	Suspended mesh cages, J-type feeders and water bottles; Can give medicated feed or water; Cull if necessary; Treat with oil-based insecticide or ivermectin	Can see with otoscope
Cheyletiella	*Cheyletiella parasitivorax* and *Listrophorus gibbus* (fur mite)		Cheyletiella may cause no signs, loose hair, erythematous patches, increased dandruff; *Listrophorus* sp. is nonpathogenic		

GUINEA PIGS

Coccidia	*Eimeria caviae*	Direct contact	Heavy infections will produce a typhlitis and colitis, which may manifest clinically by diarrhea, anorexia, lethargy, and occasionally death	Condition can be controlled by improved sanitary practices and husbandry and the use of coccidiostats	Characteristic oocysts in the feces
Ticks		Direct contact	Same as mice		
Mites	Sucking lice *Polyplax* sp. *Haemodipsus* sp. Biting lice *Gliricola* sp. *Gyropus* sp. *Chirodiscoides caviae* (fur mite) *Trixacarus caviae* (sarcoptic mite)	Posterior of animal	Signs include severe alopecia, dermatitis, pruritis on body and legs, skin thickened, dry, and scaly		

II. Procedure
    A. Add mineral oil to a slide and dip scalpel blade in it
    B. Begin scraping by holding skin between thumb and index finger of one hand and scalpel blade in the other hand
    C. While scraping, the blade must be held perpendicular to the skin
        1. Holding the blade at any other angle could result in an incision into the skin
    D. Depth of scraping depends on the suspected parasite
        1. *Sarcoptes* (burrowing mite) and *Demodex* (hair follicle mite)—scrape until blood begins to seep from the abrasion
        2. *Chorioptes* (nonburrowing mite) and *Cheyletiella* (walking dandruff)—skin is scraped superficially to collect loose scales and crusts
    E. All of the harvest (material scraped from the skin) is placed on a slide with mineral oil
    F. After adding a coverslip, examine entire slide under the 10× objective
    G. For thorough evaluation, examine at least 10 slides

Cellophane Tape Method

I. Used for mites that are primarily on skin surface and the hair (e.g., *Cheyletiella*)
II. Materials
    A. Cellophane tape
    B. Mineral oil
    C. Microscope slides
III. Procedure
    A. Using cellophane tape, lift off epidermal dermis from skin surface
    B. Place a drop of mineral oil on a slide and stick tape on top of the slide
    C. Examine slide

Glossary

acariasis Infestation of mites
anthelmintic Against worms, therefore a drug used to remove worms
arthropod Invertebrate animals having segmented external coverings and jointed legs (i.e., ticks and mites)
Baermann technique Using a funnel apparatus, soil/fecal material is deposited in cheesecloth and covered with saline overnight. A drop of fluid from the bottom of the funnel is removed and examined for larvae

cestode A group of parasites that requires two hosts for development. Adult worms are found in the final host. Larval worms are in the intermediate host. Infection with adult worms results from eating larval cyst from the intermedicate host. Commonly called "tapeworms."
efficacy The effect a drug is supposed to have against a certain organism
ELISA *E*nzyme-*l*inked *i*mmuno*s*orbent *a*ssay
final host Normal host or definitive host. Type of animal in which the adult worm is found
hexacanth Infective stage of development in a cestode egg after fertilization takes place
infective Developed to a stage capable of causing infection
intermediate host Any organism in which a parasite lives during its larval or nonreproductive stage
mange Infestation of mites
meniscus The curved upper surface of a liquid in a container
morulated A solid mass of cells clustered together
myiasis Invasion of living tissue by fly maggots
nematode A class of roundworms
noninfective Not yet developed to a stage capable of causing infection
paratenic host One in which the parasite a) does not develop to adult, b) remains alive for long periods of time, c) does not rely on host exclusively to complete its life cycle. As in transmission of infection
patent infection Worms have developed to adult, eggs are being passed, and can be diagnosed by fecal examination
PCV Packed cell volume
pediculosis Infestation of lice
prepatent infection Occurs when worms have not yet developed to adults; therefore no eggs are being shed and a diagnosis is not possible by fecal examination
prepatent period (ppp) Period of time between infection and passage of eggs in the feces
protozoa A unicelleular organism (i.e., Coccidia)
trematode A group of parasites that are hermaphroditic, have two suckers (oral and ventral), and require an intermediate host, commonly called "flukes"
zoonosis A disease acquired by an animal or shared by man and other vertebrates

Review Questions

1 ELISA tests can detect
    a. *Dirofilaria immitis*
    b. *Dirofilaria* antigen
    c. Microfilaria
    d. Only occult heartworm
2 *Eimeria stiedai* is associated with:
    a. Hepatic coccidiosis in rabbits
    b. Cecal coccidiosis in chickens
    c. Renal coccidiosis in geese
    d. Intestinal coccidiosis in dogs

3 Biting lice have which characteristic?
  a. Head wider than thorax
  b. Feed on blood
  c. Not itchy
  d. Barely move

4 Cutaneous larval migrans are caused by
  a. *Toxocara cati*
  b. *Trichuris vulpis*
  c. *Ancylostoma caninum*
  d. *Aeleurostrongylus* sp.

5 Visceral larval migrans are caused by ingestion of
  a. *Echinococcus* sp.
  b. *Toxocara* sp.
  c. *Uncinaria* sp.
  d. *Dioctophyma renale*

6 The intermediate host for the bovine tapeworm *Moniezia* sp. is
  a. Bird
  b. Pasture mite
  c. Snail
  d. Mudworm

7 *Eimeria* spp. when sporulated contain;
  a. 4 sporocysts with 2 sporozoites
  b. 2 sporocysts with 4 sporozoites
  c. 1 sporocyst with 3 sporozoites
  d. None of the above

8 The term *Pediculosis* means:
  a. Infestation by mites
  b. Invasion of living tissue by fly maggots
  c. Intense itching and hair loss
  d. Infestation by lice

9 Which of the following is *not* true about ticks?
  a. Often carry disease-causing organisms
  b. Are generally picked up from wooded areas
  c. Feed on blood
  d. Are microscopic

10. The prepatent period for *Dirofilaria immitis* is:
  a. 6.5 weeks
  b. 3 months
  c. 8 months
  d. 6.5 months

BIBLIOGRAPHY

Coles EH: *Veterinary clinical pathology,* ed 3, Pennsylvania, 1980, W.B. Saunders.

Georgi JR: *Parasitology for veterinarians,* ed 3, Pennsylvania, 1974, W.B. Saunders.

Harkness and Wagner: *The biology and medicine of rabbits and rodents,* ed 3, Philadelphia, 1989, Lea & Febiger.

Ivens et al. *Principal parasites of domestic animals in the U.S.:* 1989, University of Illinois.

Lautenslager P: 1982, Notes in veterinary parasitology for animal health technicians.

Noble and Noble: *Parasitology,* ed 4, Philadelphia, 1976, Lea & Febiger.

Pratt WP: *Laboratory procedures for veterinary technicians,* ed 3, St. Louis, 1997, Mosby.

Sloss & Kemp: *Veterinary clinical parasitology:* Ames, Iowa, 1978, Iowa State University Press.

Williams et al: *Diagnosis of GI parasitism in dogs and cats,*

CHAPTER 18

Diagnostic Microbiology and Mycology

Sandy Skeba

OUTLINE

Purpose
Equipment
  Light Microscope
  Incubator
  Sterilizing Heat Sources
  Media
  Miscellaneous Equipment
Bacteriological and Fungal Media
  Basic Media
  Specific Types of Media
Types of Specimens
  Sterile Areas
  Nonsterile Areas
  Abscessed Areas
Collection and Culture of Specimens
  Swab Specimen

Liquid Specimen
Solid Specimen
Urine Specimen
Blood Specimen
Fecal Cultures
Fungal Cultures
Bacterial Identification
  Gram-positive Cocci
  Gram-negative Cocci
  Gram-negative Rods
  Gram-negative Spirochetes
  Gram-negative Coccobacilli
  Gram-positive Rods
Fungal Identification
  Identification
  Dermatophytes

Saprophytes
Yeast
Dimorphi Fungi
Basic Diagnostic Tests
  Gram Stain
  Catalase Test
  Oxidase Test
  Bile Esculin
  API 20E Test
  Kirby-Bauer Sensitivity
  Streaking for Isolation
  Acid-fast Stain

LEARNING OUTCOMES

After reading this chapter you should be able to:

1. List and describe equipment needed to perform diagnostic microbiology.
2. Describe and list the purposes of various bacterial and fungal media.
3. Describe the types of samples that may be obtained from the body for microbiological culture.
4. Describe the collection of specimens.
5. Explain bacterial identification procedures for gram-positive and gram-negative bacteria.
6. Explain fungal identification.
7. Describe how to perform various diagnostic tests to identify specific bacteria and fungi.

Microbiology is the study of microscopic organisms. Clinical microbiology is the identification of these organisms, including bacteria, fungi, parasites, and viruses, that cause clinical illness. In this chapter we will explore the fundamental components of a working clinical microbiology laboratory, the most common causes of bacterial and fungal diseases of domestic animals, and how to use this information to assist the veterinarian in the diagnosis and treatment of these diseases.

PURPOSE

The purpose of a veterinary clinical microbiology laboratory is to:

1. Assist the veterinarian in the diagnosis and treatment of bacteriological and fungal disease
2. Provide accurate identification of causes of infections

3. Provide useful information about the organisms cultured (i.e., antibiotic sensitivity)
4. Maintain cost-and-time effectiveness while presenting all of the above
   a. Many practices send out cultures to commercial labs, since their low volume of samples makes keeping media impractical
   b. Competent staff must be available to perform microbiological procedures
   c. Clients may benefit from the quick turnaround time of an in-house lab

EQUIPMENT
Light Microscope

I. Probably the single most expensive piece of equipment needed
II. Parts of a light microscope
   A. Eyepiece(s): one in a monocular microscope; two in a binocular microscope. The eyepiece(s) magnify the viewed field 5, 10, or 15 times (most are 10×). A binocular microscope is more expensive but is preferred due to ease in viewing and increased clarity
   B. Light source: an attached, internal light bulb with a variable intensity best illuminates the viewed slide
   C. Light condenser: another means of increasing or decreasing the amount of light on the slide; most good microscopes have two—one directly above the light source and one under the stage
   D. Stage: the platform on which the slide is placed for viewing; most stages are movable by means of two knobs on the side of the microscope—one for horizontal movement and one for vertical movement
   E. Objectives: magnify the specimen
   F. Focus: most microscopes have two types of focus adjusting knobs—a coarse focus for initially viewing the specimen and a fine focus for sharpening the image
III. Many different models available; for use in a clinical microbiology lab, must have at least three objectives
   A. 10× (dry): used for scanning the slide
   B. 40× (dry): used to identify fungal elements
   C. 100× (oil immersion): used to differentiate stained bacteria

Incubator

An incubator allows an organism to be grown under controlled conditions. There are many different types of incubators available but for most clinical microbiology labs all that is needed is an incubator that keeps the specimens at 37° C (98.6° F), which is human body temperature, and room air oxygen concentration

I. Most cultures are grown overnight and held at least 48 hrs
II. Most veterinary cultures are grown at 37° C, (98.6° F), including reptile and amphibian cultures
   A. Even though reptiles and amphibians are poikilothermic (that is, their bodies stay at ambient temperature) any organisms present will grow at 37° C (98.6° F)
   B. This temperature is especially critical when performing such standardized tests as the Kirby-Bauer sensitivity tests

Sterilizing Heat Sources

I. Bunsen burner
   A. Attaches to gas wall outlets
   B. Allows flame to be ignited with a spark striker
   C. Quickly sterilizes the metal loop used for transferring microorganisms to be inoculated into growing media
   D. Also used to heatfix slides for staining procedures
II. Electric heating element
   A. Usually ceramic, an enclosed heater that sterilizes metal loops
   B. Eliminates the need for a natural gas source
   C. Cannot be used to heatfix slides
III. Alcohol lamps
   A. Usually a small glass lamp with a wick that extends into alcohol in the base
   B. Wick must be ignited with another flame source (i.e., matches)
   C. Does not sterilize metal loops as quickly or thoroughly as a bunsen burner
   D. Less expensive than above options

Media

I. Must choose appropriate type of media for isolation needs
   A. Nutritive media grow all types of bacteria (and some fungi)
   B. Selective media grow only certain types of bacteria (e.g., gram negatives or gram positives) or fungi
   C. Differential media contain elements that differentiate certain types of bacteria (e.g., lactose fermenters or hydrogen sulfide producers)

II. All media must be examined for accidental bacterial/fungal contaminants before use

III. All media plates are incubated upside down (media side up) to prevent condensation from dripping onto cultures

Miscellaneous Equipment

I. Metal loop: for transferring bacterial or fungal specimens onto media or slides; many sizes are available

II. Glass microscope slides: for placing a specimen to be examined under the microscope

III. Wooden applicator sticks: disposable; used when preforming quick identification tests

IV. Sterile cotton-tipped applicators: many uses, including applying specimens to media or microscope slide

V. Wax markers: to identify specimens on media or slides

BACTERIOLOGICAL AND FUNGAL MEDIA ▬▬

Basic Media

I. Agar: a semisolid media

II. Broth: a liquid media

III. Plate: a flat, round container of agar

IV. Tube: a screw-top container; can contain broth or agar

V. Slant: a tube of agar that has been allowed to gel at an angle

VI. Selective media: contain compounds that inhibit growth of certain types of organisms

VII. Differential media: contain compounds that identify certain characteristics of organisms grown on the media

Specific Types of Media

I. Trypticase soy agar with 5% sheep blood (TSA) or blood agar plate (BAP)
   A. General, nutritive media for cultivation of fastidious microorganisms
   B. Used for the observation of bacterial hemolytic reactions

II. MacConkey II agar (MAC)
   A. Selects for gram-negative organisms using crystal violet as a gram-positive bacterial inhibitor
   B. Differentiates between lactose and nonlactose fermenting (NLF) organisms using a neutral red indicator that produces red coloration in the presence of lactose-fermenting colonies
   C. Designed to inhibit the swarming of *Proteus* bacteria

III. Columbia colistin-nalidixic acid agar (CNA) with 5% Sheep Blood
   A. Selects for gram-positive organisms using colistin and naladixic acid

IV. *Salmonella-Shigella* agar (SS)
   A. Plated media that selects pathogenic enteric gram-negative bacteria
   B. Differentiates on the basis of lactose fermentation (see MacConkey)
   C. Differentiates hydrogen sulfide (H_2S) producing bacteria by use of ferric citrate in the formula, which produces black pigment in their presence

V. Mueller-Hinton agar (MH)
   A. A general use media specially formulated to give standardized results during antibiotic sensitivity testing
   B. Can be enriched with blood for more fastidious organisms

VI. *Campylobacter* agar with five antimicrobics and 10% sheep blood (Campy BAP)
   A. A highly selective media for use in a microaerophilic environment for the growth of *Campylobacter* species from fecal specimens

VII. Thioglycollate broth (THIO) without indicator-135C
   A. General use broth that grows most bacterial organisms, including anaerobes, and some fungi

VIII. Trypticase soy broth (TSB)
   A. A general use media that grows most bacteria, particularly fastidious organisms
   B. Used primarily in blood cultures and sterility testing

IX. Gram-negative broth (GN)
   A. A selective enrichment media for *Salmonella* and *Shigella* used in fecal culturing

X. *Campylobacter* thioglycollate medium (Campy THIO) with five antimicrobials
   A. A selective broth used in a microaerophilic environment to isolate *Campylobacter* from fecal specimens

XI. Brain-Heart infusion broth (BHIA)
   A. An enriched broth used to bring bacteria to a certain turbidity level when performing diffusion antibiotic sensitivity testing

XII. Bile-esculin agar (BEA)
   A. A slanted media used to identify bacteria that hydrolize esculin, especially enterococci

B. A positive reaction is indicated by ferric citrate, which reacts by producing a dark brown color

XIII. Sodium chloride 0.85% (NaCl 0.85%)

A. A sterile solution used for diluting gram-negative bacteria for API testing

XIV. Motility test media

A. Semisolid media used to demonstrate motility of bacteria

XV. Dermatophyte test medium (DTM)

A. A solid tubed media, supplemented with gentamycin and chlortetracycline; to isolate pathogenic fungi

B. Differentiation is provided by phenol red, which causes a color change in the presence of acid-producing, rapidly growing pathogenic fungi

XVI. Mycosel agar

A. A selective fungal media that contains cyclohexamide and chloramphenicol to inhibit bacterial growth

XVII. Nutrient agar (NA)

A. Media used for the cultivation and transport of nonfastidious organisms

XVIII. Oxidation-Fermentation medium with dextrose (OF)

A. Semisolid media used to determine dextrose utilization in gram-negative bacteria

XIX. Urea agar slant (Urea)

A. Used to determine urease production of bacteria

B. A positive result is indicated by the presence of a phenol red indicator

TYPES OF SPECIMENS

There are three types of areas of the body to consider when obtaining a specimen for microbiological culture.

Sterile areas

I. Body areas or cavities that do not normally contain bacteria or fungi. Any bacteria encountered in these specimens should be considered abnormal. The samples most commonly cultured include:

A. Blood
B. Urine
C. Spinal fluid
D. Joint fluid
E. Solid organs
F. Milk
G. Lower respiratory tract

Nonsterile areas

I. Body areas that, when healthy, contain resident bacteria and fungi, called normal flora, that must be distinguished from disease-causing organisms. These areas include:

A. Hair/fur
B. Skin
C. Sputum or saliva
D. Intestinal tract/feces
E. Ears
F. Upper respiratory tract, including nares and trachea

Abscessed areas

I. Areas that the body has filled with exudative material in response to inflammation or irritation

A. Sterile abscesses have no bacterial etiology and their culture will result in no growth

B. Primary infection abscesses usually contain only one type of pathogen (the cause of the original infection)

C. Secondary infection abscesses contain multiple opportunistic pathogens that invaded after the original infection (especially fungi)

COLLECTION AND CULTURE OF SPECIMENS

Swab Specimen

I. (Culturette or sterile cotton-tipped swab)

A. Commonly used when culturing ears, nares, abscesses

B. A liquid specimen may be squirted onto, then submitted, on a swab

C. Prepackaged sterile swabs may contain a small amount of liquid or gel used as a transport media, which keeps the organisms viable while in transit (usually for up to 48 hours)

D. Use swab to inoculate one third of each plate: BAP, CNA, MAC

E. Place remaining swab into THIO broth. If swab is plastic or wood, break off cleanly against side of tube so that specimen end of swab is immersed in media (break off at a low enough height so that swab end doesn't protrude from tube). If swab is metal, use utility scissors to cut swab off at a good site and *flame* cut end of swab before allowing to rest in broth

F. Streak inoculated plates for isolation

G. A gram stain can be made from the swab if a flamed, sterile slide is used before the swab is placed in the broth or the swab is only "swished" in the broth, then used on the slide. It's best to get a second swab for gram staining

H. Incubate overnight

Liquid Specimen

I. (Aspirate in syringe, sterile tube, etc.)

A. Typically, liquid specimens presented are abscess material, tracheal wash, broncheal wash, nasal discharge, joint fluid, spinal fluid

B. Inoculate each plate (usually BAP, MAC, and CNA) with a small drop of specimen

C. Inoculate thioglycollate broth with a few drops of specimen (more or less, depending on expected bacterial load)

D. Use flamed, cooled loop to spread inoculant on one third of each plate; streak for isolation

E. Gram stain specimen from syringe/tube

Solid Specimen

I. Solid specimens include hard abscess material and tissue samples, including organs, skin, and scales

II. Usually the best way to culture these materials is to place a small amount in broth overnight, then subculture the broth

III. Use aseptic technique when collecting tissue samples, especially at necropsy

Urine Specimen

I. The best urine specimen for culture is obtained by cystocentesis; sterile catheterization may also be used. A specimen obtained by free catch may contain normal flora from the skin and genital area

II. Use a sterile, calibrated, nonreusable loop to inoculate 100 μL of urine on a BAP

III. Spread inoculant evenly over entire surface of plate. Any colonies that grow will be counted; the results times 10 will give bacteria per mL of urine

IV. Inoculate MAC and CNA plates as for liquid specimens

V. A urine sample is generally not placed in THIO due to high incidence of false positives from contamination (even cystocentesis)

Blood Specimen

I. Mammal

A. Disinfect tops of two TSB tubes and venipuncture site with a surgical preparation solution

B. Collect blood directly into TSB tube from venipuncture (i.e., with Vacutainer). One tube is vented to allow aerobic growth; one is left sealed for anaerobic growth

C. If patient/vein size does not allow venipuncture, place noncoagulated blood into broth via syringe (use clean needle if possible or remove needle from syringe before inoculating)

D. If two tubes are inoculated, one is vented using aseptic technique with a Vacutainer needle (leave needle in place with cover on loosely)

E. Tubes should be observed every day for hemolysis/cloudiness. Anaerobic activity may be indicated if lid pops off tube

F. If signs of growth are observed, treat tubes as liquid specimens and subculture/gram stain

G. Keep tubes at least eight days, after which subculture to BAP and gram stain to confirm negative

II. Avian/reptile/amphibian/fish

A. Most of these patients are small; if large enough, follow mammal protocol

B. Place at least five drops of aseptically drawn blood into THIO broth

C. Observe tube daily. Treat as liquid specimen if signs of growth occur

D. These specimens tend to look positive due to presence of RBC nuclei; require subculture to verify

E. Confirm negatives at eight days as for mammals

Fecal Cultures

I. All fecal cultures are inoculated onto MacConkey agar and SS plates and into GN broth

II. The GN broth, regardless of plate findings, is subcultured onto an SS plate at 24 or 48 hrs

III. Be aware of species specific pathogens when looking for possible pathogenic colonies: in most carnivores and hoofstock, *Salmonella* spp. are of main concern. In primates, one must also look for *Shigella* spp. Both are nonlactose fermenters but *Salmonella* is H_2S positive and *Shigella* is not

IV. The pathogenic hydrogen sulfide (H_2S) positive organism *Salmonella* can be distinguished from the common nonpathogenic H_2S positive *Proteus* by a simple urea test (*Proteus* spp. are urea positive)

V. Also of concern in some primates and hoofstock is *Yersinia pseudotuberculosis*. This is a nonlactose fermenter (NLF) that does not produce H_2S. This bacteria is urea positive, however, and could be overlooked if urea tests are performed to rule out pathogens. For this reason, any NLF colonies encountered in a primate or hoofstock fecal sample should be fully identified

VI. Gram stain all fecal specimens; *Campylobacter* may be observed (a curved gram-negative rod, it has a pathognomotic shape) and large quantities of large gram-positive rods may indicate a clostridial problem

Fungal Cultures

I. Examine specimen for fungal elements under the microscope, if possible

II. If the specimen is to be incubated for dermatophytes (hair and/or skin samples, most often) place into a small slant tube of dermatophyte test media (DTM)

III. All other fungal cultures are placed in Mycosel slants
  A. If the sample is liquid, as in tracheal or bronchial wash, a clean needle on the syringe is used to scratch a few lines in the fungal media; then a couple drops of the specimen is placed on the media
  B. If the sample is on a swab, aseptically break the end of the swab off so it fits in the tube of media, then gently embed the swab into the agar
  C. Pieces of hair or skin can be aseptically placed on top of the media

IV. If unsure of the organism, place in both media (as in severe skin infections)

V. Cultures are placed at room temperature in a dark area and examined daily for fungal growth
  A. Dermatophyte fungi (which invade the hair and skin) will often grow within three or four days
  B. Saprophytic fungi (which are opportunistic environmental fungi) can take up to three weeks

VI. Cultures should be held for a month to confirm negatives

BACTERIAL IDENTIFICATION*
Gram-positive Cocci

Gram-positive cocci are comprised mainly of three groups: Staphylococci, Streptococci, and Micrococci. The Micrococci are not often encountered in the veterinary lab.

I. Staphylococci
  A. Note if colony causes any hemolysis on the blood agar plate (BAP) (staph are either hemolytic or nonhemolytic)
  B. The first test performed on any gram-positive colony is the catalase test (staph are catalase positive)
  C. A coagulase test is performed on the colony (generally, the coagulase-positive staph are more pathogenic)
  D. A Mueller-Hinton sensitivity test is done using BHI broth as a colony diluent
  E. Some samples (such as skin swabs) can be expected to have staph growth. It may be wise to ask the requesting veterinarian if a sensitivity test is needed
  F. Often staph colonies growing in a broth tube will resemble comets or shooting stars

II. Streptococci
  A. Streptococci are catalase negative
  B. Note any hemolysis surrounding the colonies on the BAP; streptococci hemolysis is graded into:
    1. Alpha-incomplete hemolysis: the agar surrounding the colony is greenish
    2. Beta-complete hemolysis: area surrounding the colony is clear
    3. Gamma: no hemolysis
  C. Sensitivity is performed using BHIA broth. (A Mueller-Hinton (MH) plate with 5% sheep blood is used to promote the growth of the strep)
  D. A strep that doesn't grow well on the M-H plate, especially a beta hemolytic strep, will be sensitive to most antibiotics
  E. Enterococci, or enterococcal strep, are strep that are found in the alimentary tract but are opportunistic pathogens (such as *Streptococcus faecalis*). (To determine if a colony is an *Enterococcus,* a bile esculin test is performed; enterococci are bile esculin positive)

---

*Note that these procedures are basic. They are described in greater detail in a clinical microbiology book, which is the final reference when identifying organisms.

F. Many strep will grow like stars suspended in the broth

G. Streptococci can be responsible for many illnesses in animals, including pneumonia, mastitis, and septicemia

Gram-negative Cocci

I. *Moraxella bovis:* large gram-negative cocci that sometimes resemble fat rods; they cause pinkeye in cattle

II. *Neisseria* spp.: often found as normal flora in the respiratory tract of many animals; as pathogens, the main cause for concern is in humans
A. *N. gonorrhoeae* is the cause of human gonorrhea
B. *N. meningitidis* causes human meningitis

Gram-negative Rods

I. Enterobacteriaceae, or enteric (gut) bacteria: gram-negative rod that is isolated most commonly in veterinary medicine

II. Gram-negative rods grow on the BAP and MAC plate (they will often overgrow gram-positive cocci on the BAP, which makes the CNA plate essential for recovering these)

III. Note the lactose reaction of the colony

IV. If the colony is clear (a nonlactose fermenter [NLF]), an oxidase test is performed: *all lactose fermenters (LFS) are oxidase negative*

V. The colony is prepared for API and sensitivity testing using sterile 0.85% saline

VI. If searching for fecal pathogens, *all NLFs must be identified and/or ruled out.*
A. For example: *Proteus* spp. and *Salmonella* spp. are NLF and H$_2$S positive. *Proteus,* however, is urea positive; a urea test can discount a colony within a few hours
B. *Shigella, Pseudomonas,* and *Aeromonas* look similar on a plate; to rule out suspicious colonies, perform an oxidase test: *Shigella* will be oxidase negative

VII. The API test is performed according to the directions from the package insert

VIII. The enteral bacteria are found in many infections: they are opportunistic pathogens

IX. Some of the nonenteral gram-negative rods such as *Pseudomonas* and *Aeromonas* spp. can be serious primary pathogens, especially in birds, reptiles, and amphibians

Gram-negative Spirochetes

I. *Campylobacter* spp.: bacteria found in the digestive tracts of many mammals. In hoofed mammals they can be normal flora; in others (especially primates and carnivores) they can cause a chronic debilitating diarrhea
A. The shape of *Campylobacter* is often characteristic: two small, curved gram-negative rods join end-to-end to form a "seagull" or "w." This can be difficult to see on a gram stain and other forms may be present (spiraled), so a negative gram stain is not diagnostic
B. *Campylobacter* need a microaerophilic environment to grow and are often overgrown by less fastidious organisms: so special media and growing conditions are required for culture

II. *Yersinia* spp. may be encountered in reptile/amphibian cultures or primate fecal cultures; although these bacteria are halophilic (requiring salt to grow), most media in use has enough salt to enable the bacteria to grow and be identifiable by API

Gram-negative Coccobacilli

I. The gram-negative coccobacilli include *Bordatella* spp. and *Pasteurella* spp. These organisms are of concern to the veterinary microbiology laboratory because they can cause respiratory disease, especially in dogs (*Bordatella*) and cats and rabbits (*Pasteurella*)

II. These organisms can be identified in the API system

III. Care must be taken not to misidentify these as streptococci, as they may not grow on MacConkey agar. Any flat, shiny gray colony (especially if it has no look-alike on the CNA plate) should be gram stained

IV. It can be difficult to tell coccobacilli from cocci, so it is best to work with young colonies. Older colonies of streptococci may lose their ability to hold a positive gram reaction

Gram-positive Rods

I. Most small microbiology laboratories do not attempt to identify *anaerobic* gram-positive rods

II. Their presence is noted and whether or not they have spores on gram stain

III. They will grow in THIO, toward the bottom, but not on plates. For this reason it is important to gram stain the broth

IV. The most common *aerobic* gram-positive rod encountered is *Bacillus* spp. These are large, parallel-sided rods that grow on BAP and CNA plates. The colonies often have a "grainy" appearance. Sensitivities can be done as for any aerobe but often are not necessary because *Bacillus* spp. are mostly found in culture as environmental contaminants

    A. The prominent exception is *B. anthracis,* which causes sudden death in cattle and sheep, and skin and lung lesions in humans

    B. *B. piliformis* causes acute fatal enteritis in rodents and foals

V. *Corynebacterium* spp. are small rods that are often curved and pleiomorphic, giving them a "Chinese letters" look on gram stain. In people and animals, they are often found as normal flora of the alimentary tract, especially the mouth

    A. Pathogenic *Corynebacterium* include:

        1. *C. equi* (foal pneumonia), *C. pseudotuberculosis* (caseous lymphadenitis in sheep and goats), and *C. renale* (urinary tract infections in cattle, pigs, and male sheep)

VI. *Mycobacterium* spp. are long, thin gram-negative rods that sometimes branch. These can be serious pathogens

    A. *M. tuberculosis* causes pneumonia in humans and other primates

    B. *M. avium* causes a fatal, nontreatable gastrointestinal and respiratory infection in birds. These bacteria, however, are difficult to culture—it takes months and specialized media. Their presence in sputum or tissue can be demonstrated by their ability to retain an acid-fast stain, which is a test that can be performed in most veterinary labs

FUNGAL IDENTIFICATION

Identification

I. A small piece of clear cellophane tape is pressed gently but firmly onto the colony, sticky side down, to pick up hyphae. The tape is placed, sticky side down, on a microscope slide to which a drop of saline or lacto-phenol cotton blue is added. The slide is examined under the microscope for hyphal identification

II. Other techniques can be performed for identification but these are generally more time consuming and not commonly done in small laboratories

III. The CNA plate will often grow yeast, if present in a sample. Therefore any colonies that are not easily recognized should be gram

stained (or make a wet mount with saline) and examined microscopically

IV. In very heavy fungal infections (such as avian aspergillosis) the fungus will often grow on top of the THIO and/or the surface of the BAP. These colonies are usually readily identified as fungi by their dry, fuzzy appearance

Dermatophytes

I. Found in hair, skin, nails, and claws, they are the cause of ringworm in humans and animals

II. The main dermatophytes affecting animals are *Microsporum* spp. and *Trichophyton* spp.

III. Most dermatophytes cause a color change in dermatophyte test medium (from orange to red)

IV. These fungi are distinguished by their large macroconidia, visible macroscopically

Saprophytes

I. Saprophytic fungi are found in the environment and are opportunistic pathogens

II. The saprophytes include:

    A. *Aspergillus* spp., which can cause pneumonia, especially in birds. Some species can also cause disease by their presence in feed and hay. They create a toxin known as aflotoxin, which can cause a severe imunopressive effect in animals ingesting affected feed

    B. *Mucor* spp. and *Rhizopus* spp. can cause lymph node, lung, and liver lesions in immunosupressed animals

Yeast

I. *Candida albicans* causes many diseases, especially when predisposing conditions exist such as

    A. Immunosuppression

    B. Primary bacterial infection

    C. Prolonged antibiotic use

II. *Candida* spp. can be found infecting mucous membranes, especially in the gastrointestinal tract (including the mouth), genital tract, respiratory tract, and ears

    A. *Candida albicans* can be identified by means of the germ tube test. An isolate of yeast is incubated in rabbit plasma with EDTA for a couple of hours, then examined microscopically. *C. albicans* produces germ tubes, which grow from the side of the yeast like tiny hyphae

B. Commercial agglutination tests also exist for identification of *C. albicans* and many other yeasts
III. *Cryptococcus neoformans* is an encapsulated yeast that can cause severe nasal infections in dogs and cats and meningitis in people (this is a very zoonotic organism)
    A. Cultures or nasal exudates can be examined under the microscope with an India ink preparation that highlights the thick capsule
IV. Many other yeasts are found as normal flora

Dimorphic Fungi

I. Dimorphic fungi exhibit yeast-like growth (when in animal tissue) and saprophytic fungal-type growth (in the environment)
II. These fungi are highly zoonotic and must be handled using protective measures. They are identified by their characteristic microscopic appearance. Infections can also be diagnosed by serology testing
III. Dimorphic fungi of special clinical concern
    A. *Histoplasma capsulatum:* causes respiratory tract infections in dogs, cats, and humans
    B. *Blastomyces dermatiditis:* causes blastomycosis, a respiratory and/or skin infection in dogs and humans
    C. *Coccidioides immitis:* causes respiratory disease in dogs and humans; can also affect bones and internal organs

BASIC DIAGNOSTIC TESTS
Gram Stain

I. Specimen is placed on a microscope slide
II. Colony from a plate is suspended in saline, or a flamed, cooled loop is used to transfer a drop of thioglycollate broth
III. Allow to air dry
IV. Heatfix by passing quickly through a flame, specimen slide up, about four times
V. Flood slide with crystal violet stain; let sit one minute
VI. Rinse with tap water until water runs clear
VII. Flood slide with Gram's iodine; let sit one minute
VIII. Rinse with tap water until water runs clear
IX. Flood slide with decolorizer, rock back and forth about ten seconds, then rinse slide with tap water. Repeat if specimen is very dark but try not to over decolorize

X. Flood slide with safranin counterstain, allow to sit for 30-50 seconds, then rinse with tap water until water runs clear
XI. Dry in blotting (bibulous) paper
XII. Observations under oil immersion (100×): Gram-positive bacteria stain purple or dark blue. Gram-negative bacteria stain pink. Overdecolorizing or using an old colony can cause false gram-negative reactions. Forgetting to decolorize or not decolorizing a heavy specimen may yield a false positive result

Catalase Test

I. Using a wooden applicator stick, smear a small amount of the colony to be tested on a clean glass slide
II. Place a drop of 3% hydrogen peroxide on the specimen
III. Observe for bubbling, which indicates a positive reaction

Oxidase Test

I. Using a wooden applicator stick, smear a small to moderate amount of colony to be tested on a piece of filter paper
II. Place a drop of oxidase reagent on the paper
III. The smeared sample will turn dark blue if positive (some colonies appear blue when placed on the filter paper: watch closely for color change)
IV. Many colonies will turn dark after five or more minutes, so only record immediate color change

Bile Esculin

I. Inoculate a bile esculin agar slant with *Streptococcus* colony to be tested
II. Place in incubator
III. Examine within a few hours. If agar turns black, test is positive (enterococcal strep are positive). Incubate negative result overnight to confirm

API 20E Test

I. Each little cup of the API strip is actually a separate test (tests used to be performed separately but now the results can be assessed quickly and easily)
II. The 0.85% saline of bacteria is used for setting up the Kirby-Bauer sensitivity testing
III. If the API instruction sheet is followed, the main causes for improper readouts are using

mixed colonies of bacteria, using too few colonies, or using old, nonviable colonies

Kirby-Bauer Sensitivity

I. Bacteria to be tested is diluted in 5 mL BHIA broth (or 5 mL 0.85% saline if an API strip is being set up) to match the cloudiness of a 0.5 McFarland standard

II. Using a sterile cotton-tipped applicator, the sample is inoculated onto a Mueller-Hinton plate to cover the entire surface evenly

III. Antibiotic sensitivity disks are placed on the agar surface with the antibiotic disk dispenser. If any additional disks are placed, they must be tamped lightly onto the agar surface so they adhere while the plate is being incubated

IV. Inhibition zones are read with a millimeter ruler. Several readings can be taken if the zones are unclear or irregular

Streaking for Isolation

I. Inoculate one third of agar plate, flame loop and allow to cool

II. Making a few excursions into the inoculated area with loop (more if light bacteria expected, less if heavier growth), streak another one third of plate. Flame loop and allow to cool

III. As above, streak remaining third of plate, then flame loop to disinfect

IV. Streaking for isolation is to obtain bacterial colonies that are far enough away from other colonies that they can be tested separately and identified

Acid-fast Stain

I. Make a saline or water suspension of sample on slide (not too thick); allow to air dry

II. Heatfix slide by passing through a flame, specimen side up, three to four times. Let slide cool to touch

III. Flood slide with carbol fuchsin stain; allow to sit for five minutes. Rinse with tap water until water runs clear

IV. Flood slide with malachite green counterstain; let sit for 50-60 seconds. Rinse under tap water and blot dry

V. Mycobacteria will stain as thin red or pink rods against a green or bluish background. A few yeasts will also stain pink; they are clearer and smaller

Glossary

aerobic Requiring oxygen to live

agar A semisolid media

anaerobic Requiring the absence of oxygen to live

aseptic technique Done with as little opportunity for contamination as possible

broth A liquid media

culture The deliberate growing of an organism under controlled conditions

differential media Contains compounds that identify certain characteristics of organisms grown on the media

enteral bacteria Bacteria found in the gastrointestinal tract

normal flora Organisms found in a healthy animal

opportunistic pathogen An organism able to infect an area already compromised by injury or infection

plate A flat, round container of agar

selective media Contains compounds that inhibit growth of certain types of organisms

slant A tube of agar that has been allowed to gel at an angle

tube A screw-top container that can contain broth or agar

zoonotic Capable of causing disease in animals and humans

Review Questions

1 An in-house microbiology laboratory must be:
  a. Cost effective and have the newest equipment
  b. Above all else accurate
  c. Staffed by proficient personnel and have the most up to date equipment
  d. Cost effective, staffed by proficient personnel, and aware of clients' needs

2 The oculars (or eyepieces) of a microscope:
  a. Have no magnification abilities
  b. Multiply the magnification of the objectives by ten
  c. Add ten to the magnification of the objectives
  d. Control the amount of light entering the microscope

3 Nutritive media:
  a. Select for different types of bacteria
  b. Differentiate types of bacteria
  c. Grow most bacteria
  d. Are not used for most microbiological procedures

4 MacConkey agar is an example of:
  a. A differential and selective media
  b. A general nutritive and differential media
  c. A general nutritive media
  d. A selective media

5 Sterile abscesses:
  a. Are cleaned with a disinfectant before sampling
  b. Contain only one type of organism
  c. Contain many types of organisms
  d. Contain no bacterial or fungal organisms

6 Bacterial cultures are incubated:
   a. At room temperature
   b. At the patient's body temperature
   c. At human body temperature
   d. In the refrigerator

7 The best specimen for urine culture is obtained via:
   a. Aseptic catheterization
   b. Free catch
   c. Cystocentesis
   d. Off the cage floor

8 Fungal cultures are incubated:
   a. At room temperature
   b. At the patient's body temperature
   c. At human body temperature
   d. In the refrigerator

9 A streptococcal colony on a blood agar plate with a greenish zone around it is said to be:
   a. Hemolytic
   b. Alpha hemolytic
   c. Beta hemolytic
   d. Nonhemolytic

10 Dermatophyte fungi are found:
   a. Infecting the hair and nails
   b. To commonly cause pneumonia
   c. As normal flora on most animals
   d. As free-living fungi in the environment

11 *Salmonella* can infect the gastrointestinal tract of:
   a. Humans
   b. Mammals
   c. Birds and reptiles
   d. All of the above

12 *Candida albicans* is a yeast that:
   a. Can grow on some bacteriological media and can cause opportunistic infections
   b. Is found only in the gastrointestinal tract
   c. Does not produce germ tubes
   d. Is encapsulated

BIBLIOGRAPHY

Baron and Finegold: *Bailey and Scott's diagnostic microbiology,* St. Louis, 1989, C.V. Mosby.

McCurnin DM: *Clinical textbook for veterinary technicians* ed 3, Philadelphia, 1994, WB Saunders.

Pratt PW: *Laboratory procedures for veterinary technicians,* ed 2, American Veterinary Publications, Goleta, California, 1992.

Quinn et al: *Clinical veterinary microbiology,* Europe, 1994, Mosby-Year Book Inc.

Rhode: BBL manual of products and laboratory procedures, BBL 1994, Becton-Dickenson Company.

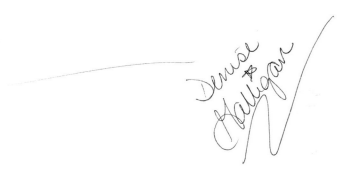

CHAPTER 19

Urinalysis, Hematology, Cytology

Bill Wade   *Marg Brown*

OUTLINE

Urinalysis
  Specimen Collection
  Evaluation
  Chemical Constituents
  Microscopic Evaluation

Hematology
  Erythrocyte Evaluation
  Erythrocyte Film Evaluation
  Leukocyte (WBC) Evaluation
  Thrombocyte (platelet) Evaluation
  Total protein
  Nonmanual Instrumentation

Cytology
  Specimen Collection
  Slide Preparation
  Staining Techniques
  Interpretation

LEARNING OUTCOMES

After reading this chapter you should be able to:

1. Explain collection and analysis of urine.
2. Explain how to perform a CBC.
3. Describe various tests for evaluation of organ function.
4. Describe how to collect, stain, and interpret cytologic samples.

Veterinarians depend on accurate laboratory results to offer the best patient care. Consistent, high-quality results provided by the veterinary technician are an essential component of this care. Many tests are routinely performed in house rather than forwarded to a reference laboratory. Values in parentheses are in SI units.

URINALYSIS

A complete urinalysis serves to provide information on the state of the kidneys and the animal's ability to normally filter and excrete metabolites. When an endocrine or metabolic disturbance occurs, a complete analysis of the urine is indicated to demonstrate any abnormalities in chemical or structural components. These tests are easily performed in most veterinary settings using a minimal amount of diagnostic equipment, time, and expense.

Specimen Collection

I. Free flow or clean catch
  A. A simple, noninvasive procedure but unsatisfactory for bacterial culture
  B. Preferably collect a midstream sample; avoid initial or end portion of the voided urine
  C. Vulva or prepuce should be cleansed before collection
II. Cystocentesis
  A. Performed by placing a needle through the ventral abdominal wall and into the urinary bladder
  B. Should be performed using aseptic technique

C. Perform on a full bladder to avoid possible damage to other abdominal organs

D. Collection by cystocentesis avoids contaminants from the lower portions of the urinary tract, making the sample suitable for bacterial culture

III. Catheterization

A. Performed by passing a rubber, plastic, or metal catheter through the urethra and into the urinary bladder

B. Type and size used depends on sex and species catheterized

C. Should be done as aseptically as possible and with caution to avoid undue trauma and erroneous test results

D. The sample is easily aspirated into a syringe attached to the exposed end of the catheter

IV. Manual expression

A. As with collecting for a voided sample, midstream collection is preferred

B. The sample is not suitable for bacterial culture

C. Vulva or prepuce should be cleansed before sample collection

D. Must be performed with care and patience; avoid excessive pressure to the bladder

E. Should never be attempted on an animal with a suspected obstruction

Evaluation

I. Sample preservation

A. Samples should be analyzed within 30 minutes for maximum valid information

B. Refrigerate for an additional 6 to 12 hours if necessary but bring to room temperature before evaluating, especially if evaluating for specific gravity and crystals

C. For cytologic evaluation, centrifuge immediately

D. Preservation of the sample can be done by the addition of formalin, toluene, or phenol but changes may occur with some chemical analyses

II. Gross examination

A. Volume may be influenced by several factors, including water intake, environmental temperature, physical activity, size, and species

1. Ideally a 24-hour urine estimation should be made

B. **Pollakiuria:** refers to frequent urination, often confused with polyuria by clients

C. **Polyuria:** increased urine output or production

1. Associated with nephritis, diabetes mellitus, and polydipsia

D. **Oliguria:** a decrease in the formation or elimination of urine

1. Occurs with shock, dehydration, water conservation, or renal failure

E. **Anuria:** complete absence of urine formation or elimination

1. Can occur as a result of renal shutdown, usually associated with obstruction

III. Color

A. In most species urine is a transparent light yellow to amber color

B. Yellow is normally due to pigments called urochromes

C. Color usually correlates with specific gravity (concentration)

1. Lighter colored urine tends to have a lower specific gravity; darker urine generally has a higher specific gravity

2. Bile pigments are likely contained in yellow-brown to greenish urine that foams when shaken

3. Red or reddish-brown urine indicates hematuria (RBCs) or hemoglobinuria (hemoglobin)

4. Brown urine may contain myoglobinuria (myoglobins from muscle cell breakdown)

D. Some species, such as rabbits, normally have a darker colored urine (orange to reddish brown)

IV. Transparency

A. Transparency is described as clear, cloudy, or flocculent

B. Cloudy urine can be associated with the presence of cellular debris such as RBCs and WBCs, and epithelial cells, crystals, bacteria, casts, mucus, semen, and lipids

1. Bacteria or crystal formation can cause standing urine to become cloudy

C. Except for horses, normal voided urine is clear

V. Odor

A. Not highly diagnostic but may be useful in detecting some bacterial growth or excessive ammonia content

B. Male cats, goats, and pigs normally have a strong urine odor

C. In some cases, a sweet or fruity odor can be indicative of ketones and is commonly associated with diabetes mellitus, pregnancy toxemia in sheep, or acetonemia in cows

1. Ammonia due to bacterial proliferation may also cause an odor to standing urine
VI. **Specific gravity:** density of a quantity of liquid as compared with that of distilled water. In practical applications it is used to assess the renal tubule's ability to concentrate or dilute filtrates from the glomerulus
   A. Refractometer method
      1. Approximately measures specific gravity or total solids of urine
      2. Place a few drops of urine on the prism cover glass
      3. Point refractometer toward bright light and read at the light-dark boundary
      4. Ensure that results are read from the S/G scale, which differs from the total protein scale
   B. Urinometer method
      1. Requires a larger volume of urine
      2. Lower weighed bulb with attached scale into cylinder containing urine sample
      3. Read results at bottom of the meniscus
      4. Urinometers are calibrated to read samples at room temperature
   C. Reagent test strips
      1. Made for use in human samples
      2. Least reliable method of determining S/G, especially if SG is greater than 1.030
      3. Place strip in sample to saturate reagent at tip
      4. Read results by comparing color changes to scale on container
   D. Changes in urine specific gravity
      1. Average specific gravity values for the following species are:
         a. Dog: 1.025
         b. Cat: 1.030
         c. Horse: 1.035
         d. Cattle and swine: 1.015
         e. Sheep: 1.030
      2. Increased specific gravity occurs with dehydration, decreased water intake, acute renal disease, and shock
      3. Decreased specific gravity occurs with increased fluid intake, renal and other diseases

Chemical Constituents

I. Urine pH
   A. Used to generally assess the body's acid-base balance. The pH expresses the hydrogen ion (H^+) concentration of the urine
   B. Reagent strips are most commonly used to determine pH. After dipping into urine sample, the color change is compared to a scale on the container
   C. pH is often affected by diet. Herbivores commonly have an alkaline pH (7-8.5), carnivores an acidic pH (cats 6-7), and omnivores may have either
   D. Loss of CO_2 occurs with samples left open and standing at room temperature, resulting in higher readings
   E. Standing urine, containing urease-producing bacteria, also increases the reading
II. Protein
   A. Proteinuria usually describes an abnormal level of proteins or protein metabolites in the urine
   B. Detection of protein levels is commonly made by use of reagent test strips (Multistix, Ames)
   C. Color comparison is made and results are recorded in mg/dl
      1. Normal should be none or trace (10 mg/dl)
   D. Results are considered semiquantitative due to variables in chemical reaction and color chart comparison
   E. Errors can occur
      1. False positives can occur when in alkaline urine
      2. If proteinuria is caused by globulins rather than albumin, false negatives can occur
      3. Depending on the reader, different values may be obtained
      4. There is a greater indication of protein loss if there is proteinuria in diluted urine than in concentrated urine
   F. Proteinuria results from several pre and post renal causes. An abnormality in the urogenital system is most often suggested
   G. Values must be taken in context with other results such as urine blood and microscopic sediment
      1. A good evaluation of protein loss in the animal can be made by comparing urine protein and urine creatinine values (should be performed at a reference laboratory)
   H. Protein values can also be evaluated by sulfosalicylic acid, which determines urine protein levels through acid precipitation
III. Glucose
   A. Detectable levels of sugar are referred to as glucosuria or glycosuria and depend on glucose levels in the blood

1. Unless the renal threshold is reached (about 170-180 mg/dl [greater than 6.8 mmol/L in dogs]), glucosuria does not usually occur

B. Testing is usually performed by using any number of reagent strips available. Clinitest (Ames) reagent tablets detect sugars in the urine. Reagent strips detect only glucose

C. Hyperglycemia along with glucosuria can be attributed to diabetes mellitus created by insulin deficiency or function
   1. For confirmation of diabetes mellitus, a blood glucose level should be evaluated

D. Other factors such as fear, stress, excitement, IV fluids with glucose, and other diseases also cause glucosuria
   1. Fasting is recommended before glucose testing to avoid higher levels after a high carbohydrate meal
   2. False positives can occur after the use of various drugs such as salicylates, ascorbic acid, and penicillin

IV. Ketones
A. Ketones include acetone, acetoacetic (diacetic) acid, and beta-hydroxybutyric acid. Acetone and beta-hydroxybutyric acid are derived from acetoacetic acid and result from the catabolism of fatty acids
   1. Ketones are produced during fat metabolism and are important sources of energy
   2. Excessive ketones are toxic, producing CNS depression and acidosis

B. In normal animals, very small amounts are found in the blood
   1. If there is increased fat metabolism, decreased carbohydrate metabolism, or both, excess ketones spill into the urine, causing ketonuria
   2. Ketonemia (ketosis) often causes ketonuria

C. In large animals ketosis is associated with hypoglycemia due to insufficient carbohydrate intake, often during lactation or pregnancy

D. Small animal ketosis occurs with diabetes mellitus
   1. Lack of insulin prevents carbohydrate breakdown

E. Ketone measurement is accomplished by using one of several reagent test strips or separate reagent tablets (Ketostix, Acetest, Ames)
   1. Color intensity is proportional to ketone concentration

2. These tests are most sensitive to acetoacetic acid

V. Bile pigments
A. Commonly detected bile pigments include bilirubin and urobilinogen
   1. Only conjugated bilirubin is found in the urine
   2. A small amount of urobilinogen, from the breakdown of bilirubin by bacteria in the intestines, is excreted into the urine

B. Bilirubinuria can be seen in several diseases, including biliary obstruction, hepatic infections, toxicity, and hemolytic anemia
   1. Light will oxidize bilirubin if urine is left standing, resulting in a false-negative reading
   2. Since the liver and kidneys of dogs and cattle have an enzyme that can conjugate bilirubin, slight bilirubinuria may be present in these species

C. Determination of bile pigments is made with reagent test strips (Bili-labstix, Multistix, Ames). Urobilinogen is not easily detected
   1. A more accurate test is the Ictotest (Ames)
   2. A rough determination of the presence of bilirubinuria can be determined if urine is shaken and a yellow foam forms

VI. Blood
A. Presence of intact RBCs in the urine is referred to as hematuria. Presence of free hemoglobin is hemoglobinuria
   1. Hematuria is usually seen as red and cloudy urine
   2. Hemoglobinuria and myoglobinuria are a red to brown color
   3. Occult blood may also be present, with no visible changes to the urine

B. Hematuria is associated with disease of the urogenital tract; hemoglobinuria indicates some intravascular hemolysis; myoglobinuria generally indicates a muscle disease

C. Besides color interpretation, blood or blood components in the urine are detected with reagent strips (Hemastix, Ames), as well as tablets (Occultest Reagent Tablets)
   1. Since these do not differentiate the cause of blood in urine, microscopic evaluation to determine RBC numbers, as well as animal history and examination, along with other tests, should be included in the evaluation process

Microscopic Evaluation

Examination of the urine sediment is a highly valuable tool used in conjunction with the interpretation of color, specific gravity, turbidity, protein, pH, and occult blood tests. Microscopic evaluation may be considered a form of exfoliate cytology.

I. Sample preparation
    A. The best sample is obtained in the early morning because it is fresh and well concentrated
    B. Refrigerate sample if it cannot be examined within 30 minutes. Room temperature storage can result in natural chemical breakdown and lysing of cells
    C. Sample is centrifuged at 1000 to 3000 rpm for 5 minutes. A 5 mL sample of fresh urine is usually adequate
    D. Note the volume of sediment. Leave about 0.3 mL of the supernatant and resuspend the sediment. Transfer a small drop to a clean microscope slide and examine
    E. Examination can be done with or without stain. Staining may be done with one drop of 0.5% New Methylene Blue or Sedi-Stain
    F. Reduce illumination, scan entire area under the coverslip under 10× (LPF) objective, and then identify through 40× (HPF) objective
    G. Crystals and cast numbers are estimated as the average per low-power field (LPF)
        1. Epithelial cells and blood cells are estimated as the average number per high-power field (HPF)
        2. Bacteria and sperm are noted as few, moderate, or many (HPF)

II. Components of sediment (Figure 19-1)
    A. WBCs (leukocytes) are normally found in very few numbers. Most cells in urine are neutrophils and appear spherical, granular,

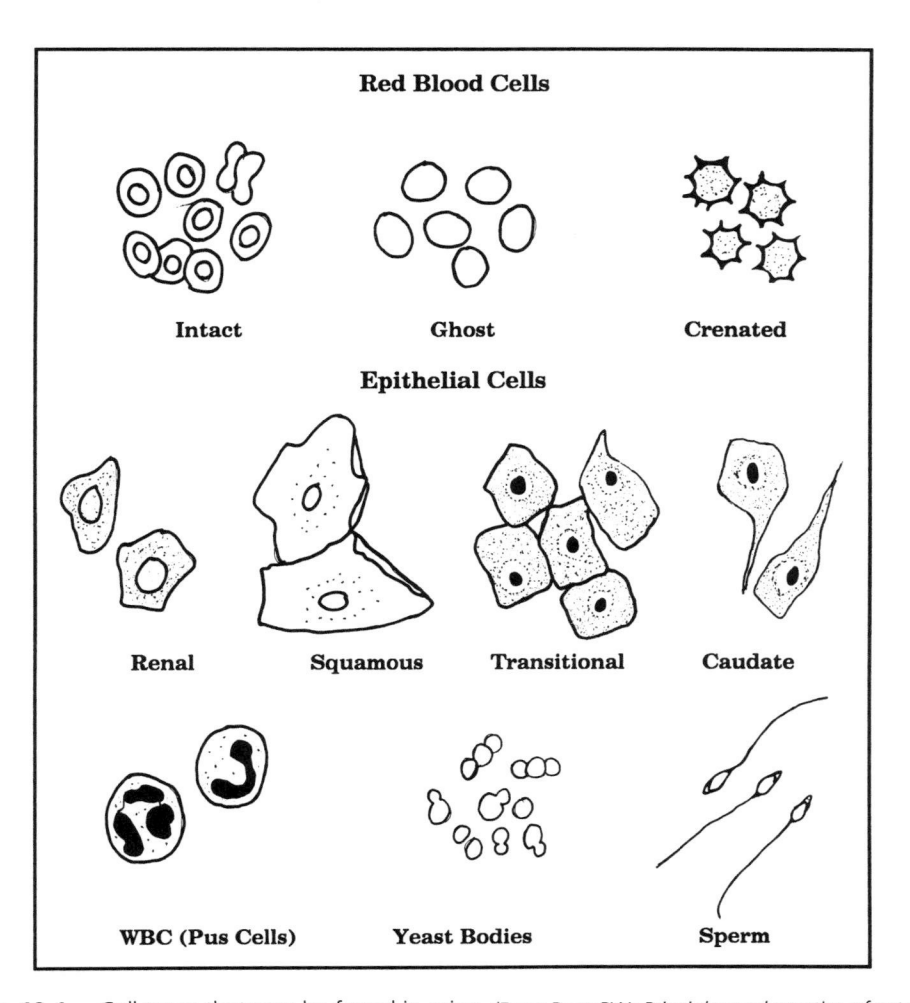

Figure 19-1   Cell types that may be found in urine. (From Pratt PW: *Principles and practice of veterinary technology*, St. Louis, 1998, Mosby.)

and larger than RBCs but smaller than epithelial cells

1. Excessive numbers are referred to as pyuria or leukocyturia
2. Increased numbers indicate active inflammatory disease along the urinary tract but can also be from the genital tract
3. More than a few (>5 HPF) should be regarded as abnormal and investigated further; note any evidence of bacteria

B. RBCs (erythrocytes) are also normally very few in number. Excessive RBCs are referred to as hematuria

1. Hematuria is associated with trauma, calculi, infection, and benign or malignant neoplasia
2. RBCs appear as pale yellow refractive disks, usually uniform in shape and smaller than WBCs. Sample manipulation can create distortion, crenation and lysis, and confusion with fat or yeast
   a. If a small amount of 2% acetic acid is added to the slide and the structures disappear, they are RBCs
3. More than a few (>5 HPF) should be noted as abnormal and investigated further

C. Epithelial cells

1. Three types usually found in urine sediment: squamous, transitional, renal

2. Squamous cells are derived from the urethra, vagina, and vulva and are largest cells found in urine sediment
   a. Appear as flat, irregularly shaped cells with angular borders and small round nuclei
   b. Usually not seen in samples obtained by cystocentesis or catheterization
   c. Their presence is not considered significant

3. Transitional cells come from the bladder, ureters, renal pelvis, and part of the urethra
   a. Wide variation in size; may be round, pear shaped, or caudate, typically with granular cytoplasm
   b. Increased numbers are associated with inflammation such as cystitis or pyelonephritis

4. Renal cells originate from the renal tubules, found in small numbers and are slightly larger than WBCs and sometimes difficult to differentiate from them
   a. Usually round with a large nucleus
   b. Increased numbers indicate renal tubular disease

D. Casts (Figure 19-2)

1. Found in the distal and collecting tubules of the kidneys. Larger numbers

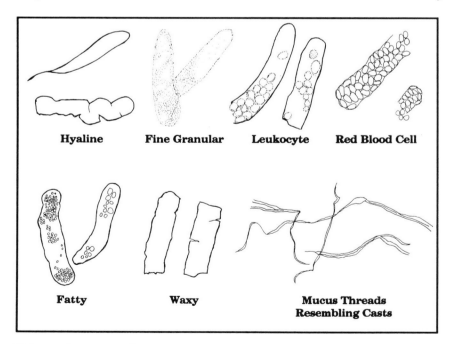

Hyaline **Fine Granular** **Leukocyte** **Red Blood Cell**

Fatty **Waxy** **Mucus Threads Resembling Casts**

Figure 19-2 Various types of casts that may be found in urine. (From Pratt PW: *Principles and practice of veterinary technology*, St. Louis, 1998, Mosby.)

of casts indicate pathology of the renal tubules
2. Hyaline casts
   a. A few may be seen in normal urine
   b. Clear, colorless, highly refractile, and composed of mucoprotein
   c. Cylindrical with symmetrical sides and rounded ends
   d. Indicates mildest form of renal irritation
3. Granular casts
   a. Most common type seen in animals
   b. Contain granules from degenerate epithelial cells and WBCs
   c. Seen in greater numbers with acute nephritis, indicate severe kidney disease
4. Epithelial, fatty, and waxy casts
   a. Epithelial casts contain cells from renal epithelium, seen in acute nephritis and renal tubule degeneration
   b. Fatty casts contain small fat droplets that are refractile. Seen in cats with renal disease and dogs with diabetes mellitus
   c. Waxy casts are wide, square ended, and have a dull appearance. More opaque than hyaline casts and indicate chronic to severe tubular degeneration
E. Crystals (Figure 19-3)
   1. May be normal or abnormal. The term *crystalline* may or may not be of clinical significance
      a. Crystal formation is influenced by pH, temperature, concentration, and medication
   2. Triple phosphates appear as classic "coffin lids": three to six sided colorless prisms found in alkaline urine
   3. Amorphous phosphate/urates
      a. Phosphates found in alkaline urine appear as granular precipitate
      b. Urates are similar but are found in acidic urine
   4. Calcium oxalate are small, colorless envelopes, sometimes dumbbell or ring formed, usually with a characteristic X form in the center
      a. Generally in acidic urine
      b. Seen in animals with ethylene glycol toxicity
   5. Leucine/cystine/tyrosine crystals may indicate hepatic disease

a. Leucine crystals are small, round, with sectioned centers
b. Tyrosine crystals appear spiculated and spindled
c. Cystine crystals are hexagon shaped (six sided)
   (1) Their presence may indicate renal tubular dysfunction
d. All three are found in acidic urine
F. Other cells that may be found in urine sediment
   1. Spermatozoa can be seen in the urine of an intact male but they are clinically insignificant
   2. Parasite ova in the urine sediment may be fecal contamination or urine parasites
   3. Fat droplets are highly refractile, spherical, and of various shapes, thus often difficult to differentiate from other cells; however, they can be stained

HEMATOLOGY

The most commonly performed hematology procedure is the Complete Blood Count or CBC. It includes determination of total red and white blood cell numbers, packed cell volume, total plasma protein, hemoglobin, RBC indices, and blood film evaluation. Normal values can be found in the listed references.

Erythrocyte Evaluation

I. Erythrocyte packed cell volume (PCV)
   A. Determines percentage of red blood cells in the circulation or blood volume
   B. Most easily measured by filling a microcapillary or hematocrit tube with fresh, anticoagulated blood
   C. Tubes are sealed and centrifuged at high speed for five minutes. Hematocrit centrifuges are often preset for speed
      1. Goat and sheep blood should be centrifuged for 10 to 20 minutes
   D. Results are determined by use of a scale on the centrifuge or a hand held alternative
   E. Results are reported as % (or L/L)
II. Erythrocyte total numbers
   A. Determined by using an automated or manual cell counting device
   B. Automated counters require calibration for cell size, depending on species
   C. Manual counts are done with a hemacytometer and are usually not as accurate
   D. Both methods require that the sample be greatly diluted before counting

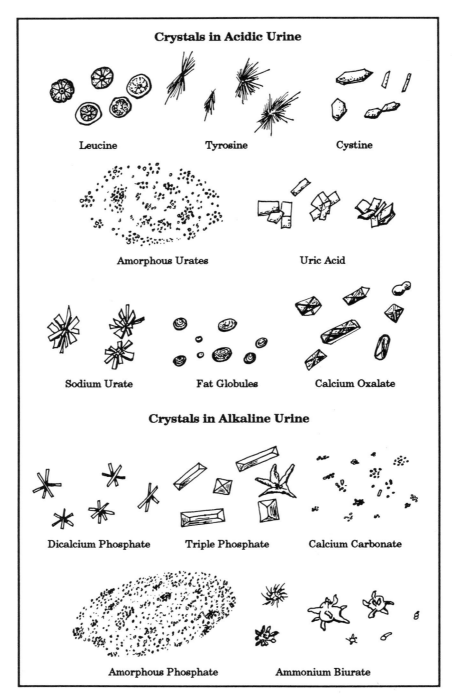

Figure 19-3 Various types of crystals that may be found in urine. (From Pratt PW: *Principles and practice of veterinary technology*, St. Louis, 1998, Mosby.)

E. Total erythrocyte count usually has no advantage over the PCV except to determine the RBC indices

F. Total RBC numbers are reported as millions per microliter ($\# \times 10^{12}$/L)

III. Hemoglobin (Hb)
  A. The part of the RBCs responsible for carrying oxygen and carbon dioxide
    1. Assists in acid-base regulation by eliminating CO_2

B. Can be measured by photometric methods or automated cell counters

C. Used for determining erythrocytic indices

D. Measured in g/dl (g/L)

E. In normal animal, hemoglobin is about one third PCV

IV. Erythrocyte indices

A. Determined by use of the total RBC numbers, Hb content, and PCV. Many electronic units automatically include these values

   1. Used to assist in classifying some anemias

B. Mean corpuscular volume (MCV) is the mean volume of a group of erythrocytes (their size)

   1. MCV is calculated by dividing the PCV (%) by the total RBC count and multiplying by 10

      a. In SI units divide the PCV (L/L) by the RBC count and multiply by 1000

   2. The MCV is recorded in femtoliters (FL); normal ranges vary among species

C. Mean corpuscular hemoglobin (MCH) is the mean weight of hemoglobin contained in the average RBC

   1. The MCH is calculated by dividing the Hb concentration by the total RBC count and multiplying by 10

   2. Results are recorded in picograms

   3. Considered least accurate of the indices because Hb and RBC counts are less accurate than the PCV

D. Mean corpuscular hemoglobin content (MCHC) is the concentration of hemoglobin in the average RBC (color of the cell)

   1. The MCHC is calculated by dividing the Hb concentration by the PCV (%) and multiplying by 100

   2. Results are reported in g/dl (g/L)

      a. In SI units divide the Hb concentration (g/L) by the PCV (L/L)

   3. Considered the most accurate of the RBC indices because it does not require the RBC count

V. Reticulocyte count

A. An expression of the percentage of RBCs that are reticulocytes or immature erythrocytes still containing the ribosomes

B. Wright's stain causes a polychromatophilic staining or diffuse, blue-gray color

C. Cats possess two forms: aggregate and punctate

   1. Only the aggregate form should be counted

   2. Similar to other species, this contains large clumps that appear polychromatophilic

D. A few drops of blood are mixed with an equal amount of New Methylene Blue stain

   1. This mixture is used to prepare a conventional blood film that shows up as granular precipitates

E. The percentage of reticulocytes per 1000 RBCs or an absolute count in reticulocytes/μL is reported

F. Useful in assessing the bone marrow response to anemia in all domestic animals except for horses because they do not release reticulocytes from the bone marrow

Erythrocyte Film Evaluation (Figure 19-4)

I. Erythrocyte size, shape, appearance, and color can vary among species of animals. These parameters can also be affected by environment, handling, technique, etc.

II. Size of the mature erythrocyte can range from 3 to 7 microns, depending on species and may be characterized as follows

A. **Macrocytosis:** an increased number of larger than normal, usually immature, polychromatic RBCs

B. **Microcytosis:** an increased number of RBCs smaller in diameter than normal, decreased MCV

C. **Normocytic:** refers to normal sized mature erythrocytes

III. Color

A. **Normochromic:** a mature cell that stains pink in color with an area of central pallor (mammals); nucleated in reptiles, birds, and amphibians

B. **Polychromasia:** cells that have a bluish tint, due to remaining organelles in the cytoplasm

   1. When stained with NMB are reticulocytes

C. **Hypochromic:** lack of or decrease in staining intensity, due to decrease in cellular hemoglobin

   1. Iron deficiency most common cause

   2. Due to large diameter, macrocytic erythrocytes may appear hypochromic

   3. True hypochromia is usually concurrent with microcytosis and determined by MCV

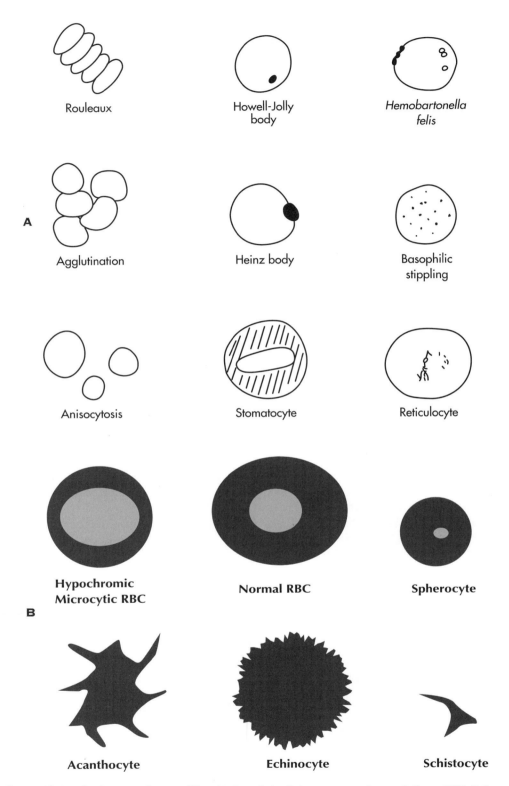

Figure 19-4 Erythrocyte abnormalities. (**A**, From Baker P: Lecture notes, Seneca College, *1997*. **B**, From Pratt PW: *Principles and practice of veterinary technology*, St. Louis, 1998, Mosby.)

IV. Shape
  A. **Acanthocyte:** cells with irregularly shaped margins/projections from the cell wall, also known as spur cells
    1. Can be due to faulty technique or disease where cholesterol concentration changes occur at the membrane
  B. **Crenation:** cells with spiny projections around the margin
    1. Often associated with slow drying of the blood film
  C. **Echinocyte** (burr cells): have spine like projections from all surfaces of the cell
    1. Appear as dark red spots when seen on top of cell
    2. Can be due to faulty technique (crenation)
    3. Observed in blood of horses after exercising or with renal disease and lymphosarcoma in dogs
  D. **Target cells:** "Mexican hat" cells
    1. Contain a central, round portion of hemoglobin inside the area of central pallor
    2. A form of leptocyte and may be called codocyte
  E. **Leptocyte:** large, thin RBC that is folded or misshapen due to increased membrane or decreased volume
    1. Common finding with regenerative anemias
  F. **Stomatocyte:** also a type of leptocyte
    1. Large thin cell that warps when passing through small blood vessels
    2. Seen in dogs with rare inherited disorders
  G. **Spherocytes:** smaller, dense, and dark staining; lack central pallor
    1. Suggestive of immune mediated hemolytic anemia
    2. Due to loss of surface membrane (partial erythrophagocytosis)
  H. **Schistocytes:** fragmented erythrocytes, also known as helmet cells
    1. Suggestive of mechanical damage or vascular occlusion (disseminated intravascular coagulation)
  I. **Poikilocytosis:** a general presence of a variation in cell shape
  J. **Rouleaux:** erythrocytes appearing as stacks of coins or rows
    1. Can indicate inflammatory changes or alteration of plasma protein
    2. A normal finding in equines (marked)

  K. **Agglutination:** an amorphous clumping of erythrocytes, typically associated with immune disease
    1. May be visibly seen: a grainy appearance on the slide
    2. If seen do not use automated RBC counting or sizing
  L. **Anisocytosis:** variation in size of RBCs
    1. Normal amount varies with species
    2. Can be due to large and/or small cells
    3. Graded as mild, moderate, or marked
V. Inclusions
  A. Howell-Jolly bodies: erythrocytes that retain small, round nuclear fragments, dark staining, intracellular bodies
    1. Noted in regenerative anemias and splenic disorders
    2. Nonrefractile when out of focus
    3. 1% of feline and equine RBCs have these
  B. Heinz bodies: small, round areas of denatured hemoglobin attached to the cell membrane
    1. Appear transparent with Wright's or Diff-Quick stain; stain blue with NMB (1 to 2 μ)
    2. Associated with oxidant drugs, lymphosarcoma, hyperthyroidism, and diabetes mellitus in cats
    3. Common in cats
  C. Basophilic stippling: small, blue staining granules (RNA) within the erythrocyte
    1. Seen in very responsive anemias in cattle, sheep, and cats
    2. Suggestive of lead toxicity
  D. Nucleated red blood cell (NRBC): slightly larger than mature RBC, darker staining cytoplasm, retained nucleus
    1. An immature cell, not normally seen in circulation, released in response to anemia (see Table 19-1 for list of precursors)

Table 19-1 Precursor blood cells in order of least immature to most mature cells

Erythrocyte precursors	Granulocyte precursors	Platelet precursors
Rubriblast	Myeloblast	Megakaryoblast
Prorubricyte	Progranulocyte	Promegakaryocyte
Rubricyte	Myelocyte	Megakaryocyte
Metarubricyte	Metamyelocyte	Platelet
Polychromatic erythrocyte	Band	

2. Nucleated RBCs are normal in birds and reptiles

VI. Blood parasites

A. *Hemobartonella felis:* small cocci or rod shaped, dark purple stained structures (with Wright's stain) at the margin of feline RBCs
   1. Often noted in secondary disease conditions

B. *Hemobartonella canis:* appear as long chains on the surface of the canine RBC; dark purple staining
   1. Rare and usually apparent in immunocompromised or splenectomized dogs
   2. Similar to *Eperythrozoon* in swine, cattle, and llamas

C. *Babesia* spp.: protozoa
   1. *B. canis* in dogs; *B. caballi* in horses
   2. Appear as fairly large, paired, teardrop shaped organisms in the RBC
   3. More noticeable in cells along feathered edge
   4. Affected cells tend to accumulate below buffy coat
   5. Can lyze cells and stain with Giemsa or diagnose through serology
   6. Transmitted by *Ixodes* ticks

D. *Cytauxzoon felis:* very rare organism found in RBCs, lymphocytes, and macrophages of cats
   1. Small, dark-staining ring forms in the cells

E. *Anaplasma marginale:* intracellular parasite of the RBC in cattle and wild ruminants
   1. Small, dark-staining cocci at the cell margin
   2. Must be differentiated from similar sized Howell-Jolly bodies

F. *Dirofilaria immitis:* heartworm of dogs, may be seen on blood films
   1. Unless present in large numbers, may be missed, best to use buffy coat
   2. Modified Knott's, filter technique or ELISA (enzyme-linked immunosorbent assay) is more accurate
   3. Must differentiate from nonpathogenic *Dipetalonema* spp. by morphology

Leukocyte (WBC) Evaluation

I. Total leukocyte counts may be done manually or with automated cell counters

A. Both methods require blood sample dilution and lysis of the RBCs before counting

B. Hemacytometer method: sample preparation using the Unopette system (Becton, Dickinson & Co) is a common method
   1. A calibrated blood sample (20 μL) is diluted at 1:100 in acetic acid diluent
   2. Sample is mixed, incubated, and placed on the hemacytometer chamber
   3. Cells are counted in the nine primary squares at $10\times$ magnification

C. Calculating total WBCs by hemacytometer method
   1. Total cells counted from both chambers is averaged
   2. Cell number is multiplied by dilution and value factors
   3. 10% of cells counted $\times$ dilution factor of 100
      a. EXAMPLE: 75 cells counted, $75 + 7.5$ $(10\%) = 82.5 \times 100 = 8250/\mu L$
      b. $(\# \times 10^9/L)$
   4. Automated counters use an electronic impulse to sense and count cells as they pass through the aperture; some calibration may be necessary
   5. Corrected WBC count: automated and manual counts include NRBCs as WBCs
      a. Corrected with use of the blood film evaluation and NRBC count
      b. A practical method is to include the NRBC in the differential count and calculate using absolute numbers
         (1) EXAMPLE: total WBC is 9000/μL $(\# \times 10^9/L)$ with 10% NRBCs or 900 absolute
            (a) $9000 - 900 = 8100$ as the corrected total
   6. Increased WBC count is leukocytosis
   7. Decreased WBC count is leukopenia

II. Leukocyte evaluation and differentiation

A. WBC evaluation and differentiation is done by examining the stained blood film
   1. Traditional stains include Wright's, Wright-Giemsa, and Diff-Quick (American Scientific Products)
   2. Techniques vary; follow manufacturer directions

B. Cells should be examined and counted in an area of the film where distribution and staining properties are best
   1. A monolayer of cells is preferable; examination is done under $40\times$ or $100\times$ oil immersion magnification
   2. Avoid the feathered edge due to increased amounts of artifacts

C. Leukocyte differential numbers should always be reported as absolutes

1. The percentage of each cell type is multiplied by the total WBC count
2. EXAMPLE: 60% neutrophils × 10,000 WBC/μL total = 6000 absolute neutrophils

D. Leukocyte morphology
1. Neutrophils: most common peripheral WBC in companion animals
   a. Irregular, segmented nucleus with coarse clumped chromatin staining dark purple
   b. Horse neutrophils show more segmentation than dog neutrophils
   c. Cytoplasm is pale pink with faint granulation
   d. Phagocytic and bactericidal properties, with an average life span of 10 hours
   e. Inflammation is usually indicated by neutrophilia with increased bands
   f. Increase may also be due to stress, exercise, glucocorticoid use, or leukemia
   g. Neutropenia may be due to decreased survival of cells, reduced or ineffective production, or sequestration
      (1) Will likely produce a degenerative left shift (more immature than mature neutrophils)
   h. Avian neutrophil is called a heterophil
2. Neutrophilic bands: immature neutrophil stage
   a. Horseshoe shaped, symmetrical nucleus with rounded ends
      (1) Increased numbers denote left shift
3. Toxic neutrophils: changes with toxicity
   a. Dohle bodies: appear as small, gray-blue cytoplasmic inclusions, indicative of mild toxemia
   b. Basophilia or blue cytoplasm and vacuoles are slightly more severe signs of toxicity
   c. Nuclear hypersegmentation implies older neutrophils
   d. More evident in many feline illnesses
   e. Other species with toxic neutrophils are often indicative of bacterial disease
4. Lymphocytes: small and large forms are recognized
   a. High nuclear/cytoplasm ratio
   b. Coarse, clumped (often round) dark staining, chromatin
   c. Slight sky blue cytoplasm surrounding nucleus of small forms with more cytoplasm in large lymphocytes
   d. Cytoplasm may contain pink-purple granules (azurophilic)
   e. Cattle tend to have more lymphocytes than neutrophils
      (1) May be large, have indented nuclei, increased cytoplasm, and granules
      (2) Difficult to separate from neoplastic lymphoid cells
   f. Reactive lymphocytes, a sign of antigenic stimulation, are shown by a pale perinuclear zone surrounded by basophilic cytoplasm and possible azurophilic granules
5. Monocytes: largest of the peripheral WBCs
   a. Variable nuclear shape (kidney bean shape, elongated, lobulated) with diffuse chromatin, not as intensely stained
   b. Blue-gray cytoplasm possibly with vacuoles and fine pink granules
   c. May be difficult to distinguish from band neutrophils or metamyelocytes
   d. Circulate briefly in blood before entering tissues as macrophages
6. Eosinophils: nuclear structure similar to neutrophils but not as coarsely clumped chromatin
   a. Distinctive red to purple staining cytoplasmic granules that vary in size and shape among species
      (1) Canine varies
      (2) Feline eosinophil granules tend to be rod shaped, small, and numerous
      (3) Horses have intense orange-red large granules
      (4) Cattle, sheep, and pig granules stain intense pink and are round
   b. An increase is noted in allergic or hypersensitive reactions
      (1) Mast cells often present
7. Basophils: a rare finding in peripheral blood
   a. Cytoplasmic granules stain blue to blue-black (lavender in felines) and may be few in number (dog) or more numerous (horse, cow)
   b. Gray-blue cytoplasm often with small vacuoles
   c. As with mast cells, involved with hypersensitivity reactions

E. *Ehrlichia canis:* an intracellular parasite of monocytes and neutrophils
1. Tropical pancytopenia; transmitted by ticks
2. Appear as small lightly stained clusters in the cytoplasm (called morulae)
3. Diagnosis through buffy coat smear or serology (best)
4. Signs include leukopenia, anemia, thrombocytopenia, increased TPP, and lymphocytosis

Thrombocyte (platelet) Evaluation

I. General information
A. Anuclear cytoplasmic fragments from bone marrow megakaryocytes
B. Vary in size, shape, and color; usually small pale blue to pink-purple in color
C. May be found in clumps (especially in cats)
D. Thrombocytes (platelets) are an important component of hemostasis
E. Adequate numbers for newer microscopes are estimated to be at 8-10 per 100×
1. Average number of platelets on 10 fields, per 100× oil immersion field, in an area where RBCs are overlapping, is multiplied by 15,000 for a rough estimate
2. With decreased estimates, platelet aggregation on the blood film or tube of blood must be ruled out before thrombocytopenia is confirmed
F. Actual counts can be done manually with the hemacytometer or an automated cell counter

Total protein

I. Combination of various proteins produced mostly by the liver
II. Abnormalities indicate diseases in tissues responsible for synthesis, catabolism, and loss
III. Total plasma or serum protein measured by total solids refractometer or chemical analysis in g/dl (g/L)

Nonmanual instrumentation

I. Quantitative buffy coat analysis (QBC)
A. Specialized equipment and capillary tubes used for measurements of PCV, total WBC count, platelet count, and limited differential
B. The buffy coat band lengths are converted to numerical readings
1. Various types and degrees of fluorescence, depending on the layers, are also observed

C. It is essential that a differential also be performed to ensure accuracy
D. Layers of cells from uppermost to lowest are platelets, mononuclear cells (monocytes and lymphocytes), eosinophils, granulocytes, reticulocytes, NRBCs, RBCs

II. Electronic cell counters
A. Various instruments ranging in costs are available
B. Many now available that automatically change instrument settings for multiple species use
C. Speed, accuracy, and reproducibility are major advantages
D. Depending on unit, will calibrate WBC and RBC count, Hb, PCV (indirectly), erythrocytic indices, and platelets
1. Some will give red cell distribution width (RDW), which is an indication of the variation in RBC size
a. The greater the variation, the higher the RDW
E. Sample must be diluted but some machines do so automatically
F. Good quality control is essential

CYTOLOGY

Microscopic examination of cells, primarily exfoliated, from tissues, lesions, fluids, and internal organs has become an increasingly valuable tool in veterinary diagnostics. Sample collection can be easily performed in most cases and special equipment required is minimal.

Specimen Collection

I. Fine needle aspiration: may be used to collect samples from the skin, lymph nodes, and internal organs
A. Recommended needle sizes range from 22 to 25 gauge, attached to a 3 to 12 mL syringe
B. Samples are collected and pushed onto clean microscope slides for staining
II. Fluid aspiration
A. Includes thoracocentesis and abdominal paracentesis when fluid accumulation is suspected
B. Usually performed with animal in standing position
C. Fluids may be centrifuged for sediment examination or submitted for bacterial culture
III. Solid mass imprinting and scraping
A. For collection and preparation of cytologic specimens *in situ*
B. Masses are cut in half, blotted dry, and several imprints are made on a clean slide

C. Scrapings are done on a freshly cut surface with a clean scalpel blade, the film is spread across a clean slide and stained

IV. Vaginal swab technique

A. Used as an aid in determining stage of estrous cycle and evaluating uterine and vaginal disease

B. Vulva and surrounding area are washed clean

C. A vaginal speculum is carefully introduced

D. Sample of the vaginal mucosa is taken with a sterile swab moistened with sterile saline

E. Samples are rolled onto clean slides for staining

Slide Preparation

I. Squash prep method

A. A small amount of aspirate is placed in the center of a clean slide

B. A second slide is placed over the sample and is carefully slid apart from the bottom slide

C. Excessive pressure can distort and rupture cells

II. Needle spread method

A. A small amount of aspirate is placed in the center of a clean slide

B. The tip of the needle is then used to pull the sample out into several projections—a starfish appearance is formed

III. Blood film technique

A. A small amount of aspirate is placed on one end of a clean slide

B. A second slide is then used to smoothly pull the sample toward the other end

C. This technique produces a film similar to that used for a whole blood differential count

Staining Techniques

I. Papanicolaou stains

A. Commonly used in human gynecologic examinations

B. Multiple steps required in staining technique

C. Excellent for accentuating nuclear detail

II. New Methylene Blue

A. Will stain nuclei, mast cell granules, and most infectious agents

B. Can be applied directly to an air dried slide

C. Selected uses include presence of nucleated cells, bacteria, fungi, and mast cells

III. Romanovsky type stains

A. Include Wright's, Giemsa, and Diff Quik

B. Provide satisfactory cytologic specimens

C. Some variation in staining quality is evident: consistent use of one type is recommended

Interpretation

I. Exfoliative cytologic interpretation refers to examination of cells shed from body surfaces

A. Vaginal cytology: readily obtained samples, as previously described, can assist in timing mating programs such as artificial insemination in small animals

1. Identification of cell populations during the estrous cycle is easily accomplished through cytologic examination

a. Anestrus

(1) Predominantly noncornified squamous epithelial cells

(2) Large cells, basophilic cytoplasm, and large round nucleus

(3) Categorized as intermediate or parabasal

(4) Some neutrophils but no RBCs

b. Proestrus

(1) Presence of noncornified squamous epithelial cells changing to cornified squamous epithelial cells

(2) Angular with jagged borders, pyknotic nucleus, eosinophilic cytoplasm

(3) RBCs increase, neutrophils decrease

c. Estrus

(1) All cornified squamous epithelial cells

(2) Many appear to be anuclear

(3) RBCs may be present but no neutrophils

d. Metestrus

(1) Noncornified squamous epithelial cells replace cornified cells

(2) Neutrophil numbers will increase

(3) RBCs generally absent

B. History and clinical signs are also important for proper interpretation

II. Proper analysis of fluid samples

A. Note gross characteristics such as ease of collection, color, and turbidity

B. Note total nucleated cell counts, total protein, cell types, and morphology

C. Other tests such as mucin clot test for synovial fluid may be performed

III. Types of effusions (an accumulation of fluid in a body cavity) can generally be classified as transudate, modified transudate, and exudate

A. There are also neoplastic, hemorrhagic, and chylous effusions

IV. Cells found in exfoliative cytology
   A. Neutrophils
      1. May resemble those in blood, be degenerative, or have undergone morphologic changes such as hypersegmentation, pyknosis, karyolysis (swollen nucleus), or karyorrhexis (nucleus broken apart)
   B. Lymphocytes
      1. Same as in blood
   C. Plasma cells
      1. Active lymphocytes with a very basophilic cytoplasm
   D. Eosinophils
      1. Same as in blood
   E. Macrophages
      1. Large (derived from monocytes)
      2. Oval to pleomorphic nucleus with lacy to condensed chromatin
      3. Abundant blue cytoplasm with vacuoles that may contain phagocytozed cells or debris
      4. May be multinucleated or giant cells (nuclei uniform in size and shape)
   F. Mesothelial cells
      1. Cells that line the pleural, peritoneal, and visceral surfaces
      2. Round, with usually one round to oval nucleus but may also be multinucleated
      3. May have nucleoli, corona (a fringe), or be seen singularly or in clusters
      4. Difficult to distinguish from macrophages once they are activated
   G. Mast cells
      1. Round to oval with round to oval nuclei
      2. Numerous blue to purple cytoplasmic granules
   H. RBCs
      1. Look for erythrocytophagia (phagocytosis of RBCs by macrophages) to confirm hemorrhage into body cavity
V. Cytology of inflammation
   A. Comprised of cells from blood, macrophages, and tissue cells
   B. Classifications
      1. Can be classified as purulent, pyogranulomatous, granulomatous, and eosinophilic
      2. Can also be classified as acute, chronic, or chronic/active
      3. Purulent (suppurative) inflammation
         a. Acute inflammation
         b. Most common type of inflammation, with the majority being caused by bacteria

         c. Over 70% neutrophils, with a few macrophages and lymphocytes
      4. Pyogranulomatous inflammation
         a. Also referred to as chronic/active
         b. Consists of macrophages and 50% to 75% neutrophils
         c. Cytologically partway between suppurative and granulomatous inflammation
      5. Granulomatous inflammation
         a. Also called chronic inflammation
         b. Greater than 70% of cells mononuclear (monocytes, macrophages, giant cells) with few neutrophils
      6. Eosinophilic
         a. Consists of greater than 10% eosinophils
         b. Often see a few mast cells, plasma cells, and lymphocytes
VI. Noninflammatory, non-neoplastic lesions
   A. Include cysts such as epidermal inclusion cysts (sebaceous cysts), hyperplasia, dysplasia, hematoma, seroma, adipocytes, and salivary mucocele
VII. Neoplasia
   A. Best indication is presence of homogenous population of cells, which may or may not be pleomorphic, in a location where they should not be
   B. May be benign or malignant and may have associated inflammation
   C. At least five criteria should be met before determining malignancy in a cytological sample
      1. Variation in cell size of same type
      2. Nucleus
         a. Most important criteria for determining malignancy
         b. Marked variation in nuclear size
         c. Marked variation in nuclear/cytoplasm ratio
         d. Chromatin irregularity
         e. Mitotic index
            (1) Small numbers normal
            (2) Abnormal if found in tissues other than bone marrow, lymph nodes, or hyperplastic tissues
         f. Abnormal mitoses such as three or more planes of division
         g. Multinucleation
            (1) Can be seen in mesothelial and transitional cells and macrophages

h. Nuclear membrane changes such as clefts, wrinkling, thickening

i. Nucleolar changes

(1) Varying sizes, shapes, and staining, or numbers, especially in a sheet of cells

3. Cytoplasm changes

a. Extreme basophilia of cytoplasmic features

b. Vacuolation, which is usually tiny

c. Boundaries may be irregular and indistinct

Glossary

absolute count Calculation of absolute cell numbers based on percentage of type multiplied by the total cell count

acanthocyte An erythrocyte with irregularly shaped margins

anemia A decrease in the PCV, RBC count, or hemoglobin below normal values

anisocytosis Variation in cell size

anuria Complete absence of urine formation or elimination

basophilia An increased number of basophils

basophilic stippling Presence of small, blue staining granules in the erythrocyte

buffy coat The layer of WBCs, platelets, and nucleated RBCs in sedimented or centrifuged blood

bilirubinuria Detectable conjugated bile pigments in the urine

crenation Erythrocytes with spiny projections on the margin of the cell

eosinopenia A decreased number of eosinophils

eosinophilia An increased number of eosinophils

erythrophagocytosis Engulfing, or phagocytosis, of the erythrocyte

erythropoiesis The production of RBCs

exfoliative cytology The study of cells shed from body surfaces such as tissues, lesions, and fluids

exudate Fluid escaped from blood vessels with a high content of protein and cellular debris

glucosuria Detectable levels of glucose in the urine (glycosuria)

granulomatous Composed of a tumorlike mass or nodule of granulation tissue

hematuria Presence of intact erythrocytes in the urine

hemoglobinuria Free hemoglobin in the urine

hemolysis Destruction of RBCs

hypersegmented A neutrophil with more than five lobes in the nucleus

hypertonic Greater than isotonic concentration

hypochromic An erythrocyte with lack or decrease in staining intensity, low cellular hemoglobin

hypotonic Less than isotonic concentration

istonic Of similar osmolality to normal plasma

ketonuria Excessive ketones (e.g., acetone) in the urine

left shift Presence of an increased number of immature (nonsegmented) neutrophils in the circulation

leukemia Neoplastic disease in which a significant number of immature blast cells are found in the bone marrow and blood

leukocytosis An increase in circulating white cell numbers

leukopenia A decrease in circulating white cell numbers

lymphocytosis An increased number of circulating lymphocytes

macrocyte An RBC that has a diameter that is larger than normal

macrocytic An increased number of large RBCs

mast cell A tissue cell having granules that contain histamine and heparin

microcyte An RBC with a diameter that is smaller than normal

microcytic An increased number of small RBCs

monocytopenia A decreased number of monocytes

monocytosis An increased number of monocytes

neutropenia A decreased number of neutrophils

neutrophilia An increased number of neutrophils

NMB New Methylene Blue, a basic dye used to stain cell nuclei and granules

normochromic A normal, pink staining erythrocyte

normocytic Adjective used to describe an RBC of normal size (volume)

NRBC Nucleated red blood cell, an immature erythrocyte

oliguria Decrease in urine formation

pancytopenia Decrease in the RBC, WBC, and platelet lines

PCV Packed cell volume or hematocrit

plasma Fluid portion of the blood in which cells are suspended

poikilocytosis A variation in general cell shape

pollakiuria Frequent urination

polychromasia Erythrocytes that have a bluish tint when stained with regular blood stains and are reticulocytes (granular precipitates) with New Methylene Blue

polyuria Increased urine production

proteinuria Abnormal level of proteins in the urine

RBC Red blood cells, or erythrocytes

right shift Presence of an increased number of hypersegmented neutrophils in circulation

rouleaux Erythrocytes formed in stacks or columns

schistocyte Fragmented erythrocyte, "helmet cell"

sedimentation rate The rate at which RBCs settle in their own plasma in a given amount of time

smudge cell A nucleated cell that has ruptured during smearing due to mechanical damage or increased fragility of the cell

spherocyte A small, dense, dark staining erythrocyte

supravital staining Use of a stain that has a low toxicity so that vital and functional processes can be studied in live cells

thrombocytopenia A decreased number of platelets (thrombocytes)

thrombocytosis An increased number of platelets (thrombocytes)

toxic neutrophils Neutrophil showing certain morphologic changes such as vacuolation, toxic granules, increased basophilia, or nuclear changes

WBC White blood cells or leukocytes

Review Questions

1 Which of the following urine collection methods is suitable for bacterial culture?
   a. Manual expression
   b. Cystocentesis
   c. Midstream
   d. Litter pan pour off

2 Pollakiuria is defined as:
   a. Complete absence of urine formation
   b. Increased urine production
   c. Frequent urination
   d. Decreased urine formation

3 Which species naturally has a darker colored urine?
   a. Dogs
   b. Cattle
   c. Rabbits
   d. Sheep

4 Which of the following chemical constituents in urine is the result of fatty acid catabolism?
   a. Acetone
   b. Bilirubin
   c. Glucose
   d. Hemoglobin

5 Which term describes cells as having spiny projections around the margin and is often the result of slow drying of the blood film?
   a. Target cells
   b. Acanthocyte
   c. Schistocyte
   d. Crenation

6 Which intracellular parasite appears fairly large, paired, teardrop shaped?
   a. *Hemabartonella felis*
   b. *Anaplasma marginale*
   c. *Babesia canis*
   d. *Hemabartonella canis*

7 A large leukocyte with variable nuclear shape with diffuse chromatin, blue-gray cytoplasm, vacuoles, and possible fine pink granules is descriptive of a:
   a. Lymphocyte
   b. NRBC
   c. Monocyte
   d. Basophil

8 The fluid portion of the blood from which fibrinogen has been removed is termed:
   a. Serum
   b. Plasma
   c. Buffy coat
   d. Packed cells

9 Which step is completed before solid mass imprinting on a glass slide?
   a. Fixing in formalin
   b. Cutting into several sections
   c. Blotting dry on paper towels
   d. Cleaning slide with alcohol

10 Cytologically, estrus may be described as which of the following?
   a. Noncornified epithelial cells with neutrophils
   b. Increased red blood cells and noncornified epithelial cells
   c. Predominately keratinized epithelial cells
   d. Increased neutrophils and red blood cells

11 Which of the following techniques should not be used to make slides for cytology examinations?
   a. Touch imprint from freshly cut tissue
   b. Imprints from formalin fixed tissue
   c. Fresh collection of fluid for making a film
   d. Squash prep of aspirated fluid

12 Which of the following will stain the nuclei of cells but not erythrocytes or eosinophilic granules?
   a. Diff-Quik
   b. Papanicolaou
   c. New Methylene Blue
   d. Wright's

BIBLIOGRAPHY

Baker P: Lecture notes, Seneca College, 1997.

Denicola DB et al: Proceedings, diagnostic cytology symposium, Purdue University, December 1987.

Elkhart modern urine chemistry, ed 1, IN, Ames Division, 1979.

Joseph SL: Urinalysis, the picture of health; Proceedings, EXPO for veterinary technicians, Washington DC, 1987.

McCurnin DM: *Clinical textbook for veterinary technicians,* ed 3, 1995, Philadelphia, Pennsylvania, W.B. Saunders.

Meyer DJ: The management of cytology specimens, *Compendium on continuing education for the practicing veterinarian,* 9:1, January 1987.

Osborne CA, Stevens JB: *Handbook of canine & feline urinalysis,* ed 1, St. Louis, Ralston Purina Company.

Pratt PW: *Laboratory procedures for veterinary technicians,* ed 3, St. Louis, 1997, Mosby.

Pratt PW: *Laboratory procedures for veterinary technicians,* ed 2, 1992, Goleta, California, American Veterinary Publications, Inc.

Rebar AH: *Handbook of veterinary cytology,* ed 1, St. Louis, Ralston Purina Company.

Rich LJ: *The morphology of canine & feline blood cells,* ed 2, St. Louis, Ralston Purina Company.

Walsh DJ, Wade WL: The differential film: errors and normal variations, *Veterinary technician* 17:7, July 1996.

CHAPTER 20

Clinical Chemistry

Joanne Hamel

OUTLINE

General Information
Kidney Function
   Creatinine
   Urea Nitrogen
   Water Deprivation/Urine Concentration Tests
Pancreatic Function
   Urine Glucose
   Serum/Plasma Glucose
   Fecal Examination for Undigested Food

Serum Amylase
Serum Lipase
TLI
Liver Function
   Bilirubin
   Urine Urobilinogen
   Total Serum/Plasma Proteins
   Albumin
   Globulins
   Enzymes
   Bile acids

Serum Cholesterol
Electrolytes and Minerals
   General Information
   Serum Sodium
   Serum Potassium
   Serum Chloride
   Serum Calcium
   Serum Phosphorus
   Serum Magnesium
Measurement of Electrolytes

LEARNING OUTCOMES

After reading this chapter you should be able to:

1. Identify common laboratory tests used to evaluate kidney, pancreatic, and liver function, as well as electrolytes and minerals, in small and large animals.
2. Understand the significance of abnormal results of these tests.
3. Provide samples required and proper conditions under which the tests are performed.
4. Identify common tests that appear in various chemistry profiles.

It is essential that all blood samples destined for biochemical analysis be collected with care, using the correct anticoagulants or no anticoagulants. One must pay close attention to any special requirements when collecting blood samples. The results are only as good as the samples tested.

Evaluation of the chemical constituents of whole blood, plasma and serum has become increasingly realistic in the practice setting. Instrumentation, equipment, and procedures have been greatly modified to allow relatively rapid and reliable diagnostics. Chemical components are routinely assayed by use of chemical reagent test strips or automated dry chemical analyses machines.

GENERAL INFORMATION

   I. Components of whole blood
      A. Whole blood: comprised of fluid and cellular components
         1. Fluid is plasma; cells are the erythrocytes, leukocytes, and thrombocytes
      B. Plasma: fluid portion of the blood in which cells are suspended; 90% water and 10% dissolved proteins, hormones, lipids, enzymes, salts, carbohydrates, vitamins, and waste materials

C. Serum: fluid portion with fibrinogen protein removed; derived when whole blood is allowed to clot

II. Sample handling
   A. The following should be kept in mind when handling samples
      1. Samples should be collected from calm, fasted patients
      2. Avoid hemolysis by selecting correct size needles and dry syringes or new evacuated tubes
      3. Serum is the sample of choice for all tests—to avoid chemical interaction with the specimen. Blood samples taken for serum separation are allowed to clot, centrifuged, and separated
         a. Samples are allowed to clot at room temperature for 20 to 30 minutes
         b. Separate the clot by "rimming" with a wooden applicator stick around the inside of the tube
         c. Blood tubes are counter balanced and centrifuged for 10 minutes at 2000 to 3000 rpm
            (1) Centrifuge as soon as possible and transfer the serum or plasma to chemically clean and properly labeled test tubes
         d. Several types of blood tubes and devices are designed to facilitate serum separation
         e. Serum is carefully pipetted or poured off into a suitable container and labeled
         f. Serum may be refrigerated or frozen; freezing may affect some test results
         g. Quality of serum
            (1) **Lipemic serum:** cloudy, excessive lipids, often due to diet, metabolic disease
            (2) **Hemolytic serum:** pink to reddish tint; caused by damage to RBCs either physiologic or iatrogenic
            (3) **Icteric serum:** yellow tinge; indicative of kidney disease
      4. Samples for whole blood or plasma should be collected with an anticoagulant. If plasma is used, be sure that the anticoagulant chosen does not interfere with the tests requested. Types of anticoagulants include:
         a. Heparin: available in sodium, potassium, lithium, and ammonium salts
            (1) Good choice for plasma samples because it interferes little with chemical assays; use at 20 units/mL of blood
         b. Ethylenediaminetetraacetic acid (EDTA): anticoagulant of choice for hematological tests because it has little effect on morphology
            (1) Should not be used for chemical assays of plasma
         c. Sodium fluoride: a glucose preservative with some anticoagulant properties
      5. Samples should be analyzed immediately
         a. When this is not possible, samples should be refrigerated until tests can be performed (return to room temperature before testing)
      6. Collect sufficient sample for the tests requested
      7. Each lab should establish a set of normal values that will reflect test procedures and conditions used

KIDNEY FUNCTION

More than 70% of the glomeruli of both kidneys must be nonfunctional before serum chemistry changes occur. The nephron parts are so closely related that malfunction in one area will eventually affect another.

Creatinine

   I. A byproduct of muscle metabolism; produced at a constant rate and filtered out almost entirely by the glomeruli
      A. A small amount is produced daily
   II. Increased serum creatinine levels are seen when there is a lack of functional glomeruli
   III. Serum creatinine concentrations are influenced by:
      A. Fluid and hydration level
      B. Pre-renal factors such as shock
      C. Post renal factors such as bladder and urethral obstructions
   IV. Used to evaluate glomerular function
   V. Sample required:
      A. Serum or plasma may be used
      B. Hemolysis does not influence the results
      C. Bilirubinemia will cause false increases

Urea Nitrogen

I. Urea is an end product of protein metabolism and is excreted primarily by the kidneys
   A. Up to 40% is reabsorbed by the tubules for reexcretion
   B. Rate of reabsorption is inversely proportional to the amount of urine output
II. Evaluates glomerular filtration and function
III. Nonrenal causes of increased serum urea nitrogen include:
   A. The amount of protein ingested and absorbed
   B. Fever
   C. Corticosteroids
IV. Levels are increased in renal insufficiency
V. Etiology of increased levels include
   A. Pre-renal factors such as shock and dehydration
   B. Post renal factors such as obstruction in the ureters, bladder, or urethra
VI. May be decreased in anorexia and liver disease
VII. Sample required
   A. Serum preferred
   B. Plasma should not be collected with ammonium oxalate
      1. False increases will be produced
   C. Plasma should not be collected with fluoride
      1. Decreases will be produced
   D. Samples should be nonlipemic
   E. It is recommended to fast the animal for 18 hours before testing
   F. Serum or plasma should be tested as soon as possible because bacterial contamination will reduce the amount of urea in the sample

Water Deprivation/Urine Concentration Tests

I. The patient is gradually deprived of water over a 3 to 5 day interval until there is a stimulus for endogenous ADH release
   A. This usually occurs at about 5% weight loss
II. If sufficient ADH, specific gravity of normal urine concentration is 1.025
III. Failure to concentrate urine over the duration of the test is indicative of insufficient ADH or tubular dysfunction
IV. This test should never be performed on animals that are dehydrated or have increased serum urea nitrogen

PANCREATIC FUNCTION

The pancreas has endocrine and exocrine functions. Pancreatic endocrine function involves the production of glucagon and insulin. Diabetes mellitus, or a deficiency of insulin resulting in hyperglycemia, is the most common endocrine disorder of the pancreas. Pancreatic exocrine function involves the production of lipase, amylase, and trypsin. Most pancreatic disturbances occur in the exocrine function of the pancreas. Dogs seem to have a greater incidence.

Urine Glucose

I. Glycosuria exists when blood glucose levels exceed the renal threshold for absorption of glucose in the proximal convoluted tubules
II. A diagnosis of diabetes mellitus is not made unless glycosuria accompanies hyperglycemia
III. Clinitest tablets (Ames) are not specific for glucose and will give a positive reaction with any reducing sugars
   A. This is considered a screening test only
IV. Reagent sticks such as Clinistix, Chemstrip, etc. are specific for measuring glucose
   A. These sticks use glucose oxidase, peroxidase, and a color indicator
V. False positives in urine may result from among:
   A. Ascorbic acid
   B. Morphine
   C. Salicylates
   D. Penicillin
   E. Tetracycline
   F. I.V. fluids containing glucose
   G. General anesthetics, etc.
VI. Sample required
   A. Freshly voided, morning sample

Serum/Plasma Glucose

I. Most test procedures use glucose oxidase, which is specific for measuring glucose in samples
II. Hyperglycemia may result from:
   A. Diabetes mellitus
   B. Several nonpancreatic causes such as stress and hyperadrenocorticism (Cushing's)
III. Hypoglycemia may result from:
   A. Malabsorption
   B. Severe liver disease
   C. Sample remaining on the cells too long
IV. Glucose tolerance tests may be used to determine how well an animal is able to utilize carbohydrates

V. Sample required
   A. Serum is preferable
      1. Sodium fluoride may be used if the plasma cannot be removed from the cells immediately
      2. It is essential to collect and treat the sample properly to get meaningful results
   B. Centrifuge sample immediately
      1. Remove plasma or serum and transfer to another test tube
   C. Blood cells will continue to utilize glucose at a rate of 7% to 10% per hour if allowed to remain in contact with the serum or plasma
   D. A fasting sample is preferred 16 to 24 hours in dogs and cats
   E. Ruminants should not be fasted

Fecal Examination for Undigested Food

I. Assessment of feces to determine pancreatic insufficiency
II. If diarrhea, rule out simple dietary, parasitic, or infectious causes
III. Microscopic examination of feces for the presence of undigested fats, starches, or proteins is performed by diluting feces and staining with Sudan III or IV
IV. For steatorrhea or neutral fats (undigested/nonsplit) use direct Sudan Stain
   A. Lipase deficiency is suggested if more than two or three globules of orange-red stained undigested fat
   B. Steatorrhea is caused by pancreatic insufficiency
V. Digested fats, use indirect Sudan Stain
   A. Acidify with glacial acetic acid; add drops of Sudan III or IV and treat with heat to view
   B. More than two or three orange-red droplets per HPF indicate steatorrhea caused by malassimilation/malabsorption
      1. Fecal protease activity should be present
VI. Starch granules in feces stain with Lugol's iodine
   A. Starch granules appear as large blackish-blue structures with a blue-green fringe
   B. Large numbers of starch granules (amylorrhea) indicate amylase deficiency
   C. Relatively insensitive test for pancreatic function

VII. Muscle fibers may be observed as blunt, striated muscle fibers in Lugol's iodine stained or unstained smears
VIII. Gelatin digestion tests for fecal trypsin
   A. X-ray film test
      1. Positive for trypsin is the clearing of the x-ray film, which is digestion of gelatin on the film
      2. False negatives can occur due to:
         a. Fluctuations in protease levels
         b. Film with indigestible gelatin
         c. Digestion using up all protease
      3. False positives can occur because:
         a. Old sample
         b. Bacteria present: digest the film
   B. Gelatin tube test
      1. Positive: failure of the tubes to solidify
      2. May also be due to old sample or digestion by bacteria

Serum Amylase

I. Amylase acts to break down starches and glycogen
II. Increased serum amylase levels are seen in:
   A. Acute, chronic, and obstructive pancreatitis
   B. Hyperadrenocorticism
   C. Liver disease
   D. Upper GI inflammation or obstruction
   E. Renal failure
III. Animals have a greater serum amylase activity level than humans (10 times greater in dog and cat) so it is recommended to dilute the serum with distilled water before testing if using tests designed for human samples
IV. Two methods of testing:
   A. Saccharogenic test: not suitable for dogs because of maltose in their serum
   B. Amyloclastic test: should be used for dogs because maltose does not influence the results
V. Amylase concentrations are not considered useful in cats
VI. Sample required
   A. Nonlipemic serum or heparinized plasma
   B. Hemolysis may elevate values

Serum Lipase

I. Lipase breaks down the long chain fatty acids of lipids into fatty acids and alcohols
II. Lipase is usually in low levels in serum but serum levels increase in cases of pancreatitis (chronic and acute)

III. Increased serum lipase is also seen in:
   A. Renal failure
   B. Hyperadrenocorticism
   C. Dexamethasone treatment
   D. Bile tract disease
IV. Manual methods for measuring lipase are cumbersome but with the newer colorimetric and new dry chemistry kits, it is easier to evaluate serum lipase levels
V. It is recommended to perform serum amylase and lipase tests on patients suspected of pancreatitis
VI. Some cats with pancreatitis do not have elevated serum lipase
VII. Sample required
   A. Nonhemolysed, nonlipemic serum or heparinized plasma

TLI

I. Trypsin-like immunoreactivity on serum
   A. Considered the test of choice
      1. A highly specific and sensitive assay for exocrine pancreatic insufficiency in dogs
   B. Trypsinogen, a trypsin-like substance, is synthesized in the pancreas and normally released in trace amounts into circulation
      1. By determining the amount of this hormone present using radioimmunoassay, it can be determined if the animal has exocrine pancreatic insufficiency (EPI)
   C. Suspect animals are fasted for 12 hours, serum is collected and sent away for analysis
      1. Normal TLI for the dog is 5.2 to 35 μg/L
      2. Dogs with EPI have levels less than 2.5 μg/L
   D. EPI may result from chronic pancreatitis, juvenile atrophy, and pancreatic hypoplasia
      1. Lack of functional tissue leads to maldigestion of food because inadequate amounts of lipase, trypsin, and amylase can be produced
   E. This condition is a common cause of malabsorption in dogs but rarely occurs in cats

LIVER FUNCTION

No one test is totally satisfactory for determining the presence or absence of liver disease. A liver profile is usually ordered, and other special tests can be done as well. Seventy percent of the liver is nonfunctional before serum chemistry changes are noted.

Bilirubin

I. Bilirubin results from the metabolism of heme by the mononuclear-phagocytic system (formerly reticuloendothelial system)
II. Hyperbilirubinemia refers to increased serum bilirubin levels
   A. Hyperbilirubinemia can cause jaundice
III. Conjugated and unconjugated forms of bilirubin are found normally in serum or plasma
IV. Increases in the total amount of bilirubin are significant
V. Total bilirubin and conjugated bilirubin are measured
   A. The amount of unconjugated bilirubin is determined by subtraction
VI. Bilirubin measured in urine is always the conjugated form
VII. Increased unconjugated serum bilirubin levels indicate prehepatic jaundice or an inability of the liver cells to take up unconjugated bilirubin
VIII. Prehepatic jaundice is due to moderate to severe hemolysis and will be accompanied by a decreased hematocrit
   A. In cattle, most hyperbilirubinemias are caused by hemolysis
   B. Unfortunately, serum bilirubin levels rarely become increased enough to aid in diagnosis
IX. Increased serum conjugated bilirubin levels are seen with hepatic jaundice or cholestasis (post hepatic jaundice)
X. A more marked rise in conjugated bilirubin is noted with post hepatic jaundice
XI. Some dogs have a lower renal threshold for bilirubin
   A. Bilirubin in the urine is considered a sensitive indicator of liver disease in dogs
XII. Cats, pigs, sheep, and horses do not normally have bilirubin in their urine
   A. Occasionally, normal cattle will exhibit biliuria
XIII. Horses will have increased unconjugated serum bilirubin in prehepatic and hepatic conditions
   A. Increased unconjugated levels also will be seen in many nonhepatic diseases (cardiac insufficiency, constipation, colic)

B. Unconjugated and conjugated serum bilirubin levels increase after fasting
XIV. In cattle, sheep, goats, and swine:
   A. Even in severe liver diseases only slight increases of total bilirubin will be noted
   B. Most increased total bilirubin levels are due to hemolytic disorders; thus serum bilirubin measurements are not useful indicators of liver disease
XV. Most testing methods for serum contain diazo reagent, which reacts specifically with bilirubin
XVI. Ictotest tablets contain diazo reagent and measure bilirubin in urine. This test:
   A. Is highly specific
   B. Is sensitive to small amounts of bilirubin
   C. Rarely produces false positives
   D. May be semiquantitative with serial dilutions of the urine
XVII. Reagent strips
   A. EXAMPLES: Ictostix, Multistix use diazo reagent
      1. Considered less sensitive to bilirubin in urine than Ictotest
   B. False positives are caused by some medications
XVIII. Samples required
   A. Nonlipemic, nonhemolyzed serum or plasma
   B. Remove serum or plasma from the clot or cells within three hours
   C. Store samples in the dark because up to 50% bilirubin will be lost in the first hour of collection if left in light
   D. Samples can be refrigerated or frozen
   E. Freshly collected urine must be tested immediately for bilirubin

Urine Urobilinogen

I. In small animals other than in cats and dogs the results are not as useful in pinpointing liver problems: testing is not routine
II. In humans and dogs, the amount of urine urobilinogen will increase in hepatocellular disease and decrease with obstructive problems
III. No urobilinogen or a decreased amount is a common finding in normal dogs
IV. Sample required
   A. Freshly voided urine sample
   B. Urine left sitting out converts to urobilin, which cannot be detected with tests used for urobilinogen

Total Serum/Plasma Proteins

I. Proteins in serum samples are easily subject to denaturation from heat, hydrolysis, exposure to strong acids or bases, enzymatic action, exposure to urea and other substances, and ultraviolet (UV) light
II. Total serum proteins (TSP) and serum albumin are measured and the serum globulins are determined by subtraction
III. Levels are affected by:
   A. Altered rates of protein synthesis in the liver
   B. Altered breakdown or excretion of proteins
   C. Dehydration or over hydration
   D. Altered distribution of proteins in the body
IV. Serum protein indicates the hydration level in the animal
   A. An animal in shock or an over hydrated animal will have decreased serum protein
   B. A dehydrated animal will have increased serum protein
V. TSP also can be used as a guide to the nutritional status of an animal
VI. The Goldberg refractometer (American Optical Company) is most commonly used to measure TSP in clinics
   A. The refractometer is considered a good screening method
   B. Results obtained are affected by electrolytes, lipids, hemolysis, urea, and glucose in the sample
   C. It is essential to have a clear, unturbid sample
VII. Wet and dry chemistry methods for measuring protein use the Biuret method for measuring serum proteins
VIII. Total dye binding is used in automated serum analysers to also measure total serum proteins
IX. Sample required
   A. Nonhemolysed, nonlipemic serum or plasma collected with EDTA or heparin
   B. Serum gives slightly lower values
   C. Avoid contact with detergents and UV light, which will denature the proteins

Albumin

I. Serum albumin levels and globulin levels change in response to several diseases
II. As a general rule, when changes occur, the albumin level decreases while the globulin level increases

III. The globulin fraction can be divided in sub-fractions

IV. Total serum protein and albumin are measured and the globulin fraction can be obtained by subtracting the smaller from the larger value

V. Albumin dye binding is used to measure serum albumin levels

VI. Increases in this fraction are rare; seen sometimes in shock

VII. Decreased albumin may occur in:
- A. Chronic liver disease
- B. Starvation/malnutrition
- C. Malabsorption
- D. Enteritis, colitis, parasites
- E. Pregnancy and lactation
- F. Prolonged fever
- G. Uncontrolled diabetes
- H. Trauma
- I. Nephritis, nephrosis
- J. Ascites, protein losing enteropathy
- K. Blood loss

Globulins

I. Globulin fractions, along with albumin, can be separated out by electrophoresis
- A. The globulin fraction of serum proteins is quite complex and can be subdivided into alpha globulins, beta globulins, and gamma globulins

II. Fibrinogen is one of the coagulation factors and is used in the clotting process
- A. Fibrinogen is part of the globulin fraction and is sometimes measured separately
  1. Plasma must be used
  2. This protein makes up about 4 g/L of the total plasma protein fraction

III. Concentration of the fraction can be measured by heat precipitation and refractometry

IV. Electrophoresis shows relative increases and decreases in the different fractions
- A. These can be related to specific diseases

V. Different species show different normal electrophoretic patterns

VI. In general, increases in this portion of serum proteins may be seen with:
- A. Inflammation/infections
- B. Antigenic stimulation
- C. Neoplasia or abnormal immunoglobulin production

VII. This fraction usually increases when albumin decreases

Enzymes

Biological enzymes are classed as plasma/serum specific (normally present in plasma/serum) and non-plasma/serum specific.

I. Nonplasma specific enzymes
- A. Assayed during clinical diagnosis, since these enzymes increase in concentration in serum if:
  1. Tissue cells are destroyed
  2. There is an increase in their production
  3. There is an obstruction of their excretory route
  4. There is a decrease in circulation
- B. Test kits should contain all required substrate, co-enzymes, and co-factors
- C. It is important to perform tests at the temperature indicated in instructions
  1. This is usually body temperature (37° C or 98.5° F)
- D. It is important to handle samples carefully, paying careful consideration to any special requirements for anticoagulants and separation
- E. Historically there have been many units of measurement used for measuring the same enzymes (e.g., SAP has been measured in Bodansky units, Bessy-Lowry-Brock units, King-Armstrong units, etc.)
  1. There is a new *International unit* of measurement for enzyme assays
    a. The new S.I. unit is the *katal,* which is defined as the amount of activity that converts one mole of substrate per second
      (1) This unit is not widely used
  2. It is advisable for labs to establish their own normal values

II. ALT
- A. Also known as alanine aminotransferase or alanine transaminase
  1. Formerly called SGPT
- B. Found in large amounts in the hepatocytes of dogs, cats, and primates
  1. Considered a useful and specific test for liver function in these species
- C. This enzyme is not present in large enough amounts in liver cells of horses, ruminants, or pigs to be of diagnostic significance
- D. Serum ALT increases if hepatocytes are damaged but the damage may not necessarily be irreversible

1. If ALT is increased but on serial tests the level declines, the increase is due to a one time event
2. If ALT remains elevated or increases, the cause is chronic in nature

E. Some drugs can cause increased ALT in dogs but not in cats
F. Sample required
1. Nonhemolyzed, nonlipemic serum or plasma collected with EDTA or sodium citrate
2. Do not freeze

III. AST
A. Also known as aspartate aminotransferase or aspartate transaminase
1. Formerly called SGOT
B. Present in all tissues of the body, especially in cardiac muscle, skeletal muscle, and in the liver
1. Not an organ specific enzyme
C. AST assays should be run in conjunction with other enzyme assays, especially ALT, when evaluating liver function
D. This enzyme is sometimes looked at as an alternative to ALT in the diagnosis of liver disease for species for which ALT is not useful
1. In this case other causes of increased AST should be ruled out before focusing on the liver
E. Horses have higher normal AST values than other species
1. The test method used should be specific for this species
2. The samples should be diluted before assaying
F. AST should be evaluated in conjunction with ALT for dogs and cats
1. Increased ALT with normal to mildly elevated AST may indicate reversible liver damage
2. Marked elevations in ALT and AST indicate hepatocellular necrosis
3. Increased AST with normal ALT may indicate the source of AST is not liver
G. Samples required
1. Nonhemolyzed, nonlipemic serum or plasma
2. The specimen should be centrifuged and removed from the cells immediately because AST will leak out of the red blood cells into the serum or plasma

IV. SAP
A. Also known as ALP, serum alkaline phosphatase
B. Present in almost all tissues of the body, especially in liver and bone
1. Used as an indication of intra- or post hepatic cholestasis
C. Increases in SAP are due to increased production of the enzyme rather than reduced excretion of the enzyme through the bile system
1. This enzyme is normally present in serum in small amounts
D. Increased SAP is common in young animals due to the increased rate of bone growth
E. Increased SAP in adult animals may be seen with bone injury or in obstructive liver disease
F. Glucocorticoids and some anticonvulsant drugs will give a marked increase in SAP for up to two weeks after administration
G. Samples required
1. Serum or heparinized plasma

V. LDH
A. Lactate dehydrogenase
B. Found in most tissues of the body, including liver, muscle, and red blood cells
C. Elevations in serum are considered nonspecific because they may be due to damage or necrosis of any tissues containing this enzyme
D. Samples required
1. Serum, plasma collected with any anticoagulant other than EDTA or the oxalates

VI. GGT
A. Gamma glutamyltransferase
B. Found in liver, pancreas, and kidney
C. Elevations in serum usually caused by liver source
1. GGT is elevated primarily in cholestasis but will be increased in all liver diseases
2. In small animals, increased GGT will usually be accompanied by increased ALT
3. Some medications also will cause an increase in GGT

VII. SD
A. Sorbitol dehydrogenase
B. Found primarily in liver cells; will be elevated in serum in cases of hepatocellular damage or necrosis

C. Sometimes used in large animals to replace ALT when diagnosing liver disease

D. *Very* unstable
   1. Much of the activity is lost within eight hours of collection of the sample
   2. This is a limiting factor if samples are being processed by out of clinic laboratories

Bile Acids

I. Formed in the liver, secreted into the bile, stored in the gallbladder between meals

II. Secreted into the intestinal tract where they aid in fat absorption and digestion

III. Most reabsorbed in the ileum, filtered from the blood by the liver, and recycled
   1. The mechanism is so efficient that normally serum values are very low
      a. Normal resting values for cats 5 μmol/L; dogs 9 μmol/L
      b. Two hour postprandial values: cats 10 μmol/L; dogs 30 μmol/L

IV. Increased serum bile acid levels are noted in all forms of liver disease because the liver cannot clear the acids from the blood

V. Decreased serum bile acid levels are noted in delayed gastric emptying and ileal disease

VI. Sample required
   A. Serum

Serum Cholesterol

I. Mostly derived from liver synthesis

II. Increases usually associated with hypothyroidism
   A. Will also occur with lipemia
   B. Associated with diabetes mellitus, hyperadrenocorticism, nephrotic syndrome, some liver diseases, bile duct obstruction, and pregnancy

III. Not a liver specific test

IV. Sample required
   A. Nonhemolyzed serum or heparinized plasma

ELECTROLYTES AND MINERALS ■■■■■■
General Information

I. Sodium, potassium, chloride, bicarbonate are the four electrolytes in plasma

II. Minerals of importance are calcium, phosphate, and magnesium
   A. These two groups are often simply called electrolytes

B. These are the anions (negatively charged ions) and cations (positively charged ions) found in the fluids of all animals

III. Electrolytes help to maintain water balance, osmotic pressure, normal muscular and nervous functions, act as activators for enzyme reactions, and function in acid-base balance

Serum Sodium

I. Cation; plays a major role in the distribution of water and the maintenance of osmotic pressure of fluids in the body
   A. If sodium is retained, water is retained
   B. The most abundant extracellular cation

II. Hypernatremia or increased serum sodium is rare unless the animal is deprived of water

III. Hyponatremia, or decreased serum sodium, is quite common and is seen in conditions such as renal failure, vomiting or diarrhea; use of diuretics, excessive ADH, congestive heart failure, water toxicity or excessive administration of fluids

IV. Sample required
   A. Nonhemolyzed serum is preferred
   B. Plasma collected with lithium or ammonium heparin is also acceptable
   C. Remove from cells as soon as possible

Serum Potassium

I. Cation; about 90% intracellular
   A. Serum levels are so low that measurement of serum potassium does not give much information about the body's potassium levels

II. Hyperkalemia or increased serum potassium will be seen in adrenal cortical hypofunction or late stage renal failure, or acidosis

III. Hypokalemia or decreased serum potassium will be seen in alkalosis, in insulin therapy, of excess fluid loss due to diuretics, vomiting, or diarrhea

IV. Samples required
   A. Nonhemolyzed serum or heparinized plasma (plasma preferred)
   B. Remove from the cells as soon as possible
      1. Especially important in cattle and horses, which have enough potassium in their red blood cells to alter serum chemistry results

Serum Chloride

I. The most abundant extracellular anion; it plays an important role in water balance, osmotic pressure, and electrolyte balance

A. Chloride concentration is regulated by the kidneys
II. There is a close relationship between sodium and bicarbonate levels
III. Hyperchloremia is increased serum chloride
    A. May be due to metabolic acidosis or renal tubular acidosis
IV. Hypochloremia is decreased serum chloride
    A. May be due to excessive vomiting, anorexia, malnutrition, diabetes insipidus, and in conjunction with hypokalemia
V. Samples required
    A. Nonhemolyzed serum preferred
    B. Also heparinized plasma
    C. Remove serum from cells as soon as possible

Serum Calcium

I. About 99% of the body's calcium is in bone
II. The remaining calcium:
    A. Maintains neuromuscular excitability and tone
    B. Acts as an enzyme activator
    C. Is important in coagulation
    D. Helps in transport of inorganic ions across cell membranes
III. Calcium and phosphorous levels are closely related and have an inverse relationship
    A. Both are regulated by PTH (parathyroid hormone), calcitonin, and vitamin D
IV. Serum calcium levels vary with serum protein and serum albumin levels
    A. These should be evaluated with serum calcium
V. Hypercalcemia or increased serum calcium seen in:
    A. Pseudohyperparathyroidism
    B. Hyperparathyroidism
    C. Excessive vitamin D intake
    D. Bony metastases
VI. Hypocalcemia or decreased serum calcium may be seen in:
    A. Malabsorption
    B. Eclampsia
    C. Pancreatic necrosis
    D. Hypoalbuminemia
    E. GI stasis or blockage in ruminants
    F. Post parturient lactation in cows, bitches, ewes, and mares
    G. Hypoparathyroidism
VII. Sample required
    A. Nonhemolyzed serum or heparinized plasma

Serum Phosphorus

I. Most of the body's phosphorus (80%) is found in bone
    A. The remaining 20% functions in the body in carbohydrate metabolism, energy storage, release and transfer, and in the composition of important structures such as nucleic acids
II. Serum calcium and serum phosphorous are closely related and have an inverse relationship
III. PTH regulates serum phosphorus
IV. Hyperphosphatemia or increased serum inorganic phosphorous may be seen in renal failure, anuria, excessive vitamin D intake, ethyl glycol poisoning, hypoparathyroidism
V. Hypophosphatemia or decreased serum inorganic phosphorous may occur in:
    A. Primary hyperparathyroidism
    B. Malabsorption
    C. Inadequate intake
    D. Hyperinsulinism
    E. Diabetes mellitus
    F. Lymphosarcoma
    G. Hyperadrenocorticism
VI. Sample required
    A. Nonhemolyzed serum or heparinized plasma
    B. Remove serum or plasma from the cells as soon as possible

Serum Magnesium

I. Magnesium (cation) is found in all body tissues and is closely related to calcium and phosphorus
II. Imbalance in the calcium-magnesium ratio can lead to muscle tetany in cattle and sheep
III. Sometimes calcium and magnesium have a reciprocal relationship; other times they have a direct relationship
IV. Sample required
    A. Nonhemolyzed serum or plasma

MEASUREMENT OF ELECTROLYTES

I. Flame photometry: serum sodium and serum potassium
II. Ion-selective electrodes: all of the electrolytes
III. Coulometric methods: serum chloride
IV. Atomic absorption: serum calcium, serum magnesium
V. Colorimetric methods: serum calcium, serum phosphorus

Table 20-1   Commonly requested clinical chemistry tests

Test	Samples used	Units
Albumin	Serum, plasma (EDTA, Heparin)	g/L g/dl
Alkaline Phosphatase	Serum, plasma (Heparin)	U/L
ALT (SGPT)	Serum, plasma (EDTA, citrates)	katal/L U/L
Amylase	Serum, plasma (Heparin)[3]	U/L Somogyi
AST (SGOT)	Serum, plasma*	katal/L U/L
Total bilirubin	Serum, plasma	μmol/L mg/dl
Urea nitrogen	Serum, plasma (any except ammonium oxalate or fluoride)	mmol/L mg/dl
Calcium	Serum, plasma (Heparin)	mmol/L mg/dl
Chloride	Serum, plasma (Heparin)	mmol/L mEq/L
Cholesterol	Serum, plasma (Heparin)	mmol/L mg/dl
Creatinine	Serum, plasma (EDTA, Heparin)	μmol/L mg/dl
Glucose	Serum, plasma, (sodium fluoride)	mmol/L mg/dl
Phosphorus	Serum, plasma (Heparin)	mmol/L mg/dl
LDH	Serum, plasma (Heparin, citrate)	katal/L U/L
Lipase	Serum, plasma (Heparin)	U/mL
Magnesium	Serum, plasma	mmol/L mEq/L
Potassium	Serum, plasma (Heparin)	mmol/L mEq/L
Sodium	Serum, plasma (Heparin, lithium, or ammonium)	mmol/L mEq/L
Protein	Serum, plasma	g/L g/dl
Triglycerides	Serum	mmol/L mg/dl
Uric acid	Serum, plasma (EDTA, Heparin)	μmol/L mg/dl

*Unless otherwise indicated, any anticoagulant may be used for the collection of plasma.

Table 20-2   Factors that interfere with chemistry results

1. Hemolysis
2. Bilirubin
3. Lipemia
4. Freezing of sample is not recommended
5. Prolonged contact between serum/plasma and cells
6. Turbidity
7. Sunlight
8. Heat, UV light, surfactant detergents, and chemicals will break down proteins and must be avoided
9. Cork stoppers can cause an increased value

Table 20-3 Summary of function tests

LIVER FUNCTION TESTS	TESTS FOR MUSCLE DISEASE
AST Aspartate aminotransferase ALT Alanine aminotransferase SAP Serum alkaline phosphatase Total serum bilirubin Direct/conjugated bilirubin Bile acids Glucose Cholesterol Urine bilirubin Urine urobilinogen Total serum protein Serum albumin Electrophoresis: protein fractionation Plasma fibrinogen Hematology	Creatine phosphokinase AST LDH

DIGESTIVE TRACT TESTS

Serum amylase
Serum lipase
Fecal trypsin
Examine feces for parasites, fat, starch, muscle fibers
Plasma turbidity test
Glucose tolerance test
Total serum protein
Hematology
Xylose absorption test
Serum folate
Serum B_{12}

KIDNEY FUNCTION TESTS

Serum creatinine
Blood urea nitrogen
Urine concentration/water deprivation tests
Endogenous creatinine clearance tests
Serum electrolytes and minerals: sodium, potassium, calcium, phosphorus, magnesium, chloride
Hematology

ENDOCRINE FUNCTION TESTS

Parathyroid gland
  Parathormone (PTH)   Serum and urine calcium
                       Serum and urine phosphorus
                       Serum alkaline phosphatase
Thyroid gland
  Thyroxine: serum T4
  Triiodothyronine: serum T3
  Serum cholesterol
  Serum protein

PANCREATIC FUNCTION TESTS

Endocrine Function
  Serum glucose
  Urinalysis; urine glucose
  Glucose tolerance tests
Exocrine function
  Serum amylase
  Serum lipase
  Fecal trypsin: gelatin digestion tests
  Fecal analysis
  Stain with Sudan III or IV for presence of fat or free fatty acids
  Stain with Lugol's iodine for presence of undigested muscle or starch
  Trypsin-like immunoreactivity assay

ADRENAL CORTEX FUNCTION TESTS

Serum glucose
Serum cholesterol
Serum alkaline phosphatase
Serum sodium
Serum potassium
Leukogram

ELECTROLYTES

Serum sodium
Serum potassium
Serum chloride

MINERALS

Serum calcium
Serum phosphorous
Serum magnesium

Glossary

amyloclastic test A method of measuring serum amylase by measuring the disappearance of a starch substrate

anion Negatively charged ions

anticoagulant Chemicals used to inhibit whole blood from clotting. The liquid portion of the sample harvested is plasma

azotemia Increased levels of urea in blood samples

bile A fluid produced by the liver and stored in the gallbladder that aids in digestion. This substance is primarily composed of bile acids or salts, bile pigments, cholesterol

cation A positively charged ion

dry chemistry A method of chemical analysis developed by Kodak. All the reagents needed for a particular test are incorporated into a multilayered film slide. These special slides are used in automated analyzers

electrolytes Ions capable of carrying an electric charge

electrophoresis The separation of ionic solutes, such as serum proteins, based on their rates of migration in an applied electric field

hemolysis The destruction of RBCs, causing release of hemoglobin

hypercalcemia Excess calcium in the blood

hyperglycemia Increased blood glucose levels

hyperparathyroidism Excessive activity of the parathyroid glands

hyperphosphatemia Excessive phosphate in the blood

hypocalcemia Blood calcium levels below normal

hypoglycemia Decreased blood glucose levels

hypoparathyroidism Underactivity of the parathyroid glands

hypophosphatemia Blood phosphate levels below normal

icterus Jaundice; result of excess bilirubin in the blood

malabsorption Impaired intestinal absorption of nutrients

malassimilation The gastrointestinal tract is unable to take up nutrients because of faulty digestion or impairment of the transport mechanisms across the intestinal mucosa

metastasis A growth of pathogenic organisms or abnormal cells distant from the primary site of development

plasma Liquid portion of blood in which proteins, cells, electrolytes, nutrients, and products of metabolism are suspended

prehepatic Before the liver

radioimmunoassay A technique that measures the rate of immune complex formation using radio labeled isotopes

saccharogenic test A method for measuring serum amylase by measuring reducing sugars that are produced as a result of amylase action

serum Liquid portion of blood that has been allowed to clot; contains all the same constituents as plasma except fibrinogen, which is consumed in the clotting process

steatorrhea Large amounts of fat in the stool

Review Questions

1 Which of the following tests is considered of least importance in a liver profile?
   a. SAP
   b. Serum glucose
   c. ALT
   d. Total serum protein
   e. Bile acids

2 For which of the following species is biliuria (bilirubin in urine) considered a normal finding?
   a. Canines and bovines
   b. Felines and canines
   c. Bovines and ovines
   d. Felines only
   e. Porcines only

3 For some species, even in severe liver disease, only minor changes will occur in total serum bilirubin levels. For which of the following species is measuring serum bilirubin of little value for determining liver disease?
   a. Cattle
   b. Sheep
   c. Horses
   d. Swine
   e. All but c

4 Which of the following statements regarding samples used for liver profiles is *not* true?
   a. Any anticoagulant can be used when collecting for the profile
   b. Serum is the sample of choice for any blood chemistry tests
   c. Samples should be separated as soon as possible, since the levels of some of the chemicals will be altered if the serum or plasma sits on the cells
   d. Commercially prepared blood collection systems are preferred over reusable syringes
   e. Not all the tests can be performed on previously frozen samples

5 Which of the serum protein fractions rarely increases in a disease state?
   a. Albumin
   b. Alpha globulins
   c. Beta globulins
   d. Gamma globulins
   e. Fibrinogen

6 Which of the following enzymes is considered a liver specific enzyme in dogs and cats?
   a. Alkaline phosphatase
   b. Aspartate aminotransferase
   c. Sorbitol dehydrogenase
   d. Alanine aminotransferase
   e. None of the above

7 Bile acids:
a. Aid in the absorption and digestion of ingested fats
b. Are usually found in high levels in the bloodstream
c. Are removed from circulating blood by the duodenum
d. Are stored in the liver
e. Decrease with all forms of liver disease

8 The anticoagulant of choice for collecting samples for electrolyte determination is:
a. Heparin
b. EDTA
c. Potassium oxalate
d. Sodium citrate
e. Sodium fluoride

9 Many of the electrolytes act closely with other electrolytes. Which of the following combinations of electrolytes are closely related?
a. Sodium, potassium, and hydrogen
b. Calcium, phosphorous, and magnesium
c. Sodium and potassium
d. Sodium and bicarbonate
e. All of the above

10 If the exocrine function of the pancreas is abnormal, one would expect to find:
a. Chronic pancreatitis
b. Acute pancreatitis
c. Hypoglycemia
d. Hyperglycemia
e. a and b

11 Clinitest tablets:
a. Measure glucose in urine
b. Measure glucose in whole blood
c. Use the glucose oxidase principle
d. Use the O-Toluidine principle
e. All of the above

12 Hyperglycemia:
a. Always leads to a diagnosis of diabetes mellitus
b. May be induced by stress
c. Often accompanies pancreatitis
d. Must be accompanied by glycosuria for a diagnosis of diabetes mellitus to be made
e. All but a

13 Undigested fats on a Direct Sudan Stain:
a. Indicate a deficiency of lipase
b. Appear as orange-red globules
c. Indicate a malassimilation problem (inability to take up fats from food)
d. Indicate a protease deficiency
e. a and b only

14 TLI (trypsin-like immunoreactivity):
a. Is highly specfic for canine exocrine pancreatic insufficiency
b. Uses EDTA anticoagulant
c. Is completed on nonfasting animals
d. Is used to determine if an animal has endocrine pancreatic insufficiency
e. Is used to check level of fecal tryspin

15 When measuring urea levels in serum or plasma these samples should be handled carefully because:
a. Ammonia in the room can produce false increases in results
b. Ammonium oxalate anticoagulant will produce false increases in results
c. Fluoride will inhibit the reaction used to measure urea
d. Hemolysis will produce false decreases in the results
e. All but d

BIBLIOGRAPHY

Bishop ML, Duben-Von Laufen JL, Fody EP, editors: *Clinical chemistry: principles, procedures, correlations,* ed 3, Philadelphia, 1985, JB Lippincott.

Canine reference intervals for blood values, 1989, Ralston Purina Co.

Duncan JR, Prasse KW: *Veterinary laboratory medicine: clinical pathology,* ed 1, Ames, 1977, Iowa State University Press.

Fenner WR: *Quick reference to veterinary medicine,* ed 2, Philadelphia, 1991, JB Lippincott.

Houston D: Lecture delivered at St. Lawrence College, 1991.

Kaneko JJ, editor: *Clinical biochemistry of domestic animals,* ed 3, New York, 1980, Academic Press.

Kaplan A, Szabo LL: *Clinical chemistry: interpretation and techniques,* ed 2, Philadelphia, 1983, Lea and Febiger.

McCurnin DM: *Clinical textbook for veterinary technicians,* ed 2, Philadelphia, 1990, W.B. Saunders.

Pratt PW: *Laboratory procedures for animal health technicians,* ed 1, 1985, American Veterinary Publications, Inc.

The principles of electrophoresis, Helena Laboratories

Simpson JW, Else RW: *Digestive disease in the dog and cat,* ed 1, London, 1991, Blackwell Scientific Publications.

Sirois M: *Veterinary clinical laboratory procedures,* ed 1, St. Louis, 1995, Mosby-Year Book.

Tietz NW, editor: *Fundamentals of clinical chemistry,* ed 1, Philadelphia, 1982, W.B. Saunders.

Virology

Patricia L. Bell

OUTLINE

Composition and Control
Viral Infections
Classification and Identification
Sampling Techniques
Collection of Specimens
Submission of Samples

Laboratory Testing of Samples
Prevention
Common Viral Diseases and
  Etiological Agents
  Bovine
  Porcine

Ovine and Caprine
Equine
Canine
Feline
Avian

LEARNING OUTCOMES

After reading this chapter you should be able to:

1. Describe the composition of a virus.
2. Describe the process of virus replication.
3. Define how viruses are classified and identified.
4. Describe sampling techniques, including the collection of specimens and submission of samples.
5. Describe various diagnostic testing procedures.
6. Explain common techniques for the prevention of contracting a virus or reducing the effects of viral diseases.

This chapter begins by reviewing the basic features of viruses, including their composition, control, replication, classification, and identification. The chapter also contains a brief summary defining common methods in studying viruses, as well as collection, culturing, and submission of clinical specimens for diagnostic laboratory analysis and laboratory diagnostic techniques. A list of a few of the most common viral diseases and their etiological agents are at the end of the chapter.

COMPOSITION AND CONTROL

  I. Viruses are not cellular
    A. Viruses consist of protein and nucleic acid; some have lipids and carbohydrates
  II. Viruses do not possess a nucleus, cytoplasm, cell membrane, or cell wall
  III. Viruses are obligate intracellular parasites
    A. Viruses depend on host cell metabolism for their reproduction
    B. Animal viruses are most commonly cultured in mice, embryonated chicken eggs, or tissue culture
  IV. Virus size is variable
    A. The largest is poxvirus ($300 \times 240 \times 200$ nm)
    B. The smallest is parvovirus (18×22 nm)
    C. Prions are considered to be smaller life forms
  V. Classification
    A. Viruses are classified:
      1. Based on their shape as seen by electron microscopy
      2. By their composition of their nucleic acid core (genome)

a. The core is contained in an inert protein shell called a "capsid"

b. The capsid protects the core while the virus is in the external environment (outside the host cell)

c. The capsid also gives the virus particle, or "virion," it's shape

d. The capsid plus the nucleic acid core are termed the *nucleocapsid*

VI. Shape

A. Three basic structural shapes

1. Icosahedron: a three-dimensional, hexagonal structure

2. Helical: having the form of a helix or spiral

3. Complex: includes all of the other shapes that do not fit into the above two categories

B. "Knobs": or surface projections that aid the virus in attachment to certain host cell membranes

1. Antibody response is directed at the "knobs"

VII. Envelope

A. The lipid membrane that surrounds the virus is termed the *envelope*

B. An "enveloped virus" has an envelope that is derived from the host cell's outer or nuclear membrane

1. Enveloped viruses are easily killed

a. Hypochlorite (common household bleach) dissolves fats

b. Freezing and thawing process will render the virus inert due to the breakdown of the envelope by frozen water molecules

C. A "naked virus" does not possess an envelope

1. Naked viruses are more refractory

2. It is more difficult to disinfect an area where these viruses have been

a. Steam sterilization is recommended to kill all viruses at the temperature of 121° C, (250° F) 15 p.s.i. for 30 minutes

b. Many commercial viricidal compounds, designed to be used in a clinical setting, are available to destroy different types of viruses

VIII. Genomes

A. Mammalian genomes are comprised of double-stranded DNA, from which various RNA are transcribed

B. Viral nucleic acid can be DNA or RNA; can also be double or single stranded

1. Viruses with an RNA nucleic acid core also possess a reverse-transcriptase enzyme to create DNA from their RNA when they infect a mammalian host cell

2. Oncogenic viruses are common in the group, which have an RNA nucleic core

C. Some double-stranded DNA viruses can incorporate their DNA sequences into host cell DNA and be replicated during mitosis

1. This does not cause cellular damage and therefore no clinical signs—these are termed *latent infections*

2. The virus may lie dormant for years until the host is stressed due to age, malnutrition, water deprivation, shipping, surgery, or trauma, when the virus reemerges to produce intact virions and disease

IX. Replication

There are four basic stages of replication for most viruses: attachment, penetration-uncoating, replication, and assembly-release.

A. Attachment

1. A virus must gain access to the host cell to which it can bind

2. This is done via the virus portal entry

3. The portal entry is usually the mucosal surface to the respiratory, urogenital, or gastrointestinal tract

4. Breaks in the integument are a rarer method of entry except when insect vectors are involved

5. The cell membrane is bound in a complementary fashion by the viral binding proteins

6. Viral binding proteins determine the species affected and the type of pathology caused

B. Penetration-Uncoating

1. Most viruses produce enzymes that degrade the host cell membrane enough to permit the nucleic acid core to enter

2. As it does so the core exits the capsid, which remains on the host cell exterior

3. The exiting of the capsid is the uncoating process and occurs simultaneously with penetration

C. Replication

1. The aim is for the virus to produce thousands of copies of itself to ensure sur-

vival, but it lacks the ability to do so on its own

2. So the virus's nucleic acid redirects the host cell DNA to ignore its own needs and produce viral components such as capsid fragments and viral nucleic acid instead

3. This results in the breakdown of the host cell membrane and this change initiates the immune response (see the immunology chapter)

4. Since the virus is hidden in the host cell the immune system is not able to respond to the virus specifically

5. The virus has already reproduced many copies of itself that readily invade other cells and begin replication before the immune system is activated

D. Assembly and release

1. After all the various components of the virus structure have attained a critical concentration, assembly occurs spontaneously

2. Viral components come together to produce virions

   a. Virions can be visualized by electron microscopy

   b. They are cytoplasmic or nuclear or both, depending on where they occur within the host cell

3. Virions almost immediately leave the cell

4. Some enveloped viruses leave the cell by a process called "budding"

   a. Budding leaves the cell intact; therefore there are no overt clinical signs

5. Most viruses exit the cell by causing it to rupture, termed the *"lysogenic cycle"*

6. The cell is destroyed and this is what causes the overall signs of disease

7. Most viruses that undergo replication are released from the host cell, spread to neighboring cells, and begin again the process of replication

8. Some viruses will be shed in secretions of the host body

X. Limitations of viruses

A. Some viruses are restricted to certain body temperatures

1. The nasal passages of a mammalian respiratory tract average 2° lower than that of the lower respiratory tract and there-

fore remain susceptible to upper respiratory tract infections

B. Some viruses are limited by the surface proteins found on certain cell types (these form localized infections)

C. Other viruses enter the systemic circulation and spread throughout the body; this is called a "viremia"

VIRAL INFECTIONS

I. Viral infections of any type can affect the host with regard to clinical signs in one of two ways:

A. Apparent infection: causes clinical disease

1. This disease may be peracute to chronic

B. Silent or unapparent infection: does not result in overt signs

1. This may result in a transient carrier state

2. Such carriers are difficult to identify. They can therefore infect a herd sometimes despite quarantine precautions

II. Examples

A. Neurons in rabies victims or the T lymphocytes in cats infected with the feline immunodeficiency virus (FIV) are cells that have become inactive or malfunction due to a virus rather than the more common lysis of the cells

B. Equine infectious anemia virus causes an immunological reaction within the host in which the immune system does more harm than the virus

III. Viral infections predispose an affected animal to secondary diseases (usually bacterial in nature) that can be worse than the primary viral disease

IV. Oncogenesis occurs with some viruses

A. Infected cells transform, resulting in neoplasm with potential for malignancy such as Marek's disease in chickens

CLASSIFICATION AND IDENTIFICATION

I. A primary criteria for classification of viruses is morphology

II. Another criteria for classification is the nucleic acid core: DNA or RNA composition

A. Despite similarities in their size or the form of their nucleic acid core, the genetic relationship between major viral family members is not always clear

III. Virus differences is the basis for subdividing viruses within families into genera

IV. Taxonomy is based on ongoing recommendations made by the International Committee on Taxonomy of Viruses

A. Viral family names end in the suffix "-viridae"

B. Viral genus names end in the suffix "-virus"

C. Names are not underlined

V. "Antigenic drift" is a process whereby new strains of viruses are created

A. Some viruses within their own genus can exchange parts of their nucleic acid cores

B. Some viruses mutate, which changes their surface antigens, such as their host cell binding receptors or enzymes

SAMPLING TECHNIQUES

I. Analysis of samples is not usually done within a veterinary practice but at a commercial, regional, or state diagnostic laboratory

II. Analysis of samples is not usually completed in time to treat the sick animal but it is used to confirm a diagnosis and for epidemiological reasons

III. Laboratory tests results are only as reliable as the quality of the samples submitted and the history provided

IV. The virus is most easily cultured from specimens just before onset of signs and for a short time afterward

V. Animals that have been showing clinical signs for a few days generally are not sampled for viruses

COLLECTION OF SPECIMENS

I. A representative animal from a herd should be sent for full examination

II. Examine ill and contact animals and sample from both because the virus concentration is highest prior to signs

III. To identify a disease antibody titer

A. Bleed at least six readily identifiable animals with early clinical signs

B. Bleed the same animals two to four weeks later

C. A change in titer means a positive diagnosis of a current disease and not immunity from previous recovery from the disease

IV. If unsure what samples to collect, take a wide range for the virologist to choose from, or call the lab and discuss sample collection with the personnel

V. Use one of the following transport media

A. Sterile Hank's balanced salt solution plus 10% bovine albumin

B. Sterile skim milk

C. Sterile charcoal transport medium, which is available commercially

VI. NOTE: A virus will survive three weeks without refrigeration and therefore will survive shipping

VII. Antibiotics may be added to control bacterial contamination

VIII. Keep specimens cool, 1 to 4° C, (34-39° F) but do not freeze

IX. Postmortem tissues collected aseptically from several areas of the body can be used for histopathology

A. The sections should be no larger than 3 to 5 mm (3/16 inch) thick

B. The sections should be fixed in 10% formalin

C. Less than 1 g of tissue in transport medium

D. Do not freeze these samples

X. Collection from a live animal

A. Heparinized plasma for immediate submission

B. Serum may also be collected, which may be frozen

SUBMISSION OF SAMPLES

Most labs will provide submission forms. The following pertinent information is needed for diagnosis.

I. Sampling information

II. Animal species

III. Age and sex of the patient(s)

IV. Size of the herd, flock, kennel involved where applicable

V. Number of animals affected

VI. Duration of the illness to date

VII. Clinical signs

VIII. Losses, if any

IX. Similar cases in the area

X. Vaccination history (if not available, note on form)

XI. Treatment given up to the time of sampling

XII. Disease suspected

XIII. Specimens submitted and labeled appropriately

LABORATORY TESTING OF SAMPLES

I. Viruses are identified initially on the basis of:

A. Clinical history

B. Specimen sample submitted

C. Immunoflourescence

D. One or a combination of histopathology, protection tests, and electron microscopy (EM)

II. The virus is then isolated by:

A. Centrifugation (sometimes requires several cycles and the use of density gradients is common)

B. Adsorption on erythrocytes

C. Extraction in fluorocarbons or cold ethanol

III. After isolation of the virus, procedures can now be started to determine what animal tissue culture cell line or lines the virus will grow in and how long it takes to cause alterations

IV. The cellular alterations are termed *"cytopathic effects"* (CPE)

   A. Can occur as inclusion bodies

      1. Round, oval, or irregular shaped formations seen intracytoplasmic, intranuclear, or both

   B. Can occur as syncytia or cell membranes, which fuse, producing large multinuclear cells

   C. Also can occur in the form of cell death

V. Final diagnosis involves results from one or more of the following tests as determined by the diagnostic laboratory's protocol

   A. Virus neutralization

   B. Hemagglutination inhibition

   C. Complement-fixation

   D. Hemadsorption inhibition

VI. Serological tests, which involve specific antibody detection and titration, include:

   A. Serum neutralization

   B. Hemadsorption inhibition

   C. Hemagglutination inhibition

   D. Complement-fixation

   E. Immunoflourescence inhibition

   F. Gel diffusion (single radial immunodiffusion, double-diffusion precipitin tests)

   G. Fluorescent antibody (FA) technique

VII. Some tests may be adapted to demonstrate presence of the suspected antigen (virus) by using a commercially purchased known antibody instead of the patient serum antibodies tested against a known viral antigen

VIII. In some instances the most commonly used techniques have been adapted to kit form so they may be used in a clinical setting or out in the field

   A. Fluorescent antibody (FA) test

      1. This test uses antibodies of known specificity that bind viral antigens

      2. The binding can then be visualized due to conjugation (labeled) with a fluorescent dye

      3. Such a procedure can be performed using frozen tissue sections, tissue imprints, tissue scrapings, and blood smears

      4. The selection depends on the viral lifecycle within the host

      5. Often such results are available rapidly (in less than an hour)

         a. Accuracy depends on the application to appropriate specimens that are in good condition (fresh with little to no autolysis)

      6. This may not be an applicable test method if the required samples can not be obtained from live animals

   B. Enzyme-linked immunosorbent assay (ELISA) test

      1. A popular test kit method in which a known specific antibody is adsorbed, usually in a small plastic well on a well plate

      2. These antibodies will have patient sample applied

      3. A common disease that is screened in this manner is feline leukemia virus (FeLV)

         a. The viral antigen, if present in the FeLV animal's serum, is tightly and specifically bound by the adsorbed antibodies

         b. Another antibody of the same specificity, which is labeled (most frequently with an enzyme), is applied to produce a sandwich formation

         c. Another alternative to the enzymatic label is a fluorescent label

         d. A very important wash step is then performed to remove any unbound labeled antibody (which would be the case if the animal does not possess the viral antigen in its serum and is therefore negative for FeLV)

         e. If the viral antigen is present, the labeled antibody will not be removed because the binding is very strong

         f. Substrate is then added—it must be one that reacts with the enzyme with which the second antibody is labeled

         g. The reaction produces a visible color change to permit the technician to recognize the unhealthy animal's state

   C. Latex agglutination (LA) test

      1. Another popular test kit; it uses the same principles as the ELISA test

      2. Antiviral antibodies are adsorbed to microscopic latex beads. If the applied sample contains the antigen (virus) it will be bound by these antibodies and produce agglutination

3. Due to the granular appearance of the latex beads in solution it is very important to run positive and negative controls simultaneously
4. Such a method can be used to detect parvovirus from fecal samples of ill dogs or rotavirus in the feces of various species suffering rotaviral diarrhea

PREVENTION

There are three major factors involved in preventing occurrence or reducing the effects of viral diseases.
I. Health measures
   A. Good hygiene
   B. Prompt disposal of dead animals
   C. Proper nutrition
   D. Clean and adequate water supply
   E. Reasonable population density to reduce stress
   F. Screening and quarantine of new animals before their entry into the household or herd
II. Immunization if possible and maintenance of current vaccinations
III. Treatment of viral disease

COMMON VIRAL DISEASE ETIOLOGICAL AGENTS

Bovine
I. Bovine leukemia: retrovirus
II. Bovine viral diarrhea: Pestivirus
III. Calf scours complex: Rotavirus and Coronavirus
IV. Infectious bovine rhinotracheitis: herpesvirus
V. Malignant cattarhal fever: Varicellavirus
VI. Parainfluenza-3: Paramyxovirus
VII. Vesicular stomatitis: Vesiculovirus

Porcine
I. Encephalomyocarditis: picornavirus
II. Hemagglutinating encephalomyelitis virus: Coronavirus
III. Pseudorabies: herpesvirus
IV. Swine influenza: orthomyxovirus
V. Swine pox: poxvirus
VI. Transmissible gastroenteritis: Coronavirus
VII. Vesicular exanthema of swine: Calicivirus

Ovine and Caprine
I. Border disease: Pestivirus
II. Bluetongue: Orbivirus
III. Contagious ecthyma: poxvirus
IV. Progressive pneumonia of sheep: Lentivirus

Equine
I. Andenoviral infection: Mastadenovirus
II. Equine encephalomyelitis: arbovirus
III. Equine influenza: orthomyxovirus
IV. Equine infectious anemia: nononcogenic retrovirus
V. Equine viral arteritis: togavirus
VI. Equine rhinopneumonitis: Varicellavirus

Canine
I. Canine coronavirus infection: Coronavirus
II. Canine distemper: Morbillivirus
III. Canine herpesvirus infection: herpesvirus
IV. Canine infectious hepatitis: adenovirus
V. Infectious tracheobronchitis: parainfluenza virus, adenovirus, Morbillivirus, and simultaneous bacterial infections
VI. Papillomatosis: Papillomavirus
VII. Parvoviral enteritis: Parvovirus
VIII. Rabies: rhabdovirus

Feline
I. Feline calicivirus infection: Calicivirus
II. Feline infectious peritonitis: Coronavirus
III. Feline leukemia: oncogenic retrovirus
IV. Feline panleukopenia: Parvovirus

Avian
I. Avian encephalomyelitis: Enterovirus
II. Avian infectious laryngotracheitis: herpesvirus
III. Avian leukosis: oncogenic retrovirus
IV. Fowl pox: poxvirus
V. Infectious bronchitis: Coronavirus
VI. Infectious bursal disease: Birnavirus
VII. Marek's Disease: herpesvirus
VIII. Newcastle Disease: Paramyxovirus
IX. Psittacine beak and feather disease: Circovirus

Glossary

altered-self Any change in the molecular configuration of one's cells and therefore attacked by the immune system. This state may be a result of viral invasion of cells, cancer, radiation, or poisoning

autoclave An instrument with a chamber in which materials are rendered sterile via a treatment with the necessary steam heat and pressure for a specific period of time

DNA The standard short form for deoxyribonucleic acid. The physical basis for the genetic code. It forms a double-stranded helix in animals. Under strict and specific physiological regulations it codes for the production of RNA. In viruses it may be single or double stranded *genome* The entire genetic complement of an organism. In animals it involves DNA and RNA but in viruses it is one or the other

heat-inactivated To render inert or nonfunctional by exposure to heat of sufficient temperature and duration

inclusion bodies Aggregations of viral proteins in the nucleus, cytoplasm, or both. This characteristic of the formation of inclusions and their location within the host cell aids in the identification of the viral disease-causing agent, as well as being used as one component in viral classification

latent A quiescent state awaiting later reactivation, which may occur years later. In the case of latent viruses, they insert their DNA into the host cell DNA to be replicated together. Frequently stress is implicated in the viruses' resurgence and resultant disease state

nucleic acid core A molecule of DNA or RNA, either of which can be double or single stranded. The term is used synonomously with viral genome

obligate intracellular parasite (see parasite)

parasite One organism that survives at the detriment of another; an obligate intracellular parasite is one that does so from within a host cell. The host cell is its only means of survival

prion Proteinaceous infectious particle, the smallest known microorganism. Still unseen by electron microscopy; laboratory tests indicate that although this microorganism does not possess any nucleic acid, it consists of protein and is capable of producing disease

PSI An old standard unit of pressure that is still widely in use; denotes pounds per square inch

RNA One form of nucleic acid of which there are three forms: ribosomal, messenger, and transfer. It codes for the assembly of proteins. Some viruses such as the retroviruses possess only RNA in their genome but due to the possession of a reverse transcriptase enzyme they can 'reverse code' for DNA

self Recognized by the immune system as one's own molecular configuration and therefore tolerated

titer Strength per volume of a volumetric test solution

tolerance The state of being tolerated by the immune system and therefore not attacked. In health this occurs to one's own body only but if it is conveyed to microorganisms it will result in an immunodeficiency

viricidal A term meaning virus killer; frequently used to describe disinfectant chemicals with this capacity

Review Questions

1 Which of the following statements is true about viruses?
a. They are microscopic, cellular, parasitic organisms
b. They are all readily destroyed by ordinary household soaps and other disinfectants
c. They are obligate intracellular parasites
d. All of the above

2 A single virus particle is termed a:
a. Capsid
b. Capsomere
c. Virus
d. Virion

3 The following statement is *false* about prions:
a. They are smaller than viruses
b. They produce disease in cattle only
c. They do not seem to possess a nucleic acid core
d. They have relatively long incubation periods

4 Which of the following is used to classify a virus?
a. Their shape, as seen via electron microscopy
b. The type of genome it possesses
c. The presence or lack of an envelope
d. All of the above

5 Autoclaving to sterilize a virally contaminated material requires the following same parameters as for a bacterially contaminated material:
a. 121° C, 15 psi for 30 minutes
b. 250° F, 150 psi for 15 minutes
c. 121° C, 10 psi, for 15 minutes
d. 250° F, 100 psi for 30 minutes

6 Complete the following statement: "viruses are spread between contacts most effectively . . ."
a. During the acute stage of the disease
b. Prior to the onset of clinical signs and for a very short time afterward
c. At the beginning of convalescence
d. None of the above

7 When submitting samples to a diagnostic laboratory virology department, it is important to:
a. Include a thorough case history
b. Use an approved shipping medium
c. Take serum samples from readily identifiable animals, now and up to four weeks later
d. All of the above

8 Viral diseases are treated by administering antibiotics:
a. True
b. Only during the viremic stage
c. Only as a supportive measure to control opportunistic infections
d. Only if the disease is due to an enveloped virus

9 Viral diagnostic tests include:
a. Fluorescent antibody test
b. Electron microscopic visualization
c. Antibody titer determination testing
d. All of the above

10 The following is an acceptable transport media for viruses:
a. Skim milk medium
b. Sterile William's solution
c. Sterile charcoal transport medium
d. Formaldehyde

BIBLIOGRAPHY

Black JG: *Microbiology principles and applications,* ed 3, New Jersey, 1996, Prentice Hall Inc.

Blood DC, Studdert VP: *Balliere's comprehensive veterinary dictionary,* London, 1990, W.B. Saunders.

Ikram M, Hill E: *Microbiology for veterinary technicians,* California, 1991, American Veterinary Publications.

Joklik WK: *Virology,* ed 2, Connecticut, 1985, Prentice Hall Inc.

Quinn PJ et al: *Clinical veterinary microbiology,* Spain, 1994, Mosby-Year Book Europe Ltd.

Roberts AW, Carter GR, Chengappa MM: *Essentials of veterinary microbiology,* ed 5, Pennsylvania, 1995, Williams and Wilkins Co.

Steinberg ML, Cosloy SD: *The Facts on File dictionary of biotechnology and genetic engineering,* New York, 1994, Facts on File Inc.

The Merck veterinary manual, ed 7, New Jersey, 1991, Merck and Company Inc.

Turgeon ML: *Immunology and serology in laboratory medicine,* USA, 1990, CV Mosby.

CHAPTER 22

Immunology

Patricia L. Bell

OUTLINE

Innate or Nonspecific Immunity
Adaptive or Specific Immunity
Immunity to Viral Infections
Antibodies
  IgM
  IgG
  IgA
  IgE

IgD
Antibody Titer
Types of Acquired Immunity
Immunopathological Mechanisms
Vaccines
  Attenuated-live/Modified-live
    (MLV) Vaccines
  Killed Vaccines

Subunit Vaccines
Vaccine Difficulties
Vaccine Precautions
Current Trends in Vaccine Produc-
  tion and Immunological Research

LEARNING OUTCOMES

After reading this chapter you should be able to:

1. Describe how the immune system defends the body from various types of infections.
2. Describe innate and adapative immunity, including the components involved.
3. List in sequential order how the body responds to a viral invasion.
4. List and describe antibody classes and their roles in the immune response.
5. Describe different types of adaptive responses.
6. Describe hypersensitivities and cell-mediated and humoral immunodeficiencies.
7. Describe the types, production, and use of vaccines.
8. Explain the newest advances in biotechnology research.

This chapter discusses how the immune system defends the body from various types of infection, including the basics on the following topics: innate and adaptive immunities (the components involved and the order of their actions), the immune response to a viral invasion, antibody classes and their roles in the immune response, and types of adaptive responses. It will also cover the basics of problems involving the immune system, including immunopathological mechanisms such as hypersensitivity reactions, and immunodeficiencies, humoral and cell mediated.

Finally, ways in which the immune system is exploited for the benefit of animal health, particularly vaccines, and the current trends in biotechnology research will be briefly covered.

INNATE OR NONSPECIFIC IMMUNITY

  I. Definition: the immunity we are born with
  II. Includes physical and chemical barriers to an antigen such as:
    A. Intact skin, stomach acids, commensal organisms, mucus production, cilia, lysozyme in tears, and body temperature
  III. Also involves the humoral and cell mediated systems
    A. They include reactions involved in the inflammatory response, wound healing, and the first defenses to contain and halt pathogen spread

IV. If the innate system is successful, the adaptive immune response will not be activated and antibody production will not occur

V. Especially important features of innate immunity

    A. Occurs immediately after an antigen's entry (which is important because antibody production takes days)

    B. Treats all antigens the same (no specificity involved)

    C. Strength and speed of the response does *not* increase with subsequent encounters with the same antigen (no memory involved)

VI. The innate response occurs as follows:

    A. An organism such as a bacterium enters via its portal of entry (broken skin or mucosal membrane) and this involves some degree (it may be minuscule) of tissue damage

    B. Platelets aggregate at the wound site to initiate healing and release serotonin

        1. Serotonin causes smooth muscle contractions and acts on mast cells to cause them to degranulate

    C. Bradykinin is also released and is responsible for pain

    D. The cell surface of the microorganism triggers the alternate complement cascade and can result in microbial cell lysis

    E. Some complement components act as chemotactic factors to guide the movement of phagocytes to the area

    F. Other complement components act as opsonins, allowing phagocytes to easily and rapidly engulf the antigens

    G. The first phagocytes to arrive (within 30-60 minutes) are neutrophils

    H. If the neutrophils fail to control antigen invasion, macrophages (mature monocytes) arrive within 4 to 5 hours

        1. Although these cells are slower to respond, they can survive a greater number of phagocytic cycles

    I. Simultaneously the antigen may be bound by IgE antibody on a mast cell surface and when this occurs these cells release their chemicals, which are full of bioactive compounds

        1. Most critical bioactive compound: histamine

        2. Histamine causes increased vascular permeability

           a. Enables phagocytes to move readily via diapedesis from the circulation to the site

        3. Clinically seen as swelling or edema because plasma leaks through

        4. Vasodilation and increased blood flow (seen as redness and felt as excess heat) permits more phagocytes to reach the area as well

        5. In some areas of the body it will also increase the release of mucus

    J. Some macrophages that arrive are specialized cells called "antigen-presenting cells"

        1. After engulfing an antigen and degrading it, these cells can select the most immunogenic particles called "epitopes" and express them on their own surface

        2. More than one type (shape) of epitope is usually expressed

        3. How this is done is not fully understood

        4. An epitope then moves via tissue fluid (lymph) to the regional draining lymph nodes where it will encounter the T and B lymphocytes that can react to that epitope

    K. This is the point at which the adaptive response begins

A viral infection is a different situation and therefore dealt with separately

ADAPTIVE OR SPECIFIC IMMUNITY

I. Definition: the response of the defences of the body to a specific substance (antigen)

II. Individuals have produced antibodies (naturally acquired immunity) or obtained antibodies (passively acquired immunity)

III. The response is highly specific

    A. Only certain cells whose receptors can bind the antigen's epitopes (a lock and key type of binding so the shapes must be complimentary) can react

IV. Adaptive immunity posesses a memory so the body's response becomes more rapid and stronger with each encounter with the same antigen

    A. Due to responding cells cloning themselves and leaving a larger population of cells ready to respond the next time

    B. These memory cells have life spans that last years and sometimes the lifetime of the individual

V. Briefly the adaptive response occurs as follows:

    A. The antigen-presenting cell (APC), having entered the lymph node, will encounter a helper T cell (T_H-lymph), whose receptor is the correct shape, and so binds the expressed epitope

B. After the helper T cell has bound, the antigen-presenting cell releases interleukin-1

    1. Interleukin-1 causes the bound helper T cell to release interleukin-2

C. Interleukin-2 causes all T cell subpopulations (including cytotoxic and suppressor T cells) that have bound this antigen to clone and produce memory cells

D. This produces an increased number of T cells of all types that are ready to defend the individual against this invader

    1. The T-suppressor cells clone more slowly than the other types of T cells

    2. This prevents their downgrading the response until the antigen has been cleared from the body

E. The cytotoxic T cells can bind the bacteria's epitopes directly (on the bacterial surface) and release perforin

    1. Perforin is a compound that punctures the cell membrane and results in the microorganism's lysis

F. Meanwhile the antigen-bound helper T cell (on the APC) internalizes the epitope and expresses it on its own surface

G. Now a B cell (B lymphocyte) of the appropriate specificity binds

H. This binding causes the helper T cell to release two important interleukins

    1. Interleukin-4 causes the B cell to clone

    2. Interleukin-6 causes the clones to be differentiated into antibody forming plasma cells, which secrete antibody, while some become memory cells

        a. The memory cells do not produce antibodies now but are ready to respond the next time this antigen attempts to invade

        b. Because this means more T and B cells will be available to defend the body after the next invasion by this microorganism, the response may be so quick and strong that the clinical signs will be reduced or nonexistent

VI. During the adaptive response, immunity is created

A. The strength that the immune system attains and therefore the individual's level of immunity reached depends on:

    1. Genetics, general state of health, the dosage of antigen, the antigen's portal of entry and persistence (rate of clearance) in the body, and the number of times it has been encountered before

VII. The antibody will bind and neutralize the antigen. The antibody provides a physical barrier between the antigen and the host cells

A. Possibly the antibody will prevent entry into the body if binding occurs in bodily secretions such as tears or mucus

B. The antibodies can also act as opsonins so the phagocytes can engulf and degrade the microorganism more readily

C. Antibodies can trigger the classical complement cascade

    1. The classical complement cascade is similar to the alternate complement cascade of the innate system (not triggered by the presence of antibody)

VIII. The end phase of the immune response includes the increase in number to produce sufficient quantities of proteins such as T-suppressor factor

A. T-suppressor factor slows and stops the immune system activities after the pathogen (antigen) has been destroyed

B. Allergy 'shots' and desensitization therapies are numerous minute doses of an allergen; they do not cause a full blown immune response

    1. Allergy shots for a short period of time cause the suppressor T cell population to increase and suppress the immunity, thereby preventing an allergic response to that material

    2. Or allergy shots may induce the formation of IgG antibodies in sufficient numbers to block the binding of the antigen (in this case an allergen) by the allergic reaction inducing IgE antibodies. This also prevents the allergic condition

    3. It is likely that the increase in the T-suppressor cell population and the blocking IgG antibody concentration occur simultaneously

IMMUNITY TO VIRAL INFECTIONS ■■■■■

I. The immune response to viral infections is a more complicated situation for the body

A. Due to the virus's ability to enter host cells the immune defenses must use other strategies as well (see Virology chapter)

II. Briefly they are as follows:

A. A virus injects its genome into the host cell, leaving its capsid on the cell's exterior

B. The virus takes over the cell's metabolic processes and directs them to make viral proteins instead of cellular proteins; therefore the cell membrane begins to degrade

C. The change in the cell membrane from healthy self (not attacked by the immune system except in cases of autoimmune disease) to unhealthy altered-self (which can be attacked) is the first signal to the immune system that something is wrong and allows it to respond

D. The infected cell secretes interferon, which activates the natural killer cells (also known as null cells) of the innate system

E. Interferon directs natural killer cells to target and destroy the infected host cell
   1. How they accomplish this is not known

F. Simultaneously cytotoxic T cells can target the infected cell, and after binding they release perforin, which punctures the membrane and lyses the cell

G. Also the usual adaptive response against the viral antigen results in the cloning of the cytotoxic T cells and the production of antibodies
   1. Here part of the viral capsid or the altered-self cellular membrane acts as the epitope

H. Antibodies can bind to the infected cell, causing complement to produce its lysis or causing phagocytes to attack
   1. If the infected cell is too large to engulf, the phagocytes will release their granules (a process known as "degranulation") that contain the degradative enzymes
   2. The enzymes will break down the cell into smaller parts to be engulfed by other phagocytes. This can cause host tissue damage ("bystander lysis") and severe inflammatory reactions

I. No matter how the infected cell is destroyed, it will prevent the production and release of millions of more viral particles and more phagocytes will come to clean up the debris

III. In most cases, the transformation of healthy cells into a neoplastic state, for an unknown reason, also causes a change from self to altered-self and permits attack by the immune system

A. It is a widely accepted theory that natural killer cells are constantly "patrolling the tissues, on the look out for such transformations"
   1. This patrol is termed *"surveillance"*; when this fails cancer can develop

ANTIBODIES

I. Definition: noncellular components (they are glycoproteins) of the adaptive immune response that bind specifically to antigenic determinants (epitopes)

II. By binding to the antigen, antibodies prevent the antigen from doing further harm (neutralizing) and they enhance other immune responses

III. Five classes of antibodies (also called "immunoglobulins" or "Ig_")

IgM

I. During the primary immune response to a particular antigen, stimulated (antigen-bound) B cells (also known as plasma or antibody-forming cells) secrete IgM antibody

A. A class of antibody that possesses ten antigen-binding sites and is therefore a large molecule

B. Has a circular shape, being comprised of five, basic Y-shaped molecules or subunits joined together

C. Due to its large size, this antibody class is confined to the vascular system and comprises about 10% of the antibody pool in most mammals

D. After a plasma cell produces IgM, intranuclear enzymes then remove the DNA gene segments that code for its production and that capability is lost forever

E. The plasma cell, depending on its location within the body, then codes for one of the other four classes of antibody

IgG

I. Most plasma cells produce IgG antibody molecules during secondary and subsequent immune responses

A. NOTE: a single plasma cell possesses specificity for only one shape of epitope and produces only antibodies with that same specificity
   1. The specificity is determined by the shape of the binding site, which is independent of the antibody class being produced. It is always the same for any given plasma cell
   2. Approximately 80% of the antibody pool in plasma is due to the single subunit molecule IgG

3. This Y-shaped molecule, being small, can escape the vascular system and enter tissue spaces to act in the body's defense

4. IgG also can cross the placental barrier in species with a lower number of placental membranes (dogs, cats, rodents, and primates) to convey short-term immunity to the newborn

5. Due to its structure IgG has only two antigen-binding sites but it acts as an opsonin and two can trigger the classical complement cascade

IgA

I. If a plasma cell resides in a lymph node that drains portals of entry such as the gastrointestinal tract, urogenital tract, or the conjunctiva of the eyes, it will produce IgA antibodies

A. Here it serves to bind the potential invader, blocking its ability to bind to the host tissue, and makes it too large to pass through the mucosal membrane

B. This class of antibody is found in body secretions, including tears, mucus, and colostrum

C. For species whose placental barrier has too many intervening membranes to allow IgG antibody to cross (pig, horse, donkey, and ruminants) it is critical to early survival that newborns nurse (receive colostrum) before their gastric secretions begin because then they can receive short-term immunity

1. After about 18 hours of life the neonate will begin to produce stomach acids and the antibodies of the colostrum will be digested, rendering them useless for immune purposes

2. Small animals also receive IgA antibody via colostrum, which supplements their immunity from the IgG antibodies that have crossed the placental barrier. So it is less critical for them to ingest colostrum but it is still important, especially regarding enteric pathogens (and the prevention of neonatal scours)

3. Remember that the dam can pass on antibodies only if she possesses immunity to the pathogen herself

a. Up-to-date vaccination protocols are very important to the dam and her progeny

IgE

I. A single Y-shaped subunit molecule that is found in minute levels in the plasma of healthy animals

A. IgE functions to boost local inflammatory reactions

B. It also plays a role in protecting animals against helminths by attracting eosinophils to the site of infestation

C. It is found on the surfaces of mast cells (tissue basophils) where if it binds to an antigen it causes these cells to degranulate, eliciting inflammation and aiding the innate response

D. If an individual produces excess IgE, such a response may become damaging to self

1. This is a hypersensitivity reaction called anaphylaxis when it acts systemically. It may induce anaphylactic shock, which can be fatal

2. When it acts locally within the body, it is known as an allergy and causes an allergic reaction, which does not cause fatality

3. Which of the two reactions occurs depends on location of the mast cells having the IgE antibody and the antigen's portal or portals of entry

IgD

I. A single subunit molecule

A. Found on lymphocyte membranes and in negligible amounts in body fluids

B. Primary role is as an antigen receptor for B cells (IgM also occasionally plays this role)

Antibody titer

I. Tests that measure the level of antibody in serum or plasma can help determine an individual's immune status to a particular pathogen

A. If an animal has an active infection the titre will increase when measured at four-week intervals

B. If the titre is significant but not increased, it generally indicates a convalescent state or a history of a previous vaccination

TYPES OF ACQUIRED IMMUNITIES ■■■■■■

I. Definitions

A. Acquired immunities: occur after birth

B. Natural immunity: without medical (human) intervention

C. Artificial immunity: medically induced immunity

D. Active Immunity: the individual's own immune system produced the antibodies (and therefore long-term immunity occurs)

E. Passive immunity: antibodies were 'donated' and therefore the individual's immune system wasn't stimulated to produce the antibodies (nor any memory cells)

　1. This involves short-term immunity because these antibodies will be quickly catabolized and cleared from the body and no replacements will be synthesized

F. Acquired natural active immunity: usually induced by disease recovery

　1. Occurs after birth

　2. No medical intervention

　3. The animal's immune system produced antibodies and memory cells

G. Acquired natural passive immunity: antibodies are passed to the fetus or neonate from the mother

　1. Across the placental barrier (species dependent)

　2. Via the ingestion of colostrum

H. Acquired artificial active immunity: the individual is induced to produce antibodies and memory cells without experiencing the disease

　1. Via vaccination

I. Acquired artificial passive immunity: antibodies produced in one animal are infused into another animal

　1. The initial animal is administered a pathogen, vaccination series, or a bacterial toxin repeatedly until that animal is "hyperimmune" (possesses a very high antibody titre)

　2. During the hyperimmune state a portion or all of the animal serum is removed and the antibodies are harvested and can be used for the following:

　　a. To produce an antiserum, which can then be given to other animals to convey short-term immunity

　　　(1) A common example is in the treatment of people after exposure to the rabies virus

　　b. To produce a toxoid (in the case of the use of a bacterial toxin on the initial animal), which can be administered to other animals

　　　(1) A common example is the antitetanus toxoid for potential *Clostridium tetani* exposure

　　　(2) It is also available for the treatment of other clostridial pathogens

IMMUNOPATHOLOGICAL MECHANISMS ■■■■

I. Disorders result from inappropriate or inadequate immune responses and are labeled as hypersensitivities, autoimmune reactions, or immunodeficiencies

II. Immunoproliferative disorders can also occur where the proliferation of the leukocytes becomes aberrant, excessive, and functional

A. EXAMPLE: lymphosarcoma, for which the theory of an oncogenic viral etiological agent has been proposed

　1. This type of pathology is usually studied as a hematological disorder even though it severely compromises the immune system's ability to function

III. Four types of hypersensitivity reactions (some of which occur in isolation but more often more than one type occurs simultaneously)

A. Type 1 involves the animal producing too much IgE antibody

　1. If this is a genetically based condition it is known as an atopy

　2. IgE is important in promoting inflammation during an innate response and is crucial to an individual's immune function

　3. When produced in excess it can produce very problematic, even fatal, conditions

　　a. Too much IgE antibody means too many mast cells degranulate and in turn too much histamine is released

　　b. This results in allergies of various forms dependent on the allergen's (an antigen that induces an allergic response) portal of entry

　　　(1) Inhalation, ingestion, or topically

　　　(2) If the reaction is systemic producing anaphylactic shock and death

　4. Unfortunately allergies are relatively common in animals and can occur to almost any compound from feedstuffs and pharmaceuticals to environmental items

　　a. Common examples: canine atopic dermatitis and contact dermatitis (classical flea bite hypersensitivity and sweet itch fit here) but the latter does not involve atopy

B. Type 2 occurs when an animal produces antibodies against its own cells that are then lysed by complement
   1. Results in an autoimmune disorder
   2. Sometimes the targeted cells are virally or neoplastically transformed but more often the condition is idiopathic
   3. EXAMPLES: autoimmune hemolytic anemia, equine infectious anemia, immune-mediated thrombocytopenia, pemphigus, and systemic lupus erythematosus
C. Type 3 occurs when antibodies bind to an antigen and form large complexes that become deposited in body tissues, often joints and vessel walls or kidneys are involved
   1. It produces inflammation and tissue necrosis at these sites
   2. Often secondary to other pathologies such as pyometra or parasitic infestations but it too is often idiopathic in nature
   3. A common example: rheumatoid arthritis
D. Type 4 is the result of the actions of stimulated T cells and macrophages
   1. They infiltrate the area in which the allergen occurs (this may involve a delay until blood vessels link the allergen with the individual's immune system, as with a tissue graft), and then redness, hard lump formation, and necrosis occur
   2. These create a granuloma
   3. EXAMPLE: flea collar sensitivities
IV. Immunodeficiencies
A. Definition: lack of a particular immune system component and/or a malfunction
B. Types
   1. Congenital, cell-mediated immunodeficiency
      a. EXAMPLE: cyclic neutropenia in gray collies and their crosses
      b. They experience a cyclic decrease of all cellular elements (most notably the neutrophils), during which time they have a very low resistance to infection
   2. Congenital, humoral immunodeficiencies include the inability to produce certain classes of antibody
      a. IgG deficiency in cattle, IgM deficiency in horses, Doberman pinschers and basset hounds, and IgA deficiency in other dogs

   3. A combined immunodeficiency can be seen in some Arabian horses and basset hounds that do not possess a thymus, no lymphoid organs, and a very low number of lymphocytes
      a. Such animals survive their first few months primarily because of the antibodies received from their mothers
      b. Usually they succumb to adenoviral pneumonia (horse) or the distemper vaccine (dog)
C. Deficiencies due to cell-mediated immunity alone is rare
D. Acquired deficiencies (occurring after birth) are common especially in cats due to feline leukemia and feline AIDS viruses
E. Animals that do not receive colostrum or that nurse from mothers with poor immunity and therefore produce low quality colostrum also have an acquired humoral immunity for a period of time
   1. These young have a difficult time surviving until their immune systems fully develop
F. Even species that obtain antibody across the placental barrier are more prone to intestinal infections resulting in diarrhea if they do not ingest the colostral IgA antibodies
G. In old age the immune system weakens and deficiencies begin to develop
H. Other general causes of inappropriate immune reactions
   1. Lack of the suppressor T cells to downgrade the response
   2. Pathogen mimicry of host cell surface molecules to avoid attack
   3. Breakdown of tolerance to usually 'ignored' material such as dust (i.e., chronic alveolar emphysema in horses, or autoimmune disease occurs)

VACCINES
Attenuated-live/Modified-live (MLV) Vaccines

I. In the production of vaccines it is common to grow a pathogenic virus in an embryonated egg or tissue culture
II. This virus can then be attenuated and injected whole, which ensures that antigenic epitopes will be injected and that those epitopes are almost similar, if not identical, to the wild strain of the same virus that causes disease
III. Such vaccinations will elicit a very rapid, strong immune reaction in the host into which

it was injected, if it doesn't kill the host itself

IV. Bacterial vaccines (bacterins) are developed in a similar way as vaccines and elicit immune reactions in the host

Killed Vaccines

I. Heat, mechanical or chemical, inactivates the pathogen before injection

II. This method risks altering the epitopes so that the antibodies mounted against these changed epitopes may bind only weakly or not at all to the wild strain of the pathogen

III. The overall immunity will be weaker, possibly useless

IV. Although the animal will not develop disease from one of these killed organisms, there is a possibility that the individual may be allergic to the compound used to destroy the pathogen

V. If a bacterial culture is used to create such a vaccine it is often termed a *bacterin*

Subunit Vaccines

I. Subunit vaccines do not use the entire microorganism, instead only an antigenic part is selected

II. This process requires identification and isolation of the most antigenic pieces while creating as little alteration as possible

III. The selection may be a polysaacharide derived from the bacterial capsule as opposed to part of the bacterial cell membrane

IV. It is possible for a material to be so small it does not react with the immune system at all

V. If creating a subunit vaccine, the selected epitopes may need to be coupled with another compound called an adjuvant

A. An adjuvant increases virus size and surface area, resists dispersal in the body (the vaccine remains at the site of injection), and therefore elicits and prolongs the inflammatory response

B. On average, the immune response to the vaccine in 500 times stronger than it would be without the adjuvant's presence

C. Commonly used adjuvants are: some salts, sugars, or oils or Freund's adjuvant that may or may not include killed *Mycobacterium* bacteria

D. Adjuvants can be the cause of allergic responses

VI. Subunit vaccines permit more than one pathogen's antigenic determinants (epitopes) to be coupled to the same adjuvant and be administered in a single dose

VII. EXAMPLE: western and eastern equine encephalitis, tetanus, and influenza vaccine

A. This 'covers' the horse for four different diseases and is therefore termed *a 4-way subunit vaccine*

B. Usually the immune response to subunit vaccines is good, with no risk of causing disease

Vaccine Difficulties

I. Vaccines are not guaranteed to work, because an individual may react to carried-over proteins from the culture environment of the virus or to chemicals used to kill it, or even the adjuvant itself

A. The adjuvant may not perform adequately or the epitopes may be altered during processing or they may not be very immunogenic in the first place

II. Usually vaccines are sold as a lyophilized powder to which a particular amount of sterile distilled water is added

A. The amount of water must be correct because the concentration is important in inducing a good response

B. The vaccine must be stored properly during shipping because temperature extremes can cause a loss of antigenicity

C. It must be handled gently after reconstitution so that no mechanical damage occurs and it must be delivered to the appropriate area in the body for which it was designed to work

1. Some are to be injected subcutaneously; others are for intramuscular injection

2. If administered incorrectly there may not be sufficient inflammation or the vaccine may be cleared so rapidly that it doesn't stimulate the immune system

3. Nonstimulation can occur with accidental intravenous administration but it could also result in anaphylaxis

4. The use of excessive quantities of alcohol at the injection site has also been implicated

III. After all proper precautions are taken, there is still no guarantee the vaccinated animal will respond appropriately

A. A young animal that is immunologically compromised may succumb to illness to a whole live vaccine or may not develop immunity to a killed or subunit vaccine

B. Even if an animal doesn't become ill from the administration of a vaccine there is no way of knowing what the animal's immune status is unless an antibody titre is done

IV. Viruses are capable of a process called "antigenic drift"

A. EXAMPLE: canine parvovirus

B. Such a virus mutates its genome and its epitopes so that preexisting antibodies from previous vaccines are now unable to bind and are therefore useless

C. As a result a previously ill and recovered animal or a previously vaccinated animal is no longer immune

Vaccine Precautions

I. Following the recommended vaccination schedule increases an animal's chances of developing a protective immunity

II. If a vaccine is given too early in life the maternal antibodies in the circulation may prevent the young animal's immune system from properly responding to the vaccine, lessening its efficacy

A. The neonate's immune system may not be sufficiently developed to respond

III. Boosters must be administered at correct times to maintain the necessarily high level of immunity to prevent disease

CURRENT TRENDS IN VACCINE PRODUCTION AND IMMUNOLOGICAL RESEARCH ▰

I. Biotechnology (genetic engineering) is instrumental in creating a new form of a more effective vaccine

II. An important part of this creation is the three new approaches to identify the pathogens' immune-stimulatory epitopes capable of inducing a protective immunity

A. Using new techniques, it is now possible to purify and obtain the amino acid sequences of epitopes designed to induce cytotoxic T cell activity

1. Inclusion of these epitopes in a vaccine will potentially confer protection against cancer and viral infections

B. New techniques permit identification and isolation of highly specific antibodies for the epitopes responsible for eliciting secondary immune responses

C. Injection of plasmid DNA encoding an antigen

1. Definition: nonchromosomal bacterial DNA that is independently self-replicating, which carries part of the pathogen's genome

2. It is usually delivered to mucosal surfaces and will be incorporated into host cells, potentially produce pathogenic epitopes, and finally elicit protective immunity in the host animal against that pathogen

3. Such a vaccine is termed *expression library immunization* or *DNA vaccine*

III. Biotechnology also has been directed at discovering ways to enhance the animal's immune response, especially to vaccines, to induce stronger, longer-lasting immunity

A. Most research has been directed at delivery of antigen to the anatomical area where T and B lymphocytes with the appropriate specificity dwell and at stimulating the necessary signals for a strong, protective response to occur

B. Because modified-live vaccines have inherent difficulties such as safety, an alternative was developed

1. The alternative uses disabled infectious single cycle (DISC) viruses

a. These viruses are generated by deleting an essential gene from the virus and inserting that gene into a 'supportive' cell line

b. As a result this virus can replicate only in the supportive cell line

c. DISC viruses are infective but can complete only a single cycle of replication in the vaccinated animal host (whose cells naturally do not contain the deleted essential viral gene)

d. It is also possible to insert genes from other pathogens into the viral vector and safely achieve multiple immunity with a single dose

C. Cytokines are hormone-like compounds responsible for providing immune stimulatory signals necessary for effective immune responses

1. Cytokines that control leukocyte migration, recruitment, and the amplification and differentiation of T and B cells have been identified and include interleukins 1, 2, 6 and interferon, etc.

2. All of these have adjuvant properties when administered with vaccines

3. These compounds often require multiple dosages to be effective and induce too strong an inflammatory response; therefore biotechnology advances are now directed at the production of cytokine inducers to accompany the vaccination process

4. Inducers are envisioned to cause the body to produce more of its own cytokines, thus bypassing the problems and obtaining the benefits of improved, safe immunity with no possibility of disease

5. It is also believed that cytokine inducers could be administered alone to stimulate increased immunity during times of low or suppressed immune responses (i.e., the neonatal period or stress of shipping)

D. Research is also studying new delivery systems that would improve current systemic, multiple-dose vaccination protocols. Their complete development, testing, and approval for use is believed to be at least a decade in the future

1. New delivery systems include polymers to allow mucosal uptake and permit oral and new intranasal administrations

2. Microencapsulation and slow release materials are being studied to provide single dosing as opposed to the multiple vaccinations needed for protective immunity

a. Unfortunately cost, long-term safety and various design issues have yet to be resolved

Glossary

allergen A material that invokes an allergic response, usually localized in an individual

antigen A material capable of eliciting an antibody response in an animal

antigenic drift A process of mutation whereby an antigen changes its epitopes, thereby rendering previous immunity (and vaccines) useless or clinically reduced. A common occurrence in influenza viruses; occurred recently in the canine parvovirus

antiserum A serum containing antibodies directed against the various epitopes of an antigen that elicited their production

autoimmune reaction Occurs when tolerance to self breaks down and the immune system attacks self; usually unhealthy

capsid The inert outer shell of a virus that protects it from the external environment while outside the host

chemotaxis Movement up a concentration gradient, usually formed by a compound released from body cells called a chemotactic factor. Such a phenomenon directs cells to the sites of their immunological functions

colostrum The "first milk" secreted by a mother. In many species it is high in proteins, including antibodies, and is therefore a form of passive natural immunity

commensal Living on or within another organism and deriving benefit while benefitting or not harming the host

complement A series of twenty or more proteins that bind the microbial surface (alternate series) or certain antibodies (classical series) and form a membrane attack complex (terminal or lytic series); a tubular structure that pierces the cell membrane and results in the microorganism's lysis

congenital Born with; possibly but not necessarily hereditary

degranulate The release of phagocyte granules and their degradative enzymes to the exterior of the cell. It permits the breakdown of materials too large to phagocytize but causes severe inflammation

diapedesis The process by which leukocytes adhere to and squeeze through vessel linings to enter tissue spaces; usually directed by chemotactic factors (see chemotaxis)

epitope A structural component of an antigen against which immune responses are made and to which an antibody binds; also called antigenic determinant

erythema Redness to the skin; often a clinical sign of a topically induced allergy

granuloma Dysfunctional tissue filled with eosinophils, fibroblasts producing scarring, and large macrophages called giant cells

idiopathic Of unknown cause

immunogen A compound that elicits an immune response; synonymous with antigen

lysis Rupture; when a red blood cell bursts it is known as hemolysis

lysozyme An enzyme that breaks down chemical bonds in the cell walls of some bacteria, especially *Staphylococcus*

macrophage A mature tissue monocyte capable of many phagocytic cycles but is slow to arrive at the site of antigenic invasion of the body

memory The ability of the immune system to respond faster and stronger to second and subsequent invasions by the same antigen; one of the hallmarks of the immune response

necrosis The breakdown and death of cells, usually a result of inflammation

neutrophil The most common leukocyte in most species, possessing a lobed nucleus and purple granules. Also called a segmented neutrophil or a polymorphonuclear neutrophil. It is capable of a few phagocytic cycles and is usually the first leukocyte at the site of antigenic invasion of the body

opsonin Any component that binds to an antigen and makes its engulfment by phagocytes more efficient

phagocytosis The process of engulfment of antigens and other material; its breakdown and release of inert waste products by phagocytic cells, primarily neutrophils, and macrophages. One episode is termed a *phagocytic cycle*

plasmid A nonchromosomal, circular strand of a bacterial genome that replicates independently from the rest of the bacteria's genetic complement. Through molecular biology it is possible to use restriction enzymes and ligase to insert pieces of a pathogen's gentic code into this plasmid. This then allows multiple copies to be made without the creation of the intact infectious microorganism. These copies can then be used in the production of vaccines without risking disease

rhinitis Inflammation in the upper respiratory tract, specifically the nose, resulting in the clinical signs of nasal discharge, congestion, and sneezing. A clinical sign of inhaled allergens

self One's own surface cells and molecules that the immune system recognizes and in health does not attack

specificity A defining property of the immune system that determines which shape of epitope an immune cell can react with, each cell having its own unique, single specificity

tolerance The lack of responsiveness by the immune system. Tolerance is healthy when it occurs to self but is immunosuppressive when it occurs to antigens; can be induced by drugs such as steroids

urticaria Clinical sign of itchiness

vesicle Blistering of the skin; a mucous membrane producing small fluid filled regions. Often occurs as a result of a type 4 hypersensitivity reaction.

Review Questions

1 Innate immunity:
 a. Involves cell-mediated but not humoral immunity
 b. Is solely created by the actions of the neutrophils
 c. Is the inborn immunity that possesses memory and specificity
 d. Is the immune system and its capabilities with which one is born

2 Which of the following is *false* regarding the immune system's property of memory?
 a. It is part of the adaptive immune response
 b. It helps to ensure that the secondary and subsequent responses to an antigen will occur faster and stronger than the primary response ✔
 c. It is due to the cloned B lymphocytes produced in the primary response
 d. It guarantees that for a particular antigen no clinical signs will occur after the primary response

3 Which of the following is a property of histamine?
 a. It causes mast cells to degranulate
 b. It causes vasodilation
 c. It acts as a chemotactic factor
 d. It is directly responsible for the sensation of pain

4 Interleukin-1 is released by:
 a. Antigen-presenting cells
 b. Antigen stimulated T_H-cells
 c. B lymphocytes
 d. Mast cells after degranulation

5 Which of the following T cell subpopulation clones more slowly?
 a. Helper T cells
 b. Cytotoxic T cells
 c. Suppressor T cells
 d. None; they all clone at the same rate

6 Cytotoxic T cells are responsible for secreting _____ , which causes _____ .
 a. Serotonin; smooth muscle contractions
 b. Complement; diapedesis of the neutrophils
 c. Interleukin-6; cloning of the B cells
 d. Perforin; lysis of the antigenic microorganism

7 Interferon functions to:
 a. Initiate inflammation
 b. Activate cytotoxic T cells
 c. Activate the natural killer cells to destroy virally infected host cells
 d. Downgrade the immune response

8 An example of acquired artificial active immunity is:
 a. Ingestion of colostrum
 b. Maternal antibodies crossing the placental barrier in cats
 c. Recovery from disease
 d. Vaccination

9 The following statement describes an allergy:
 a. It is a type 2 hypersensitivity reaction
 b. It is rare in all species of animals but when it occurs it is always hereditary in nature
 c. It is a localized reaction to an allergen in animals that produce too much IgA antibody to that compound
 d. It involves the production of IgE antibody and mast cell degranulation

10 The only antibody that can enter tissue spaces and cross the placental barrier in some species is:
 a. IgG
 b. IgA
 c. IgD
 d. IgM

BIBLIOGRAPHY

Alberts B et al: *Molecular biology of the cell,* ed 3, 1994, New York, Garland Publishing Inc.

Facts on File conference highlights agricultural biotechnology international conference, June 11-14, 1996, Saskatoon, Canada. File Inc.

Gershwin L et al: *Immunology and immunopathology of domestic animals,* ed 2, 1995, St Louis, Mosby-Year Book Inc.

Janeway CA, Travers P: *Immunobiology, the immune system in health and disease,* 1994, London, Garland Publishing Inc.

Roitt I, Brostoff J, Male D: *Immunology,* ed 4, 1996, London, Mosby-Times Mirror International Publisher Ltd.

Steinberg M, Cosloy S: *The Facts on File dictionary of biotechnology and genetic engineering,* 1994, New York, Facts on File Inc.

Tizard I: *An introduction to veterinary immunology,* ed 3, 1987, Philadelphia, W.B. Saunders.

Zoonoses

Kisha L. White-Farrar

OUTLINE

Bacterial Zoonosis
Viral Zoonosis

Parasitic Zoonosis
Mycotic Zoonosis

Other Zoonoses

LEARNING OUTCOMES

After reading this chapter you should be able to:

1. Define bacterial, viral, parasitic, mycotic, and other miscellaneous zoonotic diseases.
2. Recognize etiology, symptoms (human and animal), transmission, diagnosis, treatment, prevention, and control of various zoonotic diseases.

Zoonoses are infections or parasitic diseases that can be transmitted between humans and animals. It is beyond the scope of this chapter to address all of the known zoonoses but descriptions of many important or commonly encountered diseases are presented. Any ill or infected animal represents a potential source of zoonotic infection, but with the use of proper precautions the chances of disease transmission can be greatly reduced. People who are immunocompromised (e.g., the very young, the aged, those on chemotherapeutic regimens), splenectomized individuals, or those who are immunodeficient should avoid contact with sick animals because most pathogenic organisms can 'set up shop' in atypical host species if an individual has greatly lowered (or absent) body defenses.

Epidemiology analyzes factors that influence the incidence, distribution, and control of infectious disease. By understanding how to recognize the symptoms, transmission, diagnosis, treatment, and control of transmittable diseases, the incidence of serious illness in humans and animals can be reduced.

Table 23-1 Bacterial zoonosis

Zoonosis/etiology	Symptoms—human	Symptoms—animal	Transmission	Diagnosis	Treatment	Prevention control
Bacillus anthracis: susceptible species; all mammals, most birds	Three clinical presentations: cutaneous, intestinal, pulmonary; septicemia and/or meningitis may occur	Three clinical presentations: peracute, acute, subacute/chronic	Direct contact with infected animal or animal products; insect vectors and contaminated water possible	Culture/isolation, microscopic identification	Human: AB* therapy Animal: AB therapy (effective early in disease)	Vaccines available for humans and animals; disinfection/ sterilization of animal products; do not perform necropsy on suspected cases; incinerate or deep-bury and cover carcass with quicklime
Brucellosis (Bang's disease, undulant fever): *Brucella* spp.; susceptible species: most mammals; common in bovine, canine	Clinical presentation, from latent to chronic, may include flu-like symptoms, fatigue, weight loss, depression, meningitis, encephalitis, endocarditis; common in vocationally high risk persons	Varied, may include retained placenta, mastitis, fistulous withers, arthritis, orchitis, lymphadenopathy, sterility	Direct contact with infected animals or animal products; humans are always accidental hosts	Culture/isolation, serum agglutination, ELISA, CF (most reliable)	AB therapy	Test/slaughter, vaccinate cows and calves, protective clothing, good sanitation/hygiene, proper food handling
Campylobacteriosis (vibriosis): *Campylobacter* spp.; susceptible species: most species, common in birds	May include: abdominal pain, acute (possibly bloody) diarrhea for 3-5 days; spontaneous recovery is common, w/o AB therapy latent carriers may result	May include: 3-7 days of watery, mucoid, or bloody diarrhea, anorexia, abortions; spontaneous recovery w or w/o AB therapy, may become latent carriers	Fecal-oral, contaminated water, infected food products (animal and vegetable)	Culture/isolation, cytologic examination of feces	AB therapy—does not shorten clinical course of disease, but eliminates carrier state	Primarily good sanitation/hygiene

*Antibiotic therapy

Continued

Table 23-1 Bacterial zoonosis—cont'd

Zoonosis/etiology	Symptoms—human	Symptoms—animal	Transmission	Diagnosis	Treatment	Prevention control
Cat scratch disease: multiple bacterial species have been implicated; EXAMPLES: *Afipia felis, Bartonella henselae, Pasteurella multocida;* susceptible species: primarily feline	Primarily in children <12 years; may include identifiable primary innoculatory lesion, regional lymphadenopathy, flu-like symptoms, anorexia osteolytic lesions, oculoglandular syndrome	Felines display few, if any, clinical signs; endocarditis, usually self-limiting with no recurrence in re-covered patients	Directly or indirectly transmitted by domestic felines (bacilli may be normal oral flora—transmitted to claws during grooming), usually transmitted through bite/scratch; some evidence of flea vector	Clinical presentation/ appropriate history, primary innoculatory lesion, positive Hangar-Rose skin test, culture/isolation Most commonly from male, intact cats (<1 year), with fleas, not declawed, and indoor/outdoor access	Usually self-resolving but may require AB therapy	Declaw young felines; do not allow cats to lick open wounds; good sanitation/ hygiene, handle cats gently to prevent bites/ scratches
Listerosis: *Listeria* spp.; susceptible species: many species of mammals, fowl, fish (common in ruminants)	Several clinical presentations: depends on route of infection; may include dermal lesions, enteritis, septicemia, encephalitis, abortion/ stillbirth, birth of infected neonates	May include diarrhea, flu-like symptoms, excessive salivation, mastitis, monocytosis, septicemia, purulent/necrotic lesions of visceral organs/lymph nodes, abortion/ stillbirth, encephalitis	Exposure to infected animal/bird products contaminated silage/vegetables	Culture/isolation	AB therapy	Good sanitation/ hygiene, protective clothing
Plague: *Yersinia* spp.; susceptible species: chief reservoirs—rodents, birds, lagomorphs; also common in carnivores	Three main clinical presentations: bubonic (acute); septicemic, pneumonic; may include acute fever, painful lymphadenitis, anorexia, flu-like symptoms, dyspnea, fatigue	May include: fever, lymphadenitis/ abscess formation; some species may show high mortality rates	Flea bites, direct contact w/infected animals, inhalation of aerosolized contaminants	Culture/isolation, IFA, serological testing	AB therapy	Rodent/flea control, protective clothing, good sanitation/ hygiene

Leptospirosis (Weil's disease, Ft. Bragg fever): *Leptospira* spp.; susceptible species: wide variety mammals/reptiles but rodents are a primary reservoir	Incubation 1–2 wks, duration 1–7 days; may include flu-like symptoms, jaundice, anuria, rash, conjunctivitis, liver/kidney failure, death	Contact w/infective urine contaminated water/soil, direct contact w/infected animals	Culture/isolation (blood, urine), micro and macroagglutination, ELISA	AB therapy: treatment or prophylactic	Protective clothing, rodent control, good sanitation/hygiene, avoid contaminated water sources, vaccinate (moderately effective)
Lyme borreliosis (Lyme disease): *Borrelia burgdorferi*; susceptible species: variety of wild/domestic animals	Three clinical presentations: acute hemorrhagic, subacute, subclinical; may include (acute/subacute) high fever, septicemia, anorexia, depression, icterus, hemolytic anemia, endotoxemia, abortion, mastitis, infertility				
	May include: fever, arthralgia, arthritis, lameness, CNS involvement, encephalitis, abortion	Primarily bite from an infected tick, also oral (splashed, infective urine), placental transmission	Clinical presentation/history of tick exposure, culture/isolation, IFA and EIA available but false pos/neg results have been reported	AB therapy	Use of protected clothing, tick repellents, prevention of prolonged tick attachment, environmental tick treatment, treatment of pets for ticks. Vaccine available
	Three stages First stage: 'bulls eye' red lesion (usually at site of tick bite), maculopapular/petechial/vesicular rashes, flu-like symptoms Second stage: duration 3 days–6 wks, meningitis, encephalitis, cardiac complications, musculoskeletal pain Third stage (months–years later): CNS involvement, arthritis, chronic dermatologic complications				

Table 23-2 Viral zoonosis

Zoonosis/etiology	Symptoms—human	Symptoms—animal	Transmission	Diagnosis	Treatment	Prevention control
Arboviral encephalitis (sleeping sickness): Arboviridae spp.; EXAMPLES: EEE, WEE, VEE, St. Louis; susceptible species: many bird/wild animal (primarily rodent) reservoirs, common in equines	Usually biphasic. First phase may include headache/high fever, which may abate before disease progresses. Second phase (encephalitic): cervical stiffness, nausea/vomiting, disorientation, frequent progression to coma/convulsions	Symptoms vary but may include fever, depression, impaired vision, irregular gait, wandering, incoordination, slowed reflexes, facial/general paralysis, death	Viral reservoir is maintained by mosquito vectors	Culture/isolation, serology	AB therapy and antiviral therapy in humans	Avoid bite of mosquitoes; use protective screening/clothing; liberal use of insect repellent; use of vaccines
Herpes B viral infection: *Herpesvirus simiae*; susceptible species: primarily macaque species (principally Rhesus)	Causes an ascending encephalitis that is usually fatal—those who survive often suffer severe, permanent neurologic damage; symptoms usually occur w/in 30 days of exposure; may include vesicular skin lesions, localized neurologic symptoms, regional lymphadenopathy, fever, headaches, ataxia, encephalitis, death—usually 2-3 days after onset of clinical signs	Chiefly gingivostomatitis with buccal mucosal lesions; asymptomatic infection is believed to be common	Primarily by exposure to infected monkey saliva/tissues	Culture/isolation, serology	Thoroughly clean/disinfect all primate bite/scratch wounds; immediately report any rash/itching/numbness at wound site; evidence suggests that early administration of acylovir may aide recovery	Thoroughly clean/disinfect all bites/scratches; use protective clothing, liberal use of chemical/mechanical restraint
Poxviral disease (contagious ecthyma, bovine papular stomatitis, pseudopox): Poxviridae spp.	Usually progressive, localized skin lesions, may progress to cellular proliferation/necrosis	Same course as human	Direct contact (usually through dermal abrasion)	Clinical presentation/appropriate history, culture/isolation, CF, IFA	AB therapy for secondary bacterial infection	Use of protective clothing, use of vaccines
Rabies (hydrophobia, 'mad' dog disease); a rhabidovirus; susceptible species: all mammalian species (common in skunks, bats, canines, felines, equines)	Incubation 9 days-2+ years, clinical course usually 2-8 days; may include anxiety, hyperesthesia, hyperactivity, aerobia, increased salivation, laryngopharyngeal muscular spasms, convulsions, coma, and ultimately death	Two stages First stage: duration 1-6 days. may include behavioral changes (unusual friendliness/aggression), excitability, altered vocalizations: Second stage: duration 1-4 days, progressive paralysis and death	Primarily contamination of a wound (bite, abrasion) by infected saliva; ingestion/mucosal contact w/infected saliva	Clinical presentation/appropriate history, IFA (optimal recovery from hippocampus, brain stem, cerebellum)	Practice prophylactic treatment	Immunization of applicable species, pre-exposure prophylaxis to vocationally high risk persons

Disease/Species	Clinical signs	Clinical presentation	Transmission	Diagnosis	Treatment	Prevention
Salmonellosis (enteric fever): *Salmonella* spp.; susceptible species: almost all species (esp. prevalent in reptiles)	Incubation: 6-72 hours; primarily presents as acute gastroenteritis; may also include focal infections, chronic rheumatoid conditions, colitis, autoimmune disorders, chronic enteric hyperplastic/inflammatory conditions; shedding of infected organisms occurs for days-weeks	Four clinical presentations: subclinical, acute enteritis, subacute enteritis, chronic enteritis. Acute: may include high fever, explosive diarrhea (possibly bloody), depression, death w/in 48 hours; Chronic: may include mild symptoms, low-moderate fever, soft feces/mild diarrhea, abortion	Primarily fecal-oral route; commonly found in beef and poultry products; unthrifty appearance—stress can induce shedding of infective organisms	Clinical presentation/appropriate history, culture/isolation	AB therapy	Good sanitation/hygiene; proper cooking/handling of beef/poultry products; do not bathe animals or wash cage items in kitchen or bathroom sink
Tuberculosis (TB) *Mycobacteria* spp.; susceptible species: most species	Two clinical signs: acute, chronic. Acute: may include acute miliary TB, meningitis, secondary infections. Chronic: may include pulmonary/bone/joint lesions, meningitis, genitourinary infections, cervical lymphadenitis	May include lymphadenopathy, lesions/granulomas of organs, anorexia, weakness, wt loss, coughing/dyspnea, pleuralpneumonia, death; latent carrier state is common	Primarily fecal-oral route; ingestion of contaminated food products; contact w/infected tissues/animal products	Reaction to interdermal tuberculin test(s), culture/isolation	Human: anti-tuberculosis drug therapy/prophylaxis (for known exposure)	Intradermal tuberculin testing (animals and vocationally high risk persons), animal test/cull programs, proper preparation/handling of food
Tularemia (rabbit fever) *Francisella tularensis* sp.; susceptible species: many species of vertebrates/invertebrates	Incubation 2-3 days; several clinical presentations—depend on route of infection: ulceroglandular, typhoidal, oculoglandular, glandular, tularemic pneumonia	Usually manifests as septicemia (may show high mortality), heavy tick infestation may be concurrent	Blood/tissue of infected animals, fluids/feces of infected ticks, bites from infected ticks	Culture/isolation, FA testing, serology (later in disease)	AB therapy	Protective clothing, tick control, sanitation/hygiene

Table 23-3 Parasitic zoonosis

Zoonosis/etiology	Symptoms—human	Symptoms—animal	Transmission	Diagnosis	Treatment	Prevention control
Ancylostomiasis (hookworm disease) (cutaneous larval migrans); many species of hookworms may infect man and animals; susceptible species: most species	May include bloody diarrhea, anemia (which may lead to tachycardia, heart failure, hypoproteinemia, ascites), cutaneous infection, dermatitis, generalized edema, regional lymphadenitis, pneumonitis, corneal opacities	May include anemia, dark/tarry stools, dehydration, emaciation; fatalities are common in young animals	Fecal-oral route, cutaneous penetration by larvae	Ova on fecal flotation, clinical presentation/appropriate history	Anthelmintic therapy	Good sanitation/hygiene; treat infected animals; cover sandboxes; use protective clothing
Tapeworm infection (low pathogenicity): multiple species: Dypilidiae spp., Taeniae spp., Hymenolipiae spp.; susceptible species: most species	Common in very young children, symptoms usually mild; may include abdominal discomfort, diarrhea, pruritis, anemia, wt loss	Migrating proglottids may cause anal irritation; may include wt loss, unthrifty appearance	Ingesting infected fleas or proglottids/ova	Primarily by presence of proglottids on feces/perianally (rarely observed on fecal flotation)	Anthelmintic therapy	Flea control; treat infected animals; good sanitation/hygiene
Tapeworm infection (high pathogenicity): Echinococcal spp.; susceptible species: many species (common in canines, felines, rodents) Predator-prey cycle: predator spp. are the definitive hosts, prey spp. are intermediate hosts, man is (accidental) intermediate host	Alveolar hydatid disease; progressive onset of symptoms may include epigastric pain, malais, progressive jaundice, hepatomegaly, hepatic cysts	(see tapeworm infection-low pathogenicity)	(see tapeworm infection-low pathogenicity)	Due to small size of proglottids very difficult to detect on/in feces, indistinguishable ova (from other cestodes)	Animals: anthelmintic therapy Humans: surgical excision of cysts	(see tapeworm infection-low pathogenicity)
Toxocariasis (visceral larval migrans [VLM], ocular larval migrans [OLM]); Toxocara spp.; susceptible species: most species	VLM: larval migration through somatic tissues; may include fever, hepatomegaly, bronchiolitis, asthma, pneumonitis, CNS	Usually inapparent in adults (larval incystation in tissues); in young may include diarrhea, dehydration, intestinal distention/obstruction, exaggerated immunologic response OLM: larva enter into orbit of the eye, usually no other signs	Fecal-oral (2 wk incubation period)	Ova found on fecal flotation, clinical presentation/appropriate history, ELISA	Anthelmintic therapy	Good sanitation/hygiene, treat infected animals

Disease/Organism	Clinical signs (human)	Clinical signs (animal)	Transmission	Diagnosis	Treatment	Prevention
Toxoplasmosis: *Toxoplasma gondii*; susceptible spp.: most species but felines are definitive and intermediate hosts	Most adults show subclinical symptoms, but may include flu-like symptoms, transient cervical lymphadenopathy, myocarditis, splenomegaly, hepatomegaly, encephalitis, retinochoroiditis; congenital infections may manifest a subclinical or clinical presentation of variable severity; fatalities do occur	Most are subclinical but may include (same as human and possibly icterus, granulomatous panuveitis)	Fecal-oral, ingestion of improperly cooked meats; congenital transplacental transmission	Leukocytosis, eosinophilia, observation/isolation of tachyzoites from blood/tissues, Sabin Feldman dye test, IFA, CF, ELISA, oocyst identification from fecal flotation (requires sporulation)	Anticoccidial anthelmintic therapy	Proper handling/preparation of food, keep pet cats indoors (reduce hunting opportunities), clean litterbox regularly (ova require 3+ days incubation before infective), good sanitation/hygiene, gloves when cleaning litterbox/gardening, cover sandboxes
Sarcoptic mange (scabies): *Sarcoptes scabei* mite; susceptible species: many species	Intensely pruritic dermal lesions, may develop alopecia/skin thickening, peripheral lymphadenopathy	(same as human)	Direct contact w/ infested animal	Visualization of mites/ova from skin scraping	Anthelmintic therapy	Treat infected animals, protective clothing, regular washing/changing of animal bedding, prophylactic ivermectin

Table 23-4 Mycotic zoonosis

Zoonosis/etiology	Symptoms—human	Symptoms—animal	Transmission	Diagnosis	Treatment	Prevention control
Dermatophytosis: (ringworm, dermatomycosis); most common: *Microsporum* spp., *Trichophyton* sp.; susceptible species: most common in young mammals	Incubation 1-2 wks; superficial infections of skin/hair/nails; acute inflammatory reaction; lesions usually papulosquamous with circular/reddened borders (but may be dry/alopecic or moist/eczematous lesions)	Lesions are usually circular/crusty with/without redness/alopecia	Direct contact with an infected animal (or its hair, skin, leashes/brushes) equipment, or contaminated soil	Dermatophyte/mycologic culture/isolation, ultraviolet fluorescence (Wood's lamp), biopsy/cytology	Topical/oral antifungal therapy, vaccine (limited use)	Protective clothing, good sanitation/ hygiene, treat infected animals
Systemic mycoses; most common: Histoplasmae spp., Coccidiodae spp., Blastomycae spp., Cryptoccae spp.; susceptible species: most species	Usually begin as pulmonary infection with fever/myalgia/congestion; may progress into chronic/granulomatous pneumonia or disseminate to other organs; may develop into subacute or chronic meningoencephalitis	Similar to course of disease in human	Usually aerosolized organisms (fecal/infective soil)	Culture/isolation, ELISA	Antifungal therapy	Protective clothing (when handling infected animals or cleaning their pens/supplies)

Rocky Mountain spotted fever: *Rickettsia* spp.; susceptible species: variety of wild/domestic animals	May include abdominal pain, flu-like symptoms, rash on palms/soles, CNS abnormalities, hepatomegaly, jaundice, myocarditis, meninoencephalitis, DIC	Similar to human course of disease	Ticks (see Lyme disease)	Clinical presentation/appropriate history, CF and micro-IFA (false positive is rare but false negatives do occur)	AB therapy	(see Lyme disease)
Ehrlichiosis: *Ehrlichia* spp	May include: acute fever, flu-like symptoms, leukopenia; primarily canids	Three clinical presentations: acute, subacute, chronic thrombocytopenia, elevated hepatic enzyme activity (esp. AST, ALT) May include fever, anorexia, depression, lymphadopathy, thrombocytopenia, 'fading puppy syndrome'	(see Lyme disease)	Clinical presentation/appropriate history, IFA, isolation from tissues	AB therapy	(see Lyme disease)
Avian chlamydiosis (psittacosis, parrot fever, ornithosis); *Chlamydia psittaci*: susceptible species: primary reservoirs are birds (common in psittacines, pigeons, sea/shore birds, poultry, waterfowl)	Severity ranges from mild flu-like illness to death; may include flu-like symptoms, pneumonitis, pneumonia, myocarditis, encephalitis, thrombophlebitis	Acute or latent carriers (intermittently shedding infective organisms); stress induces disease/shedding; may include depression, anorexia, ocular/nasal discharge, dyspnea, diarrhea (green color)	Fecal-oral route; inhalation/ingestion of infected aerosolized fecal matter	Cloacal/fecal culture/isolation, serology (collected 2 wks apart)	AB therapy	Quarantine/detection/treatment of infected animals, protective clothing, dampen cage floor before cleaning (to reduce aerosolization)

Glossary

anthelmentic Chemical agent that destroys, kills, or expels parasites

CF Complement fixation (test)

ELISA Enzyme-linked immunosorbent assay (test)

epidemiology Scientific study of the factors that influence the incidence, distribution, and control of infectious diseases

FA Fluorescent antibody assay (test)

flu-like symptoms Usually sudden onset of fever, shivering, headache, myalgia, and malaise

IFA Indirect fluorescent antibody assay (test)

latent carrier State where disease-causing organisms are present but clinical disease symptoms are not manifested

miliary TB Disseminated tuberculosis, usually manifested by small, millet seed sized nodules

myalgia Muscle pain

mycotic Relating to fungi or vegetating microorganisms

proglottids Cestode segments that contain fertile, infective oocytes

typhoidal Symptoms marked by sustained high fever, severe headache, and a rash

undulant To fluctuate in wavelike patterns

Review Questions

1 Most infectious organisms have certain species that are preferred hosts. Which statement is most true about infectious organisms?
   a. They will always invade any animal, regardless of the immune status of that individual
   b. They will never invade outside their preferred host species
   c. They may invade outside their normally preferred hosts if an individual is sufficiently immunocompromised
   d. If an individual is immunocompromised, an infectious organisms will always invade the preferred host

2 The Rhabidovirus that causes 'hydrophobia' is not capable of infecting a/an _____ patient.
   a. Canine
   b. Equine
   c. Avian
   d. Feline

3 Antibiotic therapy would be indicated for a patient who has contracted
   a. Visceral larval migrans
   b. Rabies
   c. Salmonellosis
   d. Toxoplasmosis

4 Echinococcal:
   a. Proglottids are identical to the *Taenia* ssp. proglottids
   b. Ova are indistinguishable from other species of cestode ova
   c. Human infestations are treated by anthelmintic therapy
   d. In humans is considered a benign infestation

5 Ringworm infection:
   a. Is caused by a small parasite
   b. Affects only felines
   c. Commonly occurs in healthy, adult animals
   d. Is treated with a regimen of antifungal agents (topical and/or oral)

6 Cat scratch disease can be prevented in part by:
   a. Allowing a feline to lick open wounds, thus raising antibody levels
   b. Administration of vaccine to felines
   c. Administration of vaccine to humans
   d. Declawing young cats and handling them gently

7 Salmonellosis:
   a. Is transmitted by flea bites
   b. Can be prevented by a yearly vaccination
   c. Is commonly shed by latent carriers
   d. Can be transmitted in food products such as chicken or eggs

8 In humans, the first stage of Lyme disease can be diagnosed by a characteristic lesion. The lesion is similar to a/an:
   a. Bull's eye
   b. Mosquito bite
   c. A red rash
   d. An area of petechiae

9 Psittacosis can be contracted only from _____ species.
   a. bovine
   b. avian
   c. ovine
   d. equine

10 A preventive flea program is an important factor in controlling _____ infestations.
   a. *Toxascaris*
   b. Toxoplasmosis
   c. *Sarcoptes* spp.
   d. *Taenia* spp.

BIBLIOGRAPHY

Bowman DD: *Georgi's parasitology for veterinarians,* ed 6, Philadelphia, 1995, WB Saunders.

Clark WH, Dawkins B, Audin JH, editors: Zoonosis updates from *The Journal of American Veterinary Medical Association,* Schaumberg, Illinois, 1990, American Veterinary Medical Association.

Fowler ME, editor: *Zoo and wild animal medicine,* ed 2, Philadelphia, 1986, WB Saunders.

Fraser CM and Mays A, editors: *The Merck manual,* ed 6, Ratway, New Jersey, 1986, Merck & Co. Inc.

Gillespie JH, Timoney JF: *Hagan and Bruner's infectious diseases of domestic animals,* ed 7, Ithaca, 1973, Cornell University Press.

Howard JL, editor: *Current veterinary therapy, food animal practice,* ed 3, Philadelphia, 1993, WB Saunders.

Kirk RW, editor: *Kirk's veterinary therapy, small animal practice,* ed 7, Philadelphia, 1995, WB Saunders.

McCurnin DM: *Clinical textbook for veterinary technicians,* Toronto, 1985, WB Saunders.

Mills L, editor: *Current veterinary therapy in equine medicine,* Philadelphia, 1992, WB Saunders.

Pratt PW, editor: *Laboratory prodedures for veterinary technicians,* ed 2, Goleta, California, 1992, American Veterinary Publications, Inc.

Rakel RE, editor: *Latest approved methods of treatment for the practicing physician,* Philadelphia, 1996, WB Saunders.

CHAPTER 24

Small Animal Nutrition

Frances Federbush-Cheslo

OUTLINE

Basic Nutrition
Energy-producing Nutrients
   Protein
   Carbohydrates
   Fats
Nonenergy-producing Nutrients
   Water
   Minerals
   Vitamins
Daily Energy Requirements
   Feeding Methods

Nutritional Requirements for Each
   Life Stage of the Dog and Cat
   Gestation and Lactation
   Dogs
   Cats
Feline Lower Urinary Tract Disease
   (FLUTD)
Obesity
Critical Care Nutrition
   Enteral Nutrition
   Parenteral Nutrition

How to Choose a Pet Food
Pet Food
   Pet Food Label
   Guaranteed Analysis (GA)
   Ingredient Panel
   Statement of Nutritional Adequacy

LEARNING OUTCOMES

After reading this chapter you should be able to:

1. Know and explain the six basic nutrients and their role in supporting life.
2. Understand and calculate a companion animal's maintenance energy requirements based on its particular life stage.
3. Explain why different nutrient levels change with each life stage and what effects excesses or deficiencies may have.
4. Identify key factors that can prevent or help manage FLUTD.
5. Identify, understand, and assist in the manage-ment and/or prevention of an obese cat or dog.
6. Understand the role of nutritional management in the aid of the critically ill patient.
7. Identify and describe the various components of a pet food label.
8. Understand the necessary information required to help pet owners make an educated decision of which pet food to feed their animal.

9. Understand your role as a source of information for pet owners about small animal nutrition.

The most commonly asked question of a veterinary technician is "What should I feed my pet?" This chapter will allow a veterinary technician to properly and confidently counsel clients about the dietary requirements of their pets. The importance of small animal nutrition in health management has become more recognized in the past decade. The veterinary technician must be knowledgeable about the commonly used pet foods purchased by the hospital's clients to appropriately respond to questions.

BASIC NUTRITION

To understand what diet is best for a companion animal, one must first understand what nutrients are required by the body for each life stage. A basic understanding of the following six nutrients is essential in discussing small animal nutrition.

ENERGY-PRODUCING NUTRIENTS ▬▬▬▬

Protein

I. Made up of 23 amino acids, the building blocks of proteins
   A. Essential amino acids
      1. Must be present in the diet to manufacture a protein
      2. Cats specifically require taurine in their diet
         a. Taurine deficiency could result in dilated cardiomyopathy, retinal atrophy, or infertility
   B. Nonessential amino acids
      1. Amino acids that the animal can manufacture if not available in the body
      2. Dogs can synthesize 10 amino acids; cats can synthesize 11
II. Constituent of muscle, hair, blood, organs, etc. Forms hormones and enzymes
III. Excess protein will be burned for energy and can provide 4 kcal/g if energy not obtained from carbohydrates or fat
IV. Only after protein has been used for building body tissues, facilitating certain hormonal processes and other body functions, will it be used for energy. This use of protein for energy is less efficient versus energy derived from fats or carbohydrates
V. Biological value
   A. Evaluates protein usability by the body
   B. Relationship between percent of nutrient digested, absorbed, and retained to the percent of nutrients lost
   C. The greater number of essential amino acids in a protein the greater its biological value and quality
VI. Animal and plant protein vary in their composition of essential amino acids. Reciprocally, a combination of both sources of protein in a diet can be complimentary and result in a higher biological value
VII. Cats are carnivores and have a higher protein requirement than dogs because they use a certain amount of protein for energy

Carbohydrates

I. Primary function is for energy. Carbohydrates provide 4 kcal/g, same as protein; however, there are no nitrogenous end products as in protein catabolism
II. Made up of carbon, hydrogen, and oxygen chains
III. Two categories, based on digestibility
   A. Soluble: digestible carbohydrates primarily composed of monosaccharides and disaccharides such as glucose and sugar beet. They supply calories to a diet and can be used immediately for energy
   B. Insoluble: indigestible carbohydrates, primarily composed of polysaccharides such as starch, lignin, and peanut hulls (fiber). The portion of a plant that resists digestion and can provide satiety and bulk to a diet
IV. Digested through the digestive tract. Often used in the management of constipation and diarrhea due to their ability to absorb water, stimulate intestinal contractions, and normalize intestinal transit time
V. Fiber and other insoluble carbohydrates aid in regulating blood glucose levels, which is often recommended in managing diabetes
VI. Fiber is also used in pet foods to increase bulk and promote satiety during periods of weight loss and weight control
VII. Body uses carbohydrates primarily in the form of glucose. If not used, carbohydrates are stored as glycogen in the muscle or liver, or as body fat

Fats

I. Provide the most concentrated source of energy at 9 kcal/g of fat
II. Enhance palatability and caloric density of pet foods
III. Required by the fat soluble vitamins A, D, E, and K for absorption, transportation, and storage
IV. Essential Fatty Acid (EFA)
   A. The building blocks of fat
   B. Classified as saturated and unsaturated
      1. Saturated: long carbon chains without a double bond
      2. Unsaturated: One or more double bonds
   C. Essential for maintaining skin and coat
   D. Required for the synthesis of cell membranes, prostaglandins, and sex hormones
   E. Three EFAs are required for normal metabolism
      1. Linoleic acid
      2. Arachidonic acid
      3. Linolenic acid
   F. Dogs require linoleic and linolenic acid in their diet. Although one can be reconstructed by the other, the body's ability to facilitate availability is a difficult pathway; therefore, both are deemed as essential

G. Cats require dietary linoleic and arachadonic acid

V. Important in temperature regulation, protection of internal organs, and facilitates immune function

VI. Fatty acid deficiency could result in dermatological problems as well as impair wound healing

VII. Increased dietary fat requirements usually occur during periods of growth, lactation, or increased physical activity

VIII. Excess fat consumption could result in weight gain or obesity if not monitored, as well as diarrhea or steatorrhea (fatty stools) due to the body's inability to digest or absorb excess fat

NONENERGY PRODUCING NUTRIENTS ▬▬▬▬

Water

I. The most essential nutrient required by the body for survival. It is needed for almost all body metabolic processes

II. Total daily water requirements equal daily energy requirements in a thermoneutral environment

III. Requirements will vary depending on factors such as environmental temperature, physical activity, metabolism, diet, lactation, and illness

IV. Water comprises approximately 70% of adult body weight

V. Grave illness or death could result if as little as 10% of body water is lost

VI. Essential for absorption of water soluble vitamins B-complex and C

VII. Animals obtain water from metabolic processes or more importantly through ingestion by drinking or eating

VIII. Quantity of water in pet foods varies
   A. Dry kibble: 10% to 12%
   B. Semimoist: 25% to 40%
   C. Canned: 72% to 82%

IX. Animals eating canned food appear to drink less water because they obtain a large portion of daily water requirements from their diet

X. Fresh water must be available at all times. This point must be emphasized to pet owners, especially for dogs housed outside in the winter where there is a risk of water freezing

Minerals

I. Although the total percent of minerals in the body is less than 1%, they are essential for metabolic processes to take place

II. Macrominerals
   A. Dietary requirements expressed in percentages (%)
   B. EXAMPLES: calcium, phosphorus, potassium, sodium, magnesium
   C. Aid in maintaining electrolyte and water balance, skeletal integrity, muscle and nerve conduction, and cellular function

III. Microminerals
   A. Dietary requirements expressed in parts-per-million (ppm)
   B. Also known as trace minerals
   C. EXAMPLES: iron, copper, zinc, iodine
   D. Involved in the majority of biochemical reactions in the body

IV. A close inter-relationship exists between minerals. Any excess of one or more minerals could result in the deficiency of others, due to lack of absorption or imbalance

V. Mineral supplementation is contraindicated if a high quality, balanced diet is provided

VI. Minerals have many functions; any deficiencies or excesses could be harmful to an animal, as shown in Table 24-1

Vitamins

I. Function as enzymes, coenzymes, and enzyme precursors

II. Classified by solubility
   A. Water-soluble
      1. B-complex and C
      2. Not stored in the body at all
      3. Deficiency may occur during periods of excessive water loss such as polyuria, diarrhea, or GI disorders that may alter microfloral populations. Supplementation is recommended during these periods
   B. Fat-soluble
      1. A, D, E, and K
      2. Stored in fat or liver
      3. Excesses could result in toxicity

III. Cats have specific vitamin requirements that dogs do not
   A. In their diet they require preformed vitamin A, which is found in the highest constituency in animal tissue
   B. Cats also require the B vitamin niacin because they cannot convert tryptophan, an amino acid, to niacin

IV. Dogs can convert beta-carotene derived from plant sources to vitamin A, which is a characteristic of omnivores; cats cannot

Table 24-1   Mineral functions and effects of deficiency and excess

Mineral	Function	Deficiency	Excess
Calcium	Constituent of bone and teeth, blood clotting, myocardial function, nerve transmission, membrane permeability	Decreased growth, decreased appetite, decreased bone mineralization, lameness, spontaneous fractures, loose teeth, tetany, convulsions, rickets (osteomalacia—adults)	Decreased feed efficiency, decreased feed intake, nephrosis, Ca urate stones, lameness, enlarged costochondral junctions
Phosphorus	Constituent of bone and teeth, muscle formation, fat, carbohydrates, and protein metabolism, phospholipids and energy production, reproduction	Depraved appetite, decreased feed efficiency, decreased growth, dull hair coat, decreased fertility, spontaneous fractures, rickets	Bone loss, urinary calculi, decreased weight gain, decreased feed intake, calcification of soft tissues, secondary hyperparathyroidism
Potassium	Muscle contractility, transmission of nerve impulses, acid-base balance, osmotic balance, enzyme cofactor (energy transfer)	Anorexia, decreased growth, lethargy, locomotive problems, hypokalemia, heart and kidney lesions, emaciation	Rare
Sodium and chloride	Osmotic pressure, acid-base balance, transmission of nerve impulses, nutrient uptake, waste excretion, water metabolism	Inability to maintain water balance, decreased growth, anorexia, fatigue, exhaustion, dryness/loss of hair	Occurs only if there is inadequate nonsaline, good quality water available. Causes thirst, pruritus, constipation, seizures, and death. Chronic amounts may induce hypertension resulting in increased heart and renal diseases
Magnesium	Component of bone, intracellular fluids, neuromuscular transmission, active component of several enzymes, carbohydrate and lipid metabolism	Muscular weakness, hyperirritability, convulsions, anorexia, vomiting, decreased mineralization of bone, decreased body weight, calcification of aorta	Urinary calculi
Iron	Enzyme constituent: activation of O_2 (oxidases, oxygenases), O_2 transport (hemoglobin, myoglobin)	Anemia, rough hair coat, listless, decreased growth	Anorexia, weight loss, decreased serum albumin

Courtesy Dr. Karen Wedekind, Mark Morris Institute.

Continued

Table 24-1 Mineral functions and effects of deficiency and excess—cont'd

Mineral	Function	Deficiency	Excess
Zinc	Constituent or activator of 200 known enzymes (nucleic acid metabolism, protein synthesis, carbohydrate metabolism), skin and wound healing, immune response, fetal development, growth rate	Anorexia, decreased growth, alopecia, parakeratosis, impaired reproduction, vomiting, hair depigmentation, conjunctivitis	Relatively atoxic. Reported cases of Zn toxicity from consumption of die-case Zn nuts.
Copper	Component of several enzymes (i.e., oxidases), catalyst in hemoglobin formation, cardiac function, cellular respiration, connective tissue development, pigmentation, bone formation, myelin formation, immune function	Anemia, decreased growth, hair depigmentation, bone lesions, neuromuscular, enzootic ataxia, aortic rupture, reproductive failure	Hepatitis, increased liver enzymes
Manganese	Component and activator of enzymes (glycosyl transferases), lipid and carbohydrate metabolism, bone development (organic matrix), reproduction, cell membrane integrity (mitochondria)	Impaired reproduction, perosis (poultry), fatty livers, crooked legs, decreased growth	Relatively atoxic.
Selenium	Constituent of glutathione peroxidase and iodothyronine 5'-deiodinase, immune function, reproduction	Muscular dystrophy, reproductive failure, decreased feed intake, subcutaneous edema, renal mineralization	Vomiting, spasms, staggered gait, salivation, decreased appetite, dyspnea, "garlicky" breath
Iodine	Constituent of thyroxine and triiodothyronine	Goiter, fetal resorption, rough hair coat, enlarged thyroid glands, alopecia, apathy, myxedema, lethargy	Similar to deficiency. Decreased appetite, listlessness, rough hair coat, decreased immunity, decreased weight gain, goiter, fever
Boron	Regulates parathormone action, therefore influences metabolism of Ca, P, Mg, and cholecalciferol	Decreased growth, decreased hematocrit, hemoglobin, and alkaline phosphatase	Similar to deficiency. 150-200 ppm maximum tolerated level
Chromium	Potentiates insulin action, therefore improves glucose tolerance	Impaired glucose tolerance, increased serum triglycerides and cholesterol	1000 mg/d is maximum tolerated level in cats; trivalent form less toxic than hexavalent,

V. Vitamin E also functions as an antioxidant but the amount decreases as the fat is oxidized

VI. Vitamin functions, deficiencies, and possible toxicities are described in Table 24-2

DAILY ENERGY REQUIREMENTS ▬▬▬▬▬▬

How much to feed is as important as what to feed—to ensure that an animal is getting the correct amount and type of food based on its age and lifestyle. Factors that could influence daily energy requirements include growth, lactation, stress, physical exertion, breed, environmental conditions, and age.

Feeding Methods

I. Free choice
   A. Food is available at all times and the animal determines when and how much to eat
   B. Advantages
      1. Good for pets that will eat to meet their energy requirements and don't over eat
      2. Recommended method during lactation
      3. Most convenient method for pet owners
   C. Disadvantages
      1. Difficult to monitor the pet's consumption and anorexia may not be noticed immediately
      2. May lead to obesity
      3. Nutritional excesses due to overeating
      4. Economics

II. Time-restricted meal feeding
   A. An unquantified amount of food is available for the pet for a certain period of time, usually anywhere from 10 to 30 minutes
   B. Ideal choice in a multipet household where different diets must be fed
   C. This method can be repeated more than once a day

III. Food-restricted meal feeding
   A. A specific quantity of food offered at specific times during the day
   B. Beneficial for animals that have any type of digestive disorder where small frequent meals are more tolerable
   C. Recommended method for canine breeds prone to gastric dilatation/volvulus (GDV) and diabetic pets
   D. Can still meet desirable growth with this method
   E. Best feeding method

Maintenance energy requirement (MER) calculations in Table 24-3 are intended for use as a starting point and should be adjusted as necessary based on body condition and lifestyle of the pet. Owners can follow the feeding guidelines on a pet food label as a starting point.

NUTRITIONAL REQUIREMENTS FOR EACH LIFE STAGE OF THE DOG AND CAT ▬▬▬▬▬

Nutritional requirements vary greatly between each life stage and proper nutrition will result in a happier, healthier pet over its lifetime.

Gestation and Lactation

I. Nutrition is as important before breeding as it is during gestation and lactation. Poor nutrition could result in low birth weight or increased risk of neonatal mortality

II. Nutritional requirements of a pregnant bitch or queen toward the end of gestation and during lactation are similar to a neonate. Refer to Table 24-5 for specific requirements

III. The period to begin transition to a high-quality, highly digestible growth diet should be during the last three to four weeks of gestation in the bitch and from the second week of gestation in the queen

IV. It is important to calculate maintenance energy requirements at this stage to ensure that adequate nutrients are being consumed, especially during lactation

V. Cats begin to gain weight in a linear fashion from the beginning of their pregnancy; dogs have the most weight gain during the last three to four weeks of gestation

VI. Offering small frequent meals is the method of choice for dogs; free-choice feeding is recommended for cats

VII. Due to their ability to store and utilize fat, cats tend to eat less postpartum but soon regain their appetite by the third week

VIII. Fresh water should be available at all times

IX. After weaning has occurred, the cat or dog should be gradually transitioned back to a good quality, highly digestible maintenance diet

Dogs
Young Dogs

I. Neonates and puppies
   A. Neonates should be encouraged to nurse vigorously after birth to ingest colostrum
   B. Colostrum is a special milk produced within the first 24 to 48 hours after parturition that contains maternal antibodies. It is vital for the neonate because it provides a passive immunity

Table 24-2 Vitamin functions and effects of deficiency and toxicity

Vitamin	Function	Deficiency	Toxicity
FAT SOLUBLE			
Vitamin A	Component of visual proteins: rhodopsin, iodopsin. Differentiation of epithelial cells, spermatogenesis, immune function, bone resorption	Anorexia, retarded growth, poor hair coat, weakness, xeropthalmia, nyctalopia, increased CSF pressure, aspermatogenesis, fetal resorption, keratomalacia. Requirement may increase in acute infection due to urine losses (dog)	Cervical spondylosis (cat), tooth loss (cat), retarded growth, anorexia, erythema, long bone fractures
Vitamin D	Calcium and phosphorus homeostasis, bone mineralization, bone resorption, insulin synthesis, immune function	Rickets, enlarged costochondral junctions, osteomalacia, osteoporosis	Hypercalcemia, calcinosis, anorexia, lameness, others
Vitamin E	Biological antioxidant, membrane integrity through free radical scavenging	Sterility (males), steatitis, dermatosis, immunodeficiency, anorexia, myopathy, encephalomalacia (chicks), cataract (rats), hemolysis (humans)	Minimally toxic, fat soluble vitamin antagonism, increased clotting time—reversed with vitamin K
Vitamin K	Carboxylation of clotting proteins II (prothrombin), VII, IX, X, and other proteins; C, S, Z, and M. Co-factor of the bone protein osteocalcin	Prolonged clotting time, hypoprothrombinemia, hemorrhage	Minimally toxic, anemia (dogs), none described for the cat
WATER SOLUBLE			
Thiamine (B$_1$)	Component of thiamine pyrophosphate (TPP), co-factor in decarboxylase enzyme reactions in the TCA cycle, nervous system	Anorexia, weight loss, ataxia, polyneuritis, ventral flexion (cats), paresis (dogs), cardiac hypertrophy (dogs), bradycardia	Decreased blood pressure, bradycardia, respiratory arrhythmia, none described for the cat
Riboflavin (B$_2$)	Component of flavin adenine dinucleotide (FAD) and flavin mononucleotide (FMN) coenzymes, electron transport in oxidase and dehydrogenase enzymes	Retarded growth, ataxia, collapse syndrome (dogs), dermatitis, purulent occular discharge, vomition, conjunctivitis, coma, corneal vascularization, bradycardia, fatty liver (cats)	Minimally toxic, none described for cats and dogs
Niacin (B$_3$)	Component of nicotinamide adenine dinucleotide (NAD) and nicotinamide adenine dinucleotide phosphate (NADP) coenzymes, hydrogen donor/acceptor in energy releasing dehydrogenase reactions	Anorexia, diarrhea, retarded growth, ulceration of soft palate and buccal mucosa, necrosis of the tongue (dogs), reddened ulcerated tongue (cats), cheilosis, uncontrolled drooling	Low toxicity, bloody feces, convulsions, death, none described for the cat

	Function	Deficiency	Toxicity
Pyridoxine (B$_6$)	Coenzyme in amino acid reactions: transaminases and decarboxylases, neurotransmitter synthesis, niacin synthesis from tryptophan, heme synthesis, taurine synthesis, carnitine synthesis	Anorexia, retarded growth, weight loss, microcytic hypochromic anemia, convulsive seizures, renal tubular atrophy, and deposits of calcium oxalate crystals (cats)	Low toxicity, anorexia, ataxia (dogs), none described for the cat
Pantothenic acid	Precursor to coenzyme A (CoA); Acyl group carriers; Protein, fat, and carbohydrate metabolism in the TCA cycle; Cholesterol synthesis; Triglyceride synthesis	Emaciation, fatty liver, depressed growth, decreased serum cholesterol and total lipids, tachycardia, coma, lowered antibody response	Toxicity is negligible, no toxicity established in dogs or cats
Folic acid	Tetrahydrofolic acid active form, methionine synthesis from homocysteine (vitamin B$_{12}$ dependent), purine synthesis, DNA synthesis	Anorexia, weight loss, glossitis, leukopenia, hypochromic anemia, increased clotting time, elevated plasma iron, megaloblastic anemia (cats), sulfa drugs interfere with gut synthesis, cancer drugs (methotrexate) are antogonistic	Nontoxic
Biotin	Component of 4 carboxylase enzymes: (1) pyruvate carboxylase, (2) acetyl CoA carboxylase, (3) propionyl CoA carboxylase, and (4) 3-methylcrotonyl CoA carboxylase	Hyperkeratosis; alopecia (cats); dry secretions around eyes, nose and mouth (cats); Hypersalivation; Anorexia; Bloody diarrhea	No toxicity established in dogs or cats
Cobalamin (B$_{12}$)	Coenzyme function in propionate metabolism, aids tetrahydrofolate containing enzymes in methionine synthesis; leucine synthesis/degredation	Uncomplicated deficiency not described for the dog, cessation of growth (cats), methmalonic aciduria	Altered reflexes—reduction in vascular conditioned reflexes and an exaggeration of unconditioned reflexes, none described for the cat
Ascorbic acid (C)	Synthesized from D-glucose in the liver, co-factor in hydroxylase enzyme reactions, synthesis of collagen proteins, synthesis of carnitine, enhances iron absorption, free radical scavenging antioxidant pro-oxidant functionality	Liver synthesis precludes dietary requirement: therefore, no deficiency symptoms described in normal cats and dogs	No toxicity established in dogs or cats
Choline	Component of phosphatidylcholine found in membranes, the neurotransmitter acetylcholine, methyl group donor	Fatty liver (puppies), increased blood prothrombin times, thymus atrophy, decreased growth rate, anorexia, perilobular infiltration of the liver (cats)	None described for cats and dogs
QUASIVITAMINS			
Carnitine	Synthesized from the amino acid lysine, transport of long chain fatty acids into the mitochondria for use in beta oxidation	Hyperlipidemia, cardiomyopathy, muscle asthenia	None described for cats and dogs

Courtesy Mr. Chris Cowell, Mark Morris Institute

Table 24-3 Calculations for maintenance energy requirements

RESTING ENERGY REQUIREMENTS (RER)
$70 \times \text{Weight (kg)}^{0.75}$

MAINTENANCE ENERGY REQUIREMENTS (MER)		
Canine Feeding Guide		
Puppies	<4 months of age	$3 \times$ RER
	>4 months of age	$2 \times$ RER
Adult		$1.6 \times$ RER
Senior		$1.4 \times$ RER
Weight prevention		$1.4 \times$ RER
Weight loss		$1.0 \times$ RER
Gestation (last 21 days)		$3 \times$ RER
Lactation		4 to 8 $\times$ RER
Feline Feeding Guide		
Kittens		$2.5 \times$ RER
Adult		$1.2 \times$ RER
Weight prevention		$1.0 \times$ RER
Weight loss		$0.8 \times$ RER

Courtesy Hill's Pet Nutrition, Inc.

C. After the crucial first 24 to 48 hours the bitch's milk begins to change and becomes more complete to provide all the nutrients that the growing neonate requires until weaning

D. Nursing should be observed at least four to six times a day

E. Milk provides all the essential nutrients for growth and the fluids consumed help to increase the body's total circulatory volume

F. Neonates should be weighed daily for the first two weeks to ensure adequate growth; normal stool should also be observed

G. Puppies should gain 2-4 grams/day/kg or 1-2 g/day/lb of anticipated adult body weight. Puppies not achieving this growth curve should be closely monitored

H. Commercial milk replacers are necessary only when supplementing weak or premature neonates, orphans, large litters, or when a dam is unable to produce sufficient milk

II. Weaning
A. Should begin at approximately three weeks of age but can be as early as 10 to 14 days if necessary

B. A commercially prepared high quality growth diet should be prepared by blending the diet with water to form a thick soupy gruel-type mixture. This should be offered three to four times a day

C. Initially, puppies will walk and play in the food but the nutritive properties will be gained as the pups lick and play with each other

D. Puppies should be totally weaned and be eating only a moistened dry or canned growth diet by five to seven weeks for large breeds and six to eight weeks for small breeds

E. Cow's milk should not be offered because the lactose content is greater than the bitch's milk and diarrhea and dehydration could result

III. Growth
A. A growth diet should be fed from weaning until the puppy achieves skeletal maturity or 12 months

B. Characteristics of a growth diet
1. Palatable
2. High digestibility, quality, and increased caloric density (this would decrease dietary consumption and stool volume)
3. Optimum calcium:phosphorous ratio, approximately 1.2:1

C. Maintenance energy requirements should be calculated for growth (see Table 24-3)

D. Puppies should be weighed and evaluated every two weeks, using body condition scoring as described in Table 24-4, which is the best way to determine whether the amount being offered is optimal. Pet behavior can be indication as well that more or less food is desired

E. Nutritional characteristics of a growth diet are found in Table 24-5

IV. Feeding large breed puppies
A. Most common problem is overfeeding and supplementation, which can result in increased incidence of obesity, hip dysplasia, and osteochondrosis

B. Excesses or deficiencies in a diet can affect musculoskeletal development

C. Calcium excesses could result:
1. With mineral supplementation. Calcium alone is often the offending mineral and not an imbalance with the calcium:phosphorous ratio
2. In the dog becoming hypophosphatemic as well as hypercalcemic
3. In retarded bone volume, retarded bone modeling, and cartilage maturation

Table 24-4 Body condition scoring

Body score 1 Very thin	Ribs are easily palpable with no fat cover. Tailbase* has a prominent raised bony structure with no tissue between skin and bone. Bone prominences are easily felt with no overlying fat. In animals over 6 months, there is a severe abdominal tuck when viewed from the side and an accentuated hourglass shape when viewed from above
Body score 2 Underweight	Ribs are easily palpable with minimal fat cover. Tailbase* has a raised bony structure with little tissue between skin and bone. Bony prominences are easily felt with minimal overlying fat. In animals over 6 months, there is an abdominal tuck when viewed from the side and marked hourglass shape when viewed from above
Body score 3 Ideal	Ribs are palpable with a slight fat cover. Tailbase* has a smooth contour or some thickening and bony structure is palpable under a thin layer of fat between skin and bone. Bony prominences are easily felt with a slight amount of overlying fat. In animals over 6 months, there is an abdominal tuck when viewed from the side and a well proportioned lumbar waist when viewed from above.
Body score 4 Overweight	Ribs are difficult to feel with moderate fat cover. Tailbase* has some thickening with moderate amounts of tissue between skin and bone. Bony structures can still be felt. Bony prominences are covered by a moderate layer of fat. In animals over 6 months, there is little or no abdominal tuck or waist when viewed from the side and the back is slightly broadened when viewed from above. Abdominal fat apron present in cats
Body score 5 Obese	Ribs are difficult to feel under a thick fat cover. Tailbase* appears thickened and is difficult to feel under a prominent layer of fat. Bony prominences are covered by a moderate to thick layer of fat. In animals over 6 months, there is a pendulous ventral bulge and no waist when viewed from the side. The back is markedly broadened when viewed from above. Marked abdominal fat apron present in cats

*Tailbase evaluation is done only in dogs.

D. Recommended levels of calcium are 1% to 1.6% on a dry matter basis

E. Vitamin D is required in large breed puppies because:
   1. It regulates calcium metabolism and aids in the absorption of calcium and phosphorous
   2. It increases bone cell activity

F. Food-restricted meal feeding is recommended for large breed puppies based on their MER

G. Precautions in feeding a poor quality, cheaper, lower caloric density growth diet could result in:
   1. Poor appearance
   2. Inferior development
   3. Increased incidence of disease
   4. Overeating in an effort to meet caloric needs
   5. Increase in risk of obesity
   6. Higher stool volume

H. The goal of feeding large breed puppies is to decrease the rate of growth but still reach the dog's genetic potential at maturity

Adult Dogs

I. Adult maintenance
   The life style of the adult dog will determine its nutritional needs.

A. Adulthood ranges from approximately one year to seven years, depending on size of the dog. Smaller breeds mature at an earlier age than larger breeds but they also age slower

B. Diet and feeding methods should be reviewed with the pet owner; body score condition should be recorded as the dog enters adulthood

C. Supplementing with treats or table scraps should be discouraged, or, if given, they should not exceed 10% of total energy requirements. Treats can be made from the regular diet as described in Table 24-6 but the quantity per feeding should be adjusted accordingly

II. Active adult dog

A. Dogs that require increased caloric energy such as hunting, working, show, and guide dogs, or toy breeds who eat small amounts of food frequently

B. Increasing a maintenance diet is not always sufficient, since caloric needs may surpass ability to consume the appropriate volume of food (known as bulk limiting)

C. Offering a highly digestible, calorically dense food that is higher in fat is recommended

D. If caloric demand is seasonal such as in hunting or field trial dogs, a transitional pe-

Table 24-5 Life stage nutritional requirements

CANINE									
*Diet Characteristics Recommended for Dog Foods**									
Life stage	Protein	Fat	Fiber	Calcium	Phosphorus	Sodium	Potassium	Magnesium	Energy
Adult maintenance	15-28	5-20	5 max	0.5-0.9	0.2-0.8	0.1-0.4	0.4-0.8	0.04-0.15	3.5-4.5
Growth/Reproduction	28-35	15-30	5 max	1.0-1.8	0.8-1.4	0.3-0.5	0.6-0.9	0.04-0.20	4.0-5.0
Large breed growth	28-35	8-15	10 max	0.9-1.2	0.8-1.2	0.3-0.5	0.6-0.9	0.04-0.20	3.5-4.0
Geriatric	15-20	5-15	10 max	0.5-0.9	0.2-0.6	0.1-0.3	0.4-0.8	0.04-0.15	3.5-4.5
Obese-prone adult	15-28	5-15	5-17	0.5-0.9	0.2-0.8	0.1-0.4	0.4-0.8	0.04-0.15	3.0-3.5
High energy	17-30	20 min	5 max	0.6-1.0	0.2-0.9	0.1-0.5	0.45-0.9	0.05-0.20	>4.5
AAFCO Nutrient Profiles For Dog Foods									
AAFCO Growth/ Reproduction	22 min	8 min		1-2.5	0.8-1.6	0.3 min	0.6 min	0.04-0.3	3.5-4.0
AAFCO Maintenance	18 min	5 min		0.6-2.5	0.5-1.6	0.06 min	0.6 min	0.04-0.3	3.5-4.0
Nutrient Levels of Common Commercial Dog Foods									
Average can popular (14)	46	30	1.6	2.1	1.6	1.1	1.1	0.12	
Average dry popular (17)	25	13	3.2	1.3	1.0	0.4	0.6	0.15	
Average dry premium (19)	25	16	3.4	1.2	0.9	0.4	0.7	0.11	
Average can premium (9)	29	17	2.7	0.9	0.8	0.4	0.8	0.10	
FELINE									
Diet Characteristics Recommended for Cat Foods†									
Life stage	Protein	Fat	Fiber	Calcium	Phosphorus	Sodium	Potassium	Magnesium	Energy
Adult maintenance	30-45	10-30	5 max	0.5-1.0	0.3-0.8	0.2-0.6	0.5-1.0	0.04-0.1	4.0-5.0
Growth/Reproduction	35-50	18-35	5 max	1.0-1.6	0.8-1.4	0.3-0.6	0.6-1.0	0.08-0.15	4.0-5.0
Obese-prone adult	30-45	8-17	5-15	0.5-1.0	0.3-0.8	0.2-0.6	0.5-1.0	0.04-0.1	3.3-3.8
Geriatric	30-45	10-25	10 max	0.6-1.0	0.3-0.7	0.2-0.5	0.6-1.0	0.05-0.1	3.5-4.5
AAFCO Nutrient Profiles For Cat Foods									
AAFCO growth/ Reproduction††	30 min	9 min		1.0 min	0.8 min	0.2 min	0.6 min	0.08 min	4.0-4.5
AAFCO Maintenance	26 min	9 min		0.6 min	0.5 min	0.2 min	0.6 min	0.04 min	4.0-4.5
Nutrient Levels of Common Commercial Cat Foods									
Average can popular (17)	54	26	1.2	1.7	1.4	1.1	1	0.11	
Average dry popular (12)	35	12	2.2	1.3	1.2	0.4	0.8	0.13	
Average dry premium (12)	35	17	2.6	1.1	0.9	0.4	0.7	0.09	
Average can premium (9)	47	27	2.4	0.9	0.9	0.3	0.9	0.07	

Courtesy Dr. Phil Roudebush, Mark Morris Institute.
*Nutrients are expressed as % dry matter. Energy is expressed as kcal ME per gram dry matter.
†Nutrient levels of commercial foods are based on averages of manufacturers published values or analyticals performed in December 1995.
††AAFCO nutrient profiles presume 3.5 kcal ME/g in dog food and 4.0 kcal/g in cat food. Levels should be corrected for higher energy density.

riod should take place anywhere from seven days to three weeks before the event, with any physical conditioning of the dog

E. Small frequent meals and fresh water should be offered to avoid dehydration, hypoglycemia, and binging due to hunger

Geriatric Dogs

I. Small breeds begin their geriatric years at about age 7; large and giant breeds begin around age 5
II. Visual and physiological changes begin to occur
   A. Decreased activity level
   B. Cataracts

Table 24-6 Homemade treats

CANNED FOOD
1. Cut canned food into bite sized pieces
2. Place in the microwave on high for 2-3 minutes or bake at 350° for approximately 25-30 minutes until desired texture
3. Allow to cool before offering to pet, or refrigerate

DRY FOOD
1. Grind kibbles into a flour
2. Mix enough water to form a dough and shape into cookies
3. Bake at 350° on cookie sheet for 25-30 minutes until crispy
4. Allow to cool; refrigerate unused portion

C. Greying muzzle

D. Internally, organs cannot tolerate nutrient excesses or deficiencies as before

III. Re-evaluate the dog's diet and life style with the pet owner. It is important that pet owners understand an aging pet's changing nutritional requirements

IV. Maintenance energy requirements should be recalculated for the geriatric patient (see Table 24-3)

V. Characteristics of a geriatric diet should include:
   A. Reduced fat and calories—to avoid weight gain
   B. Decreased sodium, protein, and phosphorous—reduces workload on the cardiovascular system and kidneys
   C. Increased EFA and zinc—for skin and coat
   D. Increased fiber—slows intestinal transit time, improves nutrient absorption, and regulates bowel movements
   E. Increased palatability and digestibility—due to decrease in olfactory senses and appetite

VI. Elevated protein quality is crucial when dietary protein restriction is recommended

VII. Owners should be encouraged to maintain a daily exercise regime to maintain muscle tone and circulation

VIII. Avoid supplementing with high sodium treats and high-fat table scraps

IX. Complete physical examination by the veterinarian should be performed, including oral cavity and dental examination, baseline biochemistry panel, and urinalysis to ensure proper functioning of the internal organs

Cats

Cats are true carnivores; they possess typical dietary characteristics of other carnivores.
   I. Protein requirements are much higher than for dogs because cats catabolize it for energy; omnivores use fats or carbohydrates primarily
   II. Require two amino acids: arginine and taurine
   III. Require EFA arachadonic acid because like other carnivores cats cannot convert it from linoleic acid
   IV. Require vitamins niacin, pyridoxine (vitamin B_6), and preformed vitamin A, of which the two former are found in animal tissue

Kittens

   I. Care and management for kittens is similar to care and management for puppies
   II. Kittens should be observed nursing vigorously after birth to ensure they receive colostrum
   III. They should be weighed daily for the first two weeks of life and should gain approximately 90 to 100 grams (3 oz.) per week, which basically means doubling their birth weight
   IV. Nutrient requirements of the kitten can be reviewed in Table 24-5
   V. A good quality highly digestible kitten food can be introduced at approximately three weeks of age (in the same fashion as puppies). Kittens may not accept the slurry, so offering canned or dry without water is acceptable
   VI. Kittens should be free-choice fed during growth
   VII. Kittens should be weaned between 8 to 10 weeks of age but not earlier than 6 weeks

Adult Cats

   I. Cats by nature are nibblers but their MER should be calculated and the appropriate amount be left available throughout the day or divided into frequent meals
   II. Providing a cat with a premium quality, highly digestible, calorically dense diet will reduce the risk of disease such as FLUTD
   III. It's important that cat owners understand the phrase "cats aren't born finicky, they are made finicky"
   IV. Consistency is important to avoid any type of behavioral problems or to prevent problems with a cat that is a finicky eater

Geriatric Cats

   I. Cats enter their senior years at approximately six years of age

Table 24-7 Some risk factors reported in cats with lower urinary tract disease

Factor	Comment
Age	Uncommon in cats younger than 1 year. Most common between 1 and 10 years, with peak between 2 and 6 years
Sex	Urethral obstruction most commonly in males. Males and females have a similar risk for nonobstructive forms of the disease
Neutering	Increased risk of disease in neutered males and females, regardless of age of neutering
Diet	Consumption of an increased proportion of dry food in the daily ration is associated with increased risk of disease
Feeding frequency	Increased frequency of feeding associated with increased risk of disease, regardless of diet
Excessive weight	Obesity associated with increased risk of disease
Water consumption	Decreased daily water consumption associated with increased risk for disease
Sedentary life style	Lazy cats at increased risk of disease
Spring or winter season	Seasonal variation implicated as a risk factor by some investigators, but not others
Indoor lifestyle	Cats using indoor litter boxes for micturation and defecation have increased risk for disease

Courtesy of Williams & Wilkins.

Table 24-8 Mineral composition of 6,335 feline uroliths evaluated by polarized light microscopy and x-ray diffraction methods

Predominant mineral type	Uroliths	
	Number	Prevalence (%)
Struvite	3413	53.9
Newberryite	16	0.3
Calcium oxalate	2037	37.2
Calcium phosphate	68	1.1
Urate	432	6.8
Cystine	22	0.3
Xanthine	9	0.1
Silica	0	0.0
Mixed*	118	1.9
Compound†	115	1.8
Matrix	106	1.7
Total	6336	105

*Urolith did not contain at least 70% of mineral type listed; no nucleus or shell detected.
†Uroliths contained an identifiable nucleus and one or more surrounding layers of a different mineral type.
Courtesy of Veterinary Practice Publishing Company and Hill's Pet Nutrition Proceedings on Geriatric Health and Nutrition, Orlando, Florida, 1996.

II. Less information is available about nutritional and physiological changes that occur in aging cats
III. Geriatric work-up should be done to verify organ function and oral health
IV. Most dietary recommendations for cats are based on research on rats, dogs, or humans
V. Lower urinary tract disease and urolithiasis is uncommon in geriatric cats. However, calcium oxalate urolithiasis is more common in older cats

VI. Nutritional requirements for geriatric felines can be viewed in Table 24-5

FELINE LOWER URINARY TRACT DISEASE (FLUTD)

This disease can be frustrating and potentially devastating for cat owners. Prevention is the most important information a veterinary technician can relay to owners.

I. One percent to six percent of feline cases seen in a veterinary hospital are reported to be due to FLUTD. Incidence of new cases is approximately 0.5% to 1.0% per year
II. The exact etiology of FLUTD has not yet been determined. Cause could be multifactorial but is commonly related to urolithiasis, viral urinary tract infections, or inherited, genital, or acquired disorders
III. Clinical signs often include:
   A. Dysuria
   B. Hematuria
   C. Pollakiuria
   D. Urethral obstruction
   E. Inappropriate urination (urinating outside the litter box)
   F. Frequent squatting in the litter box
   G. Loss of appetite
IV. Risk factors associated with FLUTD are described in Table 24-7
V. The importance of dietary management with follow-up urinalyses and radiographs must be emphasized to the cat owner to reduce risk of recurrence
VI. Incidence and mineral composition of the most common feline uroliths can be found in Table 24-8

OBESITY

A veterinary technician has a vital role in helping clients manage and understand obesity in cats. Client education is the key to successful management, and more importantly prevention, of this disease.

   I. Approximately 25% to 44% of companion animals are obese

  II. An obese animal is one who weighs greater than 15% of its ideal body weight

 III. The first objective in helping clients deal with this situation is making the pet owner aware that the dog or cat is obese

    A. The pet owner should also be aware of risk factors involved

      1. Risk factors can include diabetes mellitus, neoplasia, hypertension, dermatosis, bacterial and viral infections

 IV. In cats, obesity can increase the risk of feline hepatic lipidosis

  V. The veterinary technician can counsel the client about:

    A. Benefits of weight loss, including increased activity, health, longevity, and alertness of their companion animal

    B. Identifying any inappropriate feeding behavior that could have been the cause of obesity

    C. Modifying any inappropriate feeding behavior of the pet and the pet owner

    D. Obtaining entire household cooperation and understanding of the pet's situation. This should result in a successful weight loss program

 VI. Another goal of a weight loss program other than having the pet lose weight is to start the pet on an exercise regime that will improve cardiovascular conditioning and improve skeletal support

 VII. Goals should be realistic and achievable to be successful. Subgoals are recommended so that pet owners can visualize benefits of their hard work, providing reinforcement to continue until the goal weight is achieved

VIII. Before beginning any weight loss program for a pet a complete physical examination by the veterinarian should be performed to rule out any medical cause for the obesity. If any illness is identified, it should be treated before a weight loss program is initiated

 IX. Determine the ideal weight of the patient and the required kilocalories per day for the patient to achieve that weight. Calorie restriction should be approximately 60% to 70% of the pet's maintenance energy requirements (see Table 24-3)

   X. Ideal rate of weight loss

    A. Cats: 0.25 lb/week (115 g)

    B. Small dogs: 0.5 lb/week (230 g)

    C. Medium dogs: 1.0 lb/week (500 g)

    D. Large dogs: 1.5 lb/week (750 g)

  XI. Charting weight loss is a useful tool for clients to see the success of their efforts

 XII. Dogs should be weighed monthly; cats should be weighed bimonthly

XIII. Have scheduled weigh-in periods in your hospital

    A. Post a chart on all patients involved in a "weight loss" program

    B. Plan weekly meetings that allow pet owners to discuss with other owners how their pets are doing

    C. Competition tends to encourage pet owners to stick with the program and your recommendations

    D. Cat owners should be cautioned about too quick a weight loss because cats can develop hepatic lipidosis

 XIV. Feeding small frequent meals throughout the day reduces begging

  XV. Acceptable treats while on a reducing diet include ice cubes, ice chips, low-calorie vegetables such as carrots or celery, or taking a portion of the prescribed diet and making homemade treats as described in Table 24-6

 XVI. Recording a cat's or dog's body condition score throughout its life is the best way to prevent obesity or to identify it in a new client

CRITICAL CARE NUTRITION

The need for nutritional therapy is emerging as an important factor in treating critically ill patients

   I. Trauma, disease, sepsis, and stress will increase an animal's metabolism, therefore increasing its energy requirements

  II. Protein-energy malnutrition may affect depletion of energy stores, wound healing, and pulmonary, cardiovascular, and gastrointestinal function

 III. The body eats 24 hours a day whether the gut is fed or not

 IV. After a patient is identified as requiring nutritional therapy, the simplest method for administering it should be chosen

Enteral Nutrition

   I. Coaxing: warming the food, hand feeding, etc.

  II. Appetite stimulants: drugs

 III. Force feeding by syringe

IV. Orogastric intubation
V. Nasogastric/Nasoesophageal intubation
VI. Esophagostomy tube feeding
VII. Gastrostomy tube feeding
VIII. Enterostomy tube feeding

Parenteral Nutrition

I. Direct intravenous infusion with basic constituents of dextrose, crystalline amino acids, and lipid emulsion
II. Option if enteral unsuccessful or contraindicated

Calculating Illness Energy Requirements (IER)

I. MER is rarely met if pet is in a debilitated state
  A. Canine IER = 1.25-$1.50 \times$ MER
  B. Feline IER = 1.10-$1.25 \times$ MER
II. If the diet chosen is tolerated, the product should be introduced gradually
  A. Suggested guidelines
    1. One third total calories on day one
    2. Two thirds of the total on day two
    3. Total calories on day three
  B. If human products are used, nutritional supplementation is required

HOW TO CHOOSE A PET FOOD ▄▄▄▄▄

I. Pet owners often seek knowledge and guidance from a member of the veterinary health care team about the best diet for their companion animal
II. It is important to be familiar with premium pet foods sold in the area, as well as products sold or endorsed by the hospital
III. Remember that the pet food label will never give a true reflection of the quality or nutritional value of its contents
IV. Calculating the daily feeding cost (Table 24-9) is beneficial when comparing a poor quality, low density product versus a premium calorically dense product. Often the cost per day is less on the premium food and the food lasts longer because of the caloric density and digestibility

PET FOOD ▄▄▄▄▄
Pet Food Label

I. A pet food label should include:
  A. Product name
  B. Designation: cat or dog food
  C. Net weight
  D. Name and address of manufacturer
  E. Guaranteed analysis
  F. Ingredient panel
  G. Nutritional adequacy statement or purpose of product

Table 24-9 Calculating daily feeding costs

Step	Description	Diet A	Diet B
A	Cost per 40 lb. bag (640 oz)	$16.00	$31.50
B	Cost per pound of diet (A/40)	$0.40	$0.79
C	Cost per ounce (B/16 oz)	$0.025	$0.49
D	Ounces/cup (by weighing one cup of food)	3.5 oz	3 oz
E	Feeding amounts in ounces/day (based on MER or feeding guide on bag)	17.5 oz (5 cups)	7.5 oz (2.5 cups)
F	Days bag will last (640 oz bag/E)	37	85
G	Cost per day (C × E)	$0.44	$0.37
H	Cost per year (G × 365 days)	$161.00	$135.00

  H. Feeding guidelines
  I. Date of manufacture or expiry code
II. In Canada, Consumer Packaging and Labelling Act and Regulations dictate that only product identity, product net quantity, dealer's name, and principal place of business be on the label
III. Regulated by the Food and Drug Administration, Department of Agriculture, U.S. law dictates that the following must be on the label: product name, designator, net weight, ingredients, guaranteed analysis, nutritional adequacy statement, feeding guide, manufacturer or distributor
IV. American Association of Feed Control Officials (AAFCO) is an association established by animal feed control officials as a regulating body to develop standards for uniformity of: definitions, policies for manufacturing, labeling, distribution, and sale of animal feeds
V. National Research Council (NRC) is a nonprofit organization that was the recognized authority for substantiation of pet food claims for nutrient requirements before 1990

Guaranteed Analysis (GA)

I. Provides minimum or maximum percentages of certain nutrients that the manufacturer claims the product meets
II. The following nutrients are required to be on the GA. Other nutrients added to the label are at the discretion of the manufacturer
  A. Crude protein—expressed as minimum %
  B. Crude fat—expressed as minimum %

C. Crude fiber—expressed as maximum %
D. Moisture—expressed as maximum %
III. Crude: term used to describe the analytical procedure used to estimate the nutrients
IV. Guaranteed analysis should not be used to compare products because values indicated do not reflect exact amounts but only minimums or maximums of a nutrient
V. The GA also includes the moisture content of the product; therefore the nutrient value indicated is diluted in moisture, so a canned food may appear to have a lower percent of nutrients than a dry product due to amount of water
VI. Dry weight analysis
A. Approximate percent of a nutrient based on dry matter of the product
B. Converting nutrients to dry matter allows for a more accurate comparison of products with different moisture levels (Table 24-10)
C. Manufacturers should provide nutrients listed on a dry matter basis (DMB) for comparison and accurate values

Ingredient Panel

I. Listed in descending order by weight, beginning with heaviest ingredient
II. Ingredients with a high water content will appear higher on the panel, even if they might be of poor nutrient value, than one with less water content
III. Terms used must be common in the feed industry or be assigned by AAFCO
IV. Manufactures can alter ingredients so that a more desirable ingredient will appear higher on the ingredient panel
V. The same ingredient may be described in various forms such as wheat being broken down into wheat middling, cracked wheat, whole wheat, flaked wheat. This can make an ingredient appear to be in smaller quantities in the diet even though when combined it forms a large percentage of the diet
VI. AAFCO determines what is meant by terms such as meat byproducts but it is difficult to know what ingredients were actually used unless one contacts the manufacturer directly. Meat byproduct could be anything such as liver, lungs, udders, or tongues
VII. The ingredient panel should not be used as a mode of comparison because two ingredient panels could be identical and there is no way to determine the quality or digestibility of the ingredients that each manufacturer uses

Table 24-10   How to calculate the dry weight analysis

Guaranteed analysis from can:
Water 75%
Protein 10%
Other dry matter 15%

Calculation of dry weight analysis:
1. Dry matter % = 100% − % moisture
= 100% − 75% = 25%
2. % Nutrient ÷ % dry matter × 100
EXAMPLE: Protein = 10/25 = 0.4 × 100 = 40% protein

Thus dry weight analysis is:
Protein 40%
Other dry matter 60%

VIII. Formulas can be fixed or variable
A. Fixed formula: every bag purchased has the same ingredients as the previous. Products in this category tend to be of higher quality, more expensive, and have more digestible ingredients
B. Variable formula: ingredients may change from batch to batch, based on ingredient availability and market price

Statement of Nutritional Adequacy

I. AAFCO established guidelines that U.S. manufactures attempt to meet for nutrient profiles for cats and dogs (see Table 24-5)
II. "Complete and Balanced" refers to a diet that contains all essential nutrients in concentrations that are proportional to the energy density of the food
III. Nutritional adequacy statements are based on feeding trials such as AAFCO's or through a calculation method
IV. Veterinary technicians should recommend products that have undergone feeding trials
V. Statements about "meeting or exceeding" standards without feeding trials are based on a chemical analysis and do not verify the digestibility or true adequacy of a product
VI. Statements help determine if the product is for a specific purpose as in "complete and balanced for puppies" or all purpose as in "meets the requirements for the life of your cat." A product with the latter statement on it could have nutrient deficiencies or excesses for a particular life stage because it was formulated for every life stage
VII. Snacks, treats, and therapeutic diets do not require nutritional statements

Glossary

AAFCO American Association of Feeding Control Officials; the regulating body of pet food manufacturers in the United States

carbohydrate A nutrient that provides energy for body tissues

dry matter basis Describes nutrient amounts in percentages as found in the dry weight of a product when the moisture is removed

essential amino acids Amino acids the body requires through diet because it cannot manufacture them

Guaranteed analysis Describes nutrients in minimum or maximum percentages that a pet food manufacturer claims the product meets

ingredient A food that delivers nutrients to the body

MER Maintenance Energy Requirements; the estimated amount of calories required per day for maintenance of a particular life stage

nutrient A food characteristic that provides nourishment to the body

protein A nutrient composed of 23 amino acids

taurine An essential amino acid that only cats require in their diet

Review Questions

1 Energy producing nutrients are:
   a. Protein, fats, water
   b. Carbohydrates, fats, protein
   c. Fats, protein, vitamins
   d. Vitamins, minerals, water

2 Biological value
   a. Pertains to the value of carbohydrates in the diet
   b. Describes the quantity of plant and animal protein sources in a diet
   c. Evaluates protein usability by the body
   d. Pertains to the value of fat in the diet

3 Which nutrient aids in the management of diarrhea and constipation?
   a. Minerals
   b. Fat
   c. Water
   d. Carbohydrates

4 The maintenance energy requirements (MER) for an 8-month-old, 22 kg (48.5 lbs) mastiff is:
   a. 1460 kcal/day
   b. 740 kcal/day
   c. 2190 kcal/day
   d. 3140 kcal/day

5 Characteristics of a canine geriatric diet include:
   a. Low fiber and sodium and higher fat
   b. Decreased sodium and essential fatty acids
   c. Restricted protein, phosphorous, and increased fiber
   d. Increased fiber, calories, and restricted essential fatty acids

6 Possible clinical signs associated with FLUTD may include:
   a. Frequent defecation
   b. Increased hunger
   c. Weight gain
   d. Hematuria

7 An animal is considered obese when its weight exceeds what percent of its ideal weight?
   a. 5%
   b. 10%
   c. 15%
   d. 25%

8 Manufacturers are required to include which percentage of the following in the guaranteed analysis?
   a. Maximum crude protein and fat
   b. Minimum crude protein and fat
   c. Minimum minerals and ash
   d. Minimum crude fiber and moisture

9 A pet food claim that is formulated to meet the AAFCO cat food nutrient profile for growth and lactation means that the food:
   a. Also meets the nutrient profile for adult maintenance
   b. Meets NRC standards
   c. Has undergone AAFCO feeding trial testing growth and lactation
   d. Has been chemically analysed only to meet the standards

10 The best way to compare the actual nutrients of two pet food labels is by:
   a. Guaranteed analysis
   b. Ingredient panel
   c. Nutritional adequacy statement
   d. Dry weight analysis

BIBLIOGRAPHY

Allen TA, Roudebush P: Canine geriatric nephrology, *Compendium on continuing education for the practicing veterinarian* 12(7):909-917, 1990.

American Association of Feed Control Officials, Official Publication, Atlanta, Georgia, 1996.

Armstrong PJ: Enteral feeding of critically ill pets: the choices and techniques, *Veterinary Medicine,* 9:900-909, 1992.

Bartges JW: Lower urinary tract disease in older cats: what's common, what's not, *Proc. Health and Nutrition of Geriatric Cats and Dogs,* 1996.

Case LP, Carey DP, Hirakawa DA: *Canine and feline nutrition, a resource for companion animal professionals,* St. Louis, 1995, Mosby.

Chandler ML, Greco DS, Fettman MJ: Hypermetabolism in illness and injury, *The Compendium,* 14(10):1284-1289, 1992.

Codner EC, Thatcher CD: Nutritional management of skin disease, *The Compendium* 15(3):411-423, 1993.

Colgan M, Brune C: *Hill's health care connection,* Topeka, Kansas, 1995.

Ettinger SJ, Feldman EC: *Textbook of veterinary internal medicine,* vol 1, Ch. 55, Developmental Orthopedics: nutritional influences in the dog, Philadelphia, 1995, W.B. Saunders.

Ettinger SJ, Feldman EC: *Textbook of veterinary internal medicine,* vol 1, Ch. 55, Enteral and parenteral nutritional support, Philadelphia, 1995, W.B. Saunders.

Guide to the Consumer Packaging and Labelling Act and Regulations, Industry Canada, March 1994.

Hand MS, Armstrong PJ, Allen TA: Obesity: occurrence, treatment, and prevention, *Veterinary Clinics of North America* 19(3):447-474, 1989.

Hefferren JJ, Boyce E, Bresnahan J: Aging and oral health, *Proc. health and nutrition of geriatric cats and dogs,* 1996.

Hill's veterinary nutritional consultant program, Topeka, Kansas, 1991.

Kealy RD et al: Effects of limited food consumption on the incidence of hip dysplasia in growing dogs, *JAVMA* 201(6):857-863, 1992.

Lewis LD, Morris ML, Hand MS: *Small animal clinical nutrition* III, Topeka, 1987, Mark Morris Associates.

McCurnin DM: *Clinical Textbook for Veterinary Technicians,* ed 2, Philadelphia, 1994, W.B. Saunders.

Norris MP, Beaver BV: Application of behaviour therapy techniques to the treatment of obesity in companion animals *JAVMA,* 202(5):728-730, 1993.

Osborne CA et al: *Consultations in feline internal medicine,* Ch. 46, Feline lower urinary tract disease: relationships between crystalluria, urinary tract infection, and host factors, Philadelphia, 1994, W.B. Saunders.

Osborne CA et al: Feline lower urinary tract disease: state of the science, Proceedings of 16th Waltham/OSU Symposium.

Osborne CA, Finco DR: *Canine and feline nephrology and urology,* Pennsylvania, 1995, William & Wilkins.

Remillard RL: Clinical aspects of nutrition, AAHA Proc., 1994.

Roudebush P: How to read and interpret pet food labels, Proc. 9th ACVIM Forum, New Orleans, May 1991.

Tennant B, Willoughby K: The use of enteral nutrition in small animal medicine, *The Compendium* 15(8):1054-1068, 1993.

Twedt DC: Dietary fiber in gastrointestinal disease, Proc. 11th ACVIM Forum, Washington, May 1993.

White PD: Essential fatty acids: use in management of canine atopy, *The Compendium,* 3:451-457, 1993.

Large Animal Nutrition and Feeding

Sandy Hass

OUTLINE

Feeding Dairy and Beef Cattle
  Feeding Factors
  Ruminant Digestion
  Nutrients
  Feeds Available
  Life Stages
Feeding Sheep and Goat
  Nutrients

Feeds Available
Life Stages
Feeding Swine
  Environmental Factors
  Nutrients
  Preparation and Feeding of Grains
  Life Stages

Feeding Equine
  Feed Sources
  Nutrients
  Life Stages

LEARNING OBJECTIVES

After reading this chapter you should be able to:

1. Understand the importance of nutrients in feeding large animals.
2. Differentiate the basic requirements of animals in their various life stages.
3. Learn the effects that environment has on nutrient requirements.

Improper nutrition can be related to as much as 90% of animal health related disease in large animals. Reasons for this include inadequate training, improper emphasis on prevention and prophylaxis, and lack of consultation by owners. It is advantageous for the veterinary team to combine preventive feeding with herd health. The increased requirements for growth, breeding, and lactation are different from maintenance levels. Ration formulation, a science best left to specially trained individuals in that field, is not covered in this unit.

FEEDING DAIRY AND BEEF CATTLE

Feeding Factors

   I. Environmental differences
     A. Temperature variations
       1. Cold stress requires more energy
       2. Warmer temperatures decrease appetite
     B. Wind, precipitation, sun exposure
     C. Consult district agrologist for specific area requirements
  II. Location concerns
     A. Industrial leaching and increased population will affect feed quality
       1. Feed tests provide valuable information
       2. Consult the nutritionist and use services of the district agrologist for specific area requirements

Ruminant Digestion

   I. Cattle, sheep, and goats are ruminants
  II. Ruminants are herbivores with a diet composed mainly of plants with high fiber (cellulose) content
 III. Ruminants can convert forage unfit for direct human consumption into a consumable product
     A. Accomplished through symbiotic relationship with bacteria, fungi, and protozoa

1. Byproducts of digestion are volatile fatty acids, methane, and CO_2 absorbed by the host and used for energy, amino acids, and vitamins

IV. The stomach is composed of four chambers: reticulum, rumen, and omasum, which make up the forestomach, and the abomasum
  A. **Reticulum:** "honeycomb" forces fluid material into the rumen
  B. **Rumen:** main fermentation vat; microbial products available for digestion and absorption
  C. **Omasum:** filled with laminae or "leaves" to squeeze fluid out of the ingesta and grind solids
  D. **Abomasum:** true glandular stomach
    1. Corresponds to stomach of monogastrics
    2. Process of peptic digestion of proteins begins here

V. Sugars and starches (e.g., concentrates) are fermented more rapidly than cellulose (e.g., forages)

VI. Intraruminal pH is generally between 6 and 7.5, depending on the diet

VII. Conversion of protein, starches, and lipids by microorganisms results in nutrients for the host. Vitamins B and K are also synthesized by microorganisms

VIII. Microorganisms can utilize poor quality protein and nonprotein nitrogen (NPN) compounds such as urea for amino acids and energy
  A. Microbial protein passes into the abomasum and is similarly digested to other dietary protein
  B. Microbial protein can form a significant amount of ruminant dietary protein but the intake of NPN compounds should be carefully monitored
  C. Dietary fiber is required to keep the microbial fermentation chambers active

IX. With proper microbial population, ruminants require proper feed, appropriate feeding intervals (fermentation is continuous), regurgitation of cud (bolus of food), rechewing (remastication) and reswallowing (deglutition), continuous churning, eructation, outflow to the rest of the tract, and sufficient water

Nutrients

For further information on functions, effects, deficiency, and toxicity see Tables 24-1 and 24-2 in Chapter 24: Small Animal Nutrition. The essential nutrients for beef and dairy cattle are:

I. Proteins
  A. Contain nitrogen, sulfur, carbon, hydro-gen, and oxygen. Some also contain phosphorus
  B. Used for growth, reproduction, lactation, repair of body tissues, formation of enzymes, antibodies and certain hormones, and for energy
  C. Depending on life stage, protein quality may not be important. However, even though total protein intake may be adequate, digestible protein may be insufficient
  D. In order from highest to lowest percent of protein digestibility there are protein supplements, common grains, alfalfa hays and grass hays
    1. Highly digestible proteins are considered high in TDN (total digestible nutrients) and low in fiber
  E. Deficiencies may result in limited growth, decreased milk and reproduction, and possible depressed appetite with weight loss and unthriftiness
  F. Excesses may also affect reproduction

II. Vitamins
  A. Fat-soluble vitamins are A, D, E, and K
  B. Water-soluble vitamins include ascorbic acid and the B complex vitamins
    1. Ruminants require water-soluble vitamins when they are ill because of a reduced ability to synthesize them
  C. Fat-soluble vitamins are stored in the body in large amounts; therefore excess in one or more of them can result in a toxic effect
  D. Deficiency in any one of these vitamins can result in severe health problems
  E. Normal, healthy ruminants do not require a dietary source of vitamin B complex, C, and K because they are synthesized by the ruminal microflora or tissues
    1. If not enough Vitamin B_1 (thiamine) is produced, polioencephalomalasia will result
  F. Vitamin A deficiency may occur if limited or poor quality forages are fed. Deficiency signs include reproductive failure, night blindness, skin ailments, and weak offspring
  G. Vitamin E deficiency along with selenium may result in white muscle disease, especially in calves
  H. Sun cured hay is the only natural food with a high vitamin D content—the leafier the better
    1. An hour a day exposure to sunlight is sufficient to meet daily vitamin D needs

III. Minerals

A highly complex relationship exists among the minerals. It has been shown that calcium, iron, and copper can interfere with the metabolism of other minerals and nutrients. Minerals that are lacking in the diet can be forcefed by supplements combined with common salt. Other than for common salt, animals apparently do not have any ability to select needed minerals. Mineral blocks should be provided.

A. Calcium and phosphorus make up over 70% of the minerals in the body
  1. They are closely tied to vitamin D and the parathyroid gland
  2. Important for skeletal growth and bone strength
  3. A large excess of either interferes with absorption of the other
  4. High quality roughages, especially legumes, are high in calcium but often low in phosphorus
    a. Concentrate feeds used for dairy cattle are relatively deficient in calcium
    b. Common supplements are bone meal, defluorinated phosphates, and dicalcium phosphate
      (1) In Europe bonemeal has been considered a possible cause of "Mad Cow Disease"
  5. Generally, a Ca:P ratio of 1.4:1 to 2:1 should be provided by the total ration
  6. Low calcium levels may cause rickets in young animals and osteomalacia in adults
  7. Excess calcium during the late dry period may lead to milk fever (parturient paresis)
    a. The parathyroid gland becomes hyporesponsive and vitamin D is decreased
    b. Bone calcium reserves are then not readily available at onset of lactation

B. Sodium and chlorine
  1. Hydrochloric acid, a substance rich in chlorine, which is obtained from salt, is essential in the digestive processes
  2. Salt must always be supplied to animals in addition to the amounts contained in the usual well-balanced ration
  3. Good livestock management provides free access to salt at all times for ruminants and horses
  4. Increased salt intake results in increased water intake
  5. In severe deficiencies, animals may experience muscle cramps, weight loss, decrease in milk production, and rough hair coat
  6. Most animals can tolerate large excesses of salt if the water supply is adequate. If the water is contaminated with excess salt this can cause anorexia, weight loss, and eventually physical collapse

C. Iodine
  1. As a rule, iodine levels in the soil are sufficient to supply adequate amounts by means of vegetation
  2. If the soil is deficient in iodine, incorporate small amounts into the salt blocks
    a. Small amounts in the blocks do not cause any harm
  3. Low levels of iodine can cause goiter, hairlessness in the young, and retarded growth and maturity
    a. In some cases deficiency can be caused not by deficiency in the feeds but by thyroid function
  4. Toxicities include anorexia, coma, and death

D. Iron and copper
  1. Necessary for the formation of hemoglobin in red blood cells
    a. Copper is necessary for iron absorption
  2. In newborn calves there is usually a sufficient amount of both minerals stored in the liver to last until the calves start to eat other foods
  3. Milk is a poor source of iron and copper so care must be taken to ensure that there is no deficiency
    a. For young animals that are fed milk replacer, care must be taken to ensure that they have an adequate supply of forage free choice
    b. Calcium and phosphorous mineral supplements and meat and fish meals also contain high levels of iron
  4. Low levels of copper can cause achromatrichia (lack of pigmentation in the hair). Iron deficiencies can show reduced hemoglobin, listlessness, and pale mucous membranes

5. Copper toxicity may predispose an animal to anemia, decreased growth, and impaired reproduction

E. Magnesium

1. Magnesium is allied with calcium and phosphorus in the body
2. Care has to be taken to avoid a magnesium deficient diet
   a. Young calves can become deficient with a restricted milk diet
   b. A more common form is hypomagnesemic tetany (grass tetany), which occurs with beef cows during initial stages of lactation. This occurs if pastures or forages are low in magnesium
3. Lactating cows are more susceptible, though other stock can be afflicted
4. Magnesium deficient cattle exhibit anorexia and reduced dry matter digestibilities. Young stock may have defective bones and teeth
5. Toxicity is rare

F. Zinc

1. Necessary for the operation of certain enzyme functions such as protein synthesis and carbohydrate metabolism
2. A deficiency results in impaired growth, swollen feet, and dermatitis. The relation to calcium and phosphorus is important

G. Manganese

1. Requirements believed to be low
2. Rations containing high calcium and phosphorus increase the level of manganese needed
3. Deficiencies lead to degenerative reproductive failure in males and females, bone malformations, and deterioration of the central nervous system
4. Excess manganese can affect iron and copper levels

H. Cobalt

1. An essential part of the vitamin B_{12} molecule
2. Cobalt deficient soil occurs in many parts of the world
   a. Cattle grazing these areas will appear normal for several weeks or months
   b. As Vitamin B_{12} stores are depleted, physical signs include loss of weight, muscular wasting, and severe anemia

c. Legumes are generally higher in cobalt than forages
3. Signs of high toxic levels of cobalt: excessive urination, defection, and salivation

I. Selenium

1. An essential element in all livestock rations
2. Important interrelationship with vitamin E
3. Deficiencies in selenium are widespread due to the selenium status in the soil
   a. Causes white muscle disease, which is characterized by white muscle, weakness, heart failure, and paralysis
4. General signs of toxicity include loss of appetite, loss of tail hair, sloughing of hoofs, and eventual death

J. Molybdenum

1. Found in nearly all body cells and fluids
   a. Concentration is high in skeletal muscle
2. Requirements are not established
   a. Molybdenum and sulfur interfere with copper metabolism
3. Molybdenum excess can cause copper deficiency

IV. Water

A. Adequate water intake is essential for life
B. A loss of 10% of total water content seriously distresses the animal; a loss of 20% will cause death
C. It is essential to dissolve all food before it may be utilized by the body
   1. The waste product of the body is removed by water as urine and the refuse of the digestive tract cannot be removed until it has been softened by water
D. Except for very young calves, water should be offered free-choice
E. Because of ruminal fermentation, cattle need two to three times more water per day than horses
   1. A cow at peak lactation may need up to 45 gallons (180 L) per day, depending on various factors
      a. Dairy cows require 3 to 5 gallons (12-20 L) of water to produce 1 gallon (4.5 L) of milk

V. Energy
   A. Measured as a calorie, or a joule
      1. One calorie equals approximately 4.184 joules
      2. This is the approximate amount of heat required to raise the temperature of 1 g of water from 16.5° C to 17.5° C (60° F to 63.5° F)
   B. Kilogram calorie and megacalorie are mostly used with animal feeding standards
   C. Energy requirements for maintenance, breeding, growth, etc. differ
   D. Formulas are available for measuring energy of feedstuffs

Feeds Available

I. Roughages or forages include pastures, range plants, plants fed green, silages and dry forages such as hay (alfalfa, brome, timothy, native grasses, etc.), and straw
   A. Forages generally have large amounts of fiber, low TDN (total digestible nutrients) and energy density, and high bulk (low weight per unit volume)
      1. This is due to the plant cell wall material of cellulose, hemicellulose, lignin, and other compounds
   B. Protein content depends on the type of plant and stage at harvesting
      1. The more mature the plant, the greater the fiber content but there is less protein, energy, and digestibility
   C. Hays are divided into legumes (such as alfalfa, clover, birdsfoot trefoil) and grass (such as timothy, brome, sorghum, blue grass, native grasses)
      1. Legumes have higher protein content than grass hays
      2. Some legumes such as alfalfa and clover may cause bloat in cattle
      3. Hay quality is determined by:
         a. The mixture of grasses (e.g., brome, alfalfa or bluegrass, and clover)
         b. The stage of maturity when cut
         c. Method and speed of harvesting
         d. Spoilage and loss during feeding and storing
   D. Silage is roughage that is preserved by ensiling
      1. The most common silages are corn silages and grass or legume silages (also called haylage, which is an example of low moisture silage)
      2. Silage with a water content of 55% to 75% has the least loss of nutrients from harvesting and storage

II. Concentrates or cereal grains include corn, barley, wheat, oats, and screenings (left over from grain processing)
   A. The way a grain is processed affects its digestibility
   B. Concentrates are fed primarily for energy and/or protein
   C. Grains contain 60% to 80% starch
   D. Fats and oils of plant or animal origin have 2.25 greater energy density than carbohydrates
   E. Corn is the most common grain
   F. Other than cereal grains, molasses, root crops, and milling byproducts can also be used as energy concentrates

III. Any concentrates that are more than 20% crude protein are classified as protein supplements

Life Stages

I. Nutrient requirements for maintenance of beef and dairy animals
   A. Maintenance requirements relate to an area where there is no loss or gain in body energy

II. Nutrient requirements of pregnant and lactating beef and dairy animals
   A. Factors to consider before a ration is developed include availability, quality, and cost of feedstuffs
   B. The energy source is the most important part of the ration
      1. Until the energy requirement is met, protein, minerals, and vitamins may not be well utilized
   C. Cow size does not seem to have much effect on the efficiency of milk production so it is more important to feed cows on the basis of their potential
      1. Referred to as challenge feeding
   D. Judge individual cow or heifer requirements by body score
      1. A condition of 3 is desirable prior to calving to help with the birth and the subsequent rebreeding (see Table 25-1)
   E. It is desirable that in the last trimester the cow gain an equal amount of weight to what will be lost at calving
   F. Fat is as undesirable as underweight because cows may be predisposed to ketosis, along with other problems

Table 25-1 Body condition scoring classification for livestock

Body condition scoring scale*			Generalized animal description†
1.0	1	Emaciated	All bones obviously protruding; no subcutaneous fat is evident
1.5	2	Very thin	Bones visible and easily palpated; minimal subcutaneous fat
2.0	3	Thin	Thin, flat musculature; prominent ribs, pelvic bones, and spinal processes
2.5	4	Moderately thin	Minimal subcutaneous fat; individual ribs not obvious
3.0	5	Moderate	Smooth musculature; bones not visible but palpable
3.5	6	Moderate fleshy	Fat palpable; soft fat over ribs and covering pelvis
4.0	7	Fleshy	Fat visible; ribs difficult to palpate; rounded appearance to pelvis
4.5	8	Fat	Thick neck; ribs difficult to palpate; rounded appearance to pelvis
5.0	9	Grossly obese	Bulging fat all over; patchy pads around tailhead

Reprinted from Grosdidier SR et al: Nutrition. In Pratt PW, editor: *Principles and practice of Veterinary Technology,* St. Louis. 1998, Mosby.
*The body condition scoring scale used depends on the species. Dairy cattle, sheep, pigs, and goats are generally scored on a scale of 1 to 5. Beef cattle and horses are usually scored on a scale of 1 to 9.
†Base the body condition score on the amount or lack of fatty tissue over the neck, ribs, spine, and pelvis without reference to body weight and frame size.

G. The last trimester and lactation are the most important stages, with lactation often exerting the most severe strain

H. Beef cows can utilize poor quality forage fairly well, if they are supplemented to meet nutrient requirements for the stage of pregnancy
   1. In cow-calf management systems, cows produce calves that form part of the breeding herd or are sent to feedlots
      a. They are usually fed forages with supplements as needed

I. The same considerations apply for pregnant dairy cattle, especially during lactation
   1. Cows in good condition fed good quality hay or pasture require no extra concentrates until two weeks before calving
   2. For lactating cattle a fully balanced ration with the proper dry matter intake (DMI) is essential for optimum milk production
      a. Greatest energy is supplied by the concentrate but a proper proportion is important to prevent overweight, digestive problems, and decreased milk production
      b. The cow's body type and ability to achieve maximum milk production are considered
      c. Generally dairies use good quality forages and grains at the correct mixture to achieve the best production that they can without losing body condition on the cow

III. Feeding replacement/breeding animals
   A. Replacement animals are those used in the breeding herd after they come of age
   B. Calving females will still be growing at the time of first parturition
   C. Energy intake of breeding animals, males and females, should be controlled so they will not become too fat
   D. Beef calves should be 'creep fed,' which is feeding small amounts of grain in a location that the dam cannot get to
      1. This aids in lowering weaning stress and enables the calves to start to digest food stuff they will be eating in their post weaning life stage
      2. Beef calves are usually weaned at six to eight months
      3. Creep fed calves will generally show a 50 lb. (22.5 kg) weight advantage at weaning
   E. Dairy calves should be pail or bottle fed milk until at least one month of age
      1. A good quality calf starter ration and hay should be fed to encourage rumination while receiving milk
      2. Longer periods (up to two months) of liquid feeding may be beneficial under some conditions because it results in decreased disease and death loss
      3. Proper sanitation of pails and bottles is important to prevent scours
   F. Forages and concentrates should be fed in large enough amounts to ensure continuous growth

IV. Animals fed for consumption
   A. Slaughter usually occurs between 13 and 18 months of age
   B. Beef animals not raised as breeding stock can be fed two ways

1. Weaned calves can be "backgrounded." The calves are fed enough feed to gain between 1 and 1.5 pounds (0.75 to 1 kg) a day through the winter and fed on pasture through the summer as yearlings
   a. Then they are slowly fed a ration increasing in grain until they are butcher weight
2. Weaned calves can also be put directly on a ration increasing in grain until slaughtered
   a. This is usually done in a feedlot, although some ranchers keep them on the range
   b. Feedlots usually hire a nutritionist for ration consulting; ranchers will sometimes use whatever feed is readily available and not necessarily in the correct amounts
3. Weather (drought) and availability of feedstuffs are factors to consider in choosing which method is best for feeding beef calves
4. Economics is the overriding factor in this decision

V. Nonbreeding dairy calves
   A. Can be raised as "dairy beef": usually not pastured and fed a ration in a feedlot to finish operation
   B. Can be fed as veal: fed a total liquid diet to keep the meat low in hemoglobin so that it stays a white color (anemia)

There is no "magic" amount of food that can be calculated to feed each life stage of the bovine. Nutritionists factor quality and type of food and available nutrient levels into the ration for each cow in the herd. This has to be done by calculation using some of the terms listed in the glossary.

FEEDING SHEEP AND GOAT

The number of veterinarians in sheep practice are few; there are less sheep than cattle and their value is considerably less. Goats are becoming more popular as a source of meat and milk. Sheep and wool or meat goats are managed similarly to beef cattle. Dairy goats are managed more intensely because of high nutritional requirements for milk production.

I. Adequate nutrition is important for the economical soundness of sheep and goat rearing. As with cattle, definitions for nutritional requirements in all life stages can be difficult because of the wide variety of environmental conditions in which sheep and goats are maintained

A. Different stages include:
   1. Increased lamb and kid crop
   2. Continuous and rapid growth of lambs and kids
   3. Heavy weaning weights
   4. Heavy fleece weights
   5. Milk production

Nutrients

An adequate diet should include water and feeds containing energy, proteins, minerals, and vitamins.

I. Water
   A. Ad lib for mature animals
      1. Generally drink 1 to 1.5 gallons (4.5-6 L) per day
   B. One half gallon (2 L) per day for fattening lambs and kids
II. Energy
   A. Requirements are greater 8 to 10 weeks after start of lactation
   B. This requirement must be met with a good grain source and high quality forage for lactation
III. Protein
   A. Good quality pasture and forage will usually provide adequate protein
   B. Sheep do not digest poor quality proteins as well as cattle
   C. Sometimes a supplement is indicated
IV. Minerals
   A. Include sodium, chlorine, calcium, phosphorus, magnesium, sulfur, potassium, and the trace minerals: cobalt, copper, iodine, iron, manganese, molybdenum, zinc, and selenium
      1. Salt
         a. Best fed free choice
         b. Adults will consume 10 g of salt daily
         c. Salt is important for general thriftiness
      2. Calcium and phosphorus
         a. Legumes and high quality forage are high in calcium
         b. Phosphorus availability is influenced by content in the soil
         c. Mature brown summer forage and winter range can be deficient in phosphorus
         d. A deficiency in calcium can occur on high grain diets (e.g., corn silage)
         e. Phosphorus deficiency results in slow growth, poor appetite, and unthriftiness in young animals. In lactating

animals, milk production declines, bones become fragile, and feed intake is poor

 f. Calcium deficiencies are more rare but can be corrected with the addition of limestone to the feed

 g. Phosphorus deficiencies can be corrected with a phosphorus supplement

3. Iodine

 a. Deficiencies can be prevented by feeding stabilized iodized salt

 b. Most important in pregnant animals

4. Cobalt

 a. Feed with the trace mineralized salt

 b. Deficiency develops rapidly because very little is stored

 c. Deficiency shows up as anemia, loss of appetite, retarded growth, general emaciation, rough hair coat, and a loss of milk production

5. Copper

 a. Pregnant animals require 5 mg of copper daily

 b. Molybdenum and inorganic sulfates can affect copper absorption

 c. Signs of deficiency include anemia, brittle or fragile bones, loss of wool or hair pigment

 d. A balance of sulfates will generally correct a deficiency problem

 e. Copper can be added to the trace mineralized salt

 f. Sheep are susceptible to copper toxicity

6. Selenium

 a. Levels vary in soil

 b. Supplementation can be provided by injections, oral feeding, or adding to trace mineralized salt

 c. Deficiency can cause nutritional muscular dystrophy and white muscle disease in lambs

 d. Toxicity results in loss of appetite, loss of hair, sloughing of hoofs, and eventual death

7. Zinc

 a. Higher levels are required for normal testicular development

 b. High calcium intake increases the need for zinc

 c. Deficiency signs: slipping of wool, swelling and lesions around hooves and eyes, excessive salivation, anorexia, wool-eating, general listlessness, and reduction of growth

 d. Zinc can be added to trace mineralized salt

V. Vitamins

 A. Vitamin A

  1. Very low levels are present at birth

  2. If dams are deficient, young may be born dead or so weak they die within a few days; females may abort during the latter stage of pregnancy

  3. Injury to the optic nerve may occur in growing animals, cerebrospinal fluid pressure is elevated, and a staggering gait may develop

  4. Immediate action is required in the form of vitamin A injections and a corrective diet

 B. Vitamin D

  1. Essential for the absorption of calcium and phosphorus

  2. Deficiency leads to swollen leg joints and beaded ribs (rickets)

  3. Deficiency is extremely rare because vitamin D requirements are met by 1 to 2 hours of sunlight a day

 C. Vitamin E

  1. Oxidation rapidly destroys vitamin E

  2. Old hay or ground grain are poor sources

  3. Deficiency is recognized as a common cause of white muscle disease

  4. This vitamin is of practical importance only to the young

  5. Vitamin E interacts with selenium

 D. Vitamin K

  1. Synthesized by rumen bacteria

  2. Becomes toxic in moldy sweet clover

 E. B complex vitamins

  1. Milk replacers should be fortified

  2. Deficiency may result if animal goes "off feed" for a long period of time

   (a) May become lethal rather rapidly

 F. Vitamin C

  1. Not required; ruminants synthesize their own vitamin C

Feeds Available

I. Good hay is a highly productive feed; poor hay, no matter how much is available, is suitable only for maintenance

II. Grains can include barley, oats, wheat, bran, beet pulp, soybean, and corn

Life Stages

I. Breeding and pregnant animals
   A. The period of weaning to breeding is critical because a high rate of twinning and milk production is desired
   B. Females should not be allowed to become excessively fat
   C. There should be a slight daily weight gain from weaning to breeding
   D. After mating, females can be maintained on good pasture
   E. During the last six to eight weeks of pregnancy, growth of the fetus is rapid, therefore nutrition should be increased gradually. This can be achieved by the addition of supplements

II. Lactating animals
   A. Good pasture is fine for grazers
      1. Dairy goats are browsers and should be offered high quality hay and a complete grain ration to maximize milk production
   B. If it is winter and the animal is confined, a good grain and forage ration with the addition of trace mineralized salts should be fed

III. Feeding lambs and kids
   A. Newborns nurse or are bottle fed colostrum and then milk or milk replacer for approximately two months
   B. At two weeks of age they should have free access to creep (ground coarse or rolled grain and hay)
   C. They should be creep fed until pasture comes available
   D. If they are not to be pastured they should be finished in a dry lot
   E. Slowly convert to whole grain in small amounts at first, then increase until the animal is on full feed
   F. In addition to grain, the animal is fed a complete diet of hay with a supplement
   G. Market weight is reached in three and one half to four months of age

IV. Orphan young
   A. Orphans should be raised on extra milk or milk replacers
   B. Ensure they receive the first colostrum
      1. Keep an extra supply of frozen colostrum for orphans
   C. Give water to drink in addition to the milk when they are put on creep at nine to ten days of age

   D. They can be weaned at four to five weeks of age if consumption of creep feed is at a reasonable level

Raising sheep and goats can be a relatively low maintenance operation if done properly; however, it is important to find the best feedstuff available in your area. Keep in mind that because of the size and constitutions of sheep and goats, deficiencies or toxicities can develop rather quickly—death loss can be high as a result.

FEEDING SWINE

I. Swine are omnivores and as such can accommodate some dietary fiber
II. Swine exhibit a better rate of gain from concentrates, which are fortified with energy, protein, and mineral and vitamin supplements to form the normal diet
III. Advanced technology is highly evident in many swine operations today
   A. Formulation of diets is more precise and economical with synthetic nutrients, high quality byproducts, and new feeds
   B. Swine operations use the technology of their feed supplier to meet nutritional needs of all pigs in the herd
   C. This is done by feeding a premix in their regular grain ration
   D. Nutrient deficiencies of these grains are corrected by the premix
   E. All life stages are met with different premix formulations

Environmental Factors

I. Stress conditions
II. Availability of nutrients
III. Variability in animals

Nutrients

I. Water
   A. Best given free-choice with easy access
II. Energy (chiefly carbohydrates and fat)
   A. Energy content in a diet controls the amount eaten
   B. Fiber corresponds directly with fat
   C. High energy diets are fed during lactation
III. Protein and amino acids
   A. Amino acids are essential for maintenance, growth, gestation, and lactation
   B. Amino acids indispensable for growing pigs are: arginine, histidine, isoleucine, leucine, lysine, methionine, phenylalanine, threonine, tryptophan, and valine

1. The three of greatest importance are lysine, tryptophan, and threonine

IV. Minerals
  A. Calcium and phosphorus
    1. Primarily for skeletal growth
    2. Play important metabolic roles in the body
    3. Adequacy is essential to gestation and lactation
    4. Easily supplied by usage of tankage, meat meal, meat and bone and fish meal, limestone, and oyster shell
  B. Sodium chloride
    1. Recommended salt allowance is 0.25% of the total diet
    2. Supplied by animal and fish byproducts in the diet
  C. Iodine
    1. Used by the thyroid gland to produce thyroxine
    2. Supplied as iodized salt
  D. Iron and copper
    1. Necessary for hemoglobin formation and to prevent nutritional anemia
    2. Milk is severely deficient in iron
    3. Iron can be fed to baby piglets orally but the preferred method is by IM injection. Sow's udder can be painted with iron
    4. Feeding lactating sows increased levels of iron does not seem to pass high enough levels to piglets
  E. Cobalt
    1. Present in the B_{12} molecule
  F. Manganese
    1. Essential for normal reproduction and growth
  G. Potassium
    1. Requirements are met in the feedstuffs
  H. Magnesium
    1. Essential for growing swine
  I. Zinc
    1. In swine nutrition zinc is interrelated with calcium
    2. Supplemented zinc is recommended to prevent parakeratosis
  J. Selenium
    1. Vitamin E is interrelated with selenium
    2. Selenium requirement depends on soil conditions where crop for feed is grown. Most swine today are raised in total confinement

V. Vitamins
  A. Vitamin A
    1. Use of stabilized vitamin A is common
    2. Natural vitamin A tends to get destroyed under normal environmental conditions
  B. Vitamin D
    1. Necessary for proper bone growth and ossification
    2. Vitamin D needs can be met by exposing pigs to direct sunlight for a short period of time each day
    3. Sources: irradiated yeast, sun-cured hays, activated plant or animal sterols, fish oils, vitamin A and D concentrates
  C. Vitamin E (tocopherol)
    1. Required by swine of all ages
    2. Interrelated with selenium
    3. Green forage, legume hays, and cereal grains all contain appreciable amounts of vitamin E
  D. Vitamin K
    1. An antihemorrhagic fat-soluble vitamin, necessary for blood clotting to convert fibrinogen to fibrin
    2. Supplement vitamin K for added insurance
  E. Thiamin, riboflavin, niacin
    1. Thiamin is not of practical importance in the diet
    2. Riboflavin is a requirement of breeding stock and lightweight pigs
      a. The crystalline form of riboflavin (and niacin) is added to premixes
    4. Riboflavin is naturally found in green forage, milk byproducts, brewer's yeast
    5. Natural sources of niacin include fish and animal byproducts
  F. Pantothenic acid
    1. Especially important for female (reproduction)
    2. Crystalline form is added in premixes
    3. Natural sources include green forage, legume meals, milk products, brewer's yeast
  G. Pyridoxine (vitamin B_6)
    1. Present in plentiful quantities in feed ingredients usually fed to swine
  H. Choline
    1. Essential for normal functioning of liver and kidneys
    2. Supplementing choline has shown to increase litter size

3. Naturally found in fish solubles, fish meal, soybean meal
I. Vitamin B$_{12}$
1. Required by the young pig for growth and normal hemopoiesis
2. Present in animal, marine, and milk products
3. The crystalline form is added to premixes
J. Biotin, folic acid, ascorbic acid
1. Biotin and folic acid are essential for growth
2. There is no evidence to indicate the need to supplement

Preparation and Feeding of Grains

I. Improvements in gain and feed efficiency can be expected from grinding grain but if grain is ground too fine digestive problems can be created
II. Grain should be reduced to a medium-fine particle size
III. Common grains are corn, oats, wheat, barley, and sorghum

Life Stages

I. Management of sows and litters
A. Preventing baby pig fatalities is a challenge in all pig operations
B. The more vigorous a baby pig is, the better its chance at survival. To produce healthy pigs, the gestation diets must be adequate in all nutrients
C. Sows are normally limit fed through gestation, with a return to appetite after she farrows. This controls constipation problems
D. Care should be taken that each piglet has nursed
E. Anemia prevention program should be in place
1. Injection of iron dextran immediately after birth
F. A palatable pig starter diet should be available from two weeks of age until weaning, usually between three and five weeks of age
II. Management of growing swine
A. Nutritional needs of growing-finishing pigs are best met by a program of full-feeding
B. Housing and space are very important aspects in growing swine

A veterinary technician's role in a swine facility involves herd health and piglet care. Nutritional needs and problems are met by the feed supplier with premixes and rations tailored to each individual operation and life stage of the pig.

FEEDING EQUINE

Horses are hindgut fermenters. The stomach has a relatively small capacity and contributes little to the digestion of the feed. Horses must eat frequently. Enzymatic digestion similar to dogs and cats occurs in the small intestine. Any ingested food that reaches the large intestine undergoes microbial fermentation. There is no gallbladder for storage and bile is excreted continuously.

Feed Sources

I. The equine consumes most of its nutritional requirements in the form of forages such as hay and pasture
A. Quality of dry roughage depends greatly on the stage of maturation at harvesting, and weather conditions during harvest
B. Soil quality also has an effect
C. Ensiled forage is not generally fed because of the sensitivity of horses to molds and mycotoxins that may be in silage
II. Ideal forages include grass hay (bromes and timothy), legume hay (alfalfa), and grazing pastures
A. Straw is not recommended as a feed because of its low nutritional value and the risk of compaction if too much is consumed
B. Hay and grasses contain variable amounts of cellulose and starch, depending on their maturity
C. It is important for horses that all forages are clean and dry with no mold or dust present, have good leafiness and lack of stems showing lack of excessive weathering, and that they also have a green color
III. Grains are used as a supplement to any forage feeding program
A. Amount of grain will be indicated by horse's life stage and or work load
B. Corn, barley, and oats are common grain supplements
C. Fat supplementation has been suggested to provide energy for growing, lactating, and working horses
D. Fermentable fiber byproducts such as rice, bran, and beet pulp are becoming more popular

Nutrients

I. Carbohydrates supply 80% to 90% of dietary energy for horses and are available in the forms of grains, forages, and supplements. The interaction of minerals and vitamins and their availability in the grains and grasses grown can be complex

II. Minerals and vitamins
  A. Maximum daily requirements of all minerals vary according to age, weight, and work of the horse
  B. Minerals and vitamins for the horse are essentially the same as for the bovine, listed at the beginning of the chapter
  C. If feedstuff is deficient in minerals, a mineral supplement may be fed free choice
    1. If a mineral deficiency is suspected, do not overlook the resources of the local diagnostic laboratory
    2. Any deficiency is often the result of anorexia or poor quality feed
  D. Over supplementation generally occurs inadvertently by well meaning owners
  E. For ease of definition for horse feeding, minerals can be divided into two groups: macro-minerals and micro-minerals
    1. Macro-minerals
      a. Macro-minerals are constituents of bones and structural proteins
      b. Expressed as parts per hundred
      c. Potassium: most forages have this available
      d. Calcium and phosphorus: for bone and cell function
        (1) Ratio is about 2:1
        (2) Deficiency can cause abnormal bone growth and thin weak bones. Mild deficiencies may cause subtle lameness
        (3) Excess calcium may impair trace mineral and phosphorus absorption. Excess phosphorus can cause nutritional secondary hyperparathyroidism
      e. Magnesium
        (1) Deficiency is very uncommon but if present will cause staggering, nervousness, and convulsions
      f. Sodium chloride (salt) is necessary for cell function and water balance
        (1) Salt is typically fed in a block
        (2) Horses lose 30 grains of salt in every pound of perspiration; working horses require additional salt in their grain rations
        (3) Salt added to a ration does not take care of the other minerals *if* the forage and grain is deficient
    2. Micro-minerals
      a. Referred to as trace minerals; Only small amounts needed by the horse
      b. Measured as parts per million (mg/kg)
      c. Iodine
        (1) Produces the hormone thyroxine, which is needed in fetal development
        (2) Deficiencies can cause serious fetal abnormalities
          (a) Foals will be born weak and prone to infections; may not suckle or stand; thyroid glands can be enlarged
          (b) Mares may have goiter, a longer gestation, and retained placenta
        (3) Excess can cause same symptoms as deficiency
      d. Copper
        (1) Important for cartilage, bone and pigment formation, and utilization of iron
      e. Iron
        (1) Necessary to form hemoglobin
        (2) A deficiency causes anemia
        (3) Overuse of iron injectable can cause iron toxicity
      f. Manganese and zinc
        (1) Zinc deficiency may cause hair loss and poor wound healing
        (2) Zinc excess can cause bone problems and lameness
      g. Selenium
        (1) Needed with vitamin E
        (2) Deficiency causes white muscle disease. Foals are born weak and unable to stand, suckle, or breathe normally. Mares have reduced fertility and increased incidence of retained placentas
        (3) Excess causes serious health problems. Overdose can cause sudden excitability and difficulty breathing. Chronic high intakes cause lameness, loss of mane or tail hair, and hoof deformity

III. Protein
    A. Feeding excess protein is wasteful. A strong ammonia odor exists in stables where horses are fed excess protein
        1. Alfalfa hay will cause stronger ammonia smell than grass hay due to increased nitrogen
    B. Protein deficient diets are very harmful
        1. Signs can be low weight gains or weight loss and skeletal stunting in young horses
IV. Water is vital
    A. The horse's body is made up of 70% water
    B. Horses drink 2 to 4 litres water/kg dry matter feed eaten (1 gal/2 lb of dry feed). A 1000 lb. horse fed hay will drink about 40 to 50 litres (10-12 gal) daily
    C. Intake also depends on size of horse, amount and type of diet fed, outdoor temperature, and amount of work being done

Life Stages

I. Feeding programs are based on:
    A. Age, depending on weanling, yearling, two-year old, mature adult, senior
    B. Current weight and ideal for age
    C. Function: idle, working, or breeding
    D. Feeds available in the area
    E. Management, including housing conditions and overcrowding
II. Feed consumption
    A. Weather is factor in amounts of feed consumed
    B. A proper horse feeding program provides adequate water and energy to ensure proper body condition (see Table 25-1)

C. Calculations are generally based on horse's weight and the amount of feed required per 100 lbs (45 kg) of horse
    1. An adult at maintenance requires about 1.2% body weight in dry matter of forage
    2. Energy for any increase in exercise is generally supplied by concentrates
    3. Pregnancy demands an increase in energy of 20% to 30%, depending on the stage
    4. Peak lactation may need 75% increase in energy
    5. Ribs should be felt but not seen in young horses

Consult the district agrologist for types of feeds and nutrient levels in your area. There are usually pamphlets available on the care and feeding of horses that pertains to the climate and area in which you are situated. All horses are individuals and feeding programs should stress that. The diet must be balanced for proteins, minerals, and vitamins.

Ruminant, swine, and equine feeding is a science that should be practically met whenever possible in agricultural operations. Large animal veterinarians that have a herd health practice will rely heavily on nutritional diagnosis. The importance of the technician is to be able to take accurate descriptions of feeding programs, know where discrepancies may occur, and know what mineral and vitamin deficiencies occur in the area. A technician in a large animal practice will have to answer questions regarding feeding programs and it helps to have some common knowledge of basic nutrition.

Table 25-2 Relative nutrient content of various feedstuffs for livestock

		Relative nutrient content					
			Minerals		Vitamins		
Feedstuff group	Protein	Energy	Macro	Micro	Fat-Sol.	B-complex	Fiber
High quality roughage	+++	++	++	++	+++	+	+++
Low quality roughage	+	+	+	+	−	−	++++
Cereal grains	++	+++	+	+	+	+	+
Grain millfeeds	++	++	++	++	+	++	++
Fats and oils	−	++++	−	−	−	−	−
Molasses	+	+++	++	++	−	+	−
Fermentation products	+++	++	+	++	−	++++	±
Oil seed proteins	+++	+++	++	++	+	++	+
Animal proteins	++++	+++	+++	+++	++	+++	+

Reprinted from Grosdidier SR et al: Nutrition. In Pratt PW, editor: *Principles and practice of veterinary technology,* St. Louis. 1998, Mosby.

Glossary

additive An ingredient or combination of ingredients added to the basic feed to fulfill a specific need

background Feed a calf to gain 1 to 1.5 pounds (½ to 1.2 kg) of weight a day

concentrates A classification of a feedstuff. Concentrate feeds include corn, milo, cotton seeds, barley, wheat, etc. Concentrates are feeds that are low in fiber. A concentrate is divided into two categories: protein or energy concentrates

digestible energy (DE) The gross energy of a food minus the energy lost in the feces. This measurement can have a tendency to overestimate the available energy of high-fiber feedstuffs. This is where TDN (a similar measurement) can be used

dry matter intake Percentage of dry matter that an animal consumes. A very important criterion for formulating rations

ensiling Harvesting process by which a forage is chopped and placed in a storage unit (e.g., silo) that excludes oxygen. Through fermenting, lactic acid is produced

feedlot Where a beef or dairy animal is fed to slaughter. Feed resources must be known to calculate a balanced ration

feedstuff Also called feed; any dietary component that provides some essential nutrient

gross energy (GE) Related to chemical composition. It has no real value in assessing feed but has to be used in determining the energy value of feedstuffs

legumes Leafy hay such as alfalfa, red and white clover, birdsfoot trefoil, and vetch

metabolizable energy (ME) A measure of the dietary energy available for metabolism after energy losses that occur in the urine (UE), and the combustible gases are subtracted from digestible energy. DE and ME are correlated

nutrient A substance that can be used as food

premix A total ration mixed with various feedstuffs at the feedmill

ration Amount of total feed provided to one animal over a 24-hour period for the desired productive purpose

replacement heifer A female calf placed in the breeding herd at 24 to 30 months of age when she has her first parturition

roughages or forages Consist of most or all of the plant such as pasture and hay

tankage The act or process of storing or putting in a tank; animal residues left after rendering fat in a slaughter house used for fertilizer or feed

total digestible nutrients (TDN) Attempts to measure digestible energy in weight units. The basis is rather simple: every feed has a total energy; after it has been through the animal, measure what comes out. What is left over is the TDN.

Review Questions

1 Geographical factors that affect nutrition and feeding in large animals are:
   a. Environment
   b. Temperature variations
   c. Wind, precipitation, sun exposure
   d. All of the above

2 The fermentation vat in ruminants is the:
   a. Omasum
   b. Abomasum
   c. Rumen and reticulum
   d. None of the above

3 Proteins are important for all of the following *except:*
   a. Growth and reproduction
   b. Lactation
   c. Prevention of digestive problems
   d. Repair of body tissues

4 The purpose of creep feeding is to:
   a. Allow young access to grain that the dams are denied
   b. Allow dams access to grain that the young are denied
   c. Increase ovulation before breeding
   d. Improve lactation capacity of dairy cattle

5 Vitamin A deficiency in cattle results in all *except:*
   a. Rickets
   b. Reproductive failure
   c. Night blindness
   d. Poor hair coat

6 A mineral that should be provided as free access for ruminants and cattle is:
   a. Copper
   b. Calcium and phosphorus combination
   c. Salt
   d. Manganese

7 The greatest energy demand for most species occurs during:
   a. First trimester of pregnancy
   b. Last trimester of pregnancy
   c. Peak lactation
   d. Growth as a yearling

8 Ruminants do not require:
   a. Vitamins B, C, and K
   b. Vitamins A, D, E, and K
   c. Vitamins A, B, and C
   d. A source of protein

9 An injection given routinely to piglets at birth is:
   a. Seven-way clostridial injection
   b. Iron
   c. Vitamins A, D, and E
   d. Selenium

10 Suitable feed sources for horses are:
   a. NPN source of protein
   b. Hay and grasses
   c. Barley
   d. Molasses

11 Carbohydrates supply what percent of the dietary energy in the equine?
a. 80%-90%
b. 60%-70%
c. 50%-60%
d. 10%-20%

12 Examples of macro-minerals that are required in equine feeding include:
a. Magnesium, iodine, and selenium
b. Sodium, chloride, magnesium, and selenium
c. Magnesium, calcium, and potassium
d. Zinc, copper, and maganese

BIBLIOGRAPHY

Baker, Greer: *Animal health: a layman's guide to disease control*

Church D: *Livestock feeds and feeding,* Oregon, 1977, Schultz/Wack/Weir.

Grosdidier SR et al: Nutrition. In Pratt PW, editor: *Principles and practices of veterinary technology,* St. Louis, 1998, Mosby.

McCurnin D: *Clinical textbook for veterinary technicians,* Philadelphia, 1994, W.B. Saunders.

Merck veterinary manual: Rathway, New Jersey 1986, Merck and Company Inc.

National Research Council: *Nutrient requirements of beef cattle,* ed 7, Washington, DC, 1996, National Academy Press.

National Research Council: *Nutrient requirements of dairy cattle,* ed 6, Washington, DC, 1988, National Academy Press.

National Research Council: *Nutrient requirements of goats: Angora, dairy, and meat goats in temperate and tropical countries,* ed 5, Washington, DC, 1996, National Academy Press.

National Research Council: *Nutrient requirements of horses,* ed 5, Washington, DC, 1996, National Academy Press.

National Research Council: *Nutrient requirements of sheep,* ed 6, Washington, DC, 1985, National Academy Press.

National Research Council: *Nutrient requirements of swine,* ed 9, Washington, DC, 1988, National Academy Press.

Naylor J, Ralston S: *Large animal clinical nutrition,* St. Louis, 1991, Mosby.

CHAPTER 26

Emergency and First Aid

Sally Powell   Elisa Petrollini

OUTLINE

Triage
Systemic Approach to Triage
    Respiratory System
    Cardiovascular System
    Central Nervous System
    Renal System
    Life-threatening Wounds
Monitoring Status of Emergency Patients
    Respiratory Status

Cardiovascular Status
Renal Status
Neurological Status
Miscellaneous Monitoring
Respiratory Emergencies
Cardiovascular Emergencies
Endocrine Emergencies
Gastrointestinal Emergencies

Central Nervous System Emergencies
Renal System Emergencies
Reproductive System Emergencies
Toxic Substance Emergencies
Cardiopulmonary Resuscitation (CPR)

LEARNING OUTCOMES

After reading this chapter you should be able to:

1. Describe triage and the guidelines for executing triage.
2. Describe how to monitor respiratory, cardiovascular, renal and neurological status of the emergency patient.
3. Describe the clinical signs, treatment and monitoring of patients with respiratory, cardiovascular, central nervous system, renal and reproductive system emergencies.
4. Describe emergencies caused by the ingestion of toxic substances by defining the clinical signs and treatment.
5. Describe cardiopulmonary resuscitation (CPR).
6. List equipment/supplies that may be needed to perform first aid and CPR.

Clinical evaluation of the emergency patient should initially focus on four major organ systems: respiratory, cardiovascular, central nervous, and renal. It is essential for the veterinary technician to understand how to rapidly evaluate each system to provide emergency care and monitor the critically ill patient. This chapter discusses guidelines for triage initial evaluation. It also outlines in chart form the common disease processes that affect the four major organ systems, including clinical signs, initial treatment, and parameters that should be monitored. A brief outline on CPR concludes the chapter.

TRIAGE

Triage is the initial assessment of the emergency patient. It is performed immediately on presentation and should take less than five minutes. Triage is the evaluation of the four major organ systems while simultaneously obtaining a capsule history. Acquiring the history can be the most difficult step. Conversation should be limited to salient points only, avoiding irrelevant details. The history should include the primary complaint, duration of the problem, and any current drug therapy.

After triage the patient is categorized as stable or unstable, allowing appropriate prioritization of care.

SYSTEMIC APPROACH TO TRIAGE

Respiratory System

I. Airway: determine patency of airway
   A. Upper airway noise (stridor/stertor)
   B. Distress with inspiration associated with stridor
II. Breathing
   A. Assess respiratory rate
      1. Tachypnea: increased respiratory rate
      2. Apnea: no respirations
   B. Assess respiratory effort
      1. Labored inspiration
      2. Labored expiration
      3. Labored inspiration and expiration
   C. Postural indications of dyspnea
      1. Stand rather than sit
      2. Abducted elbows
      3. Abdominal movement
      4. Extended neck

Cardiovascular System

I. Mucous membrane color
   A. Pink: normal
   B. Muddy or gray: poor perfusion
   C. Pale or white: anemia or poor perfusion
   D. Brick red (hyperemic): septic shock (not to be confused with severe periodontitis)
   E. Dark blue (cyanosis): hypoxia
   F. Yellow (jaundice): hepatic problems, hemolysis of red blood cells or biliary obstruction
   G. Brown: methemoglobinemia (most commonly seen with acetaminophen toxicity)
II. Capillary refill time (CRT)
   A. Normal: 1 to 2 seconds
   B. Prolonged: greater than two seconds; indicates poor perfusion
   C. Rapid: less than one second; indicates hyperdynamic state or hemoconcentration
III. Normal pulse rate
   A. Canine: 70 to 140 beats per minute (bpm)
   B. Feline: 110 to 140 bpm
IV. Pulse quality
   A. Strong and synchronous with heart rate
   B. Weak: indicates poor perfusion
   C. Hyperdynamic (snappy or bounding): anemia or sepsis

Central Nervous System

I. Gait, behavior
II. Muscular twitching
III. Head trauma
IV. Nystagmus: rapid eye movement
V. Head tilt

Renal System

I. Assessed with abdominal palpation when urinary blockage is suspected

Life-threatening Wounds

I. Open or penetrating chest wounds
II. Wounds to upper airway
III. Open or penetrating abdominal wounds
IV. Wounds affecting major blood vessels

MONITORING STATUS OF EMERGENCY PATIENTS

Frequent and perceptive evaluation of physical examination parameters are the fundamental basis of emergency and critical care monitoring. The four major organ systems should be closely monitored at all times.

Respiratory Status

I. Postural indications for dyspnea
II. Respiratory rate
   A. Tachypnea: increased respiratory rate
   B. Apnea: no respiratory rate
III. Respiratory effort
   A. Labored inspiration
   B. Labored expiration
   C. Labored inspiration and expiration
IV. Auscultation of lungs
   A. Dull lung sounds ventrally
   B. Dull lung sounds dorsally
   C. Harsh lung sounds
   D. Rales
V. Blood gas analysis

Cardiovascular Status

I. Mucous membrane color
II. Capillary refill time
III. Pulse rate
IV. Pulse quality
V. Blood pressure reading
   A. Direct arterial pressure readings
   B. Indirect pressure readings by
      1. Oscillometric pressure monitor
      2. Doppler

Renal Status

I. Urination
   A. Monitor urination
   B. Measure urine output

1. Indwelling urinary catheter with closed collection system
   2. Normal values are 1 to 2 mL/kg/hr
C. Central venous pressure: evaluates ability of the right ventricle to handle fluid therapy
   1. An early indicator of fluid overload

Neurological Status

I. Behavior
   A. Response to greeting
   B. Response to touch
   C. Response to noxious stimuli
II. Pupillary reflexes
   A. Blink
   B. Menace
   C. Pupillary light response
      1. Direct
      2. Consensual
III. Pupil size
   A. Miosis: pinpoint
   B. Anisocoria: asymmetrical or unequal
   C. Mydriasis: dilated
IV. Eye movement/position
   A. Nystagmus
      1. Horizontal eye movement
      2. Vertical eye movement
   B. Strabismus: abnormal eye position
V. Spinal cord compression
VI. Conscious proprioception
VII. Voluntary motor
VIII. Superficial pain
IX. Deep pain

Miscellaneous monitoring

I. Temperature
   A. Hypothermic due to poor perfusion, anesthesia, exposure to cold
   B. Hyperthermic due to infection, sepsis, heat prostration, malignant hyperthermia, seizures, upper airway obstruction
II. Fluid losses
   A. Vomiting
   B. Diarrhea
   C. Blood loss
   D. Effusions
   E. Edema
   F. Respiratory losses: excessive panting

RESPIRATORY EMERGENCIES

Patients in respiratory distress are often very unstable; minimizing stress to the animal is extremely important. Physical examination, diagnostics, and treatments are performed in stages to allow the patient to rest and breathe oxygen. It may be necessary to rule out primary heart disease before sedation in some cases.

Patient monitoring should include respiratory status, cardiovascular status, renal status, and temperature (Table 26-1).

CARDIOVASCULAR EMERGENCIES

Emergencies affecting the cardiovascular system are due to failure of the heart to pump blood throughout the body or an inappropriately low blood volume. The mainstay of therapy for hypovolemic, septic, neurogenic, and anaphylactic shock is aggressive fluid therapy. In contrast, fluid therapy can be fatal in the patient with heart failure. Therefore it is essential to differentiate between these conditions. Monitoring devices such as direct and indirect blood pressure and ECGs are necessary; however physical examination parameters are most important.

Patient monitoring should include respiratory status, cardiovascular status, neurological status, renal status, temperature, serial packed cell volume, total solids, dipstick BUN, dextrose (database), serial electrolyte analysis (sodium, potassium, ionized calcium, chloride), and ECGs (Table 26-2).

ENDOCRINE EMERGENCIES

Patient monitoring should include respiratory status, cardiovascular status, renal status, temperature, serial database readings, serial electrolyte analysis, serial pH analysis, serial glucose analysis, and an ECG (Table 26-3).

GASTROINTESTINAL EMERGENCIES

Patient monitoring should include respiratory status, cardiovascular status, renal status, serial database readings, serial electrolyte analysis, and an ECG. For gastric dilation or volvulus, serial measurement of abdominal girth may be performed (Table 26-4).

CENTRAL NERVOUS SYSTEM EMERGENCIES

Emergencies of the central nervous system (CNS) may affect the brain and/or the spinal cord. It is important to rule out hypoglycemia as a cause of seizures in patients presenting with continuous seizure activity. Behavior, pupillary reflexes, pupil size, and eye movement are used to evaluate the brain. The spinal cord is assessed by noting conscious proprioception, voluntary motor, superficial and deep pain (Table 26-5).

The causes of seizures include congenital/hereditary factors; inflammatory disease processes; viral, bacterial, fungal, protozoal, or rickettsial organisms; metabolic or

Table 26-1 Respiratory emergencies

Clinical signs	Treatment
COLLAPSING TRACHEA (most commonly seen in small breed dogs)	
Loud goose honk cough with expiration, +/− postural indications of dyspnea	Supply oxygen, calm with sedation when necessary (rule out primary heart disease before sedation), +/− surgical intervention
LARYNGEAL PARALYSIS (most commonly seen in large breed dogs)	
Noisy breathing, distress with inspiration, postural indications of dyspnea	Supply oxygen, calm with sedation, endotracheal intubation, +/− surgical intervention
FOREIGN BODY	
Noisy breathing, distress with inspiration, acute onset of gagging with severe respiratory distress, postural indication of dyspnea	Supply oxygen, remove obstruction
SOFT TISSUE SWELLING—ALLERGIC REACTION	
Facial swelling, +/− generalized urticaria (hives) +/− noisy breathing, +/− distress with inspiration, +/− postural indications of dyspnea	Dexamethasone sodium phosphate (anti-inflammatory agent), diphenhydramine HCl (inhibits histamine release)
SOFT TISSUE SWELLING—TUMOR	
Noisy breathing, distress with inspiration, postural indications of dyspnea	Supply oxygen, calm with sedation, +/− intubation, +/− tracheostomy
BRACHYCEPHALIC OCCLUSIVE SYNDROME (elongated soft palate, stenotic nares, hypoplastic trachea, everted laryngeal saccule)	
Upper airway stertor, distress with inspiration, postural indications of dyspnea	Supply oxygen, calm with sedation, +/− intubation, +/− surgical intervention
SMALL AIRWAY DISEASE—FELINE ASTHMA	
Dyspnea (prolonged expiration), postural indications of dyspnea, expiratory wheeze	Supply oxygen, bronchodilator, corticosteroids

nutritional deficiencies; trauma; a central vascular system breakdown; neoplasia; epilepsy; or toxicity.

RENAL SYSTEM EMERGENCIES

The etiology of renal system emergencies include acute and chronic renal failure, urethral obstructions, ruptured ureter/bladder, and urethral tears. Patients with renal disease should be monitored by measuring urine production, serum creatinine, blood urea nitrogen (BUN), electrolytes (sodium, potassium, phosphorus, calcium) and acid-base parameters on a pretreatment basis. Respi-

ratory status, cardiovascular status, neurological status, temperature, serial database readings, serial electrolyte analysis should also be monitored (Table 26-6).

REPRODUCTIVE SYSTEM EMERGENCIES

Patient monitoring should include respiratory status, cardiovascular status, renal status, temperature. Note vomiting/diarrhea, serial database readings, and serial electrolyte analysis. The patient should also be closely observed for active contractions, vaginal discharge, and delivery (Table 26-7).

Table 26-1   Respiratory emergencies—cont'd

Clinical signs	Treatment
PARENCHYMAL LUNG PROBLEMS	
Tachypnea, dyspnea (inspiration and expiration), postural indications of dyspnea, +/− pyrexia, +/− cyanosis, lung auscultation (harsh sounds), +/− rales	Supply oxygen (100% initially), 40% oxygen is suggested for long-term therapy (100% oxygen for more than 12 hours can result in pulmonary oxygen toxicity), appropriate antibiotic therapy, nebulize, coupage, +/− positive pressure ventilation
CONTUSIONS	
Tachypnea, dyspnea, postural indications of dyspnea, evidence of recent trauma, +/− shock, +/− cyanosis, +/− hemoptysis, lung auscultation (harsh lung sounds), +/− rales	Supply oxygen, fluid therapy, +/− positive pressure ventilation
PULMONARY EDEMA	
Tachypnea, dyspnea, +/− cyanosis, +/− burns in mouth (suggestive of electric shock), ongoing fluid therapy (suggestive of fluid overload), harsh lung sounds, +/− rales, +/− heart murmur	Supply oxygen, diuretics, +/− positive pressure ventilation
PULMONARY NEOPLASIA	
Tachypnea, dyspnea, +/− cyanosis, harsh lung sounds, +/− rales	Supply oxygen, +/− positive pressure ventilation
PNEUMOTHORAX	
Tachypnea, dyspnea, (rapid and short inspirations and expirations), +/− cyanosis, postural indications of dyspnea, decreased/muffled lung sounds dorsally, evidence of recent trauma	Supply oxygen, evacuate air (chest tap), +/− chest tube (placed when negative pressure is not achieved or when it is necessary to tap chest repeatedly)
PLEURAL EFFUSION (hemothorax, pyothorax, chylothorax and serous effusion)	
Tachypnea, dyspnea, postural indications of dyspnea, +/− cyanosis, decreased muffled lung sounds ventrally	Supply oxygen, evacuate fluid (chest tap), +/− chest tube
DIAPHRAGMATIC RUPTURE	
Tachypnea, dyspnea (paradoxical abdominal movement), postural indications of dyspnea, +/− cyanosis, +/− evidence of trauma, +/− auscultate borborygmi in thorax, decreased/muffled lung sounds, cardiac displacement	Supply oxygen, surgical correction

TOXIC SUBSTANCE EMERGENCIES

Patient monitoring should include respiratory status, cardiovascular status (ECG), renal status, vomiting/diarrhea, bleeding disorders (epistaxis, melena, hematemesis, hematuria), and neurological status (Table 26-8).

CARDIOPULMONARY RESUSCITATION (CPR)

CPR can be performed by a team only and therefore the first step should always be to alert the veterinarian and other technicians of an emergency situation involving cardiac arrest.

I. A common memory cue for the steps to perform CPR is ABCD.

A	Alert, assess, and airways
B	Breathing
C	Cardiac
D	Drugs

A. Alert veterinarian and other staff members and assess patient
  1. Assess animal by checking heart rate, respiratory rate, mucous membrane color, and pupil size

Table 26-2   Cardiovascular emergencies

Clinical signs	Treatment
HYPOVOLEMIC SHOCK	
Pale, gray, or muddy mucous membrane color; prolonged capillary refill time; rapid pulse rate, weak pulse quality; +/− evidence of acute blood loss; +/− evidence of fluid loss (vomiting, diarrhea); +/− evidence of fluid sequestration	Shock fluid therapy (isotonic crystalloid, hypertonic crystalloids, blood products, artificial colloid), +/− corticosteroids, +/− oxygen supplementation
SEPTIC, NEUROGENIC, OR ANAPHYLACTIC SHOCK	
Brick red mucous membrane color, hyperdynamic, rapid capillary refill time (less than 1 second), tachycardia, bounding pulse quality, +/− hyperthermia, +/− hypoglycemia	Shock fluid therapy, +/− blood culture (for septic shock), +/− antibiotics for septic shock, +/− corticosteroids for anaphylactic shock, +/− diphenhydramine for anaphylactic shock
CARDIOGENIC SHOCK—CONGESTIVE HEART FAILURE, PERICARDIAL TAMPONADE	
Pale or muddy mucous membrane color, prolonged capillary refill time, rapid pulse rate, weak pulse quality, +/− tachypnea/dyspnea, +/− postural indications of dyspnea, +/− cyanosis, +/− evidence of trauma	Oxygen supplementations, +/− diuretics, inotropics, vasodilators, +/− fluid therapy (very conservative; minimize stress levels), caution when performing stressful procedures

Table 26-3   Endocrine emergencies

Clinical signs	Treatment
ADDISONIAN CRISIS (hypoadrenocorticism)	
Hyponatremia, hyperkalemia (causing bradycardia), +/− hypovolemic shock, hypoglycemia, hypercalcemia, vomiting, diarrhea, PU/PD	Fluid therapy: normal saline, glucocorticoid (dexamethasone most commonly used) will not interfere with ACTH stimulation test, correct acidosis (if severe give sodium bicarbonate, supply oxygen)
DIABETIC KETOACIDOSIS	
PU/PD, vomiting, diarrhea, dehydration, +/− hypovolemic shock, hyperglycemia, glucosuria, ketonuria, acidemia, tachypnea	IV Fluid therapy, insulin therapy

B. Breathing
   1. Tracheal intubation
   2. Mouth to endotracheal tube if there is no oxygen supply
   3. Mouth to muzzle if needed
   4. Resuscitation bag connected to oxygen supply or anesthesia machine 30 to 60 breaths per minute
     a. No more than 20 cm of H_2O pressure for dog (if using anesthesia machine)
     b. No more than 15 cm of H_2O pressure for cat (if using anesthesia machine)
C. Circulation
   1. Continuous ECG monitoring
   2. Chest compressions (external cardiac massage)
     a. Animal should be in right lateral recumbency except for large round-chested dogs and cats, who should be in dorsal recumbency
     b. Count four to six rib spaces or use point of the elbow to locate the heart
     c. Using two hands in large dogs press down on the chest with heal of the lower hand
       (1) For cats and small dogs, squeezing the chest between the index finger and thumb is adequate
     d. Compress the chest for 1 second and release for 1 second
D. Drugs
   1. Intravenous access
     a. Intravenous fluids (isotonic crystalloid)

Table 26-4 Gastrointestinal emergencies

Clinical signs	Treatment
GASTRIC DILATION AND/OR VOLVULUS	
Abdominal distention; nonproductive retching; pale, muddy, or gray mucous membrane color; prolonged capillary refill time; tachycardia; weak pulse; +/− tachypnea; dyspnea	Fluid therapy (rapid IV bolus), decompression (trocharization or gastric intubation/lavage), corticosteroids, abdominal radiographs (right lateral most important), surgical intervention if torsion
GASTROINTESTINAL OBSTRUCTION (foreign body, intussusception, tumor)	
Vomiting; diarrhea; red, pale or gray, or muddy mucous membrane color; fast or prolonged capillary refill time; abdominal pain, +/− pale mucous membranes; prolonged CRT; tachycardia; weak pulse quality; dehydration; tachypnea; dyspnea	Shock fluid therapy, +/− endoscopy, +/− surgical intervention
PERITONITIS (gastrointestinal perforation, ruptured prostatic abscess)	
Hyperemic: brick-red mucous membrane, rapid capillary refill time, tachycardia, bounding pulse quality, hyperthermia, +/− hypoglycemia, abdominal pain	Fluid therapy, appropriate antibiotics, abdomonocentesis (obtain sample for cytology), +/− diagnostic peritoneal lavage, surgical intervention
PARVOVIRUS INFECTION	
Vomiting; diarrhea; pale, gray, or muddy mucous membrane color; prolonged capillary refill time; tachycardia; weak pulse quality; dehydration; +/− hypoglycemia; +/− hypokalemia; +/− leukopenia	Fluid therapy, antibiotics to prevent secondary bacterial infection, correct hypoglycemia, correct hypokalemia, +/− antiemetics, abdominal palpation to rule out intussusception
LIVER FAILURE	
Vomiting, +/− hematemesis; diarrhea, +/− melena; PU/PD, +/− dementia, +/− seizures; +/− jaundice; +/− anemia; +/− ecchymosis/abnormal bleeding; hypoalbuminemia; hypoglycemia; hyperbilirubinemia; hypocholesterolemia; low BUN	Fluid therapy, gastrointestinal protectants, +/− lactulose, +/− vitamin K_1, +/− antibiotics

2. Intravenous drugs
  a. Atropine sulphate
  b. Doxapram
  c. Corticosteroids
  d. Calcium gluconate
  e. Furosemide
  f. Lidocaine
3. Intratracheal drugs
  a. Epinephrine
4. Intracardiac drugs
  a. Epinephrine
  b. Isoproterenol

II. Hints for successful CPR
An arrest station or special area to conduct CPR is ideal, however many practices have "crash carts" to allow for all necessary supplies to be readily available.
A. Necessary supplies include:

1. Oxygen
  a. S-bag or anesthesia machine
2. Crash cart or emergency kit
  a. Endotracheal tubes
  b. Laryngoscope
  c. Intravenous catheters, fluids, administration sets, tape, syringes, needles, tourniquet
    (1) Venous cut down supplies: scalpel blades, catheter introducers, suture material
  d. Drugs
  e. Chart of dose rates for all drugs in the kit
  f. Clippers
  g. ECG monitor
  h. Defibrillator
  i. Suction and suction tips

Table 26-5 Central nervous system emergencies

Clinical signs	Monitoring	Treatment
EPILEPSY		
Hyperthermia, hyperdynamic state, +/− nystagmus/strabismus, +/− pupillary changes (miosis, mydriasis, anisocoria)	Respiratory status (potential for aspiration during seizure), cardiovascular status, neurological status (mental status: alert and responsive, depressed, stupor, coma and pupillary light response), renal status, body temperature	Diazepam (good anticonvulsant activity, must give to effect), phenobarbital, pentobarbitol (heavy anesthesia)
HEAD TRAUMA		
Depression, +/− stupor, +/− coma, +/− convulsions, +/− pupillary changes (miosis, mydriasis, anisocoria), +/− nystagmus/strabismus, +/− blood in aural canal, +/− hyphema, +/− scleral hemorrhage, +/− skull/facial fractures	Respiratory status (trauma to the brain stem can cause altered ventilatory status, important to keep carbon dioxide levels normal to low, increased carbon dioxide will cause increased intracranial pressure), cardiovascular status, neurological status, renal status	Corticosteroids, +/− mannitol (osmotic agent, can decrease intracranial pressure through its osmotic effects), elevate head (place patient on flat board and elevate board to approx. 30° in attempt to decrease intracranial pressure), +/− ventilation (to decrease carbon dioxide levels)
ACUTE PARESIS/PARALYSIS		
Loss of conscious proprioception, loss of voluntary motor function, loss of superficial pain, loss of deep pain	Respiratory status (patients with tetraparesis can experience loss of function to intercostal muscles), cardiovascular status, neurological status (conscious proprioception, voluntary motor activity, superficial pain, deep pain), renal status (upper motor neuron: hypertonic sphincter), (lower motor neuron: bladder hypotonia)	Conservative (commonly used when voluntary motor function is still present), corticosteroids, strict cage rest, surgical intervention (myelogram, laminectomy)

Table 26-6 Renal system emergencies

Clinical signs	Treatment
ACUTE RENAL FAILURE	
Vomiting, diarrhea, dehydration, +/− evidence of exposure to toxins (e.g., ethylene glycol or gentamycin)	Pretreatment (creatinine, BUN, potassium, phosphorus, calcium, PCV and total protein), fluid therapy (isotonic crystalloid solutions, urinary catheter, diuretics after rehydration), +/− mannitol, +/− peritoneal dialysis, gastrointestinal protectants
FELINE URETHRAL OBSTRUCTION	
Dysuria, +/− hematuria, vomiting, vocalizing, painful abdomen, distended bladder on abdominal palpation, +/− hyperkalemia, +/− hypocalcemia	Treat bradycardia/arrhythmia (IV calcium gluconate), pretreatment database (potassium, ionized calcium, creatinine), fluid therapy (isotonic crystalloid), relieve urinary obstruction (place catheter, empty and irrigate bladder)
URETER/BLADDER RUPTURE	
Vomiting, diarrhea, +/− hematuria, +/− evidence of trauma, +/− abdominal effusion, +/− RBC in urine, abdominal pain, +/− hypovolemic shock, +/− decreased urine output	Radiographs, urinary catheter, +/− excretory urogram, +/− retrograde urethrography/cystography, surgical intervention
URETHRAL TEARS	
+/− vomiting, +/− dysuria/hematuria, +/− anuria, +/− abdominal effusion, +/− SQ edema of hind limbs and ventral abdomen, +/− hypovolemic shock	+/− urinary catheter, +/− surgical intervention

Table 26-7 Emergencies of the reproductive system

Clinical signs	Treatment
PYOMETRA	
PU/PD, recent estrus, vomiting, +/− hyperthermia, +/− vaginal discharge (depends on whether the cervix is open or closed), +/− abdominal detention	Fluid therapy (isotonic crystalloid), antibiotic therapy, surgical intervention
ECLAMPSIA	
Muscle tremors, evidence of whelping and lactation usually 2-3 weeks prior, brick-red mucous membranes (hyperemic), tachycardia, bounding pulse quality, hyperthermia, hypocalcemia	Calcium gluconate (slow IV bolus), fluid therapy (when hyperthermia, isotonic crystalloid solution), oral calcium throughout lactation,* ECG while administering calcium gluconate. If bradycardia, arrhythmia or vomiting occur stop treatment
DYSTOCIA	
Active contractions for more than 30 minutes, more than 2 hours between deliveries, green discharge with no delivery of fetus	Rule out obstructive dystocia (digital exam, abdominal radiographs), oxytocin, +/− calcium gluconate +/− glucose, +/− surgical intervention

Table 26-8 Emergencies caused by toxic substances

Clinical signs	Treatment
ACETAMINOPHEN (TYLENOL) TOXICOSIS	
One to two hours post ingestion (salivation, vomiting, tachypnea, brown or cyanotic mucous membrane color, dark or chocolate colored blood, edema of face)	Induce emesis if less than 1 hour post ingestion (not performed if showing signs of tachypnea), acetylcysteine, ascorbic acid, fluid therapy (isotonic crystalloid), supply oxygen
ANTICOAGULANT RODENTICIDE TOXICITY	
No clinical signs of ingested recently, dyspnea, hematuria, hematemesis, epistaxis, melena, hemothorax	Induce emesis (if recently ingested, activated charcoal, vitamin K_1), prothrombin time analysis 2 days post ingestion, then prothrombin time analysis 2 days after vitamin K_1 finished, fresh whole blood or fresh frozen plasma if coagulopathy is present
CHOCOLATE TOXICOSIS (METHYLXANTHINE) (active ingredient theobromine) (LD 50 = 100 mg/kg)	
Vomiting, diarrhea, hyperactivity, muscle tremors, tachycardia, arrhythmia, hypertension, +/− seizures,	Induce emesis, +/− gastric lavage, activated charcoal, cathartics, fluid therapy (isotonic crystalloid), +/− oxygen supplementation
ETHYLENE GLYCOL TOXICITY (LD 50: dogs 4-6 mL/kg; cats 1.5 mL/kg)	
Vomiting, PU/PD, tachypnea, tachycardia, azotemia, increased serum osmolality, metabolic acidosis, hypocalcemia, oliguria, ataxia, seizures, stupor, coma	Gastric lavage, cathartics, fluid therapy (isotonic crystalloid), ethanol (7%), peritoneal dialysis, +/− methyl pyrazole
LEAD POISONING	
Vomiting, diarrhea, lethargy, abdominal pain, ataxia, blindness, seizures, evidence of nucleated RBC on blood smear with no evidence of anemia	Remove lead from gastrointestinal tract, enema, emetic, surgical intervention, remove lead from tissues and blood, calcium EDTA, penicillin, control seizures
NONSTEROIDAL ANTI-INFLAMMATORIES (NSAIDS)	
Vomiting, diarrhea, gastrointestinal bleeding (hematemesis, melena)	Fluid therapy (isotonic crystalloid, isotonic colloid, blood products, artificial colloid, gastrointestinal protectants, sucralfate, cimetidine HCl)
ORGANOPHOSPHATE TOXICITY	
Acronym: DUMBELS = Diarrhea, Urination, Miosis, Bradycardia, Emesis, Lacrimation; salivation, dyspnea, fasciculation, vomiting, diarrhea, seizures	Remove toxin (bathe with soap and water), atropine sulfate, diphenhydramine, +/− pralidoxime (2 Pam), fluid therapy (isotonic crystalloid), control fasciculation/convulsions (diazepam or pentobarbitol)

Glossary

abducted To draw away from an axis or median plane

acidemia Abnormal acidity of the blood

acidosis A state characterized by actual or relative decrease of alkali in body fluids in relation to acid content

ACTH Adrenocorticotropic hormone

anaphylactic A serious reaction (shock) brought about by hypersensitivity to an allergen such as a drug or protein, (anaphylaxis)

anisocoria Unequal or asymmetrical pupil size

anuria No urine production

apnea No respirations

ataxia Incoordination of limb movement

auscultation Listening for sounds produced within the body

azotemia Retention of renal excretory products

borborygmi Rumbling or gurgling noises produced by movement of gas in the gastrointestinal tract

cardiac tamponade Reduction of venous return to the heart due to increased volume of fluid in the pericardium

cathartics An agent that increases gastrointestinal flow

chylothorax Accumulation of milky chylous fluid in the pleural space, usually on the left side

coagulopathy Any disorder of blood coagulation

colloid A solution containing large molecules that can not pass out of blood vessels

coma State of unconsciousness with no response to external stimuli

coupage Striking the thoracic area to aid in the removal of secretions

crystalloid Solution containing small molecules that can pass out of blood vessels

cyanosis Bluish discoloration of skin and mucous membranes

cystography Radiography of the urinary bladder using a contrast medium

diuretic An agent that promotes excretion of urine

Doppler Device for measuring blood flow that transmits sound for measurement

dyspnea Difficulty breathing

dysuria Difficult urination

ecchymosis Large area of nonelevated bruising in the skin or mucous membranes

edema Accumulation of an excessive amount of watery fluid in cells, tissues, or serous cavities

effusion Escape of fluid from blood vessels or lymphatics into tissues or cavities

encephalitis Inflammation of the brain

epistaxis Nasal hemorrhage; nosebleed

fasciculation A localized involuntary muscular contraction

hematemesis Vomiting blood

hematuria Blood in urine

hemoptysis Coughing blood

hemothorax Blood in the pleural cavity

hydrocephalus A condition marked by an excessive accumulation of fluid in the brain

hyperdynamic Excessive muscular activity

hyperkalemic Abnormally high potassium levels

hyperthermia Increased body temperature

hyphema Blood in the anterior chamber of the eye

hyponatremia Deficiency of sodium in the blood

hypoplastic Underdevelopment of an organ or tissue

hypothermia Decreased body temperature

hypoxia Decrease in oxygen

indwelling (catheter) A catheter that is designed to stay in the urethra to drain urine from the bladder

intussusception Infolding of one segment of the intestine into another

isotonic Of similar osmolality to normal plasma

laminectomy Surgical excision of the dorsal arch of a vertebra

lavage Washing out or irrigating the intestinal tract or stomach

LD_{50} The dose that will kill 50% of the tested population

menace Menace reflex or menace response; tested by stabbing a finger toward an eye. Positive response is closing of the eyelids; absence of response could indicate paralysis of the eyelids or serious depression of consciousness

methemoglobinemia Presence of methemoglobin in the circulating blood

miosis Contraction of the pupil

mydriasis Dilation of the pupil

myelogram A graphic representation of cells found in a bone marrow sample

nebulization Treatment by a spray

neoplasia Pathologic process that results in the formation and growth of a tumor

neurogenic Originating in the nervous system

nystagmus A rhythmic involuntary movement of the eyeballs in a vertical, horizontal, or rotary direction

occlusive State of being closed; an obstruction or a closing

oliguria Reduced daily output of urine

osmolality The concentration of a solution in terms of osmoles or solutes per kg of solvent

paralysis Loss of power of voluntary movement in a muscle

parenchyma The distinguishing or specific cells of a gland or organ, contained in and supported by the connective tissue framework

paresis Incomplete voluntary movement

perfusion Passage of fluid through the vessels of an organ

periodontitis Inflammation of the area surrounding a tooth or the periodontium

pleura Serous membrane enveloping the lungs and lining the walls of the pleural cavity

pneumothorax Presence of air or gas in the pleural cavity

postural Pertaining to position or posture

proprioceptive Capable of receiving stimuli originating in muscles, tendons, and other internal tissues

protectant An agent that promotes defence immunity against a harmful substance

PU/PD Polyuria/polydipsia

pyothorax Empyema (pus) in the pleural cavity

pyrexia fever

rales Commonly used to denote crackling sounds heard on lung auscultation

septic Pertaining to sepsis; the presence of toxins in the blood or other tissues sequestration   Abnormal separation of a part or a whole portion by a disease process

serous   Relating to, containing or producing, or a substance having a watery consistency

shock   A stage in which the body is unable to adequately deliver oxygen to tissues

status epilepticus   Repeated seizure or a seizure prolonged for at least 30 minutes

stenotic   Abnormal narrowing or constriction

stertor   Snoring; a noisy inspiration sometimes due to obstruction of the larynx or upper airway

strabismus   Change in the visual axis. EXAMPLES: wandering eye, walleye, cross eye, squint

stridor   High pitched, noisy respiration sometimes due to obstruction of the larynx or upper airway

stupor   State of impaired consciousness with response to noxious stimuli

tachypnea   Rapid respirations

tetraparesis   Muscular weakness affecting all four extremities

torsion   The act of twisting

urogram   Radiography of any part of the urinary tract

urticaria   A vascular reaction of the skin that is a response to direct exposure to a chemical or an immunological response; wheals or hives

Review Questions

1 What are the four major organ systems that are immediately evaluated in an emergency situation?
  a. Renal, gastrointestinal, cardiovascular, respiratory
  b. Endocrine, central nervous, gastrointestinal, renal
  c. Musculoskeletal, gastrointestinal, endocrine, renal
  d. Respiratory, cardiovascular, renal, central nervous

2 What are the postural indications for dyspnea?
  a. Coughing, tachypnea, extended neck, upper airway noise
  b. Lay rather than sit, labored expiration, abdominal movement
  c. Stand rather than sit, abducted elbows, abdominal movement, extended neck
  d. Dyspnea, stertor, extended neck, abdominal movement

3 Forty percent oxygen is suggested for long-term therapy; 100% oxygen for more than __ can result in pulmonary oxygen toxicity.
  a. 6 hours
  b. 8 hours
  c. 12 hours
  d. 24 hours

4 What disease process requires nebulization as a treatment?
  a. Contusions
  b. Pneumonia
  c. Laryngeal paralysis
  d. Parenchymal lung problems

5 A capillary refill time of greater than two seconds is indicative of:
  a. Hyperdynamic state
  b. Liver problems
  c. Cerebral edema
  d. Poor perfusion

6 Emergency situations treated with vitamin K:
  a. Liver and anticoagulant rodenticide toxicity
  b. Chocolate toxicity and NSAID toxicity
  c. Acute paresis and acute renal failure
  d. Ethylene glycol and lead toxicities

7 Initial treatment for a patient in respiratory distress is:
  a. Electrocardiogram
  b. Chest radiographs
  c. Diuretics
  d. Oxygen supplementation

8 Dull lung sounds ventrally on auscultation indicate:
  a. Pneumonia
  b. Pleural effusion
  c. Pulmonary edema
  d. Pneumothorax

9 The clinical signs of anaphylactic shock are:
  a. Brick-red mucous membranes, CRT <1 second, and tachycardia
  b. Pale mucous membranes, CRT >1 second, and bradycardia
  c. Muddy colored mucous membranes, prolonged CRT, and weak pulse
  d. Pale mucous membranes, CRT >1 second, and tachycardia

10 Clinical signs for eclampsia are caused by:
  a. Hypoglycemia
  b. Hyperkalemia
  c. Hypocalcemia
  d. Hypernatremia

BIBLIOGRAPHY

Hensyl WR, editor: *Stedman's medical dictionary,* ed 25, Baltimore, 1990, Williams and Wilkins.

Kirby R et al, editor: The Veterinary Clinics of North America—small animal medicine, vol 2(6), *Emergency Medicine,* Philadelphia, 1994, W.B. Saunders.

Kirk RW et al: *Current veterinary therapy,* ed 12, Philadelphia, 1995, W.B. Saunders.

Murtaugh et al: *Veterinary emergency and critical care medicine,* St. Louis, 1992, Mosby-Year Book.

Plunkett SJ: *Emergency procedures for the small animal veterinarian,* Philadelphia, 1993, W.B. Saunders.

Laboratory Animal Medicine

Amanda Hathaway   *Jodilynn Pitcher*

OUTLINE

Mouse
Origin and Uses in Research
Characteristics—Behavioral and
Physiological
Handling and Breeding Considerations
Sampling
Signs of Pain and Distress
Health Conditions
Rat
Origin and Uses in Research
Characteristics—Behavioral and
Physiological
Handling and Breeding Considerations
Sampling
Signs of Pain and Distress
Health Conditions
Syrian Hamster
Origin and Uses in Research

Characteristics—Behavioral and
Physiological
Handling and Breeding Considerations
Sampling/Dosages
Signs of Pain and Distress
Health Conditions
Mongolian Gerbil
Origin and Uses in Research
Characteristics—Behavioral and
Physiological
Handling and Breeding Considerations
Sampling
Signs of Pain and Distress
Health Conditions
Rabbit
Origin and Uses in Research
Characteristics—Behavioral and
Physiological

Handling and Breeding Considerations
Sampling
Signs of Pain and Distress
Health Conditions
Guinea Pig
Origin and Uses in Research
Characteristics—Behavioral and
Physiological
Handling and Breeding Considerations
Sampling
Signs of Pain and Distress
Health Conditions
General Caging and Housing
Reproductive Data
Zoonosis
Laboratory Animal Allergy (LAA)

LEARNING OUTCOMES

After reading this chapter you should be able to:

1. List the research uses and characteristics of mice, rats, hamsters, gerbils, rabbits, and guinea pigs.
2. Describe handling and breeding considerations, signs of pain and distress, and health conditions of the above species.
3. List suggested injectable anesthetic drug protocols, sites, and volumes for injections and sampling.
4. Suggest appropriate housing conditions for each species.

5. Discuss zoonotic diseases and their effect on research and personnel.

Laboratory animals have been used in research for many years. In the last 40 to 50 years, growing concern from the public over the use of animals in research has led to the establishment of guidelines to promote better care and responsible use of laboratory animals. The laboratory animal section reviews the characteristics, uses in research, handling and breeding considerations, signs of pain and distress, health conditions, housing considerations, and injectable anesthetic protocols for mice, rats, hamsters, gerbils, rabbits, and guinea pigs. This information is also useful in a clinical setting when dealing with these species as pet animals.

MOUSE *(Mus musculus)* ━━━━━━

Origin and Uses in Research

  I. The laboratory mouse used today is purposely bred for research
  II. The different strains of mice in laboratories are defined by ecological and genetic characteristics
  III. Outbred, inbred, and congenic stock are strains defined by genetic characteristics
     A. **Outbred strains:** result of random matings to achieve genetic variations
     B. **Inbred strains:** result of brother/sister matings for a minimum of 20 consecutive generations
     C. **Congenic strains:** result of the introduction of a single mutant gene through back cross matings. This group includes F_1 hybrids, which are produced by mating two differently bred mice
  IV. The strains of mice defined by ecological characteristics can be divided into axenic, gnotobiotic, specific pathogen free, barrier sustained, and conventional
     A. Axenic or germfree animals are hysterectomy derived, free from any microorganisms, and maintained in a germfree isolation type housing
     B. Gnotobiotic animals are germfree mice that have been introduced to one or two known nonpathogenic microorganisms. They are housed in isolators or barrier units
     C. Specific pathogen free animals are those free from specific pathogenic organisms
     D. Barrier-sustained animals are gnotobiotic animals maintained under sterile conditions in a barrier unit. All air, bedding, water, and food must be sterilized; staff must shower and aseptically scrub and dress before entering
     E. Conventional animals are those bred with no special precautions and possess unknown and various microorganisms
  V. Mice are the most widely used vertebrate in toxicology studies and biomedical research

Characteristics—Behavioral and Physiological

  I. Mice may bite if frightened or handled improperly

  II. Mice are best housed in small groups, if they are compatible
  III. Males that have reached puberty may fight
  IV. Mice are nocturnal animals
  V. A unique anatomic feature of mice is the bone marrow of the long bones, which is functional throughout their lives
  VI. Mice also have a "hibernation gland," which is seen as fatty brown tissue located in various areas on the body

Handling and Breeding Considerations

  I. Mice should be picked up by the base of the tail, never the middle or tip of the tail
  II. For restraint, they should be placed on a wire grid so that their front feet grip the grid; then the handler should quickly but carefully grasp the loose skin on either side of the neck and over the back with the thumb and forefinger
     A. The handler can then turn his or her hand so that the mouse is lying on its back in the palm of the hand
     B. The little finger can be wrapped around the tail
  III. Tubular restraining devices can be used for performing bleeding and other simple procedures
  IV. The best methods of permanent identification of mice is ear punching or the insertion of a microchip that can be scanned for identification, along with cage card identification

Sampling

For injection routes, sites, needle sizes, and volumes, see Table 27-1.

  I. Gastric gavage can be done by placing a ball-tipped, curved dosing needle over the tongue, into the esophagus, and then into the stomach
  II. Simple blood sampling procedures (tail clip) can be done on awake but restrained mice. To obtain larger volumes or perform retroorbital sinus or cardiac puncture sampling, anesthesia must be used
  III. Collection of urine and feces can be done by placing the animal in a metabolism cage or by collecting the samples as an animal is restrained (it will often defecate and urinate)
     A. Use a microhematocrit tube to collect urine

Signs of Pain and Distress

  I. Signs of pain and distress in mice are decreased food and water intake resulting in weight loss and dehydration, increased sleeping times, decreased grooming and starring coat, hunched posture, changes in urination and defecation, sunken eyes

Table 27-1 Recommended needle sizes and sites and maximum volumes for injections/sampling

Species	SQ	IM	IP	IV	Sampling (nonlethal)
Mouse	<20g Scruff 2-3 ml	25g Quadriceps, posterior thigh 0.1 ml	23g 2 ml	<25g Lateral tail vein 0.2 ml	Retroorbital sinus: 0.5 ml (adult), 30-80 μL max, for animals <16 days old Lateral tail vein: 0.5-1.0 ml Intracardiac: (bevel needle) 23g, 0.5-1.0 ml Tail nick: <25g, small amounts only, DO NOT remove vertebrae
Rat	<20g Scruff, back 5-10 ml	23-25g Quadriceps, posterior thigh 0.3 ml	22-23g 5-10 ml	<23g Lateral tail vein, femoral vein 0.5 ml	Lateral tail vein or artery Intracardiac: bevel needle, >5 ml samples Jugular vein: <25 g Retroorbital sinus <3 ml
Hamster	<20g Scruff 3-4 ml	<23-25g Quadriceps, posterior thigh 0.1 ml	<23g 3-4 ml	<25g Femoral vein, jugular vein (cutdown) 0.3 ml	Retroorbital sinus: 0.5 ml maximum Intracardiac: bevel needle, 23g Femoral/jugular cutdown: <25g 2 ml/150 kg max
Guinea pig	<20g Scruff, back 5-10 ml	<21g Quadriceps, posterior thigh 0.3 ml	<20g 10-15 ml	<23g Ear, penile, or saphenous vein 0.5 ml	<23g Anterior vena cava: 2-3 ml Ear vein: 0.5 ml Intracardiac: 10-15 ml/300-400g Intra orbital sinus: 0.5 ml Penile, saphenous: 2-3 ml
Rabbit	<20g Scruff, flank 30-50 ml	<21g Quadriceps, posterior thigh, lumbar 0.5-1 ml	<20g 50-100 ml	<21g Marginal ear vein 1-5 ml, slowly	Marginal ear vein: 21g Central ear artery: 20g Intracardiac: 20g 9 ml/kg, no less than every 4 weeks Jugular vein: <10 ml
Gerbil	<20g Scruff 2-3 ml	<23-25g Quadriceps, posterior thigh 0.1 ml	23g 2-3 ml	<25g Femoral or jugular vein 0.3 ml	Retrorbital sinus: 0.5 ml only Intracardiac: 23g Tail vein/artery: dark in pigment and tough to penetrate, <25g, 2 ml/150g max.

1. When sampling, it is a good idea to replace equal amounts of fluid (i.e., physiological saline).
2. General anesthesia must be employed for intracardiac procedures and retroorbital bleeding.
3. In removing samples greater than 0.1 ml, use the largest bore needle possible to allow blood withdrawal and avoid collapsing the vessel and hematoma formation.
4. If body warming is used to dilate the vessel, the animal must constantly be monitored to prevent hyperthermia.
5. The use of xylene as a dilator is not recommended; it will cause skin rashes and is easily misused.

II. Mice may be aggressive and vocal initially but as pain and stress continue they become depressed and withdrawn from the rest of the group and become hypothermic due to lack of movement

III. Ocular and nasal discharge may be seen, along with increased and labored breathing
   A. These signs may be associated with latent respiratory disease

IV. Mice may be seen scratching excessively or biting at painful areas, which may lead to self-mutilation

Health Conditions

I. Respiratory disease
   A. The most common cause of respiratory disease in mice is Sendai virus, although other organisms can be involved
   B. Often latent and becomes apparent in young weanling, stressed mice, or in combination with bacterial infections
   C. Bacteria that may contribute to respiratory infections are: *Pasteurella pneumotropica, Klebsiella pneumoniae, Corynebacterium kutscheri,*

Bordetella bronchiseptica, and *Mycoplasma pulmonis*

    D. *M. pulmonis* alone may cause pneumonia

    E. Clinical signs are: weight loss, ruffled hair coat, dyspnea, chattering

    F. Treatment: antibiotics for secondary bacterial infections

  II. Mouse hepatitis virus

    A. Coronovirus that leads to encephalitis and hepatitis in mice

    B. Most commonly seen in immunosuppressed animals such as nude mice

  III. Tyzzer's disease

    A. *Bacillus pisiformis* is the bacteria involved in this condition

    B. Most commonly affects immunosuppressed animals and those kept in poor housing

    C. Dehydration, weight loss, and diarrhea are clinical signs that might lead to death

    D. Tetracycline placed in the water supply may help treat the condition

  IV. Epizootic diarrhea of infant mice (EDIM)

    A. Viral disease affecting suckling mice

    B. Clinical signs: soft yellow feces or dried feces around the anus in mice two weeks old or younger

    C. To prevent spread of this virus, filter-top cages should be used

  V. Lethal intestinal virus of infant mice

    A. Viral disease that affects suckling mice

    B. May affect mice up to 20 days of age

    C. Has a higher mortality rate than EDIM

RATS *(Rattus Norvegicus)* ▅▅▅▅▅▅
Origin and Uses in Research

  I. The rat is a rodent of the family Muridae

    A. The present day laboratory rat has been developed in North America

  II. Common outbred strains are Wistar, Sprague-Dawley, Long-Evans, and Osborne-Mendal

  III. Through selective breeding and mutations, more defined and inbred strains can be produced to suit a specific study

    A. EXAMPLES:

      1. CAR/CAS: caries resistant/susceptible

      2. BB rats: spontaneous diabetics

      3. Brattleboro rats: diabetes insipidus

      4. Zucker rat: obesity

  IV. Rats are the second most commonly used laboratory animal

  V. Rats are useful in studies of toxicology, teratology, cardiovascular research, immunology, dental studies, experimental oncology, and behavior

  VI. Laboratory rats are raised and maintained in ecologic classes: conventional, germfree, gnotobiotics, and barrier sustained

Characteristics—Behavioral and Physiological

  I. Rats are generally docile and may become tame and easily trained if handled frequently

  II. Rats can be housed communally and may share raising of their young

  III. Rats are omnivorous and generally are fed a commercially prepared pellet feed

  IV. They practice coprophagy if they have access to their feces

    A. May also cannibalize dead cage mates

  V. They display a range of behavioral traits and are intelligent, making them suitable for behavioral studies

  VI. They do not have a gallbladder

  VII. They possess a layer of brown fat distributed over the back and neck and around the kidney, called the hibernation gland, that has a role in thermogenesis

  VIII. The rat's long bone epiphyses do not become inactive; therefore adults continue to gradually increase in skeletal size throughout life

  IX. Harderian glands produce red tears under stress

  X. Rats are obligate nose breathers

Handling and Breeding Considerations

  I. Rats will bite if improperly handled

  II. Pet rats are best grasped and held by firmly placing the hand around the back and rib cage with the head resting between the thumb and forefinger, immediately behind the mandibles

  III. The rat could be picked up by the base of the tail and quickly placed on a work surface

    A. The handler's second hand should grasp the rat around the thorax, just under the forelimbs

  IV. The rat may be scruffed (described in the mouse restraint section of this chapter)

  V. Restraining devices may be used for short procedures or a towel or lab coat can be wrapped around the rat for restraint, but be aware rats may bite through these

  VI. Do not lay a rat on its back; it will strongly object

  VII. Never carry a rat by the tail; it could swing up and bite the handler or twist, causing the skin to be stripped from the tail, exposing coccygeal vertebrae

VIII. Female rats are polyestrus and can breed year round

IX. Estrus may be synchronized in a group of female rats by introducing a male into a cage—this is the "Whitten Effect"

Sampling

For injection routes, sites needle sizes, and volumes, see Table 27-1.

I. Gastric gavage can be performed by placing a ball-tipped, curved dosing needle over the tongue, into the esophagus, and then into the stomach

Signs of Pain and Distress

I. Rats may be seen licking or guarding a painful area

II. Increased scratching is a sign of chronic pain

III. Other signs of pain and distress are a hunched position, constant vocalization, struggling when handled, disrupted sleeping patterns, rough coat, untidy appearance, and decreased food and water intake, which will lead to weight loss and dehydration and increased respiration and sneezing

IV. Initially rats in pain and distress are more aggressive and resistant to handling but as the stress/pain continues they become depressed

V. As an animal's condition deteriorates, hypothermia will be noted

VI. Latent infections of chromodacryorrhea (red tears), produced by the harderian gland, may become apparent

Health Conditions

I. Chronic respiratory disease
   A. Also called murine respiratory mycoplasmosis
   B. Major organism involved with this disease is *Mycoplasma pulmonis*
   C. Clinical signs are: otitis media/interna (indicated by circling), sneezing and blood-flecked discharge associated with rhinitis
   D. In severe cases, pneumonia and genital tract infections (females only)
   E. Highly contagious and affected rats should be isolated from others
   F. Tetracycline may be given in the water to prevent secondary infections

II. Sendai virus
   A. Clinical signs are seen when animals are stressed
   B. Respiratory difficulty, chattering, weight loss, rough hair coat, decreased breeding efficiency, and variable mortality are signs seen in an infected animal

III. Sialodacryoadentitis (SDA)
   A. SDA is a common coronavirus that is highly contagious throughout rat colonies
   B. Most commonly seen in weanling and young adult rats
   C. The virus multiplies in salivary and lacrimal glands
   D. Clinical signs: squinting, blinking, eye rubbing, sneezing, nasal discharge, cervical swelling, and inflammation of the lacrimal and salivary glands
   E. Suborbital or periorbital swelling may develop in one or both eyes, along with an increased production of red tears
   F. Recommended treatment: application of topical ointments to the eyes to prevent further damage and bacterial infection of the eye

IV. Chromodacryorrhea
   A. Commonly referred to as "red tears"
   B. Porphyrin secretions from the harderian gland form a reddish crust around the eyes and nose and the color may spread to the rat's neck
   C. Amount of secretion varies with age, stress, and disease

V. Mammary tumors
   A. Neoplasms in the mammary tissue is commonly found in most strains of rats
   B. Tumors can be large but rarely metastasize
   C. They may be surgically removed but often grow back

SYRIAN HAMSTER *(Mesocricetus auratus)* ▬▬
Origin and Uses in Research

I. The Syrian or Golden Hamster is a rodent of the family Cricetidae, found widely in nature throughout North America, Europe, Middle East, Siberia, and eastward into China

II. The Syrian Hamster is the most widely spread species used in the laboratory, although predated by the Chinese hamster *(Cricetulus griseus)*
   A. The Syrian Hamster is easier to breed and establish in captivity

III. The hamster has a unique eversible cheek pouch suitable for studies on microcirculation and transplantation of neonatal, adult, and neoplastic studies

IV. Hamsters are also of use in hypothermia studies because they possess the ability to go into short periods of hibernation under temperatures of 48° F (10° C)

Characteristics—Behavioral and Physiological

I. Female hamsters are generally larger, stronger, and more aggressive than males

II. Hamsters are burrowers and like to hoard their food

III. They are solitary animals under natural conditions and are best kept separate

IV. They are expert escape artists; cages should not be made out of wood, aluminum, or soft plastic and must have tight fitting lids

V. The male has well-developed glands located on the hip. When sexually mature, he will rub this area to secrete a substance used to mark his territory

VI. Hamsters are omnivores; diets can be supplemented with fresh, clean fruits (particularly apples) and vegetables. This may result in a lesser degree of cannibalism

VII. Hamsters are fastidious nocturnal animals that choose different areas of the cage for food storage, defecation, urination, and nesting

VIII. Hamster urine has a high pH of 8, which is full of crystals, giving it a turbid, milky appearance

IX. Feces are almost black, tubular, firm, and approximately 5 mm (>1″) long

Handling and Breeding Considerations

I. Hamsters will bite if startled. A gentle warning such as blowing on the animal should be given before attempting to pick it up

II. Hamsters can be gently scooped up in the palm of the hand, or by using a plastic/metal container
  A. May also be grasped by loose skin over the neck or shoulder area
    1. Used for restraint
    2. Hamster should appear to be smiling when effectively restrained

III. Females should not be bred until they are at least six weeks of age
  A. Hand mating is preferable because the female will commonly destroy the male

IV. Cannibalism of young is common within the first 14 days of age
  A. Care must be taken not to disturb the female and her young within that time period

Sampling/Dosages

For recommended injection/sample sites, needle sizes, and volumes, see Table 27-1

I. Oral dosing can be performed with a ball-ended needle for oral gavage
  A. Medication may be placed in the cheek pouch

II. Animals should preferably be anesthetized for blood sampling and IV injection and sampling

III. Collection of urine and feces can be done by housing the hamster in a metabolism cage, or often

when picked up (restrained) they will urinate and defecate, enabling the handler to collect fresh samples

Signs of Pain and Distress

The hamster is usually a healthy and hardy animal. Key signs are weight loss, hunched appearance, increased aggression, depression, and extended sleep periods.

I. Under normal conditions, hamsters will sleep for long periods during the day and little activity will be seen

II. They often appear aggressive toward each other and emit loud screeching noises, which increase under painful or stressful stimuli

III. Ocular discharge is commonly associated with stress and may be accompanied by an increase in respiratory rate

IV. Loss of coat condition is seen in vitamin E and short chain fatty acid deficient diets

V. Constipation is unusual
  A. Diarrhea when it occurs is profuse and liquid, staining the perineal area

VI. Exploratory behavior is reduced and a hunched appearance is noted, as well as an unwillingness to move

VII. Increased depression occurs when the animal is left undisturbed
  A. Daytime sleep periods may be extended

VIII. Lateral recumbency can indicate that the animal is moribund

IX. Normal gait is affected when pain is associated with locomotion
  A. Stilted movements are sometimes associated with abdominal involvement (e.g., ascites)

Health Conditions

I. Wet tail (proliferative ileitis or transmissible ileal hyperplasia)
  A. May be predisposed by stresses of confinement and weaning with highest mortality in nursing or newly weaned animals between three to eight weeks of age
  B. Primary pathogens are thought to be *E. coli* and *Campylobacter* sp.
  C. Characterized by severe depression, high mortality, lethargy, irritability, anorexia, emaciation, with death occurring from 48 hours to one week after the initial onset of signs
  D. Treatment with neomycin is useful but not usually successful; prevention best—through a high level of hygiene and avoidance of stress
    1. Enrofloxacin (Baytril) can be toxic to the intestines

II. Antibiotic sensitivity
  A. Hamsters have predominantly gram-positive intestinal flora and tend to develop a fatal gram-negative enterotoxemia when given certain antibiotics
  B. Antibiotics of known toxicity include: penicillin, lincomycin, erythromycin, dihydrostreptomycin, and occasionally tetracycline, if not used in combination with sulfaguanidine

III. Hibernation
  A. Hibernation should always be considered in the case of an apparently dead hamster
  B. Warm the animal gradually

IV. Vaginitis
  A. Every four days female hamsters that have a regular estrous cycle produce a post ovulatory discharge that can be mistaken for vaginitis
  B. The white opaque discharge that may be seen periodically in the vagina is not an indication of vaginitis

V. Impacted cheek pouch
  A. An impacted cheek pouch should be cleaned out carefully with a pair of blunt-ended forceps and antibiotic ointment instilled into the pouch

VI. Respiratory infections
  A. Pneumonia is seen periodically in hamsters and is considered secondary in importance to Wet Tail
  B. Hamsters may be affected by *Streptococcus* and *Pasteurella pneumotropica,* giving rise to respiratory distress and ocular discharge
    1. Treatment includes gentamicin and chloramphenicol
  C. Sendai virus may produce pneumonia in suckling hamsters. Hamsters have shown to be susceptible to the pneumonia virus of mice

VII. Other viruses reported to infect hamsters
  A. Lymphocytic choriomenigitis virus (which may give rise to clinical disease in humans)
  B. Simian virus-5
  C. Reovirus 3
  D. Polyoma virus
  E. Tyzzer's disease
  NOTE: Hamsters should never be housed with other species

MONGOLIAN GERBIL
(*Meriones unguiculatus*) ▬▬▬▬▬▬
Origin and Uses in Research

I. The mongolian gerbil (most common) and the black mongolian gerbil, rodents of the family Cricetidae, are indigenous to the desert regions of North Eastern China and Mongolia

II. Gerbils are useful animals in radiation studies and experimental atherosclerosis, temperature regulation studies, and the effect of hormones on sebaceous glands

Characteristics—Behavioral and Physiological

I. Gerbils are friendly, extremely curious animals that tend to return to their cages in the event of escape

II. Gerbils are nocturnal natural burrowers that exhibit brief periods of intense activity alternating with brief periods of rest

III. By instinct they will make and hide in covered nests and sleep much of the day

IV. Some strains can be susceptible to epileptiform seizures after excitement, stress, sudden noise, etc., with spontaneous recovery and no noted ill effects

V. Gerbils have a great capacity for temperature regulation and can tolerate temperatures between 0° and 32° C (32 and 92° F)

VI. Relative humidity should be lower for these animals (30%-50%) in comparison to most laboratory animals
  A. When the humidity is over 50% the fur will stand away from the body and appear matted as opposed to its usual sleek, smooth appearance

VII. Gerbils are herbivorous and do well on good quality pelleted feed
  A. Care should be taken when feeding a mixed diet of seeds and greens because gerbils are extremely fond of sunflower seeds and will eat these to exclusion of all other food
    1. Sunflower seeds are low in calcium and high in fat

VIII. Feces are tubular, dry, and almost black in color

IX. Gerbils have a low to moderate requirement for dietary water and in turn put out very little urine, keeping odors down in comparison to other laboratory animals

X. Gerbils tend to nonaggression and can be grouped in large numbers (in accordance with housing standards) by sex at weaning

XI. Like rats, gerbils have a harderian gland in the orbit of the eye
  A. Red coloring may appear around the eyes and neck if excessive secretion occurs

XII. A sensitivity to cedar bedding (enzyme induced) may cause bloody nose

Handling and Breeding Considerations

I. Gerbils tolerate gentle handling well, and there is generally no problem associated with the handling of young litters and newborn pups

II. Gerbils do not tolerate being turned on their backs. When picking these animals up, do so at the base of the tail (grasping them away from the base will cause sloughing) and support the body with your other hand

III. Gerbils are monogamous and may not breed with another mate

IV. Male gerbils will aid in care of the young, but if separated to avoid post-partum mating he must be returned to his mate within two weeks of separation

V. Harem matings of a 2:1 ratio tend to be successful if grouped before sexual maturity

Sampling

For injection routes, sites, needle sizes, and volumes, see Table 27-1.

I. Sampling procedures are the same as described for hamsters

Signs of Pain and Distress

I. Gerbils are normally extremely active and nervous and under severe stress may temporarily collapse

II. If diarrhea occurs a low fluid intake may quickly lead to death

III. Dehydration is rarely seen

IV. Hunching and arching of the back may be accompanied with an abnormal gait, indicating locomotion or abdominal involvement

Health Conditions

I. Animals greater than two years of age show a high incidence of tumors
   A. Malignancies appear as spontaneous neoplasms involving the ovaries, ventral sebaceous glands, kidneys, adrenal glands, and skin

II. Gerbils are remarkably resistant to infectious diseases, particularly respiratory infections, pneumonia, and otitis media

III. Overgrowth of incisors is common

IV. Alopecia and inflammation of the skin around the external nares is usually due to a *Staphylococcus* organism in which topical or systemic antibacterial therapy is indicated

V. Gerbils also have a natural susceptibility to *Salmonella*

VI. Tyzzer's disease
   A. Most common fatal bacterial disease
   B. Caused by *Bacillus pisiformis*
   C. May cause diarrhea in weanling gerbils and sometimes adults, accompanied by lethargy, rough coats, and loss of weight
   D. Possible treatment: oxytetracycline and fluid therapy

RABBIT *(Oryctolagus cuniculus)* ▬▬▬▬
Origin and Uses in Research

I. Rabbits are from the order Lagomorpha
   A. Present day breeds are derived from the European rabbit

II. Most common breeds of rabbits used in research: Dutch, Polish, Californian, New Zealand Red, New Zealand White; the latter is the most common

III. Rabbits are useful in biomedical research for alimentary, aging, cancer, cardiovascular, genetic, immunology, virology, and toxicology studies, as well as many other areas

Characteristics—Behavioral and Physiological

I. Rabbits are generally docile and alert
   A. They are generally a social animal but may be housed singly in a lab situation to avoid fighting and to prevent ovulation and pseudopregnancy in females
      1. Females are induced ovulators

II. Rabbits in the wild are nocturnal

III. Aggressive or nervous rabbits will stomp their hind feet in the cage and males may spray
   A. If they panic they will scream

IV. Rabbits are herbivorous and prefer pelleted commercial food
   A. This diet may be supplemented with good quality legumes and vegetables

V. Rabbits have a higher requirement for fiber than other species: a high fiber diet will decrease the incidence of hair balls

VI. Rabbits have large highly vascularized ears allowing for easy intravenous and intraarterial access, and they serve as the rabbit's heat regulatory organ

VII. Rabbits have two pairs of upper incisors: a smaller pair (peg teeth) are found behind the larger pair
   A. Both pairs grow continuously and may need to be trimmed if not naturally worn down, otherwise leading to health conditions such as malocclusion
   B. Enamel is found on the entire tooth surface

VIII. Rabbits have a chin gland, more obvious in males
   A. Females have a dewlap

IX. Rabbit urine is unlike other species in that it is quite thick and cloudy and contains crystalline material
  A. Suckling babies and fasting adults have clear, crystal free urine
X. Daytime feces are usually hard, dark green, round pellets about 0.5 to 1 cm (0.25-0.5″) in diameter
  A. Night time feces are moist, dark brown clusters of small size pellets similar to a raspberry
    1. Coprophagy is a normal behavioral pattern of rabbits and helps increase digestibility of proteins and maintain adequate nutrition and intestinal flora

Handling and Breeding Considerations

I. Rabbits should be approached slowly and quietly so as not to startle them
II. They can be picked up by:
  A. Grasping the loose skin over the back, folding the nose between the rear legs, and lifting out of the cage backward, taking care that nails do not get caught in the mesh wire of the cage
  B. Then position in the handler's arm with head tucked under handler's elbow and back end supported by forearm and other hand
III. When placed back in the cage, they should go in back end first so they don't jump in, risking injury to their back with possible dislocation of lumbar vertebrae
IV. Never grasp rabbits by the ears: this could compromise nerves and circulation
V. Rabbits rarely bite but may charge or scratch when the cage is opened
VI. Male rabbits will be excitable (and therefore harder to handle) if placed in an area where a female has been
  A. In situations where both sexes will be handled, males should be handled first
VII. Restraining devices are available for simple procedures or rabbits may be wrapped up in a lab coat or towel, covering their eyes to keep them calm
  A. Care should be taken to not allow them to overheat
VIII. Rabbits have strong backs and sharp claws, which may cause harm to the handler
  A. If allowed to struggle or jump, they can break their backs
IX. Hypnosis can be used as a means of restraint for some minor noninvasive procedures but not as a substitute for anesthesia
  A. Achieved by carefully placing the rabbit in dorsal recumbency and gently rubbing its abdomen and top of head while speaking in a monotone voice
    1. The room must be very quiet

Sampling

For injection routes, sites, needle sizes, and volumes, see Table 27-1
I. Collection of feces and urine can be done by placing the rabbit in a metabolism cage

Signs of Pain and Distress

I. Difficult to identify signs of pain because rabbits often hide pain and stress
II. Careful examination of the animal may find decreased muscle mass over the back, decreased weight, dehydration, ocular discharge with protrusion of the nictitating membrane, inappetence, and limited movement
III. Rabbits in pain or distress may appear sleepy; if the pain/stress continues they will become depressed, unaware of the environment, and nonresponsive
IV. They may be found facing the back of the cage or facing away from a source of light
V. Other signs of pain and stress are fecal staining of the coat, interruption of night time pellet production, constipation/diarrhea, hairballs from excessive grooming, sore hocks from shifting of weight, stretching, and laying flat from abdominal discomfort

Health Conditions

I. Pasteurellosis
  A. Commonly known as "snuffles"
  B. Most common problem of rabbits—caused by *Pasteurella multocida*
  C. Animals under stress and poor health conditions will show signs of listlessness, nasal and ocular discharge, sneezing
    1. In severe cases: otitis media, torticollis, pneumonia, abscesses, genital infections
  D. Pasteurellosis may be transmitted to other rabbits by direct or indirect methods
  E. Antibiotics may be used to treat affected animals, although they are not likely to eliminate the disease
  F. Affected animals should be quarantined or culled to prevent further transmission through the colony
  G. Environmental stress should be reduced to decrease and prevent recurring infections
II. Tyzzer's disease
  A. Caused by *Bacillus pisiformis*

B. Stressful situations may precede the onset of diarrhea and may lead to death

C. High morbidity and mortality rate

D. Liver necrosis may occur

III. Intestinal coccidiosis

A. Agents of most concern are several *Eimeria* species with varying pathogenicity

B. Clinical signs are diarrhea, anorexia, inability to gain weight, "pot belly"

C. Husbandry practices should be improved to prevent recurrence

D. Signs may be eliminated if animals are medicated with sulfa drugs but there is no effective treatment

IV. Ear mites

A. Common ear infection caused by mites *Psorptes* sp. and *Chorioptes* sp.

B. Characterized by brown scaly debris in the external ear canal, which may be painful if badly infected

C. Ears should be cleaned and treated with mineral oil or a mixture of mineral oil and and acaracide

D. Inspection of the ears should be done regularly

GUINEA PIG *(Cavia porcellus [Cavy])* ▬▬▬▬
Origin and Uses in Research

I. Only member used widely in research of the rodent suborder *Hystricomorpha*

A. Other rodents in this suborder (hedgehog-like) include chinchilla and porcupines

1. Newer DNA evidence indicates that guinea pigs are not rodents but as of date they have not been reclassified

II. Indigenous to South America, Central America, and the Caribbean Islands

III. Most common strains used in research today: English guinea pig (short haired), particularly Duncan-Hartley and Hartley strains developed in the 1920s

IV. Most common pet guinea pigs: Peruvian (long haired), Abyssinian (short haired with rosettes), and English (short haired)

V. Used primarily in microbiology studies due to sensitivity to many infectious diseases that also affect man

VI. Also used in immunology, nutrition, and audiology studies

Characteristics—Behavioral and Physiological

I. Nervous but tame and easily handled

II. They may freeze at unexpected sounds or stampede at unexpected movements

III. Fighting rarely occurs

IV. Have poor jumping/climbing abilities and may be housed in low walled, open topped pens

V. Differ from gerbils, hamsters, mice, and rats in having a cellular membrane that closes over the opening of the vagina

VI. Have constantly erupting (incisor and cheek) hypsodont teeth, which may lead to malocclusion and "slobbers" (see Health Conditions)

VII. The thymus is cervically located and surgically removable

VIII. Guinea pigs are herbivorous and may be fed a commercial pelleted food supplement with hay, greens, or carrots to increase fiber intake

IX. Guinea pigs cannot synthesize enough vitamin C to meet daily requirements

A. Commercial diets must be fed between 60 to 90 days from the date of manufacture because vitamin C will expire beyond that time

1. Vitamin C must be stored in cool and dry conditions

B. If not given in the feed, ascorbic acid at a rate of 200 mg/L may be added to drinking water if using a non copper delivery system

1. Vitamin C activity decreases rapidly

C. If supplementing with dark green leafy vegetables, fruits, and hays, ensure they are clean and comprise no more than 10% to 15% of the weight of the pelleted food

X. Guinea pigs respond poorly to stress and antibiotic therapy

A. Contractions of the smooth muscles if severe in the bronchial tree. Can be lethal

XI. Females have two nipples and mammary glands, although litters of more than four offspring are common

XII. Mature males develop large seminal vesicles that resemble uterine horns, confusing pseudohermaphrodism in this species

Handling and Breeding Considerations

I. Females should be bred before six months of age (2.5-3 months) because the pubic bone may fuse leading to dystocia (pelvic lock)

II. Newborn guinea pigs are precocious and relatively mature with hair, erupted teeth, and open eyes

III. During the later stages of gestation, the sow becomes extremely heavy. Care must be taken to provide adequate support when handling and ensure easy access to food and water

IV. Guinea pigs are easily startled; they rarely bite but will produce a whistling noise and try to avoid capture. A gentle warning should be given on approach

V. Lift by grasping firmly and gently over their shoulders, with two fingers behind and two in front of the forelimbs. The rump should always be supported by the other hand when lifting

Sampling

For injection routes, doses, needle sizes, and blood volumes, see Table 27-1

I. Bleeding techniques require light anesthesia or heavy sedation

II. Oral dosing can be easily achieved by using a ball-ended dosing needle

III. Urine and fecal samples are best obtained by placing guinea pig in a metabolic cage

Signs of Pain and Distress

I. Key signs of pain and distress: withdrawal, vocalization, rough coat, and unresponsiveness

II. Acceptance to capture and restraint

III. Appear sleepy and unresponsive

IV. Eyes sunken and dull

V. Respiratory rate increases with painful/stressful stimuli and becomes increasingly labored

VI. Weight loss, diarrhea, hair loss, scaly skin, dehydration

VII. Tendency toward barbering under dietary stress accompanied by failure to eat and drink

VIII. Group aggression

IX. Excessive salivation

X. Pain associated with locomotion, lameness, careful gait

Health Conditions

I. Antibiotic sensitivity

A. Intestinal flora in guinea pigs is predominantly gram positive, and when treated with antibiotics that act on gram-positive organisms (penicillin, lincomycin, erythromycin, tylosin), the intestinal flora will be drastically altered, leading to an overgrowth of gram-negative organisms

1. This will result in fatal enterocolitis with diarrhea and death within three to seven days

2. Enrofloxacin (Baytril) is the antibiotic of choice for guinea pigs

II. Metastatic or soft tissue calcification

A. Seen in animals over one year of age; occurring in liver, heart, lung, and kidneys

B. Will lead to stiff joints and high mortality

C. Thought to be due to a dietary imbalance of calcium, phosphates, magnesium, and potassium

III. Slobbers (ptyalism)

A. Chronic drooling due to overgrowth of teeth, malocclusion, or mandibular deformity as a result of scurvy

IV. Scurvy (vitamin C deficiency)

A. Signs include unsteady gait, painful locomotion, hemorrhage of gums, swelling of costochondral junctions, and emaciation, due to inadequate requirement of dietary vitamin C

V. Muscular dystrophy

A. May result from a dietary deficiency of vitamin E

B. Signs include stiffness, lameness, and refusal to move

VI. Pregnancy toxemia (ketosis)

A. Occurs in obese guinea pigs in later stages (56th day) of pregnancy or obese guinea pigs under stress

B. Early treatment is helpful but prognosis is poor; control may be achieved by preventing obesity, avoiding stress (especially during late pregnancy) and providing high quality feed

VII. Enzootic cervical lymphadenitis

A. Signs are bilateral swellings and discharge under the jaw or neck region, which may lead to pericarditis, peritonitis, pleuropneumonia, and purulent otitis media

B. Animals exhibiting these signs must be isolated and treated with antibiotics or destroyed

VIII. Bacterial pneumonia

A. Often seen as chronic conditions and can be distinguished from acute salmonellosis by detection of hematuria

B. Antibiotic treatment and isolation is indicated

C. Prevention and control is accomplished through good husbandry and isolation procedures

IX. Salmonellosis

A. Rare, although it does occur

B. Treatment is not indicated; strict isolation and culling procedures are indicated

X. Pseudo-tuberculosis

A. Manifests as a chronic disease, with diarrhea, enlarged lymph nodes, and death occurring in three to four weeks

B. Treatment is impractical and strict isolation and culling procedures are indicated

XI. Three basic forms of alopecia

A. Scabby areas especially on the head (possible ringworm)

B. Well-defined lesions on posterior possibly due to self-barbering, which indicates dietary deficiencies

C. Diffuse hair loss over flanks and back, which usually grows back following parturition, may occur in pregnant females

D. Feeding of hay (preferably sterilized) may help the latter two conditions

XII. Anesthetic complications/considerations

    A. Innovar-Vet will cause self-mutilation

    B. Ketamine must be given as a deep intramuscular injection (not subcutaneously because it will create sloughing of the tissue). (See Appendix for other injectable anesthetics)

    C. It is very important to use atropine

    D. Muscular movements may occur during surgical anesthesia

GENERAL CAGING AND HOUSING

I. Choose size of caging appropriate to species; see Table 27-2

II. Animals should be confined securely and ensure comfort and safety, permitting normal postural and behavioral adjustments

III. Environmental enrichment should be provided for social and behavioral needs

IV. Animals that are social in nature should not be housed singly unless necessary for research protocol and approved by the appropriate body (animal care committee)

V. Provide adequate ventilation, viewing, and easy access to animal

VI. Food and water delivery systems:

    A. Must provide ready access

    B. Must not be contaminated with excrement

        1. Guinea pigs often play with waterers, which may flood the cage

VII. Housing must facilitate easy cleaning and disinfection (design and material)

VIII. Consider light intensity, noise levels, ventilation, and temperature effects on the animal's micro environment and ensure they are within recognized guidelines

REPRODUCTIVE DATA

I. See Table 27-3 for reproductive data

ZOONOSIS

I. From an occupational health standpoint, as well as animal colony management, it is important to be aware of the diseases that can be transmitted from one species to another, including humans

II. See Table 27-4

Table 27-2 Housing data

Species	Temperature* °C	°F	Relative humidity† (%)	Ventilation air changes (hour)	Light (hours)	Caging	Other conditions
Mouse	22-25	72-78	50-70	8-12	14, nocturnal	Shoebox/ suspended mesh	House same sex together; remove fighters; barbering
Rat	20-25	68-76	50-55	10-20	12-15, nocturnal	Shoebox/ suspended mesh	Noise greater than 50 decibels may be detrimental; group same sex together
Guinea pig	10-20	50-60	50-60	4-8	12-15, crepuscular	Shoebox/ suspended mesh	Ammonia concentration greater than 22 ppm is harmful; light changes should be gradual
Hamster	21-24	70-78	45-65	6-10	12, nocturnal	Shoebox	House in groups when young; may separate at reproductive age; hibernation brought on by decrease in temperature and light
Mongolian Gerbil	15-24	60-78	40-50	8-10	12-14, nocturnal/ diurnal	Shoebox	Burrowers; produce little urine, therefore less ammonia
Rabbit	16-20	62-70	40-50	10-12	12-14, crepuscular	Suspended wire mesh/shoebox	House alone or groups of same sex

From CCAG, Guide to the care and use of experimental animals, Volume 1

*From National Academy of Science: *The guide for the care and use of laboratory animals,* 1996, suggests that the range of temperature for all listed species is between 64 to 79° F and 18 to 26° C.

†The range of humidity for each is 30% to 70%.

Table 27-3 Reproductive Data*†

Species	Litter size	Weight at birth	Weanling age	Puberty	Breeding age	Estrus cycle	Mating	Gestation
Mouse	5-10	1g	21 days 10-12g	4-6 wks	6-8 wks	4-6 days, poly-estrus, Whitten and Bruce effects†‡	Harem, 1/4	19-21 days
Rat	1-20 avg	5-6g	21 days, eyes open at 14-15d	4-6 wks	2-3 months	5 days, poly-estrus	Harem, 1/6	21-23 days
Guinea pig	2-6	60-200g	3 wks	3-4 wks	3 months	16 days, poly-estrus	Harem, 1/5-10	63 days
Hamster	5-10	2g	21 days	4-6 wks	6-7 wks	4 days, poly-estrus, yeasty odor from genital area	Monogamous or harem, 1/5	16 days
Mongolian gerbil	4-5	2g	21 days	10 wks	10-12 wks	4-6 days, poly-estrus	Monogamous at weanling	22-26 days
Rabbit	6-10	40g	6-8 wks	5-9 months	6-9 months	No regular cycle, polyestrus	Hand mating, 1/10-15	30-32 days

*Ovulation: all listed species, other than the rabbit, are spontaneous ovulaters. Rabbits are induced ovulaters—mating initiates ovulation.
†Whitten effect: synchronization of estrus.
‡Bruce effect: if a pregnant mouse is exposed to a strange male within the first four days of pregnancy, the mouse will abort the pregnancy.

Table 27-4 Zoonoses

Disease	Causative organism/ distribution	Laboratory species	Outcome of infection, to humans
Salmonellosis	Bacteria Worldwide	Mice, rats, guinea pigs	Gastroenteritis (vomiting, diarrhea), headache, and fever
Campylobacter	Bacteria Worldwide	Hamsters	Abdominal pain and severe diarrhea
Lymphocytic choriomeningitis	Arena virus Worldwide	Especially hamsters, rodents	Meningitis—temporary illness with nervous symptoms or permanent disability associated with the central nervous system
Ringworm	Fungus: Microsporum, Trichophyton Worldwide	Guinea pigs, rats	Progressively itchy, weeping, chronic dermatitis
Tularemia/rabbit fever	Francisella tularersis Circumpolar in Northern Hemisphere	Rabbits, rodents	Without antibiotic treatment, fatal in 5% of cases; diagnosis by antibody identification via blood testing; signs are fever, lethargy, anorexia, coughing, diarrhea
Plague	Yersinia pestis Western USA, South America, Asia, Africa	Rodents	Fever, shivering, severe headaches, swollen lymph glands Pneumonic plague may be a complication; coughing produces bloody frothy sputum, labored breathing
Pseudotuberculosis (Yersiniosis)	Yersinia pseudotuberculosis Northern Hemisphere	Rodents	Coughing, chest pain, shortness of breath, fever, sweating, poor appetite, weight loss
Rat bite fever	Streptobaccillus Worldwide	Rodents	Inflammation at site of bite, swollen lymph nodes, bouts of fever, rash, painful joints
Tetanus	Clostridium tetani Worldwide	Herbivores	Stiffness of jaw, difficulty opening mouth, stiffness of abdominal and back muscles, contraction of facial muscles, asphyxia may result
Rabies	Lyssavirus Worldwide except Australia, New Zealand, Britain, Scandinavia, Japan, Taiwan	Carnivores	Fever, headache, loss of appetite, restlessness, hyperactivity, disorientation, seizures, attempts to drink produce violent painful spasms; coma and death 3-20 days after onset of symptoms
Letptospirosis (Weil's disease)	Leptospira spp. Worldwide	Rodents	Fever, chills, headache, muscle aches, eye inflammation, skin rash

AALAS training manual series, Volume 3.
CCAC, Guide to the care and use of experimental animals.
CCCAC, Guide to the care and use of experimental animals.

LABORATORY ANIMAL ALLERGY (LAA) ▬▬▬

I. An occupational health concern when regularly working with common laboratory animal species

II. An immediate hypersensitivity that may develop on exposure to the laboratory animal, its fur or dander, urine, saliva, serum, or other tissues
   A. Mild: upper respiratory signs, red itchy wheals on skin
   B. Severe: wheezing, shortness of breath, feeling of chest tightness or asthma

III. Measures should be taken to reduce exposure through good hygiene/sanitation, protective clothing, air ventilation/filtration, and education

Glossary

axenic Also referred to as germ free; these animals are hysterectomy derived, free from any microorganisms, and maintained in a germ free isolation type housing

barbering Occurs when one animal clips or chews the fur of another, usually around the muzzle or head to show dominance

barrier sustained Gnotobiotic animals that are maintained under sterile conditions in a barrier unit

bruce effect The manipulation of pregnancy by pheromones such as the termination of pregnancy in a recently bred mouse by placing it in a cage with a strange male

crepuscular Becoming active at twilight or just before sunrise

gavage Force feeding/medicating usually through a tube passed into the stomach

gnotobiotic Germ free animals that have been introduced to one or two known nonpathogenic microorganisms

harem mating Mating one male with more than two females

hypsodont Having prism shaped teeth with high crowns, as in many herbivorous animals

latent infection A condition or infection that may not be clinically noted in the animal, but under stress or poor health conditions it develops into a recognizable disease state

malocclusion A genetic or dietary related condition in which the apposing teeth do not meet when the jaw is closed

micro environment A small isolated habitat, usually within a cage

nocturnal Becoming active at night

SPF Specific Pathogen Free—these animals are free from specific pathogenic organisms

Whitten effect The introduction of a male into a group of females results in synchronization of the estrus cycle of the females

Review Questions

1 What species does not have a gallbladder?
a. Mouse
b. Rat
c. Guinea pig
d. Hamster

2 Which species does not practice coprophagy as a necessary nutritional supplement?
a. Mouse
b. Rat
c. Guinea pig
d. Rabbit

3 Which species is unable to synthesize vitamin C?
a. Rabbits
b. Guinea pig
c. Hamster
d. Gerbil

4 Which of the following are zoonotic diseases?
a. *Salmonella,* ringworm, lymphocytic choriomeningitis
b. *Salmonella,* ringworm, chromodacryorrhea
c. Ringworm, chromodacryorrhea, lymphocytic choriomeningitis
d. Ringworm, scurvy, chromodacryorrhea

5 Inbred strains are the result of at least how many generations of brother x sister matings?
a. 10
b. 20
c. 30
d. 40

6 Which species is known to go into hibernation if housing temperature is decreased?
a. Hamster
b. Rat
c. Mouse
d. Guinea pig

7 Which are inbred strains of rats?
a. Sprague-Dawley, Long Evans, Wistar
b. Wistar, Zucker, Brattleboro
c. Sprague-Dawley, CAR, BB
d. Zucker, Brattleboro, BB

8 Hamsters are escape artists and therefore their caging should have the following characteristics:
a. Loose fitting lid, not made of wood, aluminum, or soft plastic
b. Tight fitting lid, not made of wood, aluminum, or soft plastic
c. Tight fitting lid, made out of wood, aluminum, or soft plastic
d. Tight fitting lid, not made out of wood but made out of aluminum or soft plastic

9 Chromodacryorrhea is commonly referred to as red tears and is:
a. A zoonotic viral condition
b. A bacterial condition
c. Caused from porphyrin secretions from the harderian gland
d. Caused from a secretion from the hibernating gland

10 The gestation period of the gerbil is:
a. 19-21 days
b. 30-32 days
c. 22-26 days
d. 63 days

BIBLIOGRAPHY

Animals for research act, 1983, Government of Ontario.

Canadian Association for Laboratory Animal Science, *CALAS training manual,* Ottawa, 1977 and 1995 editions.

Canadian Council on Animal Care: *Guide to the care and use of experimental animals,* Volume 1, Ottawa, Ontario, 1993.

Canadian Council on Animal Care: *Guide to the care and use of animals,* Volume 2, Ottawa, Ontario, 1980-1984.

Cranney J, Zaja A: *A method for jugular blood collection in rabbits* 32:6, Nov 1993, p. 6.

Fox RR: "Health and benefits of animal research, the rabbit as a subject," *The physiologist* 27:6, 1984, pp. 393-40.

Gill TJ: "Health benefits of animal research, the rat in biomedical research," *The physiologist* 28:1, 1985, pp 9-17.

Harkness JE, Wagner JE: *The biology and medicine of rabbits and rodents,* ed 4, Lea and Febiger, Philadelphia, 1995.

Heim AR: "A practical technique for obtaining multiple blood samples from rabbits," *Lab animal,* January/February 1989, pp 32-33.

Holmes DD: *Clinical laboratory animal medicine,* Iowa State Press, Iowa, 1984.

Jenkins WL: "Pharmacological aspects of analgesic drugs in animals: an overview," *JAVMA,* 191(10), 1987, pp 1231-1239.

McGuill MW, Rowan AN: Biological effects of blood loss: implications for sampling, volumes and techniques, *ILAR news* 31(4), 1989, pp 5-18.

Merck veterinary manual, Merck and Company Inc., Rathway, New Jersey, 1986, pp 1602.

Morgan P: *Canadian medical association medical encyclopedia,* Readers Digest Association, Darling Kindersley Limited, London.

National Academy of Science: *The guide and care for the use of laboratory animals,* 1996, National Academy Press. Washington.

Sirois M: The pet guinea pig, *The veterinary technician,* January 1988, pp 50-55.

Stark D, Ostrow M, ed: *Association for laboratory animal science training manual series,* Vol 1, 3, Tennessee.

Stewart K, Johnstone E: Laboratory Gerbils and Hamsters, *The veterinary technician,* April 1989, pp 188-195.

Timm KI: Orbital venous anatomy of the mongolian gerbil with comparison to the mouse, hamster and rat, *Laboratory animal science* 39(3), May 1989, pp 262-264.

Williams CSF: *Practical guide to laboratory animals,* Mosby, Saint Louis, 1976.

Young S, Flecknell P, Dyson D, McDonell W: Short course notes on anesthesia of laboratory animals, Ontario Veterinary College, University of Guelph, Guelph, Ontario, September 1992.

CHAPTER 28

Avian and Reptile Medicine

Rebecca M. Atkinson

CHAPTER OUTLINE

Avian
Classification
Anatomical and Physiological
    Differences
Housing
Restraint and Handling
Nutrition: Diets and Problems
Noninfectious Diseases and
    Conditions
Infectious Diseases
    Bacterial and Bacterial-like
        Diseases
    Viral Diseases
    Mycotic Diseases

Parasites
    Ectoparasites
    Endoparasites
Reptile
Classifiction
Anatomical and Physiological
    Differences
Housing
Restraint and Handling
Nutrition: Diets and Problems
    Snakes
    Turtles
    Lizards

Clinical Conditions and Diseases
Infectious Diseases
    Bacterial and Bacterial-like
        Diseases
    Viral Diseases
    Protozoal Diseases
    Mycotic Diseases
Parasites
    Ectoparasites
    Endoparasites

LEARNING OUTCOMES

After reading this chapter you should be able to:

1. Describe the anatomical and physiological differences in avian and reptile species as compared to mammals.
2. Describe optimum housing and husbandry for reptile and avian species.
3. Describe restraint and handling for reptiles and avian species.
4. List optimum nutritional requirements for various avian and reptile species.
5. Identify noninfectious and infectious diseases by describing their etiology, clinical signs, and pathology.
6. Describe ecto and endoparasitic diseases in reptiles and avian species.

Since there are more clients with exotic pets, there has been a dramatic increase in questions regarding these species. In veterinary practices, there are now more procedures performed on reptiles and avians than in previous years. To effectively answer basic questions, the technician needs a fundamental knowledge of anatomy, physiology, nutritional requirements, and diseases of reptiles and avians. This chapter reviews these areas, as well as restraint, handling, and blood collection.

Avian

CLASSIFICATION

I. Class Aves
    A. Order Psittaformes (parrots, cockatoos, macaws, budgies, cockatiels)
    B. Order Passeriformes (songbirds)
    C. Order Anseriformes (ducks, geese, swans)
    D. Ciconiformes (cranes, herons)
    E. Falconiformes (falcons, hawks, eagles, owls)
    F. Galliformes (poultry, pheasants, peafowl)

ANATOMICAL AND PHYSIOLOGICAL DIFFERENCES

Reduction and modification of organs and organ systems to obtain the capacity for flight. Lack of teeth, hollowing of bones, shortened gastrointestinal tract, presence of air sacs, higher rate of metabolism, oviparity, and feathers are all adaptations for weight reduction and flight ability.

I. Integument
   A. Thinner and more delicate than in mammals
   B. Consists of the epidermis, dermis, and subcutaneous layers
   C. Modifications include the legs and feet, beak, cere, and cheek patches
   D. The ventral surface of the female bird can modify during breeding season to form a brood patch
   E. The dermal layer contains the feather follicles arranged in rows, called pterylae, separated by featherless rows called apteriae
   F. Smooth muscles attach to the follicles and are responsible for feather fluffing to conserve heat, similar to piloerection of hair in mammals
   G. Deficient of glands with the exception of the meibomian glands of the eyelid, uropygial gland above the tail base, and the holocrine gland of the external ear canal
   H. Feathers are epidermal structures analagous to mammalian hair and serve in insulation, thermoregulation, courtship displays, and flight
      I. Feather types
         1. Contour (e.g., body and flight feathers)
         2. Plume (e.g., down [modified as powder down in cockatoos, cockatiels, and African grey parrots])
         3. Semiplume (e.g., bristles and "hairs")
   J. Moulting is the process of shedding and regrowing of feathers. It is influenced by season, temperature, nutrition, stress, species, and sex. Moulting occurs at least yearly, systematically and gradually, never leaving the bird featherless

II. Sensory: senses of smell and taste are poorly developed; visual senses are extremely well developed
   A. Color vision: rods and cones are present (the numbers depend on species diurnal or nocturnal habits)
   B. Three functional eyelids: upper, lower, and nictitating
   C. Eyeballs are fixed in their sockets so the bird must be able to rotate its head almost 360 degrees
   D. Movement of one eye is independent of the other
   E. Sclerotic ring is the bony ring around the eye, where the cornea joins the sclera
   F. Pecten: a brown vascular fringe that projects from the lower medial wall of the eye toward the lens; assumed to provide nutrients to the avascular retina

III. Skeleton: extreme adaptations for flight
   A. Bones are pneumatic: lightweight
   B. Some of the air sacs are in direct communication with the proximal bones
   C. Fusion of bones: carpometacarpus, tarsometatarsus, and the pelvic girdle (synsacrum)
   D. Pectoral girdle consists of a tripod of bones: clavicle, coracoid, and scapula

IV. Digestive system varies with gross anatomical differences and short transit time (3-12 hours)
   A. Galliformes and psittacines possess a true crop
   B. Raptors have a poorly developed crop
   C. Piscivores (fish-eating birds) and owls lack a crop
   D. Beak is epidermal tissue and has characteristics based on the diet
   E. Oral cavity is made up of the tongue, glottis (no epiglottis), salivary glands, taste buds, and pharynx
   F. Proximal esophagus to crop, distal esophagus to stomach (glandular proventriculus and the muscular ventriculus or gizzard)
   G. Associated organs: liver and spleen
   H. Small intestine; duodenum, jejunum, and ileum
   I. Pancreas and gallbladder (absent in most psittacines) empty into the terminal aspect of the duodenal loop
   J. Large intestine; paired caeca (absent in psittacines), rectum, and cloaca
   K. Cloaca; coprodeum (digestive), urodeum (urinary), and proctodeum

V. Respiratory: unique anatomy
   A. No diaphragm
   B. Larynx: at anterior end of the trachea, complete rings, not sound producing
   C. Syrinx: at base of the trachea, sound producing
   D. Bronchi to lungs

E. Lungs: the most efficient gas exchange system among the vertebrates
  1. Compressed dorsally against the ribs, fixed, and do not expand during inspiration
  2. Unidirectional flow through the lung
  3. Crosscurrent relationship between the parabronchial gas and blood
  4. Countercurrent relationship between the blood and capillaries
  5. Increased diffusing capacity for oxygen
F. Air sacs
  1. Nine pair (based on the chicken as a model): single interclavicular, cervical, anterior thoracic, posterior thoracic, abdominal
  2. Communicate with the proximal pneumatic bones
  3. Thin-walled, one cell thick, epithelial tissue
  4. Connect to the lung directly by the primary or secondary bronchus
  5. Connect indirectly by the parabronchi
  6. Act as a bellows system using the sternum to push air through the lungs
VI. Circulatory: endurance for flight
  A. Four-chambered heart
    1. Relatively larger than the mammalian heart
    2. Faster heart rate
    3. Greater arterial pressure
    4. Lower peripheral resistance
  B. Blood cells
    1. Nucleated erythrocytes
       a. Large in comparison to mammalian cells
       b. Live 28 to 45 days
       c. Rapid turnover rate
       d. High polychromatic index
    2. Thrombocytes (similar to mammalian platelets)
    3. Heterophils (analogous to mammalian neutrophils)
    4. Eosinophils
    5. Basophils
    6. Lymphocytes
    7. Monocytes
VII. Urogenital
  A. No urinary bladder
  B. Metanephric kidneys
  C. Renal portal system (as in reptiles): blood from the caudal portion of the body passes through the kidneys via the renal portal system before entering the main vascular system
  D. Kidneys are three lobed: cranial, middle, and caudal; compressed dorsally
  E. Urine excreted as uric acid; voided with feces through the cloaca
  F. Female reproductive system
    1. Only one functional ovary and oviduct on the left, the right being vestigial
    2. Oviduct; the infundibulum receives the ovum from the follicle, the magnum adds the albumen, the isthmus adds the two shell membranes, the uterus lays down the calcium shell, and the vagina directs the egg to the cloaca
  G. Male reproductive system
    1. Paired testes: increase dramatically in size during the breeding season
    2. Vas deferens
    3. Seminal vesicles: store sperm and pass them into the cloaca
    4. Phallic organ is present in some birds (waterfowl, ostriches, rheas, emus, herons and flamingos); acts as an intromittent organ during copulation
  H. Sexual maturity age varies with species; budgies are active at 1 year (lifespan 8-10 years), canaries at 1 to 4 years (lifespan 4-8 years), cockatiels at 2 years (lifespan 10-15 years), and larger parrots at 3 to 7 years (lifespan 30-50 years for an Amazon parrot)

HOUSING

I. Clinic caging
  A. Incubators
  B. Stainless steel dog kennels
  C. Custom built isolates
  D. Commercial wire bird cages
II. "At home" caging
  A. A "natural" environment simulation
  B. Outdoor aviary
  C. Large enough to allow full body extension, as large as space allows
  D. Strong to resist dismantling by the bird
  E. Constructed of nontoxic materials (caution with lead or zinc compounds)
  F. Safe and easy for cleaning
  G. Sturdy, nontoxic feed and water bowls
  H. Perches of hardwood, nontoxic, and of varying diameters about the size of the bird's foot, set at alternate heights

    I. Avoid sandpaper-covered perches

    J. Substrate lining: newspaper, paper towel, paper liner

  III. Quarantine: new birds should be quarantined for 30 to 45 days in a separate facility or room before introduction into the home or existing flock

RESTRAINT AND HANDLING

    I. Restraint: caution not to restrict movement of the sternum, since birds breathe by sternal movement, and keep wings restrained from flapping

      A. Budgies, parakeets, cockatiels, and canaries can be caught from behind with a small towel or barehanded; hold the head between the middle and index finger, with the hand restraining the wings and body

      B. Larger psittacines should be caught from behind with a towel (gloves can be bulky and give a false sense of protection); hold the head between the thumb and index finger and the towel, with other hand supporting the body

      C. Waterfowl can be restrained carrying the body under the arms and with other hand holding the head

      D. Waterbirds (loons, cranes and herons) inflict nasty pecks with their pointed beaks; wear eye protection and restrain similar to above

      E. Raptorial species: capture from behind with a towel; grasp both legs above the talons, restrain the head, and body with the towel and other hand

   II. Blood collection

      A. Jugular (the right is slightly larger than the left)

      B. Brachioulnar (wing vein)

      C. Medial tibiotarsal (leg vein)

      D. Toenail clipping is not recommended

  III. Blood analysis: Coulter counter cannot be used for avian blood due to the nucleated red blood cells; complete blood count can be obtained by combining the Unopette system and hemocytometer count, which give an absolute heterophil and eosinophil count, with a differential count from a smear

  IV. Intravenous access sites (see those used for blood collection)

   V. Intraosseous catheter: proximal tibia or in the distal ulna (similar to an intravenous catheter)

  VI. Intramuscular injections: pectoral muscle rather than the leg due to presence of the renal portal system and possible nephrotoxicity or rapid excretion

  VII. Oral administration/tube feeding: metal or plastic feeding tube (metal is preferred for psittacines so they can't bite the tube and swallow it) inserted into the esophagus and down into the crop

 VIII. Temperature, pulse, and respirations

      A. Body temperature is 40-41° C, (105° F)

      B. Pulse rate 100-200 beats per minute (varies with size and species)

      C. Respiratory rate 20-40 breaths per minute (varies with stress and activity)

NUTRITION: DIETS AND PROBLEMS

    I. Proper psittacine diet

      A. Pelleted or extruded "complete" psittacine diets containing the 13 required vitamins (A, D, E, K, and B), minerals (calcium, phosphorous, sodium, magnesium, and chloride are required in large quantities); 18%-20% protein for an adult, 20%-25% protein for a juvenile; 4%-10% fat, carbohydrates, and fiber

      B. Fresh supply of water

      C. Grains and carbohydrates (pasta is a favorite)

      D. Legumes, fruits, vegetables

      E. Dairy products in low amounts (high in fat)

      F. Seeds should be restricted or used as treats due to the high fat component

      G. Calcium supplement can be added for breeding birds in the form of oyster shell, mineral block, or cuttlebone

      H. Budgies do not synthesize iodine and thus require iodine in their diet

      I. Grit is not necessary in most birds and need not be supplemented

   II. Waterfowl diet: commercially available

  III. Poultry diet: commercially available

  IV. Waterbirds are carnivorous: feed fish and frogs

   V. Raptorial species are carnivorous: feed mice, rats, quail, and chicks

  VI. Dietary problems

      A. Hypovitaminosis A: unhealthy mucous membranes and epithelium

      B. Hypocalcemia: "Metabolic bone disease" and nutritional hypoparathyroidism (parathyroid response leading to hypocalcemic tetany and convulsions observed in psittacines and raptors)

      C. Calcium/phosphorous imbalance: normal ratio is 1.5:1 to 2:1 (sunflower seed has a calcium/phosphorous ratio of 8:1)

D. Thiamine deficiency: stargazing and opisthotonos

E. Hypovitaminosis E and selenium deficiency: cause degeneration of skeletal muscles ("white muscle disease")

NONINFECTIOUS DISEASES AND CONDITIONS ■

I. Predisposing factors such as immunosuppression, dehydration, malnutrition, starvation, unhygienic environmental conditions, chilling, and stress can leave the bird susceptible to disease

II. Trauma: dislocations, fractures, soft tissue damage, and pododermatitis or "bumblefoot"

III. Feather conditions may occur from boredom ("feather-picking"), hypoparathyroidism, stress, improper moulting, skin allergies, or ectoparasites

IV. Egg-binding and chronic egg-laying: abdominal distention, dyspnea, and hypocalcemia

V. Regurgitation (and vomiting, although this is uncommon in birds) may be normal courtship behavior, lead poisoning, foreign body, or a GI problem

VI. Toxins

A. Fumes from household products, paints, pesticides

B. Toxic plants

C. Lead poisoning

1. Clinical signs of lethargy, depression, green diarrhea, wing paresis to paralysis and convulsions

2. Pet bird sources include stained glass, old paint, soldering, wine foil, galvanized wire, batteries, pellets, antique jewelry

3. Waterfowl ingest cast lead shot from the bottom of ponds

4. Raptorial species ingest waterfowl who carry lead shot in their muscle as a result of gunshot

5. Treatment includes chelation therapy with calcium disodium versonate and supportive care

INFECTIOUS DISEASE ■■■■■■■■■
Bacterial and Bacterial-like Diseases

I. Normal bacterial flora in the gastrointestinal tract of psittacines are gram positive

II. Normal flora for raptorial species and other carnivorous species are gram negative

III. Common diseases in psittacines, poultry, raptors, and waterfowl

A. Psittacosis or chlamydiosis

1. Rickettsial organism: *Chlamydia psittaci*

2. Clinical signs include green diarrhea, pneumonia, nasal and ocular discharge, sneezing, and lethargy, or may be asymptomatic

3. Lesions include splenomegaly, hepatomegaly, pericarditis, air sacculitis, and pneumonia

4. Zoonotic: causes flu-like symptoms in people

5. Diagnosis by fecal antigen capture test or serology

6. Treatment: tetracycline or doxycycline and supportive care

B. Avian tuberculosis

1. Cause: *Mycobacterium avium*

2. Clinical signs: chronic weight loss and lethargy

3. Diagnosis by acid-fast test on feces (if the bird is shedding it should be positive) or biopsy of the infected liver or intestinal mucosa

4. Treatment: long-term combined antibiotic therapy

5. Zoonotic potential

C. Coryza: upper respiratory disease

1. Cause: *Hemophilus* and *Mycoplasma*

2. Clinical signs: rhinitis, sinusitis, and upper respiratory signs

D. Pneumonia and air sacculitis: lower respiratory tract infections

1. Cause: several bacteria, including *Pasteurella, Yersinia* (pseudotuberculosis), *Streptococcus,* and *Staphylococcus*

2. Clinical signs: hyperpnea, dyspnea, abdominal breathing, and cyanosis

E. Avian cholera or pasteurellosis

1. Cause: *Pasteurella multocida*

2. Clinical signs: diarrhea, ataxia, septicemia, and sudden death, or asymptomatic

F. Enteritis

1. Cause: several bacteria, including *Clostridium*

2. Botulism occurs when spoiled food and algal bloom undergo anaerobic conditions

3. Clinical signs in waterfowl: weakness, "limber neck," paresis, paralysis, and death

4. Treatment: supportive care and antitoxin

Viral Diseases

The following viral diseases occur in psittacines, poultry, raptors, and waterfowl unless otherwise stated.

I. Avian influenza
  A. Cause: orthomyxovirus
  B. Clinical signs: congestion, sneezing, rhinitis, and pneumonia
II. Avian pox
  A. Cause: various pox strains, each species specific
  B. Clinical signs: crusty, raised, pox lesions around the eyes, beak, and feet
III. Hemorrhagic enteritis
  A. Cause: adenovirus
  B. Clinical signs: bloody feces and death
  C. Occurs commonly in turkeys and poultry, also reported in budgies and lovebirds
IV. Newcastle's disease
  A. Cause: paramyxovirus (nine virus types are currently identified)
  B. Clinical signs: ataxia, opisthotonos, and seizures
V. Marek's disease
  A. Cause: a herpesvirus
  B. Necropsy lesions are grey or white neoplastic lesions on various organs, especially liver
  C. Common problem in poultry
VI. Pacheco's disease
  A. Cause: a herpesvirus
  B. Clinical signs: anorexia and sudden death
  C. Occurs in outbreak conditions in psittacines
VII. Duck plague
  A. Cause: a herpesvirus
  B. Clinical signs: diarrhea and sudden death
  C. Common problem in waterfowl
VIII. Budgie fledgling disease (BFD)
  A. Cause: a polyomavirus
  B. Clinical signs: abdominal distention, hepatomegaly, and dystrophic feather formation
  C. Occurs in young birds in budgies and other psittacines
IX. Psittacine beak and feather disease (PFBD)
  A. Cause: a circovirus
  B. Clinical signs: clubbing of feather shafts, feather atypia, beak lesions, or feather loss
  C. Diagnosed by a feather biopsy and histology
X. Proventricular dilation syndrome or disease (PDS), or "wasting syndrome"
  A. Considered to be caused by a virus yet unidentified
  B. Clinical signs include weight loss although eating well and neurological signs as the disease progresses
  C. Diagnosis may be made on clinical signs, fluoroscopic examination, and biopsy of the affected area of crop, proventriculus or ventriculus

Mycotic Diseases

I. Aspergillosis
  A. Cause: *Aspergillosis fumigatus*
  B. Respiratory disease precipitated by stress
  C. Clinical signs: air sacculitis, dyspnea, lethargy, droopy wings, anorexia, mild to severe respiratory distress
II. Candidiasis
  A. Cause: *Candida albicans,* an opportunistic yeast that overgrows if normal bacterial flora are upset
  B. Clinical signs: gray to white plaque lesions in the oral cavity, esophagus, and crop
  C. Common in pigeons, raptors, and psittacines

PARASITES

Ectoparasites

I. Biting lice (Mallophaga)
II. Mites
  A. Scaly leg and face mites: *Knemidocoptes*
    1. Common in budgies and other psittacines
    2. Lesions on the beak, eyelids, and legs
  B. Tracheal mites: *Sternostoma tracheacolum*
    1. Common in finches, canaries, budgies, and poultry
    2. Clinical signs: sneezing, open-mouth breathing, dyspnea, and loss of voice
III. Ticks
IV. Hippoboscid flies are seen on raptorial birds
V. Most ectoparasites are easily treated with ivermectin or dilute carbaryl dusting powders

Endoparasites

I. Nematodes
  A. Ascarids
  B. Microfilaria
  C. Gapeworm (*Syngamus tracheae* in galliformes and *Cyathostoma* sp. in waterfowl)
  D. Several species of *Capillaria*
II. Cestodes: uncommon
III. Trematodes: uncommon
IV. Protozoa
  A. Coccidiosis
    1. Cause: *Eimeria*

2. Occurs in finches, poultry, waterfowl, and raptors
    3. Clinical signs: anorexia, lethargy, diarrhea, and wasting
  B. Histomoniasis
    1. Cause: *Histomonas*
    2. Clinical signs: "blackhead" in turkeys
  C. Trichomoniasis
    1. Cause: *Trichomonas*
    2. Clinical signs: oral plaques similar to *Candida* and *Capillaria*
  D. Hemosporidia
    1. Cause: blood protozoans *Hemoproteus, Leucocytozoan,* and *Plasmodium*
    2. Common in low densities in wild caught psittacines and most waterfowl and raptors
    3. Problem occurs only at high densities or under stress
  E. Giardiasis
    1. Cause: *Giardia*
    2. Zoonotic disease
    3. Clinical signs: soft, green mucoid feces and diarrhea

Reptile
CLASSIFICATION

  I. Class: Reptilia
    A. Order: Chelonia (turtles and tortoise)
    B. Order: Crocodilia (crocodiles, alligators, and caimans)
    C. Order: Rhyncocephalia (tuatara)
    D. Order: Squamata
      1. Suborder: Serpentes (snakes)
      2. Suborder: Sauria (lizards)

ANATOMICAL AND PHYSIOLOGICAL DIFFERENCES

  I. Lifestyle
    A. Terrestrial
    B. Aquatic (freshwater)
    C. Marine
    D. Arboreal
  II. Lifespan: wide range among species
    A. Seven years in a red-eared slider
    B. One hundred and fifty years in a Galapagos tortoise
  III. Growth and metabolism
    A. Slow metabolic rate
    B. Growth continues throughout life; growth rate slows nearing maturity
  IV. Integument
    A. Made up of scales or scutes

  B. Chelonians have a superficial layer of keratin shields, which make up the carapace dorsally and the plastron ventrally
  C. Lizards have bony plates in the dermis called osteoderms
  D. The skin is made up of the dermis and epidermis
  E. Healing is much slower due to the decreased metabolic rate
  F. Periods of ecdysis (shedding of the skin)
  G. Autonomy is the ability of a lizard to shed its tail when captured, and the tail will regrow but will be lacking vertebrae
  V. Sensory
    A. The eye in lizards has a movable eyelid but the nictitating membrane is reduced and nonfunctional
    B. The eye in snakes has no moveable eyelid or nictitating membrane; instead there is a spectacle covering the eye that maintains moisture and is shed during ecdysis
  VI. Skeletal
    A. Appendages as limbs (most species)
    B. Appendages modified as flippers (aquatic turtles)
    C. Appendages entirely lacking (snakes)
    D. Pythons and boas possess vestiges of hind limbs evident as spurs on either side of the cloaca
    E. Chelonians have their entire limb girdles housed within their ribcage (shell)
    F. Snakes and lizards have articulation of the upper jaw via the presence of a joint between the ptyeroid and the cranium, permitting the swallowing of large prey
    G. Six rows of teeth continually replaced
    H. Lizards and snakes have external ears
    I. Snakes use heat sensitive pits in their snout (pythons, vipers, rattlesnakes), the vomeronasal organ in the roof of the mouth and the tongue as "ears"
  VII. Digestive
    A. Well-developed epiglottis
    B. Glottis is located anteriorly to allow breathing while ingesting prey
    C. Esophagus, stomach, small intestine, large intestine, cloaca
    D. Cloaca is common opening for urogenital and digestive tract
  VIII. Respiratory
    A. Diaphragm absent
    B. Controlled by intercostal muscles in lizards and snakes

C. Controlled by alternating pressure within the body cavity during locomotion and pharyngeal pumping in turtles

D. Left lung in snakes is reduced or absent

E. Lizards have two saccular lungs; some species have air sacs

F. Lungs in turtles are saccular and compressed against the carapace

G. Turtles have a membranous structure that divides the pleuroperitoneal cavity but has no respiratory function

H. Tolerate higher levels of carbon dioxide and are capable of long periods of breath holding, making inhalation of anesthetics difficult

IX. Thermoregulation

A. Ectothermic (rely on environmental temperature to maintain their own body temperature and metabolic processes)

X. Circulatory

A. The first vertebrate to develop the complete interventricular septum, and therefore a four chambered heart, present in crocodiles

B. All other reptiles have a three chambered heart

1. Two atria

2. One ventricle

3. Incomplete interventricular septum prevents the mixing of oxygenated and deoxygenated blood by current flows

C. Blood cells

1. Nucleated red blood cells

2. Thrombocytes (similar to mammalian platelets)

3. Heterophils (analogous to mammalian neutrophils)

4. Eosinophils

5. Basophils

6. Lymphocytes

7. Monocytes

8. Azurophils: unique to reptiles; function thought to be similar to heterophils

XI. Urogenital

A. Metanephric kidneys

B. Some species possess a bladder

C. Terrestrial species excrete uric acid

D. Aquatic species excrete urea and ammonia

E. Renal portal system present, allows blood from the caudal portion of the body to pass through the kidneys before entering the main vascular system

F. Turtles have single extrudible penis

G. Lizards and snakes have two hemipenes

H. Reproduction by oviparity in caiman, alligators, turtles, most lizards, and some snakes

I. Reproduction by viviparity or ovoviviparity in some lizards and snakes

HOUSING

I. Clinic housing

A. Incubators

B. Stainless steel dog kennels

C. Custom built isolates

II. "At home" housing

A. Control temperature and humidity

B. Aquarium

C. Terrarium

D. Custom made cage

E. Each species has its own preferred optimal temperature ("POT"): (range from 12-21° C or 53-69° F for temperate species to 26-39° C or 75-103° F for tropical species)

F. Aquatic turtles should have an aquarium filter flow and a water temperature of 21-26° C or 70-80° F

G. The common green iguana's "POT" is 29-39° C or 85-102° F

H. Consider normal activity for the species (i.e., arboreal species need climbing trees, burrowing species need deep litter, shy species or nocturnal species need a hide box)

I. Basking area or "hot spot"

J. Substrate can be newspaper, aquarium gravel, corncob bedding, or sand litter

K. Clean shallow water dish

L. Chameleons will not drink from a water dish; they lap water droplets; so the aquarium should be sprayed every 2 to 3 hours, or they may drink from a dripping water bottle

M. Ultraviolet light source is necessary to activate vitamin D for calcium absorption and bone metabolism

N. In warm climates or during the summer months, some reptiles may be housed outdoors to obtain natural ultraviolet radiation

O. Heated rocks are not suggested; they may cause burns

P. A heating pad under the aquarium or heat lamp may be used to maintain temperature

Q. Humidity is an important factor, 50%-70% the optimum for proper moulting in snakes and lizards

R. Photoperiod of 12 hours daylight and 12 hours dark is suitable for all reptiles

S. Reptiles hibernate near 5° C (40° F) and at low temperatures. They become lethargic and anorexic, often leading to stress related diseases

RESTRAINT AND HANDLING ▬▬▬▬

I. Restraint
   A. For poisonous snakes, use extreme caution; the responsibility for capture and restraint should rest with the owner
   B. A squeeze box or bag and clear plastic tubing can be used to entice the snake out for restraint
   C. Nonvenomous snakes may also bite, so they should be restrained behind the head with one hand of the body supported with the other hand
   D. Large constrictors can suffocate a person: two people should handle large snakes (over 6 feet long)
   E. Lizards should never be grasped by the tail due to shedding of the tail: grasp behind the head and hold the pelvis and tail in the other hand; caution against claws and tail lashing in defense
   F. Short-term restraint for radiographs can be achieved in some lizards by applying mild digital pressure to the eyes, causing a quiescent state that lasts for a few minutes
   G. Turtles should be held at the rear portion of the carapace, anterior to the hind legs; may bite, and some have long claws
   H. Hypothermia historically has been used as a basic method of sedation for examination and radiology but should be avoided
II. Temperature, pulse, and respirations
   A. Normal values have been listed for body temperatures but are not useful, since body temperature depends on the environment
   B. Respiration differs among species and varies with size of the animal, ranging from 4 to 30 breaths per minute
   C. Pulse rate also differs among species and with the size of the animal, ranging from 40 to 100 beats per minute
III. Blood collection
   A. Ventral tail vein
   B. Jugular vein
   C. Dorsal and ventral buccal veins of the mouth
   D. Nail clip
   E. Dorsal venous sinus (close to dorsal tail vein) in turtles
   F. Cardiac puncture (not recommended)
IV. Blood analysis: Coulter counter cannot be used due to nucleated red blood cells; complete blood count can be obtained by combining the Unopette system and hemocytometer count, with a differential count from a smear
   V. Intravenous access: (see those used for blood collection) difficult to use jugular without cutdown
   VI. Intramuscular injection: dorsal portion of the body in snakes and the front leg in lizards and turtles; injections should not be given in the rear leg because of the potential for nephrotoxicity and rapid excretion due to the renal portal system
   VII. Oral administration/tube feeding: a metal or plastic feeding tube can be used; the plastic tube should be used with an oral speculum to prevent biting of the tube
   VIII. Subcutaneous fluids: similar to mammals
   IX. Intracoelomic fluids: no diaphragm; fluids absorbed readily

NUTRITION: DIETS AND PROBLEMS ▬▬▬▬
Snakes

I. All snakes are carnivorous, diet is species dependent
   A. Rats
   B. Mice
   C. Gerbils
   D. Chicks
   E. Fish
II. Fed once or twice weekly up to once monthly, depending on body size

Turtles

I. "Turtle flakes" and brine shrimp are often sold as a complete diet but are usually lacking in vitamin A and calcium
II. Cod liver oil is a good vitamin A source for supplement
III. Calcium carbonate or bone meal is a suitable calcium supplement
IV. Calcium-rich foods include alfalfa, broccoli, squash, yams, beet, clover, dandelion, pea pods, soybean, and turnip
   A. Carnivorous: trout chow, fish, or pinkie mice
   B. Omnivorous: a mix of the two diets
   C. Herbivorous: salad mixture of fruits and leafy greens, especially calcium and vitamin A rich foods
V. A multivitamin and mineral supplement can be given weekly

Lizards

I. Insectivorous species (geckos, chameleons, anoles and skinks): fed daily

II. Carnivorous species (monitors) feed on rats, mice, raw eggs and dog chow: fed a few times weekly; few nutritional problems

III. Omnivorous species: fed daily—vegetables, fruit, crickets

IV. Herbivorous species (common green iguana): fed daily—calcium and vitamin rich vegetables such as broccoli, squash, and parsely

V. May need to use a calcium and vitamin supplement

CLINICAL CONDITIONS AND DISEASES

I. Poor management: temperature, humidity, or housing
   A. Anorexia
   B. Hypothermia
   C. Trauma
   D. Rodent bites
   E. Dysecdysis (improper shedding)

II. Nutritional problems
   A. Herbivorous or insectivorous species commonly have dietary problems
   B. Metabolic bone disease: common in green iguana
      1. Occurs when the ratio of calcium and phosphorous is reversed (normal is 2:1 or 1.5:1) due to a poor diet or the animal lacks a UV source necessary to convert the precursor vitamin D_2 to D_3, which is essential for the absorption of calcium
      2. Clinical signs may include pathological fractures of the long bones; osteodystrophia fibrosa; swollen, soft, poorly mineralized bones; swollen jaw; and undefined bone cortices on radiographs
      3. Treatment includes calcium supplement, ultraviolet light supplementation, and diet correction
   C. Hypovitaminosis A
      1. Common in turtles
      2. Clinical signs: palpebral edema, swollen eyes, edematous bulge in the inguinal skin, anorexia
      3. Treatment consists of vitamin A injection initially, diet correction, and supplement
      4. Therapy for a secondary bacterial infection may also be required
   D. Hypovitaminosis E: rodents for reptile food are stored too long, destroying the vitamin E and promoting steatitis and fat necrosis

INFECTIOUS DISEASES

Bacterial and Bacterial-like Diseases

The bacterial diseases are listed by clinical problem rather than by specific pathogen.

I. Stomatitis or mouth rot
   A. Cause: suboptimal temperatures, unhygienic environment, malnutrition, trauma
   B. Common bacteria isolated include *Pseudomonas* and *Aeromonas*
   C. Begins as edema of the gums; may progress to osteomyelitis of the jaw if left untreated

II. Pneumonia
   A. Cause: suboptimal temperatures and low humidity
   B. Common bacterial isolates: *Aeromonas* and *Klebsiella*

III. Septicemia
   A. Cause: a variety of bacteria; common bacteria isolated: *Pseudomonas* and *Aeromonas*
   B. Clinical signs include pinpoint focal necrosis of the skin, small lumps or abscesses along the body or tail, and lethargy

IV. Septicemic cutaneous ulcer disease
   A. Identified in aquatic turtles
   B. Caused by *Citrobacter*

V. Salmonellosis
   A. Important zoonotic disease; causes bloody diarrhea and severe enteritis in humans
   B. Cause: *Salmonella:* a normal bacterial flora of many reptiles, especially aquatic turtles

Viral Diseases

Viral diseases are uncommon.

I. Paramyxovirus in snakes

II. Viral encephalitis in snakes

III. Herpesvirus in iguanas and turtles

Protozoal Diseases

I. *Cryptosporidium*
   A. Problem in snakes causing regurgitation, anorexia, and death
   B. A zoonotic disease causing diarrhea and lethargy in humans

Mycotic Diseases

I. Pneumonia caused by *Aspergillosis, Beauvaria,* and *Cladosporium*

PARASITES

Ectoparasites

I. Ticks: common on snakes

II. Mites: common on snakes and iguanas (red mites on the later)

Endoparasites

    I. Coccidia
       A. Cause enteritis and anorexia
   II. *Entamoeba*
       A. Causes gastritis and colitis
  III. Cestodes
  IV. Trematodes
   V. Nematodes
       A. Cestodes, trematodes, and nematodes may affect the oral, respiratory, gastrointestinal, and circulatory systems

Glossary

apteriae No feathers or down
carapace The dorsal shell of chelonians
cere Area at the base of a bird's beak
dysecdysis Improper shedding
ecdysis Shedding of the external skin
hemipenes Two vascular sacs, which act as a penis in snake and lizards
holocrine A type of secretion that is formed by the entire gland
intracoelomic Into the body cavity
metanephric Embryonic-like kidney
osteodystrophia fibrosa A bone disorder whereby the fibroosseus tissue replaces bone tissue
oviparous Producing eggs in which the embryo matures outside of the maternal body, as in birds
ovoviviparous Producing live young that hatch from eggs inside the maternal body, as in lizards
plastron The ventral shell of chelonians
ptyerylae Feather tracts on birds
steatitis Inflammation of the fatty tissue
stomatitis Inflammation of the mucosa of the mouth
uropygial A gland located laterally to the pygostyle that secretes oil to aid in waterproofing of feathers
viviparous Bearing live young

Review Questions

1 The digestive system in the bird includes the following anatomical structures, beginning cranial to caudal:
  a. Crop, glottis, proventriculus, gizzard
  b. Beak, glottis, crop, proventriculus, gizzard
  c. Crop, ventriculus, gizzard
  d. Beak, glottis, esophagus, crop, gizzard

2 The bird has _____ pairs of air sacs that make up the respiratory system.
  a. 4
  b. 6
  c. 9
  d. 13

3 The heterophil can be compared to a _____ in mammals.
  a. Eosinophil
  b. Neutrophil
  c. Lymphocyte
  d. Monocyte

4 Female birds have only one functional _____ and a slightly larger _____ vein.
  a. Left ovary and oviduct; right jugular
  b. Right ovary and oviduct; left jugular
  c. Right kidney; left medial tibiotarsal vein
  d. Left kidney; right medial tibiotarsal vein

5 Blood analysis in avian and reptile species cannot be conducted using a Coulter counter due to:
  a. Presence of nucleated red blood cells
  b. Small size of the cells
  c. Presence of heterophils
  d. Large size of the cells

6 Avian and reptile species have a renal portal system, therefore:
  a. Nephrotoxic drugs should not be given in the back legs
  b. Nephrotoxic drugs should be injected only in the back limbs for a 24-hour period after injections in the front limbs
  c. Any drug injected will be excreted rapidly
  d. Any nephrotoxic drug will be absorbed and slowly excreted from the animal

7 Some lizards may be restrained for radiography by:
  a. Manual restraint
  b. Pressure on their eyes
  c. Holding their tail in position
  d. Inhalation anesthetic only

8 Vitamin D and calcium absorption in reptiles depends on:
  a. Optimum temperatures
  b. An ultraviolet light source
  c. A heating pad or hot rock under the substrate
  d. Optimum humidity in the enclosure

9 Reptiles are sometimes difficult to anesthetize due to:
  a. Their size
  b. The fact that they can tolerate high levels of carbon dioxide and can hold their breath for long periods of time
  c. Their integument structure and cell formation
  d. The fact that they are ectothermic and therefore require high temperatures before induction

10 Birds and terrestrial species of reptiles excrete:
  a. Urine
  b. Ammonia
  c. Urea
  d. Uric acid

BIBLIOGRAPHY
Avian

Altman R: Perching birds, parrots, cockatoos, and macaws (psittacines and passerines). In Fowler ME, editor: *Zoo and wildlife medicine,* Toronto, 1978, W.B. Saunders.

Cooper JE: *Veterinary aspects of captive birds of prey,* ed 2, Gloucestershire, 1978, Standfast Press.

Harrison GJ, Harrison LR: *Clinical avian medicine and surgery,* Toronto, 1986, W.B. Saunders.

Humphreys PN: Waterbirds. In Cooper JE et al, editors: *Manual of exotic pets,* Glouchestershire, 1985, British Small Animal Veterinary Association.

McDonald SE: Anatomical and physiological characteristics of birds and how they differ from mammals, *Proc Assoc Avian Vet:* 372-389, 1990.

Pettingal OS: *Ornithology in laboratory and field,* ed 4, Minneapolis, 1970, Burgess Publishing Co.

Stunkard JA: *Diagnosis, treatment and husbandry of pet birds,* ed 2, Edgewater, 1984, Stunkard Publishing.

Taylor M: Companion bird management and nutrition, *Proc Assoc Avian Vet:* 409-431, 1990.

Turner T: Cagebirds. In Cooper JE et al, editors: *Manual of exotic pets,* Gloucestershire, 1985, British Small Animal Veterinary Association.

Reptile

Evans HE: Reptiles, introduction and anatomy. In Fowler ME, editor: *Zoo and wildlife medicine,* Toronto, 1978, W.B. Saunders.

Frye FL: *Biomedical and surgical aspects of captive reptile husbandry,* Kansas, 1981, Veterinary Medicine Publishing Co.

Jackson OF, Lawrence K: Chelonians. In Cooper JE et al, editors: *Manual of Exotic Pets,* Gloucestershire, 1985, British Small Animal Veterinary Association.

Jacobsen ER, Kolias GV: *Exotic animals,* New York, 1988, Churchill Livingstone.

Jacobsen ER: Diseases in reptiles. In Johnston DE, editor: *Exotic animal medicine in practice,* the compendium collection, New Jersey, 1986, Veterinary Learning Systems Co. Inc.

Lawrence K: Lizards, addendum and snakes. In Cooper JE et al, editors: *Manual of exotic pets,* Gloucestershire, 1985, British Small Animal Veterinary Association.

Marcus LC: *Veterinary biology and medicine of captive amphibians and reptiles,* London, 1981, Lea and Febiger.

Murphy JB, Collins JT: *A review of the diseases and treatments of captive turtles,* Kansas, 1983, AMS Publishing.

Personal and Professional Management Skills

Carlene A. Decker   *A. Patrick Navarre*

OUTLINE

Communication
  Overview
    Verbal Communication
    Nonverbal Communication
Listening
Special Communication Situation—
  Veterinary Medicine
    Client Communication

Co-worker Communication
Written Communication
Electronic Communication
Management
  Organizational Management
  Business Management
  Personal Management
  Career Management

Professional Obligations
  Professional Organizations
  Community Involvement
  Professionalism
  Education
Marketing
  Internal Marketing
  External Marketing

LEARNING OUTCOMES

After reading this chapter you should be able to:

1. Describe the elements of communication, including verbal, written, and electronic.
2. Describe techniques that can increase client communication and communication in the workplace.
3. Understand basic management and business principles for hospital managers and employees.
4. List personal management techniques.
5. List career management techniques and personal growth strategies.
6. Describe internal and external marketing strategies.

The work environment for many veterinary technicians has changed over the past decade. Now veterinary technicians must be skilled in the medical and technical aspects of veterinary medicine and may also take on responsibility for many of the business decisions that occur in the work place. For this reason, communication skills, management skills, and marketing have become important tools for the veterinary technician. These skills are also important for personal career planning and professional advancement.

COMMUNICATION
Overview

Communication is the process individuals or organizations use to create meaning with others.

  I. Components of communication
    A. **Sender:** the sender develops a message or thought that will be conveyed
      1. Channel is selected by which the message will be transmitted
    B. **Receiver:** individual who receives the sender's message
    C. **Message:** thoughts or ideas expressed by the sender

D. **Feedback:** response by the receiver as perceived by the sender. Feedback enables the sender to determine how much of the message was accurately understood and interpreted by the receiver

E. **Channels:** mechanisms for communication based on the five senses of sight, sound, smell, touch, and taste, including verbal, written, and electronic channels

F. **Interference:** any interruption (external or internal) that enters the communication loop
   1. Interruptions can include physical noise, receiver interpretation, incorrect grammar, electronic failure, and body language

G. **Listening:** a crucial element of verbal communication

II. Flow of communication
   A. Communication within an organization travels in at least three directions: downward, upward, and horizontal
      1. Downward: information from figures of authority to subordinates, providing instructions related to the task at hand
      2. Upward: information from subordinates to authority figures
      3. Horizontal: communication that takes place among individuals with the same status

Verbal Communication

Verbal communication is involved in many types of conversations that take place on a daily basis. Effective communication also includes nonverbal elements.

Nonverbal Communication

The unspoken elements that replace, reinforce, or contradict verbal communication; include visual, temporal, vocal, and spatial.

I. Visual cues include posture, facial expressions, eye contact, and hand gestures, among others
   A. Posture communicates mood of the sender
      1. Upright posture can imply confidence
      2. Slouched posture can indicate insecurity, sadness
   B. Facial expressions are good indicators of how messages are received
   C. Direct eye contact between sender and receiver indicates an open communication channel
      1. Indirect eye contact can imply an uneasiness in or a closure of the communication process

D. Hand gestures such as a handshake or a touch on the arm add meaning to communication

II. Temporal cues are in relation to time of day
   A. Receiving a message the first thing after arriving at work indicates urgency
   B. A message sent at the end of the day with a "see me at your convenience tomorrow" does not indicate the same level of urgency
   C. Timely response indicates a commitment to the message and sender
   D. A failure to respond indicates a lack of interest

III. Vocal cues are voice qualities that qualify verbal messages. Some vocal cues include pitch, rate, and volume
   A. Voice pitch ranges from low to high
      1. Monotone can imply disinterest in the topic
      2. Varied range or pitch implies enthusiasm and commitment to the topic
      3. A voice pitch inconsistent with the message may indicate incongruency
   B. Rate of speech
      1. Normal speech is 125 to 150 words per minute
      2. Both rapid and slow speech may loose the receiver
   C. Volume of voice
      1. Lack of volume can indicate tension, insecurity, lack of commitment to message
         a. A designed lack of volume can better illustrate a point by forcing the receiver(s) to listen more intently
      2. Too much volume can indicate enthusiasm and excitement but also tension and insecurity

IV. Spatial cues refer to the use of space often determined by culture, which significantly affects communication
   A. Personal space is the area around oneself, known as the *comfort zone*
      1. This area generally is 18″ to 4 feet
      2. Intrusion into the receiver's personal space can create interference in the message being sent
   B. Office space often dictates a professional tone of a communication
      1. If the sender is separated from the receiver by a desk, there is an implied message of an authority/subordinate relationship

2. This set-up should be reserved for formal conversations, reprimands, and negotiations

3. Informal conversations are best held in a neutral setting within the office such as around a small work table or sitting in chairs next to one another

LISTENING

Effective communication requires listening capabilities of the sender and the receiver.

I. The listening process requires total concentration on the message being sent. Barriers to effective listening can be avoided by

A. Concentrating on the message being sent with a clear, undivided mind

B. Avoiding judgment of the message sender. Do not let personal and emotional opinions distort the message

C. The mind can process information faster than it can be spoken; to effectively listen, do not get ahead of the message being sent

D. Communication flowing downward from a superior can create barriers for the subordinate listener when no avenue for upward feedback is provided. This also causes a lack of credibility of the message

II. Better listening requires practice of the following:

A. Do not interrupt the sender while the message is being delivered

B. Ask for clarification of the message if necessary

C. Ignore distractions in the environment

D. Respond to the message; provide feedback

E. Observe the sender's body language to uncover other meanings in the message

F. Do not place personal opinions or preconceived opinions into the message

SPECIAL COMMUNICATION SITUATION— VETERINARY MEDICINE
Client Communication

Communication with clients takes place in different ways such as client education, grief counseling, emergency situations, telephone conversations, and angry/hostile clients.

I. Client education is a vital component of the veterinary technician's role in the hospital

A. Technicians communicate with the client by describing routine procedures performed on pets using terminology understood by the client

B. To assist in this communication the technician often develops visual tools, including diagrams, charts, specimens, and newsletters

C. Special explanations for children can be developed to assist them in understanding procedures performed on their pets

II. Grief counseling is an important communication tool used to help clients deal with grief and emotional pain resulting from loss of a pet

A. Listening skills are an essential component of grief counseling

B. Five stages of grief a client may experience at various times (not necessarily in order)

1. Denial—usually the first stage the body goes through to prepare for emotional trauma. During this stage, the client refuses to deal with the pet's condition

a. The client needs support, understanding, and permission to grieve

b. Communicate clearly and listen actively, rephrase if necessary and avoid medical jargon

c. Remain unjudgemental; give client time to move out of the denial stage at his or her own pace

d. Allow client to feel a sense of closure such as viewing the body or saying good bye

2. Bargaining is often an irrational attempt to reverse or control a situation and may include negotiation with a higher being for the health/life of the pet

a. This phase is not seen as often in pet loss as in loss of a human

b. It is important not to become defensive, and patiently answer any questions or concerns

3. Anger often follows denial. The veterinary technician or the veterinarian may be the target of that anger as the client places the blame for the demise of their pet on the ones who were entrusted with its medical care

a. It is particularly important not to become defensive or mirror the anger

b. Give the client permission to vent anger

c. Listen actively by mirroring, maintaining eye contact, using empathetic statements

4. Guilt often accompanies this stage so relieve it by assuring the client that the best decision was made

   5. Depression is sadness that follows after anger subsides
      a. This phase begins and ends at different times for each client
      b. Allow clients to express feelings and follow up after the death of the pet
      c. Listen actively and empathetically; a touch on the forearm or shoulder may convey compassion
      d. Validate normalcy of the client's feelings
      e. This may be a good time to encourage memorialization of the pet such as planting a tree, starting a scrapbook
   6. Resolution is when the pet owner accepts the fate of the pet
III. Emergency situations require quick assessment and response to patient needs
   A. This assessment requires that appropriate instructions be given to the client for management of the emergency
   B. Clients under stress may not have appropriate listening capabilities so communications must be short, concise, and without emotion in the technician's voice tones
IV. Telephone conversations with clients are an important means of communication. Telephone etiquette includes:
   A. Professional greetings, name of the business, and name of the person answering the phone
   B. The ability to assess the caller's needs (i.e., an emergency, etc.)
   C. Appropriate voice tones
   D. Following rules associated with length of time to keep a client "on hold"
   E. Answering the phone before a predetermined number of rings
   F. Appropriate use of voice mail systems
   G. Protocol for taking and returning messages
 V. Communication with angry/hostile clients requires recognizing the potentially hostile situation before it escalates. Considerations include:
   A. A proper place for conversation with an angry client
   B. Disassociation of the problem from the person so that solutions might be more easily seen
   C. One of the best ways to diffuse a hostile situation is to use active listening skills
   D. Never argue with a dissatisfied client because the client is always right, even when wrong

   E. Use conflict resolution techniques that include recognizing and defining each piece of the problem, generating ideas to develop a resolution plan, making and implementing a decision where everyone wins, and evaluating the outcome
   F. If the client seems unreasonable, ask the veterinarian to handle the problem as quickly as possible
   G. People on drugs or alcohol could become violent and uncontrollable: be careful
      1. Law enforcement officials may have to be called if substances are used in excess

Co-worker Communication

Communication with co-workers is the key to success of the team. Positive idea exchange, the act of providing and receiving constructive criticism, is essential.
   I. Mechanisms of positive idea exchange
      A. Staff meetings provide an open forum for exchange of ideas
      B. Staff should verbally share information on work-related issues
      C. Goals of the practice should be shared so members of the organization have a clear understanding of the direction in which the organization is heading
      D. New techniques learned at continuing education meetings or seminars should be shared
      E. Clearly written manuals containing written policies and protocols, including job responsibilities, should be available
  II. Conflict resolution: handling of conflict through appropriate channels within the workplace is essential for dealing with conflict. The following are further pertinent elements of conflict resolution
      A. Face to face conversation about a problem allows all parties an opportunity to air opinions
      B. A mediated session can be held where a neutral party is identified and serves as an intermediary to observe, listen, and keep the discussion focused on issues, not individuals
      C. A written grievance can be filed, following steps accepted by the hospital
      D. Staff meetings can be a good source for conflict resolution because all variables surrounding a conflict can be discussed openly
      E. Conflict can result in positive change in the work environment in the form of constructive criticism or critique of current protocols, techniques

F. Conflict should be resolved immediately
 1. Waiting provides an opportunity for conflict to build up into a larger problem
 2. Immediate handling allows clear memory of the situation by those involved
 3. Waiting too long to address a conflict gives the "injured party" a sense that the problem is not important

WRITTEN COMMUNICATION

 I. Definition: communication through messages delivered in written form. Good writing skills are essential for the veterinary technician
 II. The technician will have to communicate in writing with co-workers and other professionals in the form of letters, memos, and reports
 III. The technician will communicate with clients and the general public via client information handouts, written take home directions, hospital newsletters, public education information in newspapers, etc.
 IV. Main components of business communications
 A. Audience should be identified and materials tailored to educational/knowledge level
 B. Correct grammar and punctuation are a must
 C. Pitfalls to avoid
 1. Wordiness
 2. Slang terms or expressions
 3. Big words, medical terminology not familiar to the reader
 4. Vague expressions: be concise and direct
 5. Condescending statements
 6. Sexist language
 7. Negative expressions
 D. All written communication should be printed on good quality paper with attention to appearance of the final document. Typographical errors must be eliminated by repeated proofreading

ELECTRONIC COMMUNICATION

 Also known as telecommunications, electronic communication is a means to transmit voice, data, and images from one location to another through the use of a host of electronic equipment.
 I. Computers have become vital in most veterinary practices for the management of information and communication
 A. Patient records, data, financial management, inventory of medical supplies, and communication with colleagues are now performed with computers

 B. Software packages specifically designed for veterinary hospitals allow word processing, database management, ordering, and inventory control
 C. Electronic communication, known as E-mail, transmits messages through telephone lines
 1. Messages are posted in the receiver's electronic mailbox in a fraction of the time of conventional methods
 2. Immediate transmission and response can occur when the receiver logs onto the computer
 D. Computer on line networks such as Network of Animal Health (NOAH) on Compuserve, Veterinary Information Network on America On Line, and the World Wide Web are examples of computer networks
 1. Latest information on veterinary related subjects is provided
 2. On line discussion also provides continuing education opportunities
 II. Telephone systems using multiple phone systems and features allow better communication with the client
 A. On hold message feature: allows client while on hold to listen to messages developed by the veterinary hospital describing services or facilities that are available
 B. Call waiting feature: signals when another call is coming in and can assure a quicker response to a client's inquiry
 C. Conference call option: allows multiple individuals to be included simultaneously in a conversation
 D. Cellular phones: send messages by using radio transmitters. These phones allow greater mobility and portability for individuals
 1. Can be used to keep communication lines open between the hospital and individuals traveling to clients by vehicle
 2. Also allow access to computer on line networks for consultations, drug formulas, and new information regarding medical issues in combination with portable computers while in the field

MANAGEMENT
Organizational Management

 I. Definition: working with and through people to accomplish organizational goals
 II. Within a veterinary hospital, managerial tasks may be delegated to a practice manager, who

may be a veterinary technician. The practice manager is involved with four functions

A. Planning: thinking through and making decisions about goals and actions in advance so that objectives can be defined and procedures established

B. Organization: the next step after planning, so that human and material resources of a practice will achieve goals of the organization

C. Leadership: directing and influencing the practice's employees to carry out the organization's objectives

D. Control: monitoring and evaluating performance

III. The understanding of certain management principles will facilitate efficiency and harmony among the employees. These include, but are not limited to, the following concepts:

A. Teamwork: the result of all members of an organization understanding their roles and working together to accomplish the goals of an organization

   1. Teamwork is an essential component of the organizational structure

     a. Each position should have specified tasks based on education and legal limits of the practice

     b. More efficiency will result if the task is given to the lowest paid qualified worker

B. Supervisory skills: involve the ability to direct a co-worker or subordinate's work to meet goals of the organization

   1. An effective supervisor motivates, provides constructive criticism and evaluates performance

C. Delegating: formally assigning responsibility for completion of a given task to a subordinate. For delegation to be effective the following rules apply:

   1. Carefully consider who should be given the assignment and which tasks can and should be delegated

   2. Provide all pertinent information about the responsibility at the time of delegation

   3. Provide a system for feedback

IV. Consistency can be facilitated by making commonly performed procedures and policies accessible to every employee

A. Policy manual: provides a written record of organization policies and includes policies that govern organization-wide actions and those that cover the actions of individuals

   1. Organization-wide activities include history, the organization's purposes and goals, mission statement, policies on community affairs, etc.

   2. Individual activities or what the employee needs to know

     a. Policies on personnel guidelines, job descriptions of all team members, scheduling, absenteeism, tardiness, injury on the job, impairment on the job, etc.

B. Procedures manual

   1. Outlines protocols for various procedures performed within an organization such as surgery, laboratory, or radiology protocols and safety procedures

   2. Helps ensure that all employees adhere to the standards of the organization

     a. Written clearly and provides suggestions on the efficient completion of tasks

     b. Highlighted governmental rules and regulations and quality control measures

Business Management

I. Definition: practices required for the successful financial operation of a facility

II. Time is often a limiting factor but without proper business policies there would be no practice

III. Various aspects of business include:

A. Records

   1. Involved in all aspects of hospital operation

   2. Many formats available but whatever format used there must not be complete obliteraton or erasure

     a. Handwritten records must be legible, accurate, and written in permanent ink

     b. Any errors should be crossed out by a single line, corrections made, dated, and initialed by the person making the entry

   3. Some records and consent forms may require client's signature

     a. A minor can not legally enter into a contract

   4. Ownership

     a. The veterinary practice, not the client, owns the records

     b. Original records are a legal document and must be retained by the practice

c. Any release of information is at the discretion of the veterinarian or practice

d. A request for transfer should be made in writing; best to mail prepared records directly to referring or new veterinarian

5. Information contained in all medical records is confidential and should not be discussed with outside parties without client's written permission

a. Exception is the reporting of certain contagious and zoonotic diseases

6. Statute of limitations requires that records be legally retained for a certain length of time, usually five to seven years (depending on the state or province) from the date of last visit or discharge

7. Many record filing systems are available; most medical records arranged alphabetically by the owner's last name

8. Any lost records should be explained to the client and a new record begun immediately

9. Medical records include:

a. Log books: contain entries of services provided and include controlled drugs (required by law), radiography, surgery, euthanasia, laboratory, and necropsy logs

b. Animal records: must be individualized and contain certain information such as signalment (owner's name, address and telephone, patient's name, sex, species, age, breed, and color), as well as date seen, chief complaint, history, clinical signs, diagnosis, prognosis, authorization records, radiographic data, laboratory reports, and vaccination and surgical records

i. Financial information may be included in medical records, but separate billing is becoming more common practice

ii. Basic formats include:

• Chronological or conventional method: events are entered as they occur

• Problem oriented method: includes separating out the problems, data base, comprehensive history and physical examina-

tion, and progress notes (divided into SOAP: S, Subjective data. O, Objective data. A, Assessment. P, Procedure for diagnosis and treatment.)

10. Vaccination and spaying/neutering certificates need to be accurate

11. Authorization or consent forms are not legal requirements but protect the veterinarian and ensure that the client understands all treatments and procedures

12. Medication labels must be complete and accurate

B. Credit and collection policies

1. Policies should be written and strictly adhered to

2. A written estimate should always be used

3. Accounts receivable should be kept to a minimum

C. Inventory control

1. Two goals

a. Have items on hand when needed

b. Minimize expense of keeping supplies in stock

2. Turnover rate should be 8 to 12 times per year; calculated by: Yearly inventory expense ÷ Average cost of inventory on hand

a. Inventory turned over close to once a month = items used up before the bills are due

b. Turnover rate can be calculated on the 80/20 rule whereby 20% of items stocked account for 75% to 85% of the expenditures

3. Elements of a good inventory system include:

a. Good record keeping that includes a reorder log, purchase order records, individual inventory records, inventory master list, and vendor files

b. Effective use of inventory control cards or computer control

c. Appropriate arrangement and storage of inventory

d. Effective monitoring of inventory levels and expiration dates

e. Smart purchasing policies, including knowledge of products

D. Accounts payable should be paid close to the due date to maximize use of capital

1. Arrange for discounts for prompt payment

2. Do not allow accounts to proceed beyond due date (credit rating may drop)

E. Consider use of a computer if the practice does not already have one
   1. Much of the hospital operation can be provided by the computer, including inventory control, medical records management, client communication and information analysis, vaccination reminders, accounting
   2. Many well-designed programs are available
   3. Research particular needs so that the proper system can be purchased

F. A fax (facsimile) is an efficient rapid mode of communication
   1. Strict confidentiality must be maintained

G. Monthly analysis should be completed to establish trends, make comparisons of past months and past years, note immediate changes, and to review fees, inventory comparisons, and credit policies

Personal Management

I. Definition: skills and techniques required of each individual member of an organization to make the team function most efficiently

II. Personal management skills allow the veterinary technician to manage within the team to the benefit of the team. Components of personal management are time management, goal setting, decision making, stress management, coping with burnout, and negotiating

Time Management

I. Effectively using available time during the workday maximizes productivity for the employee and helps alleviate stress

II. Time is a unique resource in that it cannot be accumulated and each person has the same amount

III. Time management is a personal process and must fit into one's life style and circumstances

IV. The following suggestions can be applied to almost everyone to help manage time and reduce stress
   A. Make a daily "to do" list
   B. Develop daily, weekly, and yearly lists of goals
   C. Learn to say "no"—gain control of what takes up your time
   D. Establish priorities
   E. Use technology to acquire more efficiency—computer, calculator, new laboratory equipment

F. Never handle a piece of paper more than twice

G. Learn to skim what you read

H. Keep procrastination to a minimum

I. Work at meeting deadlines

J. Exercise at least 20 minutes per day to help you focus

Goals

I. Life offers a series of choices and decisions that need to be made

II. Establishing goals allows an individual to have a choice in the course of action required to accomplish a certain task and help lead in this direction

III. Set effective goals
   A. Identify possible needs in areas such as career, personal life, financial concerns, physical fitness, community involvement, leisure time
   B. Set a goal for each identified need by describing the result
   C. Prioritize
   D. Define objectives required to achieve the goal (steps to be done to achieve the goal)
   E. Select activity to complete each objective
   F. Indicate time frame for implementation
   G. Evaluate and monitor accomplishments

IV. As much as possible, make sure the objectives set for achieving the goals are measurable, clear, realistic, and stated as required results

V. Greater success will be achieved if one:
   A. Prioritizes
   B. Draws up written plans to help achieve goals
   C. Breaks goals into smaller sequential steps that can be achieved one at a time
   D. Begins now

Decision Making

I. The process of identifying and selecting a course of action for a specific problem or situation

II. Indecision or making no choice paralyzes the ability of an organization or an individual to move forward

III. Key components to making a decision are similar to problem solving techniques and include:
   A. Listing options
   B. Evaluating options (thinking it over)
   C. Factoring in personal feelings
   D. Evaluating how the decision will affect priorities already set
   E. Making the decision and discarding other options
   F. Committing to the decision (mentally not looking back)

G. Doing everything possible to make the decision work

Stress Management

I. Stress is the feeling of tension and pressure that results when a demand can not be readily dealt with or there is a perceived threat

II. Stress is response to a force that upsets one's equilibrium; strain is the adverse effects of stress on an individual's mind, body, and actions

III. Stressor: a force that brings about stress

IV. The body's physiological and chemical changes react to the fight-or-flight response and include an increase in heart rate, blood pressure, blood glucose, and blood clotting

V. Short-term physiological changes and prolonged stress can lead to annoying and life threatening conditions and a weakening of the immune system

VI. Due to lack of control, job pressures create stress for many people

VII. Not all stress is bad; some stress leads to achieving goals and meeting or exceeding personal potential
  A. Referred to as eustress

VIII. Stress management is individual and varies from highly specific techniques to a change in life style
  A. Identify stress signals
  B. As much as possible, eliminate or modify stressors
  C. Improve work habits
  D. Physical exercise reduces tension and keeps one in good condition and more resistant to fatigue
  E. Stress can be managed through mental relaxation techniques, including relaxation response, biofeedback training, muscle monitoring, and concentration techniques

Coping with Burnout

I. Burnout is closely related to stress and is defined as a state of exhaustion, (physical, mental, and emotional) caused by involvement in situations that are demanding

II. Burnout is a set of behaviors that result from strain

III. Persons suffering from burnout exhibit many symptoms—some physical, some emotional

IV. Employer role: reduce the amount of burnout
  A. Jobs should be clearly defined and provide the employee with a sense of purpose and opportunities for growth

V. Employee role: find significance in something other than work

A. Develop new interests that provide satisfaction outside the workplace

B. Time management and goal setting might also be effective

VI. For recovery from burnout, counseling and support are needed

Negotiating/Conflict Resolution

I. Differences of opinion or situations of conflict frequently arise

II. A win-win solution is a key to being a valuable team member

III. To prepare for negotiation:
  A. Always separate the person from the problem
  B. Focus on the interest at hand, not the position taken
  C. Identify options for a viable solution
  D. Discuss options after clearly weighing all possible solutions

Career Management

I. Make career decisions that move one closer to self-fulfillment

II. Key components to finding the right job opportunity include personal finance, job search, and interview

Personal Finance

I. Step one in career planning

II. Determine the type of income that will be required to meet financial obligations
  A. Prepare a budget that will allow you to view your obligations and make correct important career decisions
    1. Budget is defined as a statement of resources allocated for specific activities over a certain period of time
    2. All income, which includes salary, return on investments, and interest income, is projected and should be listed
    3. List all expected expenses
      a. Housing, utilities, telephone, property tax, all types of insurance, automobile expenses (including loan payments, gas, and maintenance), other outstanding loan payments (including credit cards), food, household repairs, clothing, entertainment, travel, and miscellaneous expenses
    4. The goal is more income than expenses
      a. If there are more expenses, one of the categories will have to be adjusted

b. It is wise not to accept a job that will not allow you to meet current financial obligations

Job Search

A. Career choices and options for veterinary technicians are not limited to practice settings
   1. Opportunities also exist in biomedical research, specialty practice, education, universities, industry, zoos, animal husbandry related areas, military service, and humane societies
   2. Research each of the areas that interest you and note pros and cons
   3. A career choice is not necessarily a long-term decision, since changing career paths is not uncommon
B. Seek job notices in placement services, classified advertisements, and through networking
I. Resume, cover letter, references
A. Resume
   1. Summarizes your background, qualifications, and accomplishments
   2. Key components of a resume
      a. Personal identification, including name, address, and telephone number where you can be reached
      b. Career objective defines what type of job you are seeking
         (1) State clearly what you hope to achieve in your professional career
      c. Traditionally, work history in reverse chronological order
         (1) Accomplishments highlight pertinent achievements at each job
      d. Traditionally, education in reverse chronological order
      e. Personal interests are optional
         (1) May be best to include job related activities only
      f. The traditional chronological resume, functional resume, or a combined format can be used
B. Cover letter
   1. Usually read before the resume, its goal is to get you to the interview stage
   2. Key components
      a. The letter should be one page in length with approximately three paragraphs
         (1) First paragraph: introduces yourself and identifies the position you are applying for
         (2) Second paragraph: lists accomplishments that would be beneficial for the business
         (3) Third paragraph: serves as a closing and indicates your next step, which is usually a phone call in a few days
   3. Rules governing cover letter and resume
      a. Always use premium paper and matching envelopes
      b. Check very carefully for typographical errors, including spelling and punctuation
      c. Make sure the appropriate person at the prospective place of employment is addressed
      d. Keep copies of all documents you send out and a list of who they were sent to
      e. Do not include photographs or mention your race, color, creed, or political affiliation
      f. Proofread all materials several times
C. References
   1. Provided by former employers, college instructors, and clients (check with an individual before using them as a reference)
   2. Provide prospective employers with a telephone number where a reference can be contacted
   3. If a written reference is required, provide references with the correct address and background information

Interview

I. Provides a personal opportunity to impress a potential employer
II. Research your potential employer. Obtain:
A. A detailed job description
B. Background on the business, including type of practice and number of owners
C. Contact employees of the business and or company representatives
D. Gather information from the Chamber of Commerce or a local newspaper on the community in which the business is located
E. Make a list of questions you have about the job
F. Estimate the wages you will need to earn (as indicated by your budget) in order to take the job
G. Prepare a list of potential questions the interviewer may ask and format your responses

III. During the interview your objective is to gather information, as well as provide the potential employer with knowledge about you
   A. In less than ten seconds you will make a first impression on the interviewer and in less than four minutes the interviewer will acquire a lasting impression of you
   B. Personal appearance for the interview is very important
      1. Your appearance should convey a clean, conservative, and professional person
   C. Be punctual
   D. Relax
   E. Listen to and answer questions carefully
   F. Ask questions you have about the potential employment
   G. Stress your strengths as well as what you can offer
   H. Encourage the employer to make you an offer. A decision can be made later on whether to accept or not
IV. Certain questions do not have to be answered during an interview. These involve: marital status, child care, plans for having a family, arrest record, age, questions that can be construed as prejudicial
 V. Be prepared to negotiate salary and benefit packages
   A. Best to have offer presented in writing
   B. Consider the entire package, not just salary
      1. A lower salary with health insurance, life insurance, and paid vacation may be better
   C. Benefits are a vital portion of any job offer and add to value of the job. Benefits that may be offered include, but are not limited to:
      1. Health insurance/dental insurance
      2. Life insurance
      3. Bonuses
      4. Discounted pet care and uniforms
      5. Paid vacation
      6. Paid sick days
      7. Expenses for continuing education, including registration, time off, travel, lodging, and per diem expenses
      8. Professional association dues
VI. It is important to personally thank each person who was involved in your interview process at the conclusion of the interview
   A. It may also be sent in writing 24 hours after the interview is complete
VII. Wait at least one day before accepting any offer to allow time to compare all propositions

PROFESSIONAL OBLIGATIONS

 I. Definitions
   A. Profession: a vocation or occupation requiring advanced education and training, and involving intellectual skills
   B. Professional: engaged in or worthy of the high standards of a profession

Professional Organizations (see Appendix A)

Professional organizations for veterinary technicians provide members with the opportunity for career advancement by supporting groups who work to advance the entire profession.

 I. Technicians, during their careers, have obligations to their profession and professional organization, as well as themselves
 II. National/international organizations
   A. Organizations that deal with issues affecting a broad range of topics, including public image of the veterinary technician, laws and legislation governing the profession, and effective use of the veterinary technician within the veterinary health care team
   B. These organizations actively interact with other organizations, looking for ways that a collaborative effort might benefit the entire health care team
      1. Career building and professionalism are important goals of these types of associations
III. State/provincial/local organizations
   A. Provide members with information pertinent to the profession on a local level
   B. Become actively involved in laws pertinent to their specific location, providing information to residents of their area and updating members on local issues

Community Involvement

The veterinary technician has an obligation to provide information about his or her career to the general public, co-workers, and peers as a means of promoting the profession and their own career.

Professionalism

Professionalism includes demeanor, appearance at work and in the community, and ethics

 I. The perception of the entire profession can be affected
 II. Key components of professionalism
   A. Demeanor: outward behavior or conduct should always reflect positively on you, your employer, and the profession

1. A professional will always project a proper image to those around them
B. Dress: clothing, hairstyle, jewelry, etc. worn during the workday and in the community reflect a person's level of professionalism
   1. Workplace: clothing should be appropriate for the job
      a. Uniforms with a name tag identifying you as a veterinary technician are appropriate for a practice setting
         (1) The uniforms should be changed if soiled
      b. Business casual clothing are most appropriate for continuing education seminars, workshops, or presentations
         (1) T-shirts, jeans, and shorts are generally not acceptable and do not portray a sense of professionalism
C. Speech: words used to communicate with the public, clients, co-workers, and even patients reflect a level of professionalism
   1. Avoid personal problems, gossip, health, controversial social issues, politics, religion, sex, and slang phrases
   2. Maintaining confidentiality is essential when dealing with business matters. Office situations, clients, and their pets should not be discussed socially or in the presence of the general public
   3. Jokes and terminology that may be offensive to those of a certain sex, physical appearance, or ethnic origin should be avoided
D. Ethics: rules established by organizations to set guidelines for and influence behavior and actions of the group
   1. As legal agents for veterinary employers, technicians must "accept [their] obligations to practice [their] profession conscientiously and with sensitivity, adhering to the profession's Code of Ethics" (from the North American Veterinary Technician Association [NAVTA]) (see Appendix A)
      a. Veterinarians are held liable for the actions of veterinary technicians
   2. Veterinary technicians are under supervision and control of a veterinarian and must never engage in practices reserved for the veterinarian
      a. These include diagnosing, prognosing, performing surgery, and prescribing medication

b. Technicians must never complain about veterinarians or other employees to or in the presence of a client
3. As professionals the actions of technicians must be based on the best interests of patients and clients
4. The veterinary technician code of ethics:
   a. Communicates to the public and members of the profession, the profession's ideals
   b. Is a general guide for professional ethical conduct
   c. Provides disciplinary procedures to members who are not operating at an acceptable level of conduct

Education

The veterinary technician has an obligation to remain current and up to date on technical information that pertains to the job. This involves a commitment to continuing education and lifelong learning and may even require higher-level education for advancement.

I. Continuing education comes in various forms, including advanced, review, and new information
   A. Registration requirements in certain areas demand proof of attendance
   B. Lifelong learning shows a commitment to growth
II. Advanced degrees
   A. Most veterinary technicians' education consists of a two-year program in the field of veterinary technology
   B. As career plans change and job opportunities become available a bachelors or masters degree may become important
   C. Investigate all options for degrees, including those offered through computer access and special programs set up for the employed adult learner

MARKETING

I. Definition: communication to others about goods or services that are offered
   A. In veterinary medicine, marketing is the process of educating the client/public on services that can be provided for quality care
   B. Marketing consists of all activities employed to promote goods and services
   C. Veterinary technicians have an important role in these activities
   D. Marketing in a veterinary hospital can be divided into two distinctly different areas: internal marketing and external marketing

Internal Marketing

The process of marketing veterinary services to clients and potential clients. The following are areas of the veterinary hospital suited to internal marketing.

 I. Outward appearances: the initial visual image that a client/potential client sees when approaching and entering the veterinary hospital

  A. Exterior of building, parking lot, and grounds should all be well kept

  B. First impressions of the inside of the building and waiting room are important, including cleanliness and freedom from odor

  C. Consider equipment, including availability of modern equipment and computers

  D. Professional appearing staff, clean uniforms, name tags

  E. A sense of order

 II. A caring attitude should be displayed by ALL staff members at all times

  A. The staff should be positive and enthusiastic and not display anger or dissatisfaction with their jobs

 III. Client needs must be evaluated in any marketing plan, consider:

  A. Location of the practice. Clients in rural areas will require different services than those in a strictly urban environment. Goods and services should be provided accordingly

  B. The time commitment made by your client in coming to your practice. Do not minimize

   1. Today's consumer should be greeted with fast, courteous service

  C. Conveying the importance of clients and their pets will make them more eager to return to your practice for future veterinary care

  D. Client needs can be evaluated by focus groups, questionnaires, and listening to complaints

 IV. Marketing tangible products to the client can be done most effectively by identifying a need of a client and/or pet and finding a product within the hospital to fill it

  A. The veterinary technician must be knowledgeable about the products being sold to clients

  B. Improper information about a product can be hazardous to the pet and to the confidence the client has in the practice

  C. The veterinary/client/patient relationship must be considered when dispensing products

   1. This relationship means the client's animal has had contact with the veterinarian within a specified period of time

  D. Over-the-counter products vs. professional products should be handled accordingly

 V. Tangible items that can be used to market goods or services include:

  A. Client reminders—a simple postcard reminder to the client of routine vaccinations and dental and heartworm checks can go a long way to keeping clients coming back year after year. This is also seen as an extension of the caring veterinary hospital

  B. Commercial handouts—many companies provide materials that are available to describe their product and its benefits to the client and pet when used

   1. These materials provide excellent marketing of goods without expense of preparation

  C. Practice newsletters and health bulletins keep the client in contact with the practice throughout the year

   1. They can provide valuable information on seasonal needs of pets, special promotions being run by the practice, and updates on new or common diseases

   2. All newsletters must clearly indicate the hospital, be printed in a professional appropriate manner, and be free of typographical errors

  D. Sympathy communication—a very personal and caring message is sent (through a card or letter from the practice staff) when client's grief at the loss of a pet is recognized

  E. Sales point displays—often corporations will provide displays for their products for use in the clinic's waiting area

   1. Display products in a visually appealing manner

   2. Only use such displays for marketable products

  F. Animal care talks—the practice that provides puppy and kitten talks, behavior classes, etc. has opened another avenue for marketing its goods and services and for showing care

 VI. Intangible items such as services cannot be overlooked even though results are not often visually beneficial. Preventive health care programs fall into this category and may or may not be equated with veterinary care

External Marketing

External marketing activities are aimed at expanding current client activity within the practice and increase the exposure of goods and services to those who are currently not clients

I. External marketing usually involves advertising and can be done in some of the following ways

    A. External visual signs promoting the practice include use of hospital signs and distribution of business cards for the veterinarian and the veterinary technician

    B. Media routes for advertising services include telephone directories, newspaper articles or advertisements, radio and television commercials

    C. Direct mail provides information to a targeted audience via the postal service

        1. Primarily to acquaint nonclients with services

II. Community activities can be seen as gestures of good will and can be accomplished by talking to community groups about good quality pet care, by promoting the veterinary technology profession, and by participating in community service such as volunteering to judge children's animal projects at a local fair

    A. The veterinarian and the veterinary technician should volunteer their expertise to the community

Glossary

accounts payable Money owed by one business to another

accounts receivable Money owed to a business, usually owed by the clients

burnout A state of emotional, mental, and physical exhaustion in response to prolonged stress

career development A planned approach to achieving growth and satisfaction in work experiences

chronological resume A job resume that presents education, work experience, interests, and accomplishments in reverse chronological order

communication Sending, receiving, and interpretation of messages

conflict A situation in which there is disagreement, incompatibility, or mutual exclusiveness

counseling A formal discussion method, usually with a professional, in which an individual is encouraged to overcome a problem or improve his or her potential

ethics Rules established by an organization to influence actions and behaviors of the group, not enforced in a court of law

eustress A positive or good stress that rejuvenates, excites, or stimulates an individual

flight-or-fight response The body's physiological and chemical response to stressors in which the individual attempts to avoid or cope with the situation

functional resume One that organizes skills and accomplishments into the functions or tasks required for the position sought

relaxation response Lowered metabolism, heart rate, respiration, and blood pressure

stress The body's response to stressors that threaten to disturb homeostatic state

stressor Anything that causes stress

win-win conflict resolution A method of resolving conflict whereby both sides gain something of value

Review Questions

1 Feedback is from the receiver and allows the sender to:
  a. Interpret the message
  b. Interpret the interference
  c. Understand how much of the message is comprehended
  d. Understand the receiver's message

2 Body language does not include:
  a. A handshake
  b. Direct eye contact
  c. Slouched posture or upright posture
  d. A kind word in a low voice

3 "Good" communication techniques include all of the following skills *except:*
  a. Concentrating on the message
  b. Processing the information too rapidly
  c. Providing feedback
  d. Avoiding judgment of the message sender

4 The five stages of grief a client may experience are:
  a. Denial, bargaining, anger, depression, and resolution
  b. Denial, bargaining, resolution, anger, and sadness
  c. Anger, sadness, bargaining, grief, and depression
  d. Anger, sadness, grief, resolution, and depression

5 Which of the following actions diminishes a successful resolution of a problem with a staff member?
  a. A staff meeting
  b. Waiting two months before talking about the problem
  c. Allowing all parties to express opinions
  d. A written grievance filed with the manager

6 All of the following techniques may be used to increase a veterinary technician's time management abilities *except:*
  a. Make a daily list of jobs to do
  b. Establish priorities
  c. Learn to say "no" to your employer
  d. Procrastinate less and meet deadlines more

7 The best personal reference for a potential position in a large progressive veterinary practice is:
  a. Your childhood neighbor
  b. Your family physician
  c. Your college instructor
  d. A former client, who you have not seen in two years

8 An example of a tangible internal marketing tool is:
  a. An advertisement in the telephone directory
  b. An announcement of a new practice in the area
  c. A sympathy card to a client who recently lost a pet
  d. A visit to the local primary school

9 A message sent in a loud voice indicates:
   a. Tension
   b. Insecurity
   c. Enthusiasm
   d. All of the above

10 The area of personal space or "comfort zone":
   a. Depends on personal preference
   b. Is approximately 4 to 6 m (13-19 ft)
   c. Is approximately 45 cm to 1.2 m (18 inches to 4 ft)
   d. Depends on gender of the individual

BIBLIOGRAPHY

Brock SL: *Better business writing,* Los Altos, California, 1988, Crisp Publications.

Dessler G: *Personnel/human resource management,* ed 5, Englewood Cliffs, New Jersey, 1991, Prentice-Hall.

Dubrin A: *Human relations: a job oriented approach,* ed 4, New Jersey, 1988, Prentice Hall.

Haynes ME: *Personal time management,* Los Altos, California, 1987, Crisp Publications.

McCarthy EJ, Perreault WD: *Basic marketing,* ed 10, Boston, Massachusetts, 1990, Irwin.

McCurnin D: *Clinical textbook for veterinary technicians,* ed 3, Philadelphia, Pennsylvania, 1994, W.B. Saunders.

Quible ZK: *Administrative office management,* ed 4, Englewood Cliffs, New Jersey, 1989, Prentice-Hall.

Rosenberg MA: *Companion animal loss and pet owner grief,* ed 2, Lehigh Valley, Pennsylvania, 1993, Alpo Pet Foods, Inc.

Skills for success, Bristol, Vermont, 1989, Soundview Summaries.

Soner JAF, Freeman RE: *Management,* ed 4, Englewood Cliffs, New Jersey, 1989, Prentice-Hall.

Tannenbaum J: *Veterinary ethics: animal welfare, client relations, competition and collegiality,* ed 2, St. Louis, 1995, Mosby.

The Veterinary Technician Profession, Legislation, Associations, and Colleges

Barbara Pinker *Monica Tighe*

CHARACTERISTICS OF A PROFESSION

I. Identifiable membership
II. Special advanced education or preparation
III. Promotion of a body of knowledge in the field (e.g., research and theory development)
IV. Strong service orientation
V. Autonomy of practice
VI. Self-regulation
VII. Recognized authority with societal sanction
VIII. Primarily intellectual work
IX. Adherence to a code of ethics

VETERINARY TECHNICIAN DEFINITION

I. A professional who provides support services to veterinarians
II. In the United States, a graduate of a two, three, four year Veterinary Technology program or a person who is recognized by a state practice act
III. In Canada, a graduate of a two or three year Veterinary Technology program

VETERINARY TECHNICIAN PROFESSION CHARACTERISTICS

I. Special education and training
II. Continuing education components to registration
III. Adherence to prescribed code of ethics
IV. Use of a designation
   A. Licensed Veterinary Technician, Certified Veterinary Technician, or Registered Veterinary Technician
      1. In Canada, Registered Veterinary Technician or Registered Animal Health Technician is used
      2. In the United States all three designations are used

V. Regulation of professionals
   A. United States: license granted by a state agency or board
      1. Limits practice to
         a. Responsibilities/behaviors prescribed by law in the state practice act
         b. Responsibilities/behaviors delineated by rules and regulations
         c. Authorizes practice by professional meeting-specified qualifications
   B. Canada: registration status is granted by the provincial association

PURPOSE OF A VETERINARY TECHNICIAN PROFESSIONAL ORGANIZATION

I. Represent and promote the profession of Veterinary Technology
II. Provide education
III. Work with allied organizations to promote competent care and humane treatment of animals
IV. Provide direction for its members
   A. EXAMPLE: each association has objects and/or a code of ethics

OBJECTS OF THE CANADIAN ASSOCIATION OF ANIMAL HEALTH TECHNOLOGISTS AND TECHNICIANS (CAAHTT)

I. Establish a national standard of membership
II. Promote and assist in continuing education programs in Veterinary Technology
III. Promote greater communications nation wide
IV. Promote the profession of Veterinary Technology within the veterinary field and to the general public
V. Provide an information source on Veterinary Technology programs in Canada

NORTH AMERICAN VETERINARY TECHNICIAN ASSOCIATION CODE OF ETHICS

I. Veterinary Technicians shall aid society and animals through providing excellent care and services for animals.

II. Veterinary Technicians shall prevent and relieve the suffering of animals

III. Veterinary Technicians shall promote public health by assisting with the control of zoonotic diseases and informing the public about these diseases

IV. Veterinary Technicians shall assume accountability for individual professional actions and judgments

V. Veterinary Technicians shall protect confidential information provided by clients

VI. Veterinary Technicians shall safeguard the public and the profession against individuals deficient in professional competence or ethics

VII. Veterinary Technicians shall assist with efforts to ensure conditions of employment consistent with the excellent care of animals

VIII. Veterinary Technicians shall remain competent in Veterinary Technology through a commitment to lifelong learning

IX. Veterinary Technicians shall collaborate with members of the veterinary medical profession in an effort to ensure quality health care services for all animals

CONTRIBUTIONS TO THE GROWTH OF VETERINARY TECHNOLOGY AS A PROFESSION ▪

I. More than 75 accredited Veterinary Technology programs in the United States and Canada

II. In the United States, recognition and support by the American Veterinary Medical Association

III. Growth of the North American Veterinary Technician Association (NAVTA), and in Canada the Canadian Association of Animal Health Technologists and Technicians/Association Candadienne des Techniciens et Technologistes en Sante Animale (CAAHTT)

IV. Growth of the many provincial and state organizations

V. Veterinary Technician conferences offering continuing education specifically designed for Technicians

VI. Increased public awareness of the profession and the need for professionals in animal hospitals, research institutions, and humane societies

   A. National Veterinary Technician Week (NVTW) is an annual celebration recognized by many states and provinces

VII. Quality care provided for patients

VIII. The growing number of specialty organizations interested in a specific discipline

   A. The American Society of Veterinary Dental Technicians (ASDVT)

   B. The Veterinary Technician Anesthetist Society (VTAS)

   C. The Academy of Veterinary Emergency/Critical Care Technicians (AVECCT)

      1. At present, the AVECCT is the only specialty group recognized by NAVTA

IX. Establishment of the International Veterinary Nurses and Technician Association (IVNTA)

   A. Meets annually; usually in Birmingham, United Kingdom

   B. NAVTA and CAAHTT members are automatically a member of the IVNTA

OBSTRUCTIONS TO GROWTH OF VETERINARY TECHNOLOGY AS A PROFESSION ▪

I. Low self-esteem of the members

II. Low participation in state/provincial/national professional organizations

III. Lack of continuity from state to state regarding regulations and designations

IV. Poor delineation of duties between the Veterinary Technician and the Veterinary Assistant

V. Lowering educational standards for Veterinary Technicians due to budgetary restraints

VI. Poor professional attitude of some members of the profession

VII. Lack of recognition of Veterinary Technicians as a professional body by veterinary state and provincial boards

LAWS THAT GOVERN VETERINARY TECHNICIANS

I. United States

   A. A practice act governs the profession of veterinary medicine

      1. A practice act is law

      2. The practice act defines the parameters under which Veterinary Technicians work

      3. The practice act is written by veterinary state boards and enacted into law

   B. Rules and regulations

      1. Written by veterinary state boards to regulate Veterinary Technicians

         a. May include the following (each state has different regulations)

            (1) Education

(2) Continuing education requirements
(3) Certification revocation
(4) Examination competence
(5) Specify duties

II. Rules and regulations do not take precedence over the practice act

III. Duties that can be performed by Veterinary Technicians have been debated. However, every state's and province's rules and regulations include the following acts that cannot be performed by a Veterinary Technician
   A. Diagnose
   B. Prognose
   C. Prescribe medication or make therapy decisions
   D. Perform surgery

IV. Eight states, the District of Columbia, and Puerto Rico do not have laws or regulations governing the registration of Veterinary Technicians. These states are:
   A. Delaware
   B. Hawaii
   C. Idaho
   D. Montana
   E. New Hampshire
   F. Rhode Island
   G. Utah
   H. Vermont

V. In ten states certification is voluntary and laws may or may not govern activities of Veterinary Technicians
   A. Wyoming
   B. Connecticut
   C. Florida
   D. Alaska
   E. Louisiana
   F. Minnesota
   G. New Jersey
   H. Texas
   I. Vermont
   J. Colorado

VI. Canada
   A. Seven provincial associations govern Canadian Veterinary Technicians
   B. Titles
      1. In Ontario and the Atlantic provinces: Veterinary Technician
      2. In Saskatchewan: Veterinary Technologist
      3. In British Columbia, Alberta, Manitoba, and Quebec: Animal Health Technologist
   C. Two provinces have private members bills that restrict use of the title
      1. Ontario: The OAVT Act—Registered Veterinary Technician
      2. British Columbia—Animal Health Technologist
   D. In Alberta, Veterinary Technicians must be a member of the Alberta Association of Animal Health Technologists to practice in the province
   E. In Saskatchewan, Veterinary Technologists must be a member of the Saskatchewan Association of Veterinary Technologists to practice in the province
   F. Presently, the Quebec provincial association is working toward their own act, which will describe duties and limit those duties to Animal Health Technicians only
   G. In 1995 Canadian provincial associations agreed on complete reciprocity for their respective members
      1. Reciprocity allows registered members of provincial associations portability from one province to another

INFORMATION RESOURCES ▬▬▬▬▬▬▬

UNITED STATES INFORMATION ON STATE LAWS AND REGULATIONS ▬▬▬▬▬

The American Association of Veterinary State Boards
P.O. Box 1702
Jefferson City, MO U.S.A. 65102
Phone (573) 761-9937
Fax (573) 761-9938
e-mail aavsb1@socketis.net

State Agencies Responsible for Regulation of Veterinary Technicians

NOTE: Each state has its own laws concerning the certification, registration, or licensure of Veterinary Technicians

Alabama
Executive Officer
Board of Veterinary Medicine
PO Box 1767
Decatur, AL 35602
502-353-3544

Alaska
Department of Commerce &
Economic Development
Division of Occupational Licensing
PO Box 110806
Juneau, AK 99811-0806
907-465-5470

Arizona
Veterinary Medical Examining Board
Executive Director
1400 W. Washington, Rm 230
Phoenix, AZ 85007
602-542-3095

Arkansas
Executive Secretary
Arkansas Veterinary Medical
Examining Board
PO Box 5497
Little Rock, AR 72215
501-224-2836

California
Executive Officer
Board of Examiners in Veterinary
Medicine
1420 Howe Ave., Suite 6
Sacramento, CA 95825
916-263-2610

Colorado
CACVT
PO Box 24922
Denver, CO 80224

Connecticut
Connecticut Association of Animal Health
Technicians
c/o Eileen Malsick
99 Boston Post Rd. N.
Windham, CT 06256

Florida
Allen Altvater, Secretary
Florida VMA, VT Committee
46 Lake Henry Dr.
Lake Placid, FL 33852-6197

Georgia
Gregg W. Schunder
Executive Director
166 Pryor St. SW
Atlanta, GA 30303
404-656-3912

Illinois
Department of Professional
Regulation
320 W. Washington
Springfield, IL 62786
217-782-8556

Indiana
Health Professions Bureau
Ms. Barbara Sargent
402 W. Washington St., Rm. 041
Indianapolis, IN 46282
317-233-4407

Iowa
Secretary, Iowa Veterinary Medical
Examining Board
Wallace Bldg., 2nd Floor
Des Moines, IA 50319
515-281-5305

Kansas
Registration Board
KS Registered VTs
1255 S. Range
Colby, KS 67701

Kentucky
Kentucky Board of Veterinary Examiners
PO Box 456
Frankfort, KY 40602
502-564-3296

Louisiana
Louisiana Board of Veterinary Medicine
200 Lafayette St., Suite 604
Baton Rouge, LA 70801-1203

Maine
Professional and Financial
Regulations
State House Station 35
Augusta, ME 04333
207-624-8603

Maryland
Secretary, State Board of
Veterinary Medical Examiners
50 Harry S. Truman Pkwy.
Annapolis, MD 21401
410-841-5862

Massachusetts
Massachusetts VT Association
Joint Committee on VT
Certification
c/o Angell Memorial Animal
Hospital
350 S. Huntington Ave.
Boston, MA 02130

Michigan
Michigan Board of VeterinaryMedicine
Department of Commerce/BOPR
PO Box 30018
Lansing, MI 48909
517-373-3596

Minnesota
Veterinary Technician Committee
of MVMA
2469 University Ave.
St. Paul, MN 55114

Mississippi
Executive Secretary
Mississippi Board of Veterinary
Medicine
209 S. Lafayette St.
Starkvill, MS 39759
601-324-9380

Missouri
Executive Director
Missouri Veterinary Medical
Board
PO Box 633
Jefferson City, MO 65102
314-751-0031

Nebraska
Director, Bureau of Examination
Board
Department of Health
Box 95007
Lincoln, NE 68509
402-471-2115

Nevada
State Board of Veterinary Medical
Examiners
1005 Terminal Way, Suite 246
Reno, NV 89502
702-322-9422

New Jersey
NJVMA
66 Morris Ave.
Springfield, NJ 07081
201-379-1100

New Mexico
Executive Director
New Mexico Board of Veterinary
Examiners
1650 University Blvd. NE
Suite 400C
Albuquerque, NM 87102
505-841-9112

New York
Executive Secretary
Board of Veterinary Medicine
Cultural Education Center
Room 3043
Albany, NY 12230
518-474-3867

North Carolina
Executive Director
Veterinary Medical Board
PO Box 12587
Raleigh, NC 27605
919-733-7689

North Dakota
Board of Veterinary Medical
Examiners
c/o ND Board of Animal Health
600 E. Blvd. Ave., J-Wing, 1st Floor
Bismarck, ND 58505-0390
701-224-2655

Ohio
Executive Secretary
Veterinary Medical Board
77 S. High St., 16th Floor
Columbus, OH 43266-0116
614-644-5281

Oklahoma
Board of Veterinary Medical Examiners
PO Box 54556
Oklahoma City, OK 73514

Oregon
Veterinary Medical Examining Board
800 NE Oregon St. #21 Suite 407
Portland, OR 97232
503-731-4051

Pennsylvania
Secretary, State Board of Veterinary Medicine
PO Box 2649
Harrisburg, PA 17105-2649
717-783-1389

South Carolina
South Carolina Department of Labor
Licensing & Regulation
PO Box 11329
Columbia, SC 29211-1329
803-734-4146

South Dakota
Secretary/Treasurer
State Board of Veterinary Medical
Examiners
c/o State Veterinarian
411 S. Fort St.
Pierre, SD 57501
605-773-3321

Tennessee
Ms. Judy Hartman, Administrator
Board of Veterinary Medical
Examiners
283 Plus Park Blvd.
Nashville, TN 37217
615-367-6282

Texas
State MA
6633 Hwy. 290 East, Suite 201
Austin, TX 78723
512-452-4224

Virginia
Virginia Board of Veterinary Medicine
606 W. Broad St., 4th Floor
Richmond, VA 23230-1717
804-662-9915

Washington
Department of Health
Professional Licensing Services
Veterinary Board of Governors
PO Box 1099
Olympia, WA 98504

West Virginia
West Virginia Board of Veterinary
Medicine
1900 Kanawha Blvd. E.
Charleston, WV 25305-0199
304-558-2016

Wisconsin
Veterinary Examination Board
PO Box 8935
Madison, WI 53708
608-266-2811

Wyoming
Animal Technician Committee
of WVMA
Box 6573
Boise, ID 83707

CANADIAN PROVINCIAL ASSOCIATIONS FOR INFORMATION ON LAWS AND REGULATIONS ■

AHT/VT Associations of Canada

Canada
CAAHTT/ACTTSA: Canadian Association of
Animal Health Technologists and
Technicians/Association Canadienne des
Techniciens et Technologistes en Sante
Animale
Box 91
Grandora, SK S0K 1V0
(306) 329-8660

Alberta
AAAHT: Alberta Association of Animal Health
Technologists
#100 8615 - 149th St.
Edmonton, AB T5R 1B3

Atlantic Provinces
EVTA: Eastern Veterinary Technician
Association Ltd.
Box 3156
Charlottetown, PEI C1A 7N9

British Columbia
AHTA of BC: Animal Health Technologists
Association of B.C.
Box 275
Sicamous, BC V0E 2V0
(604) 836-4815

Manitoba
MAHTA: Manitoba Animal Health
Technologists Association
Box 3025
Winnipeg, MB R3C 4E5

Ontario
OAVT: Ontario Association of Veterinary
Technicians
Box 833
Guelph, Ontario N1H 6L8
(519) 836-4910
Fax (519) 836-3638

Quebec
ATSAQ: Association des Techniciens en Sante
Animale du Quebec
1120 Wolfe
St. Bruno-de-Montarville, QC J3V 3K5
(514) 582-2178

Saskatchewan
SAVT Inc.: Saskatchewan Association of
Veterinary Technologists
Box 346 RPO University
Saskatoon, SK S7N 4J8

UNITED STATES PROGRAMS IN VETERINARY TECHNOLOGY*

Programs accredited by the AVMA Committee on Veterinary Technician Education and Activities (CVTEA)

Alabama
Snead State Community College*
Boaz, 35957
(205) 593-5120

California
California State Polytechnic University†
College of Agriculture
3801 W. Temple Ave.
Pomona, 91768
(909) 869-2200

Cosumnes River College*
8401 Center Pkwy.
Sacramento, 95823
(916) 688-7355

Foothill College*
12345 El Monte Rd.
Los Altos Hills, 94022
(415) 949-7203

Hartnell College*
156 Homestead Ave.
Salinas, 93901
(408) 755-6700

Los Angeles Pierce College*
6201 Winnetka Ave.
Woodland Hills, 91371
(818) 347-0551

Mt. San Antonio College*
1100 N. Grand Ave.
Walnut, 91789
(909) 594-5611

Yuba College*
2088 N. Beale Rd.
Marysville, 95901
(916) 741-6962

Colorado
Colorado Mountain College*
Spring Valley Campus
3000 County Rd. 114
Glenwood Springs, 81601
(970) 945-7481

Bel-Rea Institute of Animal Technology*
1681 S. Dayton St.
Denver, 80231
(800) 950-8001

Front Range Community College‡
4616 S. Shields
Ft. Collins, 80526
(970) 204-0466

Connecticut
Quinnipiac College*
Mt. Carmel Ave.
Hamden, 06518
(203) 288-5251

Florida
St. Petersburg Junior College*
P.O. Box 13489
St. Petersburg, 33733-3489
(813) 341-3652
Distance Learning Program‡

Georgia
Fort Valley State College‡
Fort Valley, 31030
(912) 825-6353

Illinois
Parkland College*
2400 W. Bradley
Champaign, 61821
(217) 351-2224

Indiana
Purdue University*
School of Veterinary Medicine
West Lafayette, 47907
(317) 494-7619

Iowa
Kirkwood Community College*
6301 Kirkwood Blvd. SW
Cedar Rapids, 52406
(319) 398-5411

Kansas
Colby Community College*
1255 S. Range
Colby, 67701
(913) 462-3985

Kentucky
Morehead State University*
25 MSU Farm Dr.
Morehead, 40351
(606) 783-2326

Murray State University*
Department of Agriculture
Murray, 42071
(502) 753-1303

Louisiana
Northwestern St. University of LA*
Dept. of Life Science
Natchitoches, 71457
(318) 357-5323

Maryland
Essex Community College*
7201 Rossville Blvd.
Baltimore, 21237
(410) 780-6617

Massachusetts
Becker College*
3 Paxton St.
Leicester, 01524
(508) 791-9241

Holyoke Community College*
303 Homestead Ave.
Holyoke, 01040-1099
(413) 538-7000

Mount Ida College*
777 Dedham St.
Newton Centre, 02192
(617) 969-7000 ext. 145

Michigan
Macomb Community College*
44575 Garfield Rd.
Clinton Township, 48044
(810) 286-2169

Michigan State University*
College of Veterinary Medicine
East Lansing, 48823
(517) 353-7267

Wayne County Community College*
c/o Wayne State University Department of Lab Animal Resources
540 E. Canfield
Detroit, 48201
(313) 577-1156

Minnesota
Medical Institute of Minnesota*
5503 Green Valley Dr.
Bloomington, 55437-0064
(612) 844-0064

Ridgewater College*
2101 15th Ave. NW
Willmar, 56201
(612) 235-5114

Mississippi
Hinds Community College*
P.O. Box 10461
Raymond, 39154
(601) 857-3456

*Source: AVMA May 1997
*Full accreditation
†Provisional accreditation
‡Probational accreditation

Missouri
Jefferson College*
1000 Viking Dr.
Hillsboro, 63050
(314) 789-3951

Maple Woods Community College*
2601 N.E. Barry Rd.
Kansas City, 64156
(816) 437-3235

Nebraska
Nebraska College of Technical Agriculture*
Curtis, 69025
(308) 367-4124

Omaha College of Health Careers*
10845 Harney
Omaha, 68154
(402) 333-1400

New Jersey
Camden County College*
P.O. Box 200
Blackwood, 08012
(609) 227-7200

New York
LaGuardia Community College*
31-10 Thompson Ave.
Long Island City, 11101
(718) 482-5764

Medaille College*
18 Agassiz Cr.
Buffalo, 14214
(716) 884-0291

Mercy College*
555 Broadway
Dobbs Ferry, 10522
(914) 693-4500

State University of New York*
Agricultural & Technical College
Canton, 13617
(315) 386-7011

State University of New York*
Agricultural & Technical College
Delhi, 13753
(607) 746-4349

Suffolk Community College*
Western Campus
Crooked Hill Rd.
Brentwood, 11717
(516) 851-6700

North Carolina
Central Carolina Community College*
1105 Kelly Dr.
Sanford, 27330
(919) 755-5401

Gaston College†
201 Hwy. 321 South
Dallas, 28034-1499
(704) 922-6440

North Dakota
North Dakota State University*
Dept. of Veterinary Science
Fargo, 58105
(701) 231-7511

Ohio
Columbus State Community College*
550 E. Spring St.
Columbus, 43216
(614) 227-2569

Raymond Walters College*
University of Cincinnati
Cincinnati, 45221
(513) 558-5171

Stautzenberger College‡
5355 S. Wyck
Toledo, 43614
(419) 866-0261

Oklahoma
Murray State College*
Tishomingo, 73460
(405) 371-2371

Oregon
Portland Community College*
P.O. Box 19000
Portland, 97219
(503) 244-6111

Pennsylvania
Harcum Junior College*
Bryn Mawr, 19010
(610) 526-6055

Johnson Technical Institute‡
3427 N, Main Ave.
Scranton, 18505
(717) 342-6404

Manor Junior College‡
Fox Chase Rd. & Forrest Ave
Jenkintown, 19046
(215) 885-2360

Wilson College*
Chambersburg, 17201
(717) 264-4141

Puerto Rico
University of Puerto Rico*
Medical Sciences Campus
P.O. Box 365067
San Juan, 00936-5067
(809) 758-2525 Ext 1051, 1052

South Carolina
Tri-County Technical College*
P.O. Box 587
Pendleton, 29670
(803) 646-8361

South Dakota
National College/Allied Health Div.*
321 Kansas City St.
Rapid City, 57709
(800) 843-8892

Tennessee
Columbia State Community College*
Columbia, 38401
(615) 540-2722

Lincoln Memorial University*
Harrogate, 37752
(615) 869-6278

Texas
Cedar Valley College*
3030 N. Dallas Ave.
Lancaster, 75134
(214) 372-8164

Midland College‡
3600 N. Garfield
Midland, 79705
(915) 685-6431

Sul Ross State University*
Range Animal Science Dept.
Alpine, 79830
(915) 837-8205

Tomball College*
3055 Tomball Pkwy.
Tomball, 77375-4036
(713) 351-3357

Utah
Brigham Young University*
Provo, 84602
(801) 378-4294

Vermont
Vermont Technical College‡
Randolph Center, 05061
(802) 728-3391

Virginia
Blue Ridge Community College*
Box 80
Weyers Cave, 24486
(540) 234-9261

Northern Virginia Community College*
Loudoun Campus
1000 Harry Flood Byrd Hwy
Sterling, 22170
(703) 450-2561

Washington
Pierce College at Fort Steilacoom*
9401 Farwest Dr. SW
Tacoma, 98498
(206) 964-6665

West Virginia
Fairmont State College‡
Fairmont, 26554
(304) 367-4763

Wisconsin
Madison Area Technical College*
3550 Anderson
Madison, 53704
(608) 246-6100

Wyoming
Eastern Wyoming College*
3200 West C St.
Torrington, 82240
(800) 658-3195 ext. 8268

CANADIAN VETERINARY
TECHNOLOGY PROGRAMS*

British Columbia
The University College of the Cariboo†
P.O. Box 3010
Kamloops BC
V2C 5N3
(604) 828-5174

Alberta
Northern Alberta Institute of Technology†
11762 106th St
Edmonton, AB
T5G 2R1
(403) 477-4282

Fairview College†
Box 3000
Fairview, AB
T0H 1L0
(403) 835-6632

Olds College†
4500 50 St.
Olds, AB
T4H 1R6
(403) 556-8281

Lakeland College†
Vermilion Campus
Vermilion, AB
T0B 4M0
(403) 853-8586

Saskatchewan
Saskatchewan Institute of Applied
Science & Technology†
Kelsey Campus
Box 1520
Saskatoon, SK
S7K 3R5
(306) 933-6490

Manitoba
Red River Community College†
2055 Notre Dame Ave.
Winnipeg, MB
R3H 0J9
(204) 632-2168

Ontario
St. Clair College of Applied
Arts and Technology†
2000 Talbot Rd. W.
Windsor, ON
N9A 6S4
(519) 972-2727

Seneca College of Applied Arts and Technology
King Campus
13990 Dufferin St. N
King City, ON
L7B 1B3
(416) 491-5050

St. Lawrence College of Applied‡
Arts and Technology
P.O. Box 6000
Kingston, ON
K7L 5A6
(613) 544-5400

University of Guelph-Ridgetown Agricultural
    College†
Main St. E
Ridgetown, ON
N0P 2C0
(519) 674-1665

Quebec
CEGEP de la Pacatiere‡
140 Rieme Ave.
LaPocatiere, QC
G0R 1Z0
(418) 856-1525

College de Sherbrooke
475 rue Parc
Sherbrooke, QC
J1H 5M7
(819) 564-6187

Vanier College
821 Ste. Croix Ave
St. Laurent, QC
H4L 3X9
(514) 744-7143

College Lionel Groulx‡
100 Rue Duquet
Ste. Therese, QC
J7E 3G6
(514) 430-3120

College Lefleche‡
1687 boul. Carmel
Trois Rivieres, QC
G8Z 3R8
(819) 375-7346

CEGEP - St. Felicien‡
1105 Boul. Hamel, B.P. 7300
St. Felicien, QC
G8K 2H5
(418) 679-5412

Nova Scotia
Nova Scotia Agricultural College†
Truro, NS
B2N 5E3
(902) 893-6648

---

*Source-CAAHTT/ACTTSA December 1997
Programs accredited by the CVMA
†Accredited by the Canadian Veterinary Medical Association
‡3 year program, all other programs are 2 year programs

Medical Terminology

PREFIXES

a, ab-, abs- From; away; departing from the normal
ad- Addition to; toward; nearness
amb-, ambi- Both; ambidextrous, having the ability to work effectively with either hand
amphi- On both sides
ampho- Both
an- Negative; without or not
ana- Upper, away from
andro- Signifying man
ant-, anti- Against
ante-, antero- Front; before
bili- Pertaining to bile
brady- Slow
brom-, bromo- A stench
broncho- Relating to the bronchi
cac- Bad
cardi-, cardio- Relating to the heart
cata- Down or downward
cervico- Relating to the neck
circa- About
circum- Around
co- With or together
con- Together with
contra- Opposite; against
demi- Half
di- Twice
dia- Through
dialy- To separate
en- In
end-, endo-, ento- Inward; within
ep-, epi- On; in addition to
ex- Out; away from
exo- Without, outside of
extra- Outside of; in addition to
fibro- Relating to fibers
gaster-, gastr-, gastro- Pertaining to the stomach
hemi- Half
hemo- Relating to the blood
hepat-, hepatico-, hepato- Pertaining to the liver
heter-, hetero- Meaning other; relationship to another
homeo- Denoting likeness or resemblance
homo- Denoting sameness
hyal-, hyalo- Transparent

hyper- Above; excessive; beyond
hypo- Below; less than
ideo- Pertaining to mental images
idio- Denoting relationship to one's self or to something separate and distinct
in- Not; in; inside; within; also intensive action
infra- Below
inter- In the midst; between
intra- Within
intro- In or into
iso- Equal or alike
juxta- Of close proximity
karyo- Relating to a cell's nucleus
kypho- Humped
laryngo- Pertaining to the larynx
medi- Middle
myelo- Pertaining to the spinal cord or bone marrow
oari-, oaric- Pertaining to the ovary
omni- All
per- Through; by means of
peri- Around; about
post- Behind or after
postero- Relating to the posterior
pre- Before
pro- Before, in front of
pseudo- False
re- Back; again (contrary)
retro- Backward
semi- Half
steato- Fatty
sub- Under; near
syn- Joined together
trans- Across; over
un- Not; reversal

SUFFIXES

able, -ible, -ble The power to be
-ad Toward; in the direction of
-aemia, -emia Pertaining to blood
-age Put in motion; to do
-agra Denoting a seizure; severe pain
-algia Denoting pain
-ase Forms the name of an enzyme
-blast Designates a cell or a structure
-cele Denoting a swelling
-centesis Denoting a puncture
-ectomy A cutting out
-esthesia Denoting sensation

From Darby ML: *Mosby's Comprehensive Review of Dental Hygiene,* ed 3, St Louis, 1994, Mosby.

-facient That which makes or causes

-gene, -genesis, -genetic, -genic Denoting production; origin

-gog, -gogue To make flow

-gram A tracing; a mark

-graph A writing; a record

-iasis Denoting a condition or pathologic state

-id Denoting shape or resemblance

-ite Of the nature of

-itis Denoting inflammation

-logia Denoting discourse, science, or study of

-oid Denoting form or resemblance

-oma Denoting a tumor

-osis Denoting any morbid process

-ostomosis, -ostomy, -stomy Denoting an outlet; to furnish with an opening or mouth

-plasty Denoting molding or shaping

-rhagia Denoting a discharge; usually a bleeding

-rhaphy Meaning suturing or stitching

-rhea Meaning a flow or discharge

-scopy Generally an instrument for viewing

-tomy Denoting a cutting operation

-trophy Denoting a relationship to nourishment

COMBINING FORMS

aer-, aero- Denoting air or gas

alge-, algesi-, algo- Relating to pain

allo- Other; differing from the normal

anomalo- Denoting irregularity

arthro- Relating to a joint or joints

brevi- Short

celio- Denoting the abdomen

centro- Center

cheil-, cheilo- Denoting the lip

chol-, chole-, cholo- Relating to bile

chondr-, chondri- Relating to cartilage

chrom-, chromo- Relating to color

cole-, coleo- Denoting a sheath

colp-, colpo- Relating to the vagina

cranio- Relating to the cranium of the skull

crymo-, cryo- Denoting cold

crypt- To hide; a pit

cyano- Dark blue

cyclo- Pertaining to a cycle

cysto- Relating to a sac or cyst

cyto- Denoting a cell

dacryo- Pertaining to the lacrimal glands

dactylo- Relating to digits

dent-, dento- Relating to teeth

derma-, dermat- Relating to the skin

desmo- Relating to a bond or ligament

dextro- Right

diplo- Double; twofold

dorsi-, dorso- Referring to the back

duodeno- Relating to the duodenum

electro- Relating to electricity

encephalo- Denoting the brain

entero- Relating to the intestines

episio- Relating to the vulva

eso- Inward

esthesio- Relating to feeling or sensation

facio- Relating to the face

gangli-, ganglio- Relating to a ganglion

geno- Relating to reproduction

gero-, geronto- Denoting old age

giganto- Huge

gingivo- Relating to the gingiva or gum

gloss-, glosso- Relating to the tongue

gluco- Denoting sweetness

glyco- Relating to sugar

gnath-, gnatho- Denoting the jaw

gon- Denoting a seed

grapho- Denoting writing

hapt-, hapte-, hapto- Relating to touch or a seizure

helo- Relating to a nail or a callus

hist-, histio-, histo-, Relating to tissue

holo- Relating to the whole

hydr-, hydro- Denoting water

hygro- Denoting moisture

hyl-, hyle-, hylo- Denoting matter or material

ileo-, ilio- Relating to the ileum

ipsi- Meaning self

irido- Relating to a colored circle

iso- Equal

jejuno- Referring to the jejunum

kerato- Relating to the cornea

kino- Denoting movement

labio- Pertaining to the lips

lacto- Relating to milk

laparo- Pertaining to the loin or flank

latero- Pertaining to the side

leido-, leio- Smooth

leuk-, leuko- Denoting deficiency of color

lip-, lipo- Pertaining to fat

litho- Denoting a calculus

macr-, macro- Large; long

mast-, mastro- Relating to the breast

meg-, mega- Great; large

meli- Sweet

meningo- Denoting membranes; covering the brain and spinal cord

micr-, micro- Small in size or extent

mono- One

morpho- Relating to form

multi- Many

my-, myo- Relating to muscle

myc-, mycet- Denoting a fungus

myringo- Denoting tympani or the eardrum

myx-, myxo- Pertaining to mucus

narco- Denoting stupor

naso- Relating to the nose

necro- Denoting death

neo- New

nephr-, nephro- Denoting the kidney

normo- Normal or usual

oculo- Denoting the eye
odyno- Denoting pain
oleo- Denoting oil
onco- Denoting a swelling or mass
onycho- Relating to the nails
oo- Denoting an egg
opisth-, opistho- Backward
ophthal-, ophthalmo- Pertaining to the eye
optico- Relating to the eye or vision
orchi-, orcho- Relating to the testes
oro- Relating to the mouth
ortho- Straight; right
oscillo- Denoting oscillation
osteo- Relating to the bones
ot-, oto- Denoting an egg
palato- Denoting the palate
patho- Denoting disease
pedia-, pedo- Denoting a child
perineo- A combining form for the region between the anus
   and scrotum or the vulva
phago- Denoting a relationship to eating
pharyngo- Pertaining to the pharynx
phleb-, phlebo- Denoting the veins
phon-, phono- Denoting sound
phot-, photo- Relating to light
phren- Relating to the mind
picr-, picro- Bitter
pilo- Denoting hair
plasmo- Relating to plasma or the substance of a cell
pneuma-, pneumono-, pneumoto- Denoting air or gas
pod-, podo- Meaning foot
poly- Many
proct-, procto- Denoting the anus and rectum
psych-, psycho- Relating to the mind
ptyalo- Denoting saliva
pubio-, pubo- Denoting the pubic region
pulmo- Denoting the lung
pupillo- Denoting the pupil
pyel-, pyelo- Denoting the pelvis
pyloro- Relating to the pylorus
py-, pyo- Denoting pus
recto- Denoting the rectum
rhin-, rhino- Denoting the nose
rrhagia- Denoting abnormal discharge
salpingo- Denoting a tube, specifically the fallopian tube
schizo- Split
sclero- Denoting hardness
scoto- Relating to darkness
sero- Pertaining to serum
sialo- Relating to saliva or the salivary glands
sidero- Denoting iron
sinistro- Left
somato- Denoting the body
somni- Denoting sleep
spasmo- Denoting a spasm
spermato-, spermo- Denoting sperm
sphero- Denoting a sphere; round

sphygmo- Denoting a pulse
splen-, spleno- Denoting the spleen
staphyl-, staphylo- Resembling a bunch of grapes
steno- Narrow; short
sterco- Denoting feces
steth-, stetho- Relating to the chest
stomato- Denoting the mouth
sym-, syn- With; along
tacho-, tachy- Swift
tarso- Relating to the flat of the foot
terato- Denoting a marvel, prodigy, or monster
thoraco- Relating to the chest
thrombo- Denoting a clot of blood
toxico-, toxo- Denoting poison
tracheo- Denoting the trachea
trichi-, tricho- Denoting hair
ur-, uro-, urono- Relating to urine
varico- Denoting a twisting or swelling
vaso- Denoting a vessel
veno- Denoting a vein
ventri, ventro- Denoting the abdomen
vertebro- Relating to the vertebra
vesico- Denoting the bladder
viscero- Denoting the organs of the body
vivi- Denoting alive
xantho- Denoting yellow
xero- Denoting dryness

TERMINOLOGY FREQUENTLY USED TO DESIGNATE BODY PARTS OR ORGANS ■■■

anus Anal, ano-
arm Brachial, brachio-
blood Hem-, hemat-
chest Thoracic, thorax
ear Auricle, oto-
eye Ocular, oculo-, ophthalmo-
foot Pedal, ped-, -pod
gallbladder Chole-, chol-
head Cephalic, cephalo-
heart Cardium, cardiac, cardio-
intestines Cecum, colon, duodenum, ileum, jejunum
kidney Renal, nephric, nephro-
lip Cheil-
liver Hepatic, hepato-
lungs Pulmonary, pulmonic, pneumo-
mouth Oral, os, stoma, stomat-
muscle Myo-
neck Cervix, cervical, cervico-
penis Penile
rectum Rectal
skin Derma, integumentum
stomach Gastric, gastro-
testicle Orchio-, orchi-, orchido-
urinary bladder Cysti-, cysto-
uterus Hystero-, metra
vagina Vulvo, vaginal

Normal Values

	Feline	Canine	Equine	Porcine	Bovine	Ovine	Caprine
Temp °F	98.6-104	98.6-104	98.6	100.4-104	100.4-102.2	100.4-104	100.4-104
Temp °C	37.5-39.5	37.5-39.5	37-39	38-40	37.5-39.5	38.5-40.5	38.5-40.5
Pulse/min*	110-140	70-140	32-44	60-80	60-80	60-90	40-60
Resp/min*	0-30	10-30	8-16	8-18	10-30	12-20	12-20
Onset of puberty (months)	5-9	6-8	12-18	5-7	9-10	6-7	3-7
Gestation (days)	63-65	63-65	336	114	285	148	149
Length of estrous cycle	6 months	7-8 months	22 days	21 days	21 days	17 days	21 days
Length of estrus	4 days	5-9 days	6 days	48-55 hours	18-24 hours	10-30 hours	40 hours

*The above values are estimated for mature animals. In general, immature animals have slightly higher ranges for respiration and pulse rate.

Table of Species Names

Common name	Scientific (generic)	Male/Female terminology	Neutered male	Act of parturition	Young called
Cat	*Felis catus* (Feline)	Tom/Queen		Queening	Kitten
Cattle	*Bos taurus* *Bos indicus* (Bovine)	Bull/Cow	Steer	Calving	Calf
Chicken	*Gallus domesticus*	Rooster/Hen	Capon	Laying/ Hatching	Chick
Chinchilla	*Chinchilla laniger*				Kid
Dog	*Canis familiaris* (Canine)	Dog/Bitch		Whelping	Puppy
Ferret	*Mustela putoris furo*	Hob/Jill	Gib female—Sprite	Kindling	Kit
Gerbil (jird)	*Meriones unguiculatus*				Pup
Goat	*Capra hircus* (Caprine)	Buck/Doe	Wether	Kidding	Kid
Guinea pig (cavy)	*Cavia porcellus*	Boar/Sow		Farrowing	Pup
Hamster	*Mesocricetus auratus*				Pup
Horse	*Equus caballus* (Equine)	Stallion/Mare	Gelding	Foaling	Foal (either sex) Colt (male) Filly (female)
Llama	*Llama glama*	Bull/Cow	Gelding		Cria
Mouse	*Mus musculus*				Pup
Pig	*Sus scrofa* (Porcine)	Boar/Sow	Barrow	Farrowing	Piglet, pig
Rabbit	*Oryctolagus cuniculus*	Buck/Doe	Lapin	Kindling	Bunny
Rat	*Rattus norvegicus*				Pup
Sheep	*Ovis aries* (Ovine)	Ram/Ewe	Wether	Lambing	Lamb

Modified from McBride DF: *Learning Veterinary Terminology,* St Louis, 1996, Mosby.

Abbreviations and Symbols

A

A angstrom unit; anode; anterior

a ampere; anterior; area

āā of each

AAHA American Animal Hospital Association

ab antibody

A₂ aortic second sound

ABO three basic human blood groups

AC alternating current; adrenal cortex

a.c. before meals (ante cibum)

ACE adrenocortical extract

ACh acetylcholine

ACH adrenocortical hormone

ACTH adrenocorticotropic hormone

ad lib. as much as desired (ad libitum)

ADH antidiuretic hormone

A/G; A-G ratio albumin-globulin ratio

Ag silver

ag antigen

AIDS acquired immune deficiency syndrome

Al aluminum

Alb albumin

ALT alanine aminotransferase (formerly SGPT)

amp. ampere

ana so much of each, or āā

anat anatomy or anatomic

A-P; AP; A/P anterior-posterior

A.P. anterior pituitary gland

APHIS Animal and Plant Health Inspection Service

Aq water (aqua)

ARD acute respiratory disease

As arsenic

ASD atrial septal defect

AST aspartate aminotransferase (formerly SGOT)

AU Angstrom unit

Au gold

A-V; AV; A/V arteriovenous; atrioventricular

Av average or avoirdupois

AVMA American Veterinary Medical Association

ax axis

B

B boron; bacillus

Ba barium

Bact bacterium

BBB blood-brain barrier

BE barium enema

Be Beryllium

Bi bismuth

bid; b.i.d. twice a day (bis in die)

BM bowel movement

BMR basal metabolic rate

BP blood pressure

bp boiling point

BPH benign prostatic hypertrophy

BSA body surface area

BSP bromsulphalein

BUN blood urea nitrogen

C

C carbon; centigrade; Celsius

c̄ with

Ca calcium, cancer

CaCO₃ calcium carbonate

Cal large calorie

cal small calorie

CBC; cbc complete blood count

cc cubic centimeter

CCl₄ carbon tetrachloride

CDC Centers for Disease Control

cf compare or bring together

CFT complement-fixation test

Cg; Cgm centigram

CHCl₃ chloroform

CH₃COOH acetic acid

ChE cholinesterase

CHF congestive heart failure

C₅H₄N₄O₃ uric acid

C₂H₅OH ethyl alcohol

CH₂O formaldehyde

CH₃OH methyl alcohol

Cl chlorine

cm centimeter

CNS central nervous system

CO carbon monoxide

CO₂ carbon dioxide

Co cobalt

CPC clinicopathologic conference

CSF cerebrospinal fluid

CT; CAT computed (axial) tomography scan

Cu copper

CuSO₄ copper sulfate

CVA cerebrovascular accident

cyl cylinder

From McBride DF: *Learning Veterinary Terminology*, St Louis, 1996, Mosby.

D

D dose; vitamin D; right *(dexter)*
DC direct current
DCA deoxycorticosterone acetate
DEA Drug Enforcement Administration
Deg degeneration; degree
dg decigram
diff differential blood count
dil dilute or dissolve
dim one half
DNA deoxyribonucleic acid
DOA dead on arrival
DSH domestic short hair (cat)
Dx diagnosis

E

E eye
ECG electrocardiogram, electrocardiograph
ED effective dose
ED$_{50}$ median effective dose
EEG electroencephalogram, electroencephalograph
EENT eye, ear, nose, and throat
EKG electrocardiogram, electrocardiograph
EMB eosin-methylene blue
EMC encephalomyocarditis
EMG electromyogram
EMS Emergency Medical Service
ENT ear, nose, and throat
ER emergency room (hospital); external resistance
ESR erythrocyte sedimentation rate
Et ethyl
ext extract

F

F Fahrenheit; formula
FA fatty acid
FANA fluorescent antinuclear antibody test
F & R force and rhythm (pulse)
FBS fasting blood sugar
FD fatal dose; focal distance
FDA Food & Drug Administration
Fe iron
FeCl$_3$ ferric chloride
FIP Feline Infectious Peritonitis
Fl fluid
fld fluid
fl oz; fl. oz. fluid ounce
FLUTD Feline Lower Urinary Tract Disease
FR flocculation reaction
FSH follicle-stimulating hormone
ft foot
FUO fever of undertermined origin
FUS Feline Urological Syndrome

G

g gram
Galv galvanic

GB gallbladder
GBS gallbladder series
GFR glomerular filtration rate
GH growth hormone
GI gastrointestinal
Gm; gm gram
GP general practitioner; general paresis
gr grain(s)
GLPs good laboratory practices
GSW gunshot wound
gt drop *(gutta)*
GTT glucose tolerance test
gtt drops *(guttae)*
GU genitourinary
Gyn gynecology

H

H hydrogen
H$^+$ hydrogen ion
H & E hematoxylin and eosin stain
Hb; Hgb hemoglobin
HBC hit by car
H$_3$BO$_3$ boric acid
HCG human chorionic gonadotropin
HCl hydrochloric acid
HCN hydrocyanic acid
H$_2$CO$_3$ carbonic acid
HCT; Hct hematocrit
HDL high density lipoprotein
He helium
Hg mercury
HNO$_3$ nitric acid
H$_2$O water
H$_2$O$_2$ hydrogen peroxide
H$_2$SO$_4$ sulfuric acid

I

I iodine
^{131}I radioactive isotope of iodine (atomic weight 131)
^{132}I radioactive isotope of iodine (atomic weight 132)
IB inclusion body
ICS; IS intercostal space
ICSH interstitial cell-stimulating hormone
ICU intensive care unit
Id. the same *(idem)*
ID intradermal
IH infectious hepatitis
IM intramuscular
IP intraperitoneal
IOP intraocular pressure
IU immunizing unit
IV intravenous
IVP intravenous pyelogram
IVT intravenous transfusion
IVU intravenous urogram/urography

K

K potassium
k constant
Ka cathode or kathode
KBr potassium bromide
kc kilocycle
KCl potassium chloride
kev kilo electron volts
Kg kilogram
KI potassium iodide
km kilometer
KOH potassium hydroxide
kv kilovolt
kw kilowatt

L

L left; liter; length; lumbar; lethal; pound
lb pound *(libra)*
LCM left costal margin
LD lethal dose
LDL low density lipoprotein
LE lupus erythematosus
LFD least fatal dose of a toxin
LH luteinizing hormone
Li lithium
lig ligament
Liq liquor
LPF leukocytosis-promoting factor
LTH leuteotrophic hormone
LV left ventricle

M

M meter; muscle; thousand
m meter
Mag large *(magnus)*
μc microcurie
μμ micromicron
mcg; μg microgram
MCH mean corpuscular hemoglobin
MCHC mean corpuscular hemoglobin concentration
mCi; mc millicurie
MCV mean corpuscular volume
Me methyl
MED minimal effective dose
mEq milliequivalent
mEq/L milliequivalent per liter
ME ratio myeloid-erythroid ratio
Mg magnesium
mg milligram
mHg millimeters of mercury
MI myocardial infarction
MID minimum infective dose
ML midline
ml milliliter
MLD median or minimum lethal dose
MM mucous membrane
mm millimeter; muscles

mμ millimicron
Mn manganese
mN millinormal
MRI magnetic resonance imaging
MS mitral stenosis; morphine sulphate
MT medical technologist
mu mouse unit

N

N nitrogen
n normal
Na sodium
NaBr sodium bromide
NaCl sodium chloride
Na₂C₂O₄ sodium oxalate
Na₂CO₃ sodium carbonate
NaF sodium flouride
NaHCO₃ sodium bicarbonate
Na₂HPO₄ sodium phosphate
NaI sodium iodide
NaNO₃ sodium nitrate
Na₂O₂ sodium peroxide
NaOH sodium hydroxide
Na₂SO₄ sodium sulfate
NAVTA North American Veterinary Technicians Association
Ne neon
NH₃ ammonia
Ni nickel
NPN nonprotein nitrogen
NPO; n.p.o. nothing by mouth *(non per os)*
NTP normal temperature and pressure

O

O oxygen; oculus; pint
O₂ oxygen
O₃ ozone
OB obstetrics
OD right eye *(oculus dexter);* optical density; overdose
Ol oil *(oleum)*
OR operating room
OS left eye *(oculus sinister)*
Os osmium
OSHA Occupational Safety and Health Administration
oz ounce; ℥

P

P phosphorus; pulse; pupil
P₂ pulmonic second sound
P—A; P/A; PA posterior-anterior
P & A percussion and auscultation
PAB; PABA para-aminobenzoic acid
PAS; PASA para-aminosalicylic acid
Pb lead
PBI protein-bound iodine
p.c. after meals *(post cibum)*
PCV packed cell volume
PDA patent ductus arteriosus

PDR *Physician's Desk Reference*
PE physical examination
PEG pneumoencephalography
PET positron emission tomography
PFF protein-free filtrate
PGA pteroylglutamic acid (folic acid)
pH hydrogen ion concentration (alkalinity and acidity measure)
Pharm; Phar. pharmacy
PM postmortem; evening
PMN polymorphonuclear neutrophil leukocytes
PN percussion note
PO; p.o. orally *(per os)*
POVMR problem oriented veterinary medical records
PPB parts per billion
PPD purified protein derivative (TB test)
PPM parts per million
PRN, p.r.n. as required *(pro re nata)*
pro time prothrombin time
PSP phenosulfonphthalein
pt pint
Pt platinum; patient
PTA plasma thromboplastin antecedent
PTC plasma thromboplastin component
Pu plutonium
PZI protamine zinc insulin

Q

Q electric quantity
q.d. every day *(quaque die)*
q.h. every hour *(quaque hora)*
qid, q.i.d. four times daily *(quater in die)*
q.l. as much as desired *(quantum libet)*
qns quantity not sufficient
q.p. as much as desired *(quantum placeat)*
q.s. sufficient quantity
qt quart
Quat four *(quattuor)*
q.v. as much as you please *(quantum vis)*

R

R respiration; right; *Rickettsia;* roentgen
℞ take
Ra radium
rad unit of measurement of the absorbed dose of ionizing radiation
RAI radioactive iodine
RAIU radioactive iodine uptake
RBC; rbc red blood cell; red blood count
RE right eye; reticuloendothelial tissue or cell
Re rhenium
Rect rectified
Rep. let it be repeated *(repetatur)*
RES reticuloendothelial system
Rh symbol of rhesus factor; symbol for rhodium
Rn radon
RNA ribonucleic acid

R/O rule out
RPM; rpm revolutions per minute
RT radiation therapy

S

S sulfur
S. sacral
↔s without (sine)
S-A; S/A; SA sinoatrial
Se selenium
SD skin dose
Sed rate; SR sedimentation rate
SGOT serum glutamic oxaloacetic transaminase (see AST)
SGPT serum glutamic pyruvic transaminase (see ALT)
Si silicon
Sn tin
SOAP subjective objective assessment plan
Sol solution
SP spirit
sp. gr. specific gravity
Sr strontium
s̄ s̄ one half *(semis)*
Staph staphylococcus
Stat immediately *(statim)*
STD sexually transmitted disease
STH somatotropic hormone
Strep streptococcus
Sym symmetrical

T

T temperature; thoracic
t temporal
T₃ triiodothyronine
T₄ thyroxine
tab tablet
TB tuberculin; tuberculosis; tubercle bacillus
TE tetanus
Th thorium
tid, t.i.d. three times daily *(ter in die)*
Tl thallium
TPR temperature, pulse, and respiration
tr tincture
TS test solution
TSH thyroid-stimulating hormone

U

U uranium; unit
UA urinalysis
ung ointment *(unguentum)*
URI upper respiratory infection
UTI urinary tract infection
US ultrasonic
USDA United States Department of Agriculture
USP *U.S. Pharmacopeia*
Ut. dict. as directed *(ut dictum)*

V

V vanadium; vision
v volt
VC vital capacity
VHD valvular heart disease
VLDL very low density lipoprotein
VS volumetric solution
VSD ventricular septal defect
VW vessel wall

W

w watt
WBC; wbc white blood cell; white blood count
WL wavelength
Wt; wt weight

X

X-ray roentgen ray

Z

z symbol for atomic number
Zn zinc

Symbols

$>$ Greater than
$<$ Less than
♀ Female
♂ Male

The Metric System and Equivalents

The basis of measurement in science is a standard one, the metric system, in which the chief units are the meter, the gram, and the liter, which are always multiplied and divided by 10. Although the English system is still used in the United States, the metric system is the preferred system because of its logic and accuracy.

Units of length

Metric linear decimal scale and English (U.S.) equivalents

10 millimeters	=	1 centimeter	=	0.3937 inch
10 centimeters	=	1 decimeter	=	3.937 inches
10 decimeters	=	1 meter	=	39.37 inches (3.2808 feet)
10 meters	=	1 dekameter	=	10.936 yards
10 dekameters	=	1 hectometer	=	19.884 rods
10 hectometers	=	1 kilometer	=	0.62137 mile
10 kilometers	=	1 myriameter	=	6.2137 miles
1 inch	=	2.54 centimeters	or	25.4 millimeters
1 foot	=	3.048 decimeters	or	304.8 millimeters
1 yard	=	0.9144 meter	or	914.40 millimeters
1 rod	=	0.5029 dekameter		
1 mile	=	1.6093 kilometers		

Units of weight

Metric weights and English (U.S.) equivalents

1 milligram	=	0.001 gram	=	0.015 grain
1 centigram	=	0.01 gram	=	0.154 grain
1 decigram	=	0.10 gram	=	1.543 grains
1 gram	=	(1 gram)	=	0.035 ounce
1 dekagram	=	10 grams	=	0.353 ounce
1 hectogram	=	100 grams	=	3.527 ounces
1 kilogram	=	1000 grams	=	2.205 pounds
1 grain	=	0.0648 gram		
1 ounce	=	28.349 grams		
1 pound	=	0.453 kilogram		

Units of volume

Metric liquid measure capacity and English (U.S.) equivalents

1 milliliter (cc)			=	16.23 minims or 0.2705 fluidram or 0.0338 fluidounce
1 liter			=	33.8148 fluidounces or 2.1134 pints or 1.0567 quarts or 0.2642 gallon
1 fluidram			=	3.697 milliliters
1 fluidounce			=	29.573 milliliters
1 pint	=	16 ounces	=	473.166 milliliters or 0.473 liter
1 quart	=	2 pints	=	946.332 milliliters or 0.946 liter
1 gallon	=	4 quarts	=	3.785 liters

Temperature equivalents

Conversion rules

To convert Fahrenheit to Centigrade (Celsius), subtract 32 from the Fahrenheit temperature and multiply that figure by $\frac{5}{9}$.

To convert Centigrade (Celsius) to Fahrenheit, multiply the Centigrade temperature by $\frac{9}{5}$ and add 32 to the total.

From McBride DF: *Learning Veterinary Terminology,* St Louis, 1996, Mosby.

Answer Key

Chapter 1

1. b
2. a
3. d
4. b
5. d
6. a
7. b
8. c
9. d
10. d

Chapter 2

1. a
2. c
3. b
4. a
5. c
6. a
7. d
8. c
9. b
10. b

Chapter 3

1. b
2. a
3. a
4. d
5. c
6. c
7. a
8. a
9. a
10. b

Chapter 4

1. a
2. c
3. d
4. d
5. a
6. d
7. d
8. d
9. c
10. a
11. a
12. d
13. b
14. d
15. b
16. b
17. a
18. a
19. b
20. d
21. c
22. b
23. a

Chapter 5

1. a
2. a
3. d
4. b
5. a
6. a
7. c
8. b
9. c
10. c

Chapter 6

1. c
2. b
3. a
4. a
5. c
6. a
7. c
8. c
9. d
10. b

Chapter 7

1. c
2. b
3. c
4. a
5. a
6. a
7. b
8. a
9. a
10. a

Chapter 8

1. c
2. c
3. b
4. b
5. c
6. c
7. c
8. b
9. a
10. b
11. a
12. b
13. c
14. c
15. b
16. d
17. d
18. b
19. d
20. a

Chapter 9

1. c
2. d
3. c
4. b
5. a
6. a
7. d
8. b
9. a
10. d

Chapter 10

1. b
2. d
3. b
4. b
5. a
6. b
7. c
8. d
9. c
10. a
11. b
12. c
13. b
14. a
15. c
16. a
17. a
18. c
19. a
20. d

Chapter 11

1. d
2. b
3. d
4. a
5. d
6. b
7. c
8. c
9. b
10. d
11. c
12. c

Chapter 12

1. c
2. b
3. d

4. b
5. c
6. c
7. a
8. b
9. d
10. a
11. c
12. a
13. c
14. c
15. a

Chapter 13

1. b
2. a
3. a
4. a
5. c
6. d
7. c
8. c
9. c
10. d
11. d
12. c

Chapter 14

1. c
2. b
3. c
4. a
5. d
6. a
7. d
8. a
9. c
10. d
11. b
12. b
13. c
14. d
15. c

Chapter 15

1. b
2. b
3. d
4. a
5. d
6. a
7. c
8. b

9. c
10. c

Chapter 16

1. c
2. c
3. b
4. a
5. a
6. a
7. c
8. a
9. b
10. b

Chapter 17

1. b
2. a
3. a
4. c
5. b
6. b
7. a
8. d
9. d
10. d

Chapter 18

1. d
2. b
3. c
4. a
5. d
6. c
7. c
8. a
9. b
10. a
11. d
12. a

Chapter 19

1. b
2. c
3. c
4. a
5. d
6. c
7. c
8. a
9. c
10. c

11. b
12. c

Chapter 20

1. b
2. a
3. e
4. a
5. a
6. d
7. a
8. a
9. e
10. e
11. a
12. e
13. e
14. a
15. e

Chapter 21

1. c
2. d
3. b
4. d
5. a
6. b
7. d
8. c
9. d
10. c

Chapter 22

1. d
2. d
3. b
4. a
5. c
6. d
7. c
8. d
9. d
10. a

Chapter 23

1. c
2. c
3. c
4. b
5. d
6. d
7. d
8. a

9. b
10. d

Chapter 24

1. b
2. c
3. d
4. a
5. c
6. d
7. c
8. b
9. c
10. d

Chapter 25

1. d
2. c
3. c
4. a
5. a
6. c
7. c
8. a
9. b
10. b
11. a
12. c

Chapter 26

1. d
2. c
3. c
4. d
5. d
6. a
7. d
8. b
9. a
10. c

Chapter 27

1. b
2. a
3. b
4. a
5. b
6. a
7. d
8. b
9. c
10. c

Chapter 28

1. b
2. c
3. b
4. a
5. a
6. a
7. b
8. b
9. b
10. d

Chapter 29

1. c
2. d
3. b
4. a
5. b
6. c
7. c
8. c
9. d
10. c

Index

A

A mode; *see* Amplitude mode
AAFCO; *see* American Association of
 Feeding Control Officials
Abdomen
 bandaging, 89
 palpation for pregnancy diagnosis, 26,
  27
 small animal physical examination, 78
Abdominal ballottement, 30
Abducted, defined, 336
Abductor muscle, 6
ABE; *see* Adjusted base excess
ABG; *see* Arterial blood gases
Abomasopexy, 114
Abomasum, 9, 313
 displaced, 107-108
Abortion, 98, 110
Abscess
 dental, 117
 microbiologic culture, 223
 periapical, 124
Absolute count, defined, 247
Absorbed dose, 143
Absorption, 59
Acanthocephala, 213
Acanthocyte, 240, 241, 247
Accounts payable, 371, 378
Accounts receivable, 378
ACE; *see* Angiotensin-converting en-
 zyme
Acepromazine, 61, 177
Acetaminophen, 61
 toxicity, 335
Acetonemia, 107
Achromycin-V; *see* Tetracycline
Acid-base balance, 190-192
Acidemia, 336
Acid-fast stain, 229
Acidic pH, 233
Acidosis, 192, 336
 metabolic, 191
 respiratory, 191
 rumenal, 108
Acoustic impedance, 148, 153
Acoustic shadowing, 151

Acquired immunity, 275-276
Actinobacillosis, 108
Activated charcoal, 65
Active immunity, 276
Active transport, 3
Actual focal spot, 143
Acute renal failure, 334
Adaptive immunity, 272-273
Addisonian crisis, 332
Additive, 325
Adductor muscle, 6
ADH; *see* Antidiuretic hormone
Adipose tissue, 4
Adjusted base excess, 191-192
Administration of drugs, 58-59
 ruminant and swine, 105
 small animal, 78-79
Adrenal cortex, 15
 function tests, 260
Adrenal gland, sonographic appearance,
 152
Adrenal medulla, 15
Adrenalin chloride, 63
Adrenocorticotropic hormone, 15
ADSOL, 81, 83
Adson tissue forceps, 165
Aerobic, defined, 229
Aeromonas, 226
Aerrane; *see* Isoflurane
Afipia felis, 284
Agar, 222, 229
Agglutination, 240, 241
Aggression
 canine, 33, 53-54
 feline, 50
Agouti, 22
Air filtration for microbial control, 157
Airway triage, 327
Alanine aminotransferase, 255-256, 258
Albumin, 254-255, 259
Alcohol
 electrocardiography, 85
 microbial control, 159, 160
Alcohol lamp, 221
Aldehydes, 158-159, 160
Aldosterone, 12

Alkaline pH, 233
Alkaline phosphatase, 256
Alkalosis, 191, 192
Allantois, 14
Allele, 22
Allelomimetic animal, 41
Allergen, 280
Allergy, 276, 330, 351
Allergy shot, 273
Alligator clip, 85
Allis tissue forceps, 165
Alopecia, 91, 348-349
ALP; *see* Alkaline phosphatase
Alpha$_2$-agonists, 61, 178
ALT; *see* Alanine aminotransferase
Altered-self, defined, 268
Alveolar bone, 118, 123
Amcill; *see* Ampicillin
American Association of Feeding
 Control Officials, 304, 308, 309,
 310
Amiglyde-V; *see* Amikacin
Amikacin, 60
Amikin; *see* Amikacin
Amino acids, 295, 320-321
Aminoglycosides, 59, 60
Aminopentamide hydrogen sulfate, 65
Aminophylline, 64
Amnion, 14
Amorphous urates, 237, 238
Amoxicillin, 60
Amoxi-Tabs; *see* Amoxicillin
Amp-Equine; *see* Ampicillin
Amperage, 143
Amphiarthrosis, 6
Amphibian, 224
Amphicol; *see* Chloramphenicol
Amphogel; *see* Antacids
Ampicillin, 60
Amplitude, 148, 150
Amplitude mode, 150, 153
Amputation
 digit, 110
 tail, 90
Amylase, 10, 252, 258
Amyloclastic test, 252, 261

Anaerobic, defined, 229
Anal area, 78
Anal sac
  expression, 87-88
  preoperative hair removal, 172
Analgesia, 61-62, 192
  perioperative, 188
  ruminant and swine, 111-113
Anaphylactic shock, 91, 275, 332, 336
Anaplasma, 110, 242
Anased; *see* Xylazine
Anatomy
  defined, 1, 16
  directional terminology, 4-5
Ancef; *see* Cefazolin sodium
Ancylostoma, 196, 287
Anechoic sonographic image, 151
Anemia
  defined, 192, 247
  equine infectious, 100
  surgery and, 190
Anestatal; *see* Sodium thiamylal
Anesthesia, 176-193
  acid-base balance, 190-192
  analgesia, 188
  blood loss, 190
  breathing circuits, 183-184
  breathing systems, 182-183
  digit amputation, 110
  general, 62
  guinea pig complications, 349
  inhalation, 181
  injectable, 179-181
  monitoring, 186-188
  muscle relaxants, 188
  nitrous oxide, 181-182
  oxygenation problems, 192
  parts of anesthetic machine, 185
  preanesthetic medication, 177-179
  ruminant and swine, 111-114
  stages, 185-186
  vaporizers, 184-185
  ventilation, 188-189
Anestrus, 14
  canine, 26
  cell population identification, 245
Anger, 50
Angiotensin-converting enzyme inhibitor, 63
Anion, 261
Anisocoria, 336
Anisocytosis, 240, 241, 247
Anode, 128, 143
Anodontia, 117, 123
Anomaly, 22
Anoplocephala, 207
Antacids, 64, 65
Anterior, defined, 5
Anterior enteritis, 97
Anthelmintic, 64, 66, 218, 292
Anthrax, 110
Antiarrhythmics, 62-63

Antibiotics, 59-61
  equine gastrointestinal ailments from, 97
  sensitivity
    guinea pig, 348
    hamster, 344
Antibodies, 274-275
Antibody titer, 275
Anticholinergics, 177
Anticoagulant rodenticide toxicity, 335
Anticoagulants
  blood collection, 81, 82, 250
  defined, 261
Anticonvulsants, 61
Antidiarrheals, 64, 65
Antidiuretic hormone, 12, 15, 251
Antiemetics, 64, 65
Antifungals, 60
Antigen, 280
Antigenic drift, 266, 279, 280
Antigen-presenting cell, 272
Antihistamines, 64
Antiprotozoals, 60
Antipruritics, 64
Antipyretics, 61
Antirobe; *see* Clindamycin
Antiseptic, 162
Antiserum, 280
Antispasmodics, 65
Antitussives, 63, 64
Antiulcers, 64, 65
Anuria, 91, 232, 247, 336
Aortic arch, 8
Apex, defined, 123
API 20E test, 228-229
Apical, defined, 123
Apnea, 12, 16, 192, 336
Apomorphine, 65
Appearance; *see* General appearance
Appendicular skeleton, 5
Approach
  bovine, 40
  equine, 37
Apteriae, 363
Aptitude testing for puppy selection, 51
Aqueous humor, 15
Arachidonic acid, 295
Arachnoid, 7
Arboviral encephalitis, 286
Area in metric system, 71
Areolar connective tissue, 4
Argasid, 201
Arkansas stone, 120
Arrhythmia
  anesthesia monitoring, 187
  defined, 192
  sinus, 86
Arterial blood gases
  anesthesia monitoring, 187
  normal values, 192
Arteriole, 8
Artery, 8

Arthropod, 207, 218
Arthroscopy, 102
Articular cartilage, 5
Articulation, 6, 16
Artifacts
  radiographic, 137, 139, 143
  sonographic, 151-152
Artificial immunity, 275
Ascarid, 196, 204, 212, 215, 217
Ascorbic acid, 300, 322
Asepsis, defined, 174
Aseptic, defined, 91
Aseptic technique, 229
  operating room, 173-174
  patient preparation, 171-172
  surgical scrub, 172-173
Aspartate aminotransferase, 256, 258
Aspergillus, 227, 358
Aspicularis teraptera, 214
Aspirate, defined, 91
Aspiration
  general anesthesia, 113
  for specimen collection, 244-245
Aspirin, 61, 62
AST; *see* Aspartate aminotransferase
Asthma, 330
Asymptomatic, defined, 102
Asystole, 87
Ataxia, 91, 336
Atelectasis, 11
Atgard; *see* Organophosphate
Ativan; *see* Lorazepam
Atrial fibrillation, 86-87
Atrial flutter, 86
Atrial premature contraction, 87
Atrioventricular block, 87
Atrium, 8
Atropine, 177
Attached gingiva, 123
Attack signals, 36
Attenuated-live vaccine, 277-278
Attenuation in ultrasonography, 148, 151
Auditory, defined, 55
Auscultation, 8, 78, 91, 336
Autoclave, 160-162, 268
Autoimmune reaction, 277, 280
Autonomic nervous system, 6
Autosomal gene, 20, 22
Aversive, defined, 55
Avian medicine, 353-359
  blood specimen, 224
  chlamydiosis, 291
  common viral disease, 268
Axenic, defined, 351
Axial skeleton, 5
Azaparone, 114
Azotemia, 261, 336

B

B cell, 273
B mode; *see* Brightness mode
Babcock tissue forceps, 165

Babesia, 81, 242
Bacillary hemoglobinuria, 109
Bacillus, 110, 227, 283, 341
Bacitracin, 96
Back cross, 21, 22
Backhaus towel clamps, 165, 166
Bacterial infection
   antibiotics and, 59
   avian, 357-358
   diagnostic microbiology, 222-223,
      225-227
   pneumonia in guinea pig, 348
   reptilian, 362
   zoonosis, 283-285
Bacteriostat, 162
Bacteroides nodosus, 110
Baermann technique, 218
Bain system, 183-184
Balfour retractor, 167
Balling gun, 44, 105
Ballottement, 30
Banamine; *see* Flunixin meglumine
Bandaging, 88-90
Bang's disease, 283
Barbering, 351
Barbiturates, 62, 179
Bard-Parker scalpel handle, 169
Bark, 49
Barrier sustained, 351
Bartonella henselae, 284
Basalgel; *see* Antacids
Basophil, 243-244
Basophilia, 247
Basophilic stippling, 240, 247
Battering ram, 41, 42
Baymix; *see* Organophosphate
Baytril; *see* Enrofloxacin
Beef cattle
   nutrition, 312-318
   restraint and handling, 40
Behavior
   companion animal
      abnormal, 55
      normal, 48-50
      problems, 51-55
   emergency patient monitoring, 329
   laboratory animal
      gerbil, 344
      guinea pig, 347
      hamster, 342-343
      mice, 339
      rabbit, 345-346
      rat, 341
   restraint and handling
      bovine, 40
      canine, 33
      caprine, 42
      equine, 36-37
      feline, 35
      ovine, 40
      porcine, 43
Behavior modification technique, 52

Benadryl; *see* Diphenhydramine
Benzimidazoles, 66
Benzodiazepines, 177
Beta blockers, 63
BFD; *see* Budgie fledging disease
Bicarbonate radical, 191-192
Biguanide, 159
Bile, 261
Bile acids, 257
Bile esculin, 228
Bile esculin agar, 222-223
Bile pigment, 234
Bilirubin, 234, 253-254, 258
Bilirubinuria, 234, 247
Binding energy, 143
Biological indicator for sterilization qual-
   ity control, 162, 171
Biologicals, 67-68
Biomox; *see* Amoxicillin
Biosol; *see* Neomycin
Bio-Tal; *see* Thiamylal
Biotin, 300, 322
Bird; *see* Avian medicine
Birth; *see* Parturition
Birth canal, 13
Bisecting angle technique for dental
   radiography, 123
Bismuth subsalicylate, 65
Bite
   bovine, 40
   equine, 36
   level, 117
   normal, 116
Biting lice, 200, 217
Blackleg, 109
Bladder
   rupture, 334
   sonographic appearance, 152
Blastomyces dermatiditis, 228
Blindfold, 38
Blink in anesthesia monitoring, 186
Bloat, 108, 113
Block, atrioventricular, 87
Blood
   anatomy and physiology, 4
      avian, 355
      components, 249-250
      reptile, 360
   clinical chemistry, 249-262
      electrolytes and minerals, 257-258
      kidney function, 250-251
      liver function, 253-257
      pancreatic function, 251-253
   equine disorders, 100
   parasites, 195-203, 242
   specimen collection, 224
      avian, 356
      mice, 339
      reptile, 361
      sample handling, 250
      small animal, 81-84
   in urine, 234

Blood agar plate, 222
Blood component therapy, 83
Blood gas level
   anesthesia monitoring, 187
   normal values, 192
Blood pressure, 187
Blood transfusion, 83-84, 190
Blood vessel, 8
Blood-brain barrier, 7
   drug invasion and, 59
Bloodworm, 204
Bluetongue, 110
Boar; *see* Swine
Body condition scoring, 302, 303
Body fluid, abnormal loss of, 79
Body temperature
   avian, 356
   monitoring
      anesthesia, 187-188
      emergency, 329
   neonatal
      bovine, 28
      canine, 27
      caprine, 29
      equine, 27
      feline, 26
      ovine, 29
      porcine, 30
   parturition, 26, 27, 29
Boiling for microbial control, 157
Bone, 4, 5-6
Borborygmus, 102, 336
Bordatella, 226
Boron, 298
Borrelia bergdorferi, 81, 290
Bovine; *see* Cattle
Bovine respiratory disease complex, 109
Bovine respiratory syncytial virus, 109
Bovine viral diarrhea, 109
Bowel
   anatomy and physiology, 10
   sonographic appearance, 152
Bowie Dick test, 162
Bowman's capsule, 12
Brachycephalic, defined, 192
Brachycephalic dog, 35
Brachycephalic occlusive syndrome, 330
Brachygnathism, 117, 123
Bradycardia, 86, 187, 192
Bradykinin, 272
Brain, 7
Brain stem, 7
Brain-heart infusion broth, 222
Breathing; *see* Respiration
Breathing circuits during anesthesia,
   183-184
Breathing systems during anesthesia,
   182-183
Breeding
   bovine, 27-28
   canine, 26-27
   caprine, 28-29

Breeding—cont'd
  equine, 27
  feline, 25-26
  genetics in, 21-22
  gerbil, 345
  guinea pig, 347-348
  hamster, 343
  mice, 339
  nutritional requirements, 317, 320
  ovine, 29
  porcine, 29-30
  rabbit, 346
  random, 21
  rat, 341-342
Brethine; *see* Terbutaline sulfate
Brevital; *see* Methohexital
Bricanyl; *see* Terbutaline sulfate
Brightness mode, 150
Bronchi, 11
Bronchiole, 11
Bronchodilators, 63, 64
Broth, 222, 229
Brown-Adson tissue forceps, 165, 166
Bruce effect, 351
Brucellosis, 110, 283
BSRV; *see* Bovine respiratory syncytial
    virus
Buccal, defined, 123
Buck jar, 28
Budgie fledging disease, 358
Buffy coat, 203, 244, 247
Bull; *see* Cattle
Bundle of His, 84
Bunostomum, 209
Bunsen burner, 221
Burnout, 373
Burr cell, 241
Business management, 370-371
Butorphanol, 61, 64, 178
Butting, 39-40
BVD; *see* Bovine viral diarrhea

C

Caging
  avian, 355-356
  laboratory animal, 349
Calcification, soft tissue, 348
Calcitonin, 15
Calcium
  nutritional requirements
    bovine, 314
    caprine and ovine, 318-319
    equine, 323
    porcine, 321
    small animal, 298, 302-303
  serum, 258, 259
  milk fever, 107
Calcium borogluconate, 107
Calcium channel blockers, 63
Calcium oxalate, 237, 238
Calcium tungstate phosphor, 130
Calculus, defined, 123

Calf
  castration and dehorning, 111
  restraint, 41
California Mastitis Test, 106-107
Caliper, 143
Calving, 107-108
Campylobacter
  microbiology identification, 225, 226
  vibriosis, 110
  zoonosis, 283, 350
Campylobacter agar, 222
Campylobacter thioglycollate medium,
    222
Canaliculi, 5
Cancellous bone, 5
Candida, 227-228, 358
Canine; *see* Dog
Canine tooth, 94, 119, 122, 123
Cannibalism, 343
Canthi, 16
Capillary, 8
Capillary refill time
  anesthesia monitoring, 187
  defined, 91
  small animal physical examination,
    77-78
  triage, 327
Caprine; *see* Goat
Capsid, 264, 280
Capsule administration, 78-79
Capture
  caprine, 42-43
  equine, 37
  ovine, 42
Capture pole, 34
Carafate; *see* Sucralfate
Carapace, 363
Carbohydrates, 295, 310, 322-323
Carbon dioxide
  rebreathing systems during anesthesia,
    182-183
  respiration, 11
  respiratory acidosis and alkalosis, 191
Carbon dioxide absorber of anesthetic
    machine, 185
Carbon dioxide partial pressure, 192
Carborundum stone, 121
Carcinoma, oral, 117
Cardiac arrest, 87
Cardiac cycle, 8
Cardiac muscle, 4, 6
Cardiac tamponade, 336
Cardiogenic shock, 332
Cardiopulmonary resuscitation, 331-333
Cardiovascular system
  anatomy and physiology, 7-8
    avian, 355
    reptilian, 360
  drug therapy, 62-63
  emergencies of, 329, 330-331
  monitoring
    anesthesia, 187
    emergency patient, 328

Cardiovascular system—cont'd
  small animal physical examination, 78
  triage, 327
Cardoxin; *see* Digoxin
Career development, 378
Career management, 373-375
Caries, 118, 123
Carmilax; *see* Laxatives
Carnassial tooth, 120, 123
Carnitine, 300
Carnivore, 9, 16
Carparsolate; *see* Thiacetarsemide
    sodium
Cartilage, 4, 5
Cassette, radiographic, 130
Casting, 44, 90
Castration
  behavior intervention, 52
  bovine, 111
  preoperative hair removal, 171-172
  restraint techniques, 42, 43
Casts, urinary, 236-237
Cat, 76-93
  accessory sex glands, 12
  anal sac expression, 87-88
  asthma, 330
  bandaging, 88-90
  behavior
    characteristics, 35
    hostility, 35
    normal, 49-50
    problems, 51-52, 54-55
  blood collection and transfusion, 82-
    84
  breeding, reproduction, and neonatal
    care, 25-26
  dentition, 119
  drug administration, 78-79
  electrocardiography, 84-87
  enemas, 88
  fluid therapy, 79-81
  gestational period, 14
  heart rate, 8
  lower urinary tract disease, 306
  nutrition; *see* Nutrition
  parasites of, 196-202
  penis, 13
  pet selection, 51
  physical examination, 77-78
  preoperative hair removal, 171, 172
  respiratory rate, 11
  restraint and handling, 35-36
  sinus bradycardia, 86
  sinus tachycardia, 86
  skeletal system, 6
  tortoiseshell, 20-21
  ultrasonography, 152
  urethral obstruction, 334
  urine specific gravity, 233
  viral disease, 268
  X-linked heredity, 20-21
Cat bag, 36
Cat scratch disease, 284

Catalase test, 228
Catalepsy, 192
Catecholamine, 63
Cathartic, 336
Catheterization, 232, 336
Cathode, 127-128, 144
Cation, 261
Cattle
  anesthesia, 111-112, 113
  behavioral characteristics, 40
  breeding, reproduction, and neonatal
    care, 27
  dentition, 119
  diseases of, 107-109
    preventable, 109-110
  drug administration and sample
    collection, 105, 106
  gestational period, 14
  milk sampling, 106-107
  nutrition, 312-318
  parasites in, 208-211
  penis, 13
  physical examination, 104-105
  restraint and handling, 39-41
  surgical procedures, 110-111
  urine specific gravity, 233
  venipuncture, 105-106
  viral disease, 268
Caudal
  defined, 4
  radiographic terminology, 142
Caudal auricular venipuncture, 106
Caudal spine, 6
Caudocranial, radiographic terminology,
    144
Caveman pet, 36, 39, 44
Cecum, 10
Cefazolin sodium, 60
Cell
  ionizing radiation damage, 140-141
  microscopic examination, 244-247
  movement in and out, 3
  structure and physiology, 2-3
Cell membrane, 2
Cellophane tape method for parasite
    identification, 218
Cells of Leydig, 12
Cellular phone, 369
Cementoenamel junction, 118, 123
Cementum, 118, 123
Central Haversian canal, 5
Central nervous system
  anatomy and physiology, 6, 7
  emergencies of, 329-330, 334
  triage, 327
Central vascular system, 8-9
Centrine; *see* Aminopentamide hydrogen
    sulfate
Cephalosporin, 60
Ceramic stone, 121
Cere, 363
Cerebellum, 7
Cerebrospinal fluid, 7

Cerebrum, 7
Cervical line lesion, 117
Cervical spine
  enzootic lymphadenitis, 348
  formula for designation, 6
Cervix, 13
Cestex; *see* Epsiprantel
Cestode
  bovine and ovine, 210
  canine and feline, 197-198
  defined, 218
  equine, 207
  porcine, 213
  rabbit, 216
CF; *see* Complement fixation
Chain shank, 39
Chain twitch, 38
Charcoal, activated, 65
Check valve of anesthetic machine, 185
Cheek pouch impaction, 344
Chelonian; *see* Reptile
Chemical indicator for sterilization qual-
    ity control, 162, 171
Chemicals for microbial control, 157-160
Chemotaxis, 280
Chest lead, 85
Cheyletiella, 202, 217
Chirodiscoides caviae, 217
Chlamydiosis, 291, 357
Chloral hydrate, 113
Chloramphenicol, 59, 60
Chloride
  metabolic alkalosis, 192
  serum, 257-258, 259
  small animal nutrition, 299
Chlorine
  for microbial control, 159
  nutritional requirements, 314
Chlorpromazine, 177
Chocolate toxicosis, 335
Choker collar, 34
Cholera, 357
Cholesterol, 257, 259
Choline, 300, 321-322
Chorion, 14
Chorioptes, 202, 218
Choroid, 15
Chromium, 298
Chromodacryorrhea, 342
Chromosome, 22
Chronological resume, 378
Chute, 40
Chylothorax, 336
Chyme, 10
Chymotrypsin, 10
Cide, 162
Cidex; *see* Glutaraldehyde
Cimetidine, 65
Circle system, 183
Circulation
  cardiopulmonary resuscitation, 332
  coronary, 8, 16
  fetal, 8-9

Circulation—cont'd
  pulmonary, 7-8
  systemic, 8
CITE Heartworm Test Kit, 203
Clavamox; *see* Potentiated amoxicillin
Clawing, 50
Clean catch urine collection, 231
Client communication, 367-368
Clindamycin, 60
Clostridial infection, 96, 97, 109, 110
Clotting factor, 83
CMT; *see* California Mastitis Test
CNS; *see* Central nervous system
Coagulopathy, 336
Cobalamin, 300
Cobalt, 315, 318-319, 321
Coccidia
  bovine and ovine, 210
  canine and feline, 199
  equine, 207
  guinea pig, 217
  porcine, 213
  rabbit, 215, 347
Coccidioides immitis, 228
Coccobacilli, 226
Cochlea, 16
Codeine, 61
Codeine phosphate, 64
Codominance, 19, 22
Coffin bone, 100
Coggins test, 100
Colace; *see* Dioctyl sodium sulfosuc-
    cinate
Colibacillosis, 110
Colic, 95
Colitis, 95-96
Colitis X, 96
Collagenous connective tissue, 4
Collar, 34
Collection policy, 371
Collimation, radiographic, 130
Colloid, 81, 91, 336
Colon, 10
Colostrum, 30, 275, 280, 299
Columbia colistin-nalidixic acid agar,
    222
Columnar epithelia, 4
Coma, 336
Comet tail, 152
Comfort zone, 366
Commensal, defined, 280
Communication, 365-369, 378
  canine, 49
  client, 367-368
  co-worker, 368-369
  electronic, 369
  feline, 49-50, 51
  listening, 367
  nonverbal, 366-367
  verbal, 366
  written, 369
Community involvement, 375
Compact bone, 5

Companion animal behavior, 48-56
  abnormal, 55
  normal, 48-50
  problems, 51-55
Complement, 280
Complement fixation, 292
Complete blood count, 237
Computer, 369
Concentration of solution, 72-73
Conditioning for behavior modification, 52
Conflict, defined, 378
Conflict resolution, 368-369, 373, 377
Congenic strain of mice, 339
Congenital, defined, 280
Congestive heart failure, 332
Conjunctiva, 15, 16, 91
Connective tissue, 4
Conspecifics, 55
Consumer Packaging and Labeling Act and Regulations, 308
Contact ulcer, 117
Contagious ecthyma, 110
Continuous wave transducer, 148
Contrast
  radiographic, 135-137, 143, 144
  sonographic, 149
Controlled drug, 58
Contusion, respiratory, 331
Cooperia, 208
Coping with burnout, 373
Copper, 298, 314-315, 318-319, 321, 323
CornBot; *see* Organophosphate
Cornea, 15, 16
Corneal reflex, 186
Cornell block, 112
Cornual nerve block, 112
Coronal, defined, 123
Coronary circulation, 8, 16
Corpus luteum, 13-14, 30
Corrective mixture; *see* Bismuth subsalicylate
Corticosteroids, 62
Corynebacterium, 227
Coryza, 357
Cotton suture, 170
Cotyledonary placentation, 30
Cough, 63
Cough suppressant analgesic, 64
Counseling
  defined, 378
  grief, 367-368
Counter conditioning in behavior modification, 52
Coupage, 336
Cover hair, 15
Cover letter, 373
Cow; *see* Cattle
Co-worker communication, 368-369
CPE; *see* Cytopathic effects
CPR; *see* Cardiopulmonary resuscitation
Cradle, 39, 44

Cranial
  defined, 4
  radiographic terminology, 142
Cranial vena cava, 106
Crash cart, 333
Creatinine, 250, 259
Credit policy, 371
Crenation, 241, 247
Crepuscular, defined, 351
Crevicular fluid, 119, 123
Crile forceps, 165
Critical care nutrition, 307-308
Cross tying, 38, 44
Crossbite, 117
Crown of tooth, 123
CRT; *see* Capillary refill time
Cryptococcus, 228
Crystalloid, 81, 189, 336
Crystals
  sonographic, 148-149
  urinary, 237
CSF; *see* Cerebrospinal fluid
Ctenocephalides canis, 200
Ctenocephalides felis, 200
Cuboidal epithelia, 4
Culture
  defined, 229
  microbiologic, 223-225
Curet scaler, 120
Curettage, subgingival, 124
Cusp, 123
Cyanosis, 336
Cyathostomes, 205
Cyclohexamine, 178
Cystine crystals, 237, 238
Cystocentesis, 231-232
Cystography, 336
Cytauxzoon felis, 242
Cytokines, 279-280
Cytology, 244-247
Cytopathic effects, 267
Cytoplasm, 2
Cytoskeleton, 3
Cytotoxic T cell, 273, 274

D

Dairy cattle
  displaced abomasum, 107-108
  milk sampling, 106-107
  nutrition, 312-318
  restraint and handling, 40
Darbazine; *see* Prochlorperazine isopropamide
Darkroom techniques, 133-134
Date in metric system, 71
DCT; *see* Distal convoluted tubule
DEA; *see* Drug Enforcement Administration
Dead space, 11, 16
Deafness, 16
DEC; *see* Diethylcarbamazine

Deciduous tooth, 119
  defined, 123
  dental interlock, 117
  numbering, 120
  retained, 117
Decision making, 372
Declawing, 172
Degranulation, 280
Dehorning, 43, 111, 112
Dehydration, 79-80
Delayed lethal gene, 22
Delegation, 370
Deletion in genetics, 22
Demerol; *see* Meperidine
Demodex, 201, 218
Dense bone, 5
Density, radiographic, 135, 136
Dental formula and care, equine, 94-95
Dental problems, 117-118
  gum disease, 121-122
  interlock, 117
  malocclusions, 116-117
  oral lesions, 117
Dental procedures
  instruments, 120-121
  prophy, 121
  radiography, 122-123
  restraint, 38
  safety, 121
Dental quadrant, 123
Dentin, 118, 123
Dentition, 119
Deoxyribonucleic acid, 3, 268
  antibiotics and, 61
  ionizing radiation damage, 140
  vaccine, 279
  viral, 265
Depolarization, 84
Depression, 35
Depressor muscle, 6
Dermatophyte test media, 223
Dermatophytes, 227, 289
Dermis, 14
Desensitization in behavior modification, 52
Detail, radiographic, 144
Detergent for microbial control, 158
Detomidine, 61, 178
Developer in film processing, 134
Dexamethazone, 62
Dextrose, 223
Diabetic ketoacidosis, 332
Diagnostic microbiology; *see* Microbiology
Diapedesis, 280
Diaphragm
  respiration, 11
  rupture, 331
Diaphysis, 5
Diarrhea
  antibiotic and nonsteroidal antiinflammatory drug therapy, 97

Diarrhea—cont'd
  bovine viral, 109
  infant mice, 341
  neonatal in farm animals, 108-109
Diarthrosis, 6
Diastole, 8
Diastolic blood pressure, 187
Diazepam, 61, 177
Dictyocaulus amfeldi, 206
Dictyocaulus viviparus, 209
Diencephalon, 7
Diestrus, 14
Diethylcarbamazine, 66
Differential media, 221, 222, 229
Diffuse placenta, 30
Diffusion, cellular, 3
Di-Fil, 203
Difil Tabs; *see* Diethylcarbamazine
Digestible energy, 325
Digestive system
  anatomy and physiology, 9-10
    avian, 354
    reptilian, 359
    ruminant, 312-318
  function tests, 260
Digit amputation, 110
Digoxin, 63
Dihybrid cross, 19-20, 22
Dilution calculations, 72-73
Dioctophyma renale, 196
Dioctyl sodium sulfosuccinate, 65
Dipetalonema reconditum, 195-203
Diphenhydramine, 64
Diploid, 22
Diprivan; *see* Propofol
Dipylidium caninum, 197
Direct parasitic smear, 195
Directional terminology in anatomy and
    physiology, 4-5
Dirocheck, 203
Dirocide; *see* Diethylcarbamazine
Dirofilaria immitis, 195-203, 242
Disabled infectious single-cycle virus,
    279
Disal; *see* Furosemide
Disbudding, 44
DISC; *see* Disabled infectious single-
    cycle virus
Disinfection, 155-163
Displaced abomasum, 107-108
Disposaject; *see* Dioctyl sodium
    sulfosuccinate
Distal, defined, 5, 123
Distal convoluted tubule, 12
Distension, defined, 91
Distraction techniques, 36, 38-39, 40-41
Di-trim; *see* Potentiated sulfa
Diuretics, 63, 336
Diuride; *see* Furosemide
DNA; *see* Deoxyribonucleic acid
Dobutamine, 63
Dobutrex; *see* Dobutamine

Docking, 42
Docusate sodium, 65
Dog
  accessory sex glands, 12
  anal sac expression, 87-88
  bandaging, 88-90
  behavior
    characteristics, 33
    normal, 48-49
    problems, 51-54
    vicious or aggressive, 33, 34
  blood collection and transfusion, 81-
    82, 83-84
  breeding, reproduction, and neonatal
    care, 26-27
  dentition, 119
  drug administration, 78-79
  electrocardiography, 84-87
  enemas, 88
  fluid therapy, 79-81
  gestational period, 14
  heart rate, 8
  nutritional requirements, 299-305
  parasites of, 196-202
  penis, 13
  pet selection, 51
  physical examination, 77-78
  preoperative hair removal, 171
  respiratory rate, 11
  restraint and handling, 33-35
  sinus bradycardia, 86
  sinus tachycardia, 86
  skeletal system, 6
  ultrasonography, 152
  urine specific gravity, 233
  viral disease, 268
Dominant gene, 20, 22
Domitor; *see* Medetomidine
Donor, blood, 81, 82
Doppler, defined, 336
Dormosedan; *see* Detomidine
Dorsal
  defined, 4
  radiographic terminology, 142
Dorsal recumbency, 101
Dorsopalmer, radiographic terminology,
    144
Dorsoplantar, radiographic terminology,
    144
Dorsoventral, radiographic terminology,
    144
Dosage calculation, 72
Dosimeter, 144
Downey position, 85
Drape, packing of, 170-171
Draschia megastoma, 206
Drench, 105
Dress, 376
Dressing forceps, 165
Drip rates, 73
Droncit; *see* Praziquantel
Droperidol, 61, 114

Drug Enforcement Administration, 58,
    81
Drugs
  administration, 58-59
    ruminant and swine, 105
    small animal, 78-79
  anthelmintics, 64, 66
  antibiotics, 59-61
  basic terminology, 58
  behavior intervention, 52
  cardiopulmonary resuscitation,
    332-333
  cardiovascular, 62-63
  defined, 57
  euthanizing agents, 68
  gastrointestinal, 64, 65
  general anesthetics, 62
  hormones and endocrine, 64-67
  oncological agents, 68
  pharmacokinetics, 58-59
  respiratory, 63-64
  topical, 68
  vaccines, 67-68
Dry animal, 44
Dry chemistry, 261
Dry heat for microbial control, 156-157
Dry matter basis, 309
Dry weight analysis, 309
Dry weight intake, 325
Drying for microbial control, 157
Duck plague, 358
Ductus deferens, 12
Duodenum, 10
Duplication in genetics, 22
Dura mater, 7
Dursban products; *see* Organophosphate
Dwarf tapeworm, 214-215
Dyrex; *see* Organophosphate
Dysecdysis, 363
Dysentery, 110
Dyspnea, 12, 116, 327, 336
Dystocia, 14, 16, 335
Dystrophy, muscular, 348
Dysuria, 336

E

EAE; *see* Enzootic abortion in ewes
Ear
  anatomy, 16
  as behavior indicator, 37
  small animal physical examination, 77
Ear mite, 202, 347
Earth phosphor, 130
Eastern equine encephalomyelitides, 99,
    286
Ecchymosis, 336
Ecdysis, 363
ECG; *see* Electrocardiography
Echinococcus granulosus, 197
Echinocyte, 240, 241
Echoic sonographic image, 150, 153
Eclampsia, 335

Ecthyma, contagious, 110
Ectoparasite
    avian, 358
    bovine and ovine, 211
    canine and feline, 200-202
    reptilian, 362
Edema
    defined, 91, 336
    malignant, 109
    pulmonary, 331
EDIM; *see* Epizootic diarrhea of infant mice
EDTA; *see* Ethylenediaminetetraacetic acid
Education, 376
EEE; *see* Eastern equine encephalomyelitides
EFA; *see* Essential fatty acids
Effective focal spot, 144
Efficacy, defined, 218
Effusion, defined, 336
Ehrlichia
    blood collection, 81
    leukocyte evaluation, 244
    Potomac horse fever, 96
    zoonosis, 291
EHV; *see* Equine herpes virus
EIA; *see* Equine infectious anemia
Eimeria, 207, 210, 213, 216, 217
Ejaculation, 13
EKG; *see* Electrocardiography
Elastase, 10
Electrical circuit for x-ray tube control, 129
Electrical current in metric system, 71
Electrocardiography, 8, 84-87
Electrolytes, 257-258, 260, 261
Electromagnetic radiation, 127, 144
Electron, 144
Electron beam, 144
Electronic communication, 369
Electrophoresis, 261
Elevators, 169
Elimination problems, feline, 54-55
E-mail, 369
Emasculatome, 111
Emergency
    cardiopulmonary resuscitation, 331-333
    cardiovascular, 329, 332
    central nervous system, 329-330, 334
    endocrine, 329, 332
    gastrointestinal, 329, 332
    patient monitoring, 328-329
    renal, 330, 334
    respiratory, 329, 330-331
    toxic substance, 331, 335
    triage, 327-328
Emetics, 64, 65
EMP; *see* Equine protozoal myeloencephalitis
Enacard; *see* Enalapril maleate
Enalapril maleate, 63

Enamel, 118, 123
Enamel hypoplasia, 117
Encephalitis, 336
Encephalomyelitides, 99, 286
Endocardium, 7
Endochondral bone, 5
Endocrine system
    anatomy and physiology, 4, 14, 15, 16
    drug therapy, 64-67
    emergencies, 329, 332
    function tests, 251, 260
    influence on excretory system, 12
Endocytosis, 3
Endometrium, 13
Endoparasite, 358-359, 363
Endoplasmic reticulum, 2
Endosteum, 5
Endotracheal tube, 113
Enema, 88
Energy
    binding, 143
    bovine requirements, 316
    caprine and ovine requirements, 318
    cell movement, 3
    digestible, 325
    nutrients producing, 295-296
    porcine requirements, 320
    small animal requirements, 299, 302
        during illness, 308
Enhancement, sonographic, 151
Enrofloxacin, 60
Enrofloxin, 61
Ensiling, 325
Enteral bacteria, 229
Enteral nutrition, 307-308
Enteric disease, 110
Enteritis, 97, 286, 357, 358
Enterococci, 225
Enterotoxemia, 109
Enucleation, 110-111, 114
Environmental factors
    behavior intervention, 52
    nutrition, 312, 320
Enzootic abortion in ewes, 110
Enzootic cervical lymphadenitis, 348
Enzyme-linked immunosorbent assay, 203, 267
Enzymes, 10, 255
EO; *see* Ethylene oxide
Eosinopenia, 247
Eosinophil, 243, 246
Eosinophilia, 247
Eosinophilic ulcer, 117
Epidemiology, 292
Epidermis, 14
Epididymis, 12
Epidural block, 112
Epidural space, 7
Epiglottis, 11
Epilepsy, 334
Epinephrine, 15, 63
Epiphyseal cartilage, 5
Epiphyses, 5

Epistasis, 19-20, 22
Epistaxis, 336
Epithelia, 4
Epithelial casts, 237
Epithelial cells in urine, 235, 236
Epizootic diarrhea of infant mice, 341
Epsiprantel, 66
Epulis, 117, 123
Equigard; *see* Organophosphate
Equine; *see* Horse
Equine encephalomyelitides, 99
Equine herpes virus, 98-99
Equine infectious anemia, 100
Equine protozoal myeloencephalitis, 98
Equipment
    dental radiographical, 122
    diagnostic microbiology, 221-222
    restraint, 34-35, 36
Eqvalan Liquid; *see* Ivermectin
Erection, 13
Erosion, dental, 123
Erysipilas, 110
Erythema, 280
Erythro-100; *see* Erythromycin
Erythro-200; *see* Erythromycin
Erythrocyte; *see* Red blood cell
Erythromycin, 60
Erythrophagocytosis, 247
Erythropoiesis, 247
Escherichia coli, 110
Esophagus, 9
Essential amino acids, 295, 310
Essential fatty acids, 295-296
Estrogen, 13, 15, 64
Estrous cycle, 13, 16
    bovine, 28
    canine, 26
    caprine, 28
    cell population identification, 245
    equine, 27
    feline, 26
    ovine, 29
    porcine, 30
    progestins for regulation, 64
Estrus
    cell population identification, 245
    signs of, 26, 27, 28, 29, 30
Ethics, 376, 378
Ethylene glycol toxicity, 335
Ethylene oxide, 159-160
Ethylenediaminetetraacetic acid, 250
Eukaryote, 2-3
Eupnea, 12, 16
Eustachian tube, 11
Eustress, 378
Euthanasia, 68, 100
Euthansol; *see* Pentobarbital
Euthanyl; *see* Pentobarbital
Ewe; *see* Sheep
Examination; *see* Physical examination
Excitement, house soiling and, 533
Excretory system; *see* Renal system
Exfoliative cytology, 246, 247

Exhaust valve, 185
Exocrine function, 251
Exocrine gland, 4, 16
Exocytosis, 3
Expectorant, 63, 64
Expiration, 11
Expiratory reserve volume, 11
Explorer, 120
Expression library immunization, 279
Extensor muscle, 6
External respiration, 11
Extinction in behavior modification, 52
Extirpation, 114
Extracellular, defined, 3, 16, 91
Extra-label usage, 58
Exudate, 247
Eye
    anatomy, 15
    enucleation, 110-111
    equine surgery, 101
    monitoring
        anesthesia, 113, 186
        emergency, 329
    physical examination
        bovine, 41
        small animal, 77
    reptilian, 359
Eyelid press, 39

F

Facial expression
    canine, 53
    feline, 50
Facilitative diffusion, 3
Family generation, 22
Far side of horse, 44
Farrowing, 45
Farrowing crate, 43
Fasciculation, 102, 336
Fasciola hepatica, 210
Fat, dietary, 295-296
Fat-soluble vitamins, 296, 300
Fatty acids, 295-296
Fatty casts, 237
Fear, 50, 53
Fecalyzer, 195
Feces
    culture and examination, 224-225
        pancreatic function, 252
        parasitic, 194-195
    equine postoperative care, 102
    feline scent marking, 50
    specimen collection in mice, 339
Feed
    bovine, 316
    caprine and ovine, 319
    equine, 322
    nutrient content, 324
    porcine, 322
Feedback in communication, 366
Feeding; *see* Nutrition
Feedlot, 325
Feline; *see* Cat

Feline leukemia virus, 267
Feline lower urinary tract disease, 306
Feline urethral obstruction, 334
FeLV; *see* Feline leukemia virus
Female reproductive system, 13-14
    avian, 355
Fenbendazole, 66
Fentanyl, 61, 114
Fermentation vat, 9
Fertilization, 14
Fetal circulation, 8-9
Fetal membranes, 14
FFD; *see* Focal-film distance
Fiber, dietary, 295
Fiberglass cast, 90
Fibrillation, 86-87
Fibrinogen, 255
Fibrosarcoma, 117
Filament, x-ray, 144
Filarassay F Heartworm Diagnostic Kit,
    203
Filaribits; *see* Diethylcarbamazine
Filing of radiographic film, 133
Film, radiographic, 132-133, 134, 144
Filtration, 3
    microbial control, 157
    radiographic, 129-130
Finance, personal, 373
Fine needle aspiration, 244
Finochetto retractor, 167
First aid; *see* Emergency
First pass effect, term, 59
First-degree atrioventricular block, 87
Fish, 224
Fistula
    defined, 174
    oronasal, 117, 124
Fixer in film processing, 134
Flagyl; *see* Metronidazole
Flank restraint, 41, 43
Flat bone, 5
Fleas, 200
Flexor muscle, 6
Flight-or-fight response, 378
Floating tooth, 95
Flotation technique in parasitology, 195
Flowmeter, 185
FLU; *see* Influenza
Fluid aspiration, 244
Fluid balance, normal, 79
Fluid filtration for microbial control, 157
Fluid therapy
    before anesthesia, 189-190
    equine salmonellosis, 96
    small animal, 79-81
Fluke, 198
Flu-like symptoms, 292
Flunixin meglumine, 61, 62
Fluorescent antibody test, 267
Fluoride application, 121
Fluothane; *see* Halothane
FLUTD; *see* Feline lower urinary tract
    disease

Flutter, atrial, 86
Focal-film distance, 138
Focusing, sonographic, 149-150
Focusing cup, 128
Fogging, radiographic, 133-134, 144
Folic acid, 300, 322
Follicle-stimulating hormone, 13, 15
Food and Drug Administration, 308
Food animal medicine, 58, 317-318
Food in digestive process, 10
Foot
    bovine
        danger potential, 40
        restraint for examination, 41
    equine
        ailments, 100-101
        kicking potential, 36
        picking up, 39
Foot rot, 110
Forages, 316, 322, 325
Forane; *see* Isoflurane
Forceps, 165-167
Foreign body aspiration, 330
Formaldehyde, 159
Formicide; *see* Formaldehyde
Fort Bragg fever, 289
Four point block, 112
Fracture, 102
Francisella tularensis, 285
Frazier-Ferguson tip, 169
Free flow urine collection, 231
Free gingiva, 123
Free gingival margin, 123
Freer elevator, 169
Frequency, sonographic, 148, 153
Fresh frozen plasma, 83
Fresh whole blood, 83
Frick's speculum, 41, 105
Frothy bloat, 108
FSH; *see* Follicle-stimulating hormone
Fulvicin-U/F; *see* Griseofulvin
Functional resume, 378
Fungal infection, 222-223, 225, 227-228
Fur mite, 217
Furcation, 123
Furniture scratching, 55
Furosemide, 63

G

GA; *see* Guaranteed analysis
Gait
    defined, 91
    small animal physical examination, 78
Gallbladder
    anatomy and physiology, 10
    sonographic appearance, 152
Gamma glutamyltransferase, 256
Gamma radiation, 157
Garacin; *see* Gentamicin
Garasol; *see* Gentamicin
Gas bloat, 108
Gasterophilus, 207
Gastric gavage, 339, 342

Gastroenteritis, 110
Gastrointestinal system
    drug therapy, 64, 65
    emergencies, 329, 332
    equine ailments, 95-97
    nematodes, 208-209
    small animal physical examination,
        77-78
Gauntlet, 36
Gauze muzzle, 34-35
Gavage
    defined, 351
    gastric, 339, 342
Gecolate; *see* Guaifenesin
Gelatin digestion test, 252
Gelatin tube test, 252
Gelpi retractor, 167
Geminis; *see* Xylazine
Gene, 22
General anesthesia, 62, 113-114
General appearance, 77
Generic drug, 58
Genetics, 18-24
    breeding, 21-22
    chromosomal abnormalities, 22
    defined, 22
    dihybrid cross, 19-20
    monohybrid cross, 18-19
    X-linked inheritance, 20-21
Genitalia, 78
Genitourinary system
    anatomy and physiology
        avian, 355
        reptile, 360
    small animal physical examination, 78
Genome, 264, 269
Genotype, 22
Gentamicin, 60
Gentocin; *see* Gentamicin
Geometric unsharpness, 144
Gerbil, 344-345
    dentition, 119
    housing, 349
    needle size and site for injection and
        sampling, 340
    reproductive data, 350
    zoonoses, 350
Geriatric animal
    nutritional requirements, 304-306
    restraint, 33-34
Gestation, 14
    bovine, 28
    canine, 26-27
    caprine, 28
    defined, 30
    equine, 27
    feline, 26
    nutritional requirements, 299
    ovine, 29
    porcine, 30
GGT; *see* Gamma glutamyltransferase
Giant kidney worm, 196
Giardia, 199, 359
Gingiva, 117, 118-119, 123

Gingival sulcus, 119, 123
    dental prophy, 121
Gingivitis, 121
Glandular epithelia, 4
Glans penis, 13
Glial cell, 7
Gliricola, 217
Globulins, 255
Glomerulus, 12
Glove; *see* Gauntlet
Gloving, 173
Glucagon, 15
Glucocorticoids, 15
Glucose
    ketosis, 107
    serum, 251-252, 259
    urinary, 233-234, 251
Glucose tolerance test, 251
Glucosuria, 247
Glutaraldehyde, 159
Glycerol guaiacolate, 64
Glycopyrrolate, 177
Glycosuria, 233-234, 251
Gnotobiotic, defined, 351
GnRH; *see* Gonadotropin-releasing hor-
    mone
Goals, 371-372
Goat
    anesthesia, 112-113
    behavior characteristics, 42
    breeding, reproduction, and neonatal
        care, 28-29
    castration, 111
    dehorning, 111
    dentition, 119
    digestion, 312-318
    diseases of, 107-109
        preventable, 110
    drug administration and sample
        collection, 105, 106
    nutrition, 318-320
    physical examination, 104-105
    restraint and handling, 42-43
    teat laceration repair, 110
    venipuncture, 106
    viral infection, 268
Goldberg refractometer, 254
Golgi complex, 2-3
Gonadocorticoids, 15
Gonadotropin-releasing hormone, 30
Gown, packing of, 170-171
Gowning, 173
Grain feed, 322
Grain overload, 108
Gram stain, 228
Gram-negative broth, 222
Gram-negative organisms, 226
Gram-positive organisms, 225-227
Granular casts, 237
Granulocyte precursors, 241
Granuloma, 280
Granulomatous, defined, 247
Gravity displaced autoclave, 160-161
Grey, 141

Grid, radiographic, 130-131, 144
Grief counseling, 367-368
Grifulvin; *see* Griseofulvin
Grisactin; *see* Griseofulvin
Griseofulvin, 60, 61
Groove director, 169
Gross energy, 325
Growl, 49
Growth and development, 302, 303, 304,
    322
Growth hormone, 15
Grunt test, 108
Guaifaxin; *see* Guaifenesin
Guaifenesin, 64, 113
Guaranteed analysis, 308-309, 310
Guinea pig
    dentition, 119
    housing, 349
    as laboratory animal, 347-349
    needle size and site for injection and
        sampling, 340
    parasites, 217
    reproductive data, 350
    zoonoses, 350
Gums
    disease, 121-122
    physical examination, 77, 121
Gun, balling, 44
Gyropus, 217

H

Habituation in behavior modification, 52
Habronema microstoma, 206
Habronema muscae, 206
Haemodipsus, 217
Haemonchus contortus, 208
Haemonchus placei, 208
Haemophilus somnus, 109
Hair
    anatomy and physiology, 15
    preoperative removal, 171
Halogen, 159, 160
Halothane, 62
    general anesthesia, 113, 114
    inhalation anesthesia, 181
Halsted mosquito forceps, 165, 166
Halter, 37, 40, 42
Hamster
    dentition, 119
    housing, 349
    as laboratory animal, 342-344
    needle size and site for injection and
        sampling, 340
    reproductive data, 350
    zoonoses, 350
Handling, 32-47
    avian, 356
    bovine, 39-41
    canine, 33-35
    caprine, 42-43
    equine, 36-39
        salmonellosis and, 96
    feline, 35-36
    gerbil, 345

Handling—cont'd
  guinea pig, 347-348
  hamster, 343
  mice, 339
  ovine, 41-42
  porcine, 43-44
  rabbit, 346
  rat, 341-342
Haploid, defined, 22
Hardware compartment, 9
Hardware disease, 108
Harem mating, 22, 351
Harness, 35
Haversian system, 5
hCG; *see* Human chorionic gonadotropin
Head
  bandaging, 88-89
  danger potential, 39-40
  restraint, 40, 43
  trauma, 334
Headgate, 45
Hearing, 16
Heart; *see* Cardiovascular system
Heart attack, 87
Heart rate, 8
  anesthesia monitoring, 187
Heart sounds, 8
Heartguard; *see* Ivermectin
Heartworm, 197
Heat for microbial control, 156-157
Heat-activated, defined, 269
Heel effect, 144
Heinz body, 240, 241
Helper T cell, 272-273
Hemacytometer, 242
Hematemesis, 336
Hematology, 237-244
  erythrocyte evaluation, 237-242
  leukocyte evaluation, 242-244
Hematuria, 234, 236, 247, 336
Hemipenes, 363
Hemobartonella canis, 81, 242
Hemobartonella felis, 82, 240, 242
Hemoglobin, 238-239
Hemoglobinuria, 234, 247
  bacillary, 109
Hemolysis, 247, 261
Hemolytic serum, 250
Hemoptysis, 336
Hemorrhagic enteritis, 286, 358
Hemorrhagic enterotoxemia, 109
Hemorrhagic shock, 91
Hemosporidia, 359
Hemostatic forceps, 165-167
Hemothorax, 336
Heparin, 250
Hepatic system; *see* Liver
Hepatitis, 109, 341
Herbivore, 9, 16
  urinary pH, 233
Hering-Breuer reflex, 11
Hernia, inguinal, 111
Herpes virus
  equine, 98-99
  zoonosis, 286

Heterosis, 21, 22
Heterozygous, defined, 18-19, 22
Hexacanth, 218
Hibernation, 344
Histamine, 272
Histomoniasis, 359
Histoplasma, 228, 289
Hobble, 41, 45
Hog panel, 44
Hog snare, 44, 45
Hohmann retractor, 167
Holocrine, 363
Homemade treat, 303, 305
Homozygous, defined, 18-19, 22
Hookworm, 196, 209, 287
Hormones
  anatomy and physiology, 4, 14, 15
  defined, 16
  drug therapy, 64-67
  influence on excretory system, 12
Horns
  bovine removal, 111
  danger potential, 39-40
Horse
  accessory sex glands, 12
  behavioral characteristics, 36-37
  blood disorders, 100
  breeding, reproduction, and neonatal
    care, 27
  dentition, 94-95, 119
  foot ailments, 100-101
  gastrointestinal ailments, 95-97
  gestational period, 14
  neuromuscular disorders, 97-99
  normal values, 94
  nutrition, 322-324
  parasites in, 204-207
  respiratory disease, 99-100
  respiratory rate, 11
  restraint and handling, 36-39
  surgery, 101-102
  urine specific gravity, 233
  viral disease, 268
Host, 218
Hot air oven for microbial control,
    156-157
Hot water for microbial control, 157
House soiling, 53-54
Housing
  avian, 355-356
  laboratory animal, 349
  reptile, 360-361
Howell-Jolly body, 240, 241
Howl, 49
Human chorionic gonadotropin, 30
Human voice, 35
Humane twitch, 38
Hurdle, 44
HW; *see* Heartworm
Hyaline casts, 237
Hybrid, defined, 22
Hybrid vigor, 21
Hydrocephalus, 336
Hydrophilic, defined, 162

Hymenolepis nana, 214
Hyostrongylus rubidus, 212
Hyperbilirubinemia, 253
Hypercalcemia, 258, 261
Hypercapnia, 192
Hyperchloremia, 258
Hyperechoic sonographic image, 151,
    153
Hyperglycemia, 234, 251
Hyperimmunity, 276
Hyperkalemia, 257, 336
Hyperkalemic periodic paralysis, 97
Hypernatremia, 257
Hyperparathyroidism, 261
Hyperphosphatemia, 258, 261
Hyperplasia, gingival, 117
Hypersegmented neutrophil, 247
Hypersensitivity reaction, 275, 276-277
Hypertension, 192
Hyperthermia, 188, 336
Hyperthyroidism, 67
Hypertonic solution, 3, 16, 247
Hyperventilation, 187, 192
Hyphema, 336
Hypnotics, 62
Hypoadrenocorticism, 332
Hypocalcemia, 258, 261, 356-357
Hypocalcemic parturient paresis, 107
Hypochloremia, 258
Hypochromic red blood cell, 239, 240,
    247
Hypoderma bovis, 211
Hypoderma lineatum, 211
Hypoechoic sonographic image, 151, 153
Hypoglycemia, 251, 261
Hypokalemia, 257
Hyponatremia, 257, 336
Hypoparathyroidism, 261
Hypophosphatemia, 258, 261
Hypoplasia, enamel, 117
Hypoplastic, defined, 336
Hypoproteinemia, 83, 91
Hypotension, 192
Hypotensive, defined, 91
Hypothalamus, 7
Hypothermia, 188, 336
Hypothyroidism, 67
Hypotonic solution, 3, 16
Hypoventilation, 187, 192
Hypovitaminosis, 356-357, 362
Hypovolemia, 192
Hypovolemic, defined, 91
Hypovolemic shock, 91, 332
Hypoxia, 192, 336
HYPP; *see* Hyperkalemic periodic
    paralysis
Hypsodont, 351

I

IBR; *see* Infectious bovine rhinotrach-
    eitis
Ibuprofen, 62
ICSH; *see* Interstitial cell stimulating
    hormone

Icteric serum, 250
Icterus, 261
Ictotest tablet, 254
Identification, radiographic, 133
Idiopathic, defined, 280
IER; *see* Illness energy requirements
IgG; *see* Immunoglobulin G
Ileitis, 343
Ileum, 10
Ileus, 102
Illness energy requirements, 308
IM; *see* Intramuscular
Immiticide; *see* Melarsomine
Immunity, 271-281
    acquired, 275-276
    adaptive or specific, 272-273
    antibodies, 274-275
    immunopathological mechanisms, 276-277
    innate or nonspecific, 271-272
    vaccines, 277-280
    to viral infection, 273-274
Immunodeficiency, 277
Immunogen, 280
Immunoglobulin G
    immune response, 274-275
    neonatal diarrhea, 109
    placental crossing, 30
Immunoglobulins, 274, 275, 276
Immunopathological disorder, 276-277
Impaction, dental, 117
In utero, defined, 102
Inbred strain of mice, 339
Inbreeding, 21, 22
Inbreeding depression, 21-22, 22
Incineration for microbial control, 156
Incisal, defined, 123
Incisor, 119, 122
Inclusion bodies, 269
Incomplete dominance, 19, 22
Incubator, 221
Inderal; *see* Propranolol
India stone, 121
Indigestion, 108
Indirect fluorescent antibody assay, 292
Indwelling catheter, 336
Infection
    avian, 357-358
    bacterial; *see* Bacterial infection
    fungal, 222-223, 225, 227-228
    latent, 265, 351
    parasitic; *see* Parasites
    patent, 218
    prepatent, 218
    protozoal; *see* Protozoa
    reptilian, 362
    viral; *see* Viral infection
Infectious bovine rhinotracheitis, 109
Infectious necrotic hepatitis, 109
Infective, defined, 218
Inflammation, 246
Influenza, 99-100, 358
Ingredient, defined, 309
Inguinal hernia, 111

Inhalation anesthesia, 181
Inhalation/exhalation flutter valve, 185
Injury; *see* Trauma
Innate immunity, 271-272
Inner ear, 16
Innovar-vet; *see* Fentanyl
Inotropes, 63
Inspiration, 11
Inspiratory reserve volume, 11
Instruments
    dental, 120-121
    sterilization in autoclave, 161
    surgical, 164-170
Insulin, 15
Insulin therapy, 67
Integumentary system; *see* Skin
Intensifying screen, radiographic, 130
Intercellular, defined, 3, 16
Interceptor; *see* Milbemycin oxime
Interdental, defined, 123
Interferon, 274
Interleukins, 273
Intermediate host, 218
Intermediate inheritance, 19, 22
Intermittent positive-pressure ventilation, 188-189
Internal respiration, 11
International Committee on Taxonomy of Viruses, 265
Interstitial cell stimulating hormone, 13, 15
Interview, 374
Intestine
    anatomy and physiology, 10
    digestive process, 10
    equine clostridial infection, 96
    sonographic appearance, 152
Intracellular, defined, 3, 16, 91
Intracoelomic, defined, 363
Intradermal, defined, 91
Intramedullary, defined, 91, 174
Intramedullary fluid administration, 80
Intramembranous bone, 5
Intramuscular drug administration, 79, 106
Intraperitoneal, defined, 91
Intravenous administration, 80
Intussusception, 336
Inventory control, 370-371
Inverted L block, 112
Iodine, 298, 314, 318-319, 321, 323
Ionizing radiation, 127, 143
    hazards, 140-141
    microbial control, 157
IPPV; *see* Intermittent positive-pressure ventilation
Iris, 15
Iron, 297, 314-315, 321, 323
Irregular bone, 5
Isoechoic sonographic image, 151, 153
Isoflurane, 62, 181
Isospora, 199, 213
Isotonic solution, 3, 16, 91, 336
IV; *see* Intravenous

Ivermectin, 66
Ivornec; *see* Ivermectin
Ixodid, 201

J

Jacking, 41, 45
Jacobs chucks, 169
Jaundice, prehepatic, 253
Jaw
    anesthesia monitoring, 186-187
    equine, 94-95
Jejunum, 10
Job search, 373-374
Joint, 6
Jugular vein venipuncture, 105, 106
Jumping, caprine, 42
Juvenile period behavior, 49

K

Kao-Forte; *see* Kaolin/pectin
Kaolin/pectin, 65
Kaopectolin; *see* Kaolin/pectin
Karyotype, 22
Kefsol; *see* Cefazolin sodium
Kelly forceps, 165
Kern forceps, 169
Ketalean; *see* Ketamine
Ketamine, 62, 113, 114, 178, 180-181
Ketaset; *see* Ketamine
Ketoacidosis, 332
Ketoconazole, 61
Ketones, urinary, 234
Ketonuria, 247
Ketosis, 107, 234
Kicking potential, 36, 40
Kid
    castration, 111
    nutrition, 320
Kidney
    acid-base balance and, 190-191
    anatomy and physiology, 12
    drug excretion, 59
    emergencies of, 330, 334
    emergency patient monitoring, 328-329
    pulpy, 109
    sonographic appearance, 152
    triage, 327
Kidney function tests, 250-251, 260
Killed vaccine, 278
Kilovoltage peak, 135, 137, 144
Kirby-Bauer sensitivity test, 229
Kitten
    nutritional requirements, 305
    pet selection, 51
Knott's technique, modified, 195-203
K-P-Sol; *see* Kaolin/pectin
kVp; *see* Kilovoltage peak

L

Label
    pet food, 308
    prescription, 73-74

Labial, defined, 123
Labor; *see* Parturition
Laboratory animal allergy, 351
Laboratory animal medicine, 338-352
   caging and housing, 349
   dentition, 119
   guinea pig, 347-349
   Mongolian gerbil, 344-345
   mouse, 339-341
   parasites in, 214-217
   rabbit, 345-346
   rat, 341-342
   reproductive data, 349, 350
   Syrian hamster, 342-344
   zoonosis, 349, 350
Lacrimal apparatus, 15, 16
Lactase, 10
Lactate dehydrogenase, 256, 259
Lactation, 14, 16
   defined, 45
   nutritional requirements, 299
      bovine, 316-317
      ovine and caprine, 320
Lacunae, 5
Lamb
   castration, 111
   nutrition, 320
   restraint, 42
Lamellae, 5
Laminae, 16
Laminectomy, 336
Laminitis, 96, 100
Langbeck elevator, 169
Lanoxin; *see* Digoxin
Laparotomy, 110, 171, 174
Large intestine
   anatomy and physiology, 10
   sonographic appearance, 152
Laryngopharynx, 11
Larynx
   anatomy, 11
   paralysis, 330
Lasix; *see* Furosemide
Latent, defined, 269
Latent carrier, 292
Latent image, 132, 144
Latent infection, 265, 269, 351
Lateral
   defined, 5
   radiographic terminology, 142
Lateral recumbency, 101
Latex agglutination test, 267-268
Lavage, 336
Laxatives, 64, 65
Laxatone; *see* Laxatives
LDA; *see* Left displaced abomasum
LDH; *see* Lactate dehydrogenase
Le Systeme International d'Unites, 70
Lead poisoning, 335, 357
Lead shank, 38-39, 45
Leading horse, 37
Leash, 34, 36
Left displaced abomasum, 107-108
Left shift, 247

Leg; *see* Limb
Legume, 325
Length measurement, 71, 74
Lens, 15
Leptocyte, 241
Leptospirosis, 110, 290
Lethal gene, 22
Leucine crystals, 237, 238
Leukemia, 247, 267, 268
Leukocyte; *see* White blood cell
Leukocytosis, 247
Leukopenia, 247
Levator muscle, 6
Level bite, 117
LH; *see* Luteinizing hormone
Lice, 200, 217
Lidocaine, 62, 63
Lifting, porcine, 44
Ligating, defined, 174
Light microscope, 221
Limb
   bandaging, 89-90
   preoperative hair removal, 172
   restraint, 36, 41
Lincocin; *see* Lincomycin
Lincomycin, 60
Lincosamide, 59, 60
Line breeding, 21, 23
Linear scanner, 149, 153
Linen pack sterilization, 161
Linen suture, 170
Lingual, defined, 123
Linoleic acid, 295
Linolenic acid, 295
Lip examination, 121
Lipase, 10, 252-253, 259
Lipemic serum, 250
Lipophilic, defined, 162
Liquid
   measurement, 74
   specimen, 224
   sterilization, 161
Listening, 367
Lister bandage scissors, 165, 166
Listeriosis, 110, 284
Littauer scissors, 165
Litter box problems, 54-55
Liver
   anatomy and physiology, 10
   drug absorption, 59
   sonographic appearance, 152
Liver fluke, 210
Liver function tests, 253-257, 260
Lizard; *see* Reptile
LLA; *see* Laboratory animal allergy
Local anesthesia, 111-113
Lockjaw, 97-98
Locus, defined, 23
Long bone, 5
Long latitude film, 136-137
Loop of Henle, 12
Lorazepam, 177
Lufenuron, 66
Lugol's iodine, 252

Lumbar spine, 6
Lung; *see* Respiratory system
Lung fluke, 198
Lungworm, 206, 209, 213
Luteinizing hormone, 13, 15
Lyme disease, 289
Lymphatic system, 10, 78
Lymphocyte, 243, 246
Lymphocytosis, 247
Lysis, defined, 280
Lysogenic cycle, 265
Lysosome, 3
Lysozyme, 280

M

M mode; *see* Motion mode
Maalox; *see* Antacids
MacConkey II agar, 222
Macracanthorhynchus hirundinaceus,
   213
Macrocyte, 247
Macrocytosis, 239
Macrolide, 59, 60
Macrominerals, 296, 323
Macrophage, 246, 272, 280
Mad cow disease, 314
Mad dog disease, 286
Magnalax; *see* Antacids
Magnesium
   nutritional requirements
      bovine, 315
      equine, 323
      porcine, 321
      small animal, 299
   serum, 258, 259
      milk fever, 107
Magnet therapy, 108
Maintenance energy requirements, 299,
   302, 310
Malabsorption, 261
Malassimilation, 261
Male reproductive system, 12-13, 355
Malignant edema, 109
Mallophaga, 200
Malocclusion, 91, 116-117, 123, 351
Maltase, 10
Mammary tumor, 342
Management skills, 365-378
   business, 370-371
   career, 373-375
   communication, 365-369
      client, 367-368
      co-worker, 368-369
      electronic, 369
      listening, 367
      nonverbal, 366-367
      verbal, 366
      written, 369
   marketing, 376-378
   organizational, 369-370
   personal, 373
   professional obligations, 375-376
Mandible, 117, 122, 123
Manganese, 298, 315, 321, 323

Mange, 218, 288
Mannitol, 63
Manometer, 185
Marek's disease, 358
Marketing, 376
mAs; *see* Milliampere-seconds
Mass in metric system, 71
Mast cell, 246, 247
Master gland, 15
Mastitis, 106-107, 109
Mathieu needle holder, 167
Mating, harem, 351
Maxilla, 117, 122, 123
Maximum permissible dose, 141, 144
Mayo scissors, 164, 165
Mayo-Hegar needle holder, 167, 168
MCH; *see* Mean corpuscular hemoglobin
MCHC; *see* Mean corpuscular
    hemoglobin content
MCV; *see* Mean corpuscular volume
Mean corpuscular hemoglobin, 239
Mean corpuscular hemoglobin content,
   239
Mean corpuscular volume, 239
Mebendazole, 66
Mechanical sector transducer, 149
Mechanical ventilation, 188-189
Medetomidine, 178
Media
   diagnostic microbiology, 221-223
   radiographic, 142
Medial
   defined, 5
   radiographic terminology, 142
Medulla oblongata, 7, 11
Medullary cavity, 5
Meiosis, 23
Meissner's corpuscle, 14
Melanocyte, 14
Melanoma, 117
Melarsomine, 66
Melophagus ovinus, 211
Menace reflex, 336
Meninges, 7, 16
Meningitis, 110
Meniscus, 218
Meperidine, 61, 178
MER; *see* Maintenance energy require-
   ments
Meriones unguiculatus, 344
Mesial, defined, 123
Mesothelial cell, 246
Metabolic acidosis, 191
Metabolic bone disease, 362
Metabolite, 59
Metabolization of drugs, 59
Metabolizing energy, 325
Metanephric, defined, 363
Metastasis, 261
Metastrongylus apri, 213
Metestrus, 13-14, 26, 245
Methemoglobinemia, 336
Methimazol, 67
Methohexital, 179, 180

Methoxyflurane, 62, 181
Methylated oxybarbiturates, 179
Methylxanthine toxicity, 335
Metoclopramide, 65
Metofane; *see* Methoxyflurane
Metric system, 70-72, 74
Metronidazole, 60, 61, 66
Metzenbaum scissors, 164
Mexican hat cell, 241
Meyerding retractor, 167
Micro environment, 351
Microbial resistance and control,
   156-162
Microbiology, 220-230
   bacterial identification, 225-227
   basic diagnostic tests, 228-229
   equipment, 221-222
   fungal identification, 227-228
   media, 222-223
   purpose, 220-221
   specimen types, 223
Microcyte, 247
Microcytic red blood cell, 239, 240, 247
Microminerals, 296, 323
Microorganism, defined, 162
Microscope, 221
Microsporum, 227, 289
Midazolam, 177
Midbrain, 7
Middle ear, 16
Milbemycin oxime, 66
Miliary tuberculosis, 292
Milk, surgical, 170
Milk fever, 107
Milk of Magnesia; *see* Laxatives
Milk sampling, 106-107
Milk vein in venipuncture, 106
Milliampere-seconds, 144
Mineralocorticoids, 15
Minerals
   function tests, 257-258, 260
   nutritional requirements
      bovine, 314-315
      caprine and ovine, 318-319
      equine, 323
      porcine, 321
      small animal, 296, 299-303
Minimal alveolar concentration, 192
Miosis, 336
Mirror image, sonographic, 151
Mite, 201, 217
Mitochondria, 2
Mitosis, 23
Mixed lesion, 153
MLV; *see* Modified-live vaccine
Mobitz type I, 87
Modified Knott's technique, 195-203
Modified-live vaccine, 277-278
Moist heat for microbial control, 157
Molar, 120, 123
Molybdenum, 315
Monestrous, 13, 16, 30
Mongolian gerbil, 344-345
Moniezia, 210

Monitoring
   anesthesia, 186-188
   emergency patients, 328-329
Monocyte, 243
Monocytopenia, 247
Monocytosis, 247
Monohybrid cross, 18-19, 23
Monotocous, 16
Moraxella bovis, 226
Morphine, 61, 178
Morulated, defined, 218
Mosquito, 99
Motility test media, 223
Motion mode, 150, 153
Mouse
   dentition, 119
   housing, 349
   as laboratory animal, 339-341
   parasites, 214-215
   reproductive data, 350
   zoonoses, 350
Mouth
   anatomy and physiology, 9
   physical examination, 77, 121
   wry, 117
MPD; *see* Maximum permissible dose
Mucogingival, defined, 124
Mucor, 227
Mucous membrane
   anesthesia monitoring, 187
   bandaging assessment, 89
   small animal physical examination, 77
   triage, 327
Mueller-Hinton agar, 222
Multiceps serialis, 216
Mus musculus, 339
Muscle, 4
Muscle disease tests, 259
Muscle relaxant, 64, 188
Muscle tone in anesthesia monitoring,
   186-187
Muscular dystrophy, 348
Musculoskeletal system
   anatomy and physiology, 5-6, 78
   avian, 354
   reptile, 359
Muzzle, 33, 34-35, 36
Myalgia, 292
Mycobacterium, 227, 285
Mycoptes muscalinis, 215
Mycosel agar, 223
Mycotic, defined, 292
Mycotic disease, 289, 358, 362
Mydriasis, 336
Myeloencephalitis, 98
Myelogram, 336
Myiasis, 218
Myobiomusculi, 215
Myocardium, 7, 16, 91
Myoglobinuria, 234
Myometrium, 13
Myositis, 102
Mystery swine disease, 109

N

Naked virus, 264
Naltrexone, 61
Naoplura, 200
Narcan; *see* Naxolone
Narcotics, 61
Nares, 10, 77
Nasal cavity, 10
Nasogastric, defined, 102
Nasogastric tube, 102
Nasopharynx, 10
National Committee on Radiation Protec-
    tion and Measurement, 141
Natural immunity, 275
Navicular syndrome, 100-101
Naxolone, 61
N/d2/DO; *see* Anesthesia
Near side of horse, 45
Nebulization, 336
Neck bandaging, 88-89
Neck of tooth, 124
Necrosis, 280
Needle
    intramuscular injection, 106
    laboratory animal sampling, 340
    surgical, 169-170
    venipuncture, 106
Needle holder, 167, 168
Needle tooth, 43, 45
Negative pressure relief valve, 185
Negative reinforcement, 52
Negotiation, 373
Neisseria, 226
Nemacide; *see* Diethylcarbamazine
Nematode
    bovine and ovine, 208-209
    canine and feline, 196-197
    defined, 218
    equine, 204-206
    porcine, 212-213
Nematodirus, 209
Nembutal; *see* Pentobarbital
Nemex; *see* Pyrantel pamoate
Neomycin, 60
Neonatal, defined, 30
Neonatal care
    bovine, 28
    canine, 27
    caprine, 29
    equine, 27
    feline, 26
    ovine, 29
    porcine, 30
Neonatal porcine colibacillosis, 110
Neonate
    behavioral development, 48, 49
    diarrhea in ruminant and swine,
        108-109
    immunity, 275
    nutritional requirements, 299-302
Neoplasia
    defined, 336
    exfoliated cytology, 246-247
    gerbil, 345

Neoplasia—cont'd
    mammary, 342
    oral, 117
    pulmonary, 331
    soft tissue swelling, 330
Nephron, 12
Nervous system
    anatomy and physiology, 6-7
    emergencies of, 329-330, 334
    emergency patient monitoring, 329
    small animal physical examination, 78
    tissue of, 4
    triage, 327
Neurectomy, 102
Neurogenic, defined, 336
Neurogenic shock, 332
Neuroglial cell, 7
Neuroleptanalgesics, 179, 180
Neuromuscular disorders, 97-99
Neuron, 7
Neutropenia, 247
Neutrophil
    defined, 280
    exfoliated cytology, 246
    innate immunity, 272
    toxic, 247
    white blood cell evaluation, 243
Neutrophilia, 247
Neutrophilic band, 243
New Methylene Blue stain, 245, 247
Newcastle's disease, 358
Newsletter, 377
Niacin, 298, 321
Nictitating membrane, 15
Nitro-bid; *see* Nitroglycerin
Nitroglycerin, 63
Nitrol; *see* Nitroglycerin
Nitrong; *see* Nitroglycerin
Nitrostat; *see* Nitroglycerin
Nitrous oxide, 181-182
NLF; *see* Nonlactose fermenting
    organism
NMB; *see* New Methylene Blue
Nocturnal, defined, 351
Nodular worm, 209, 212
Noninfective, defined, 218
Nonlactose fermenting organism, 222
Nonspecific immunity, 271-272
Nonspontaneous ovulator, 16
Nonsteroidal antiinflammatory drugs, 61,
    62
    equine gastrointestinal ailments from,
        97
    toxicity, 335
Nonverbal communication, 366-367
Norepinephrine, 15
Normal flora, 229
Normochromic red blood cell, 239, 247
Normocytic, defined, 239, 247
Nose bot, 211
Nose lead, 411
Nostril, 10
Notoedres, 202, 215
NRBC; *see* Nucleated red blood cell

NSAIDS; *see* Nonsteroidal antiinflam-
    matory drugs
Nucleases, 10
Nucleated red blood cell, 241-242, 247
Nucleic acid core, 269
Nucleocapsid, 264
Nucleus
    anatomy and physiology, 2-3
    ionizing radiation damage, 140
Numorphan; *see* Oxymorphone
Nutrient
    defined, 310, 325
    total digestible, 325
Nutrient agar, 223
Nutrition
    avian, 356-357
    bovine, 312-318
    caprine and ovine, 318-320
    equine, 322-324
    porcine, 320-322
    reptile, 361-362
    small animal, 294-311
        basic nutrition, 294-295
        critical care, 307-308
        daily energy requirements, 299, 302
        energy-producing nutrients,
            295-296
        feline lower urinary tract disease,
            306
        life stage requirements, 299-306
        nonenergy-producing nutrients,
            296-299, 298-299, 302-303
        obesity, 307
        pet food, 308-309
Nutritive media, 221
Nystagmus, 91, 336

O

Obedience training, 51-52
Obesity, 304, 307
Object film distance, 139, 144
Oblique, radiographic terminology, 142
Obsessive/compulsive disorder, 55
Obstruction, feline urethral, 334
Occlusal, defined, 124
Occlusion, 116-117
Occlusive, defined, 336
Occult blood, 234
Ocular larval migrans, 287
Odontoblast, 124
Oesophagostomum, 209, 212
Oestrus ovis, 211
OFD; *see* Object film distance
Olfaction, defined, 55
Olfactory communication, 49, 50
Oligodontia, 117, 124
Oliguria, 232, 247
OLM; *see* Ocular larval migrans
Olsen-Hegar needle holder, 167
Omasum, 9, 313
Omentopexy, 114
Omnivore, 9, 16
    urine pH, 233
Oncological agents, 68

Oncotic pressure, 91
Operant conditioning for behavior modifica-tion, 52
Operating room, 173-174
Opioids, 61-62, 178
Opossum, 98
Opportunistic pathogen, 229
Opsonin, 280
Oral administration, 78-79, 80
Oral lesions, 117
Organ of Corti, 16
Organizational management, 369-370
Organophosphate, 66
    toxicity, 335
Oronasal fistula, 117, 124
Oropharynx, 11
Orphan young nutrition, 320
Orthopedic surgery, 169, 172
Oryctolagus cuniculus, 345
Osmolality, 336
Osmosis, 3
Ossification, 5
Osteodystrophy fibrosa, 363
Osteogenesis, 5
Osteology, 5, 16
Ostertagia circumcinta, 208
Ostertagia ostertagi, 208
Otodectes, 202
Outbred strain of mice, 339
Outbreeding, 21, 23
Outer ear, 16
Ovariohysterectomy, 171, 174
Ovariohysterectomy hook, 167, 169
Ovary, 13, 15
Ovassay, 195
Ovatector, 195
Oviduct, 13
Ovine; *see* SHeep
Oviparous, 363
Ovoviviparous, 363
Ovulation, 13, 26, 30
Oxidase test, 228
Oxidation for microbial control, 156-157
Oxidation-fermentation medium with dextrose, 223
Oxybarbiturates, 179
Oxygen flush valve, 185
Oxygen partial pressure, 192
Oxygen therapy
    anesthesia, 113, 114, 182-183
    cardiopulmonary resuscitation, 333
Oxygenation problems during anesthesia, 192
Oxymorphone, 61, 62, 178
Oxytetracycline, 96
Oxytocin, 15, 67
Oxyuriasis, 205, 214, 216

P

P wave, 8, 84, 85
Pacheco's disease, 358
Pacinian corpuscle, 14

Packed cell volume, 237, 247
    dehydration and, 80
    during surgery, 190
Packed red cell transfusion, 83
Pain
    anesthesia monitoring, 186
    signs of
        gerbil, 345
        guinea pig, 348
        hamster, 343
        mice, 339-340
        rabbit, 346
        rat, 342
Palatal, defined, 124
Palate, 124
Palmar, radiographic terminology, 142
Palpation
    abdominal, 26, 27
    defined, 91
Palpebral reflex, 186
Panacur; *see* Benzimidazoles
Pancreas
    anatomy and physiology, 10
    hormones of, 15
    sonographic appearance, 152
Pancreatic amylase, 10
Pancreatic enzymes, 10
Pancreatic function tests, 251-253, 260
Pancreatitis, 91
Pancytopenia, 247
Panmycin; *see* Tetracycline
Pantothenic acid, 300, 321
Papanicolaou stain, 245
Paragonimus kellicotti, 198
Parainfluenza III, 109
Paralumbar block, 112
Paralumbar fossa, 114
Paralysis
    as central nervous system emergency, 334
    defined, 336
    hyperkalemic periodic, 97
    laryngeal, 330
Parascaris equorum, 204
Parasites, 194-219, 242, 269
    avian, 358-359
    blood collection and examination, 81, 195-203
    bovine and ovine, 208-211
    canine and feline, 196-202
    equine, 204-207
    external identification, 203-218
    feces examination, 194-195
    in laboratory animals, 214-217
    porcine, 212-213
    reptile, 362
    zoonosis, 287-288
Parasympathetic nervous system, 6
Parasympatholytics, 177
Paratenic host, 218
Parathormone, 15
Parathyroid gland, 15

Paravertebral block, 112
Parenchyma, 336
Parenchymal lung problem, 331
Parenteral, defined, 91
Parenteral drug administration, 79
Parenteral nutrition, 308
Paresis, 334, 336
Parrot fever, 291
Parturition, 14
    bovine, 28
    canine, 26-27
    caprine, 28
    defined, 17, 30
    equine, 27
    feline, 26
    ovine, 29
    porcine, 30
Parvovirus, 110
Passive immunity, 276
Passulurus ambiguus, 216
Pasteurella, 109, 226, 284, 346, 357
Patent infection, 218
Pathogen, defined, 162
Paw bandaging, 90
PCT; *see* Proximal convoluted tubule
PCV; *see* Packed cell volume
PDS; *see* Proventricular dilation syndrome
Pecten, 354
Pedal reflex, 186
Pedicle, defined, 174
Pediculosis, 218
Pedigree chart, 21, 23
Peg tooth, 345
Penetrance in genetics, 23
Penicillin, 60
Penis, 12-13
Pentobarbital, 62, 68, 179
Pentothal; *see* Thiopental
Peptidase, 10
Pepto-Bismol; *see* Bismuth subsalicylate
Percent concentration, 73
Perfusion, defined, 334, 336
Periapical abscess, 124
Pericardial tamponade, 332
Pericardium, 7
Perimetrium, 13
Perineal, defined, 174
Perineal urethrostomy, 172
Perineum, 174
Period, sonographic, 148
Periodontal disease, 121-122
Periodontal ligament, 118, 124
Periodontal probe, 120
Periodontitis, 336
Perioperative care, 101-102, 171-172
Periosteal elevator, 169
Periosteum, 5
Peripheral, defined, 91
Peripheral nervous system, 6
Peristalsis, 9
Permanent teeth, 119, 120

Peroxisome, 3
Peroxygen compounds, 159
Personal finance, 373
Personal management, 372
Pet food, 308-309
    nutritional requirements, 304
    water quantity, 296
Pet selection, 51
Peterson eye block, 112
Pethidine; *see* Meperidine
PFBD; *see* Psittacine beak and feather
        disease
pH
    acid-base balance and, 190-191
    normal values, 192
    urinary, 233
Phagocyte, 272
Phagocytosis, 3, 280
Pharmaceutical calculations, 70-75
Pharmacokinetics, 58-59
Pharmacology, 57-69
    analgesics/sedatives, 61-62
    anthelmintics, 64, 66
    antibiotics, 59-61
    basic terminology, 58
    cardiovascular drugs, 62-63
    definitions, 57
    euthanizing agents, 68
    gastrointestinal drugs, 64, 65
    general anesthetics, 62
    hormones and endocrine drugs, 64-67
    oncological agents, 68
    pharmacokinetics, 58-59
    respiratory drugs, 63-64
    topical drugs, 68
    vaccines, 67-68
Pharynx, 9, 10-11
Phased array sector scanner, 149
Phencyclidines, 178
Phenobarbital, 61, 179
Phenols, 158, 160
Phenothiazine, 61, 177
Phenotype, 23
Phenylbutazone, 62
PHF; *see* Potomac horse fever
Phosphor crystal, radiographic, 130
Phosphorus
    nutritional requirements
        bovine, 314
        caprine and ovine, 318-319
        equine, 323
        porcine, 321
        small animal, 299
    serum, 258, 259
Photon, 144
Physical examination
    equine, 38
    ruminant and swine, 104-105
    small animal, 77-78
Physiology, defined, 1, 17
Pia mater, 7
Piezoelectric effect, 149, 153

Pig; *see* Swine
Piglet
    castration, 111
    danger potential of teeth, 43
    enteric disease, 110
    nutrition, 322
Pigmentation, 14
Piloerection, 55
Pinocytosis, 3
Pinworm, 205, 214, 216
Pipa-Tabs; *see* Piperazine
Piperazine, 66
Pituitary gland, 15
Placenta, 14, 30
Placentation, 30
Plague, 284, 350, 358
Plantar, radiographic terminology, 142
Plaque, dental, 121, 124
Plasma, 247, 249, 261
Plasma cell, 246
Plasma glucose, 251-252
Plasma membrane, 2
Plasma proteins, 254
Plasma transfusion, 83
    during surgery, 190
Plasmid, 280
Plaster of Paris cast, 90
Plastron, 363
Plate in diagnostic microbiology, 222,
        229
Platelet
    innate immunity, 272
    microscopic evaluation, 244
    precursors, 241
    transfusion, 83
Play, feline posture, 50
Pleura, 336
Pleural effusion, 331
Pleuritis, 11
P/M; *see* Oxymorphone
Pneumatic bone, 5
Pneumonia, 11, 348, 357, 362
Pneumothorax, 11, 189, 331, 336
PNS; *see* Peripheral nervous system
Poikilocytosis, 241, 247
Poison, defined, 57
Poisoning; *see* Toxicity
Pole, rabies or capture, 34
Polishing of tooth, 121
Pollakiuria, 232, 247
Poloxalene, 65
Polychromasia, 239
Polychromatic beam, 144
Polydontia, 117
Polyestrous, 13, 17, 30
Polyflex; *see* Ampicillin
Polygenic trait, 19, 23
Polyplax, 217
Polytocous, 17
Polyuria, 91, 232, 247
Pons, 7, 11
Poole tip, 169

Porcine; *see* Swine
Porcine reproductive and respiratory
        syndrome, 109, 110
Positioning
    general anesthesia, 113
    radiographic, 142-143
        dental, 122
    sonographic, 152
    surgical, 101, 110-111
Positive inotropes, 63
Posterior, defined, 5
Posterior crossbite, 117
Postmortem tissue sample, 266
Postoperative care, 102
Postural, defined, 336
Posture, feline, 50, 51
POT; *see* Preferred optimal temperature
Potassium
    metabolic alkalosis, 192
    nutritional requirements
        equine, 323
        porcine, 321
        small animal, 299
    serum, 257, 259
Potentiated amoxicillin, 60
Potentiated sulfa, 60
Potomac horse fever, 96
Potter-Bucky diaphragm, 130, 131
Pouch pack sterilization, 161
Pounds per square inch, 269
Poxiviral disease, 286, 358
PPP; *see* Prepatent period
PR interval, 84, 85
Praziquantel, 66
Preanesthetic medication, 177-179
Prednisone, 62
Preferred optimal temperature, 360
Pregnancy
    diagnosis, 26, 27, 28, 29, 30
    nutrition, 316-317, 320, 322
    physiology, 14
    restraint, 34
    toxemia, 107, 348
Prehepatic, defined, 261
Premature ventricular contraction, 87, 91
Premix, 325
Premolar, 120, 124
Preoperative care, 101, 171-172
Prepatent infection, 218
Prepatent period, 218
Prepping for equine surgery, 101
Prescription labels, 73-74
Pressure reducing valve, 185
Prevacuum autoclave, 161
Primary teeth, 124
Princillin; *see* Ampicillin
Prion, 269
Probran; *see* Organophosphate
Procedures manual, 370
Prochlorperazine isopropamide, 65
Proestrus, 13, 26, 245
Professional obligation, 374-376

Professionalism, 375
Progesterone, 15
Progestin, 64-67
Proglottid, 292
Prognathism, 116, 124
Program; *see* Lufenuron
Prokaryote, 2
Prolactin, 15
Proliferative ileitis, 343
Promace; *see* Acepromazine
Propagation artifact, 151
Propofol, 62, 180
Propranolol, 62, 63
Proprioceptive, defined, 336
Pro-spot; *see* Organophosphate
Prostaglandins, 67
Prostate, 152
Protamine zinc insulin, 67
Protectant, 336
Protein
    barbiturate binding to, 179
    nutritional requirements
        bovine, 313
        caprine and ovine, 318
        equine, 324
        porcine, 320-321
        small animal, 295, 310
    plasma, 254, 259
    serum, 254, 259
    total, 244
    urinary, 233
Proteinuria, 233, 247
Proteus, 225
Protozoa
    bovine and ovine, 210
    canine and feline, 199
    defined, 218
    equine, 207
    equine protozoal myeloencephalitis,
        98
    porcine, 213
    reptile, 362
Proventricular dilation syndrome, 358
Proximal, defined, 5, 124
Proximal convoluted tubule, 12
PRRS; *see* Porcine reproductive and
    respiratory syndrome
Pruritis, 91
Pseudomonas, 226
Pseudorabies, 110
Pseudostratified epithelia, 4
Pseudotuberculosis, 348, 350
PSI; *see* Pounds per square inch
Psittacine beak and feather disease, 358
Psittacosis, 291, 357
Psoroptes cuniculi, 217
Psychoactive drug, 55
Ptyalism, 348
Ptyerylae, 363
Puberty, 25-26, 27, 28, 29, 30
Pulmonary edema, 331
Pulmonary system; *see* Respiratory
    system

Pulp, dental, 118, 124
Pulpy kidney, 109
Pulse
    anesthesia monitoring, 187
    avian, 356
    neonatal, 26, 27, 28, 29, 30
    parturition, 27
    triage, 327
Pulsed wave transducer, 148
Punishment in behavior modification, 52,
    53
Punnett square, 18, 23
Pupil, 15
    monitoring
        anesthesia, 186
        emergency, 329
    small animal physical examination, 78
Puppy
    nutritional requirements, 299-306
    pet selection, 51
    restraint, 34
    sinus tachycardia, 86
Purina liquid wormer; *see* Piperazine
Purulent, defined, 91
Purulent inflammation, 246
PVC; *see* Premature ventricular
    contraction
Pyometra, 335
Pyothorax, 336
Pyrantel pamoate, 66
Pyrantel tartrate, 66
Pyrethrin, 66
Pyrexia, 102, 336
Pyrexic, defined, 91
Pyridoxine, 300, 321

Q

QRS complex, 8, 84, 85
Quality, radiographic, 134-137, 138, 139,
    140, 144
Quality control, 162
Quantitative buffy coat analysis, 244
Quantity
    metric system, 71
    radiographic, 144
Quantum mottle, 144
Quarantine, 356
Quasivitamin, 300
Quaternary ammonium compounds, 158,
    160
Quinolones, 60

R

Rabbit
    dentition, 119
    housing, 349
    as laboratory animal, 345-346
    needle size and site for injection and
        sampling, 340
    parasites, 216-217
    reproductive data, 350
    zoonoses, 350
Rabbit fever, 285, 350

Rabies, 98, 286, 350
Rabies pole, 34
Radiation
    defined, 127
    measurement, 141
    microbial control, 157
    safety, 140-141
    types, 127
Radiodense, 144
Radiography, 126-146
    contrast, 143
    darkroom and processing techniques,
        133-134
    defined, 144
    dental, 122-123
    image receptors, 131-133
    positioning techniques, 142-143
    pregnancy diagnosis, 26
    quality, 134-137, 138, 139, 140
        contrast, 135-137
        defined, 134-135
        density, 135, 136
        detail or definition, 137, 138, 139,
            140
    safety, 140-142
    technical errors and artifacts, 137, 139
    technique chart development, 137-140
    x-ray machine, 129-131
    x-ray production, 127
    x-ray tube, 127-129
Radioimmunoassay, 261
Radiology, defined, 144
Radiolucent, defined, 144
Radiopaque, 144
Rales, 336
Ram
    penis, 13
    puberty, 29
    teaser in pregnancy diagnosis, 29
Random breeding, 21
Ranitidine, 65
Rapinovet; *see* Propofol
RAS; *see* Reticular activating system
Rat
    dentition, 119
    housing, 349
    as laboratory animal, 341-342
    needle size and site for injection and
        sampling, 340
    parasites, 214-215
    reproductive data, 350
    zoonoses, 350
Rat bite fever, 350
Ration, 325
Rattus norvegicus, 341
RDA; *see* Right displaced abomasum
Reagent test strip, 233
Rebreathing bag of anesthetic machine,
    185
Rebreathing system during anesthesia,
    182-183
Recessive gene, 20, 23
Recording thermometer, 162

Rectification, defined, 144
Rectum, 10
Recumbency
    bovine general anesthesia, 113
    equine surgery, 101
    porcine, 44
Red blood cell, 247
    evaluation, 237-239
    exfoliated cytology, 246
    film evaluation, 239-242
    in urine, 234, 235
Red stomach worm, 212
Red tears, 342
Reduction forceps, 169
REE; see Resting energy requirements
References, 374
Reflex
    anesthesia monitoring, 186
    emergency patient monitoring, 329
    menace, 336
Refraction, sonographic, 151
Refractometer, 233, 254
Regional anesthesia, 111-113
Reglan; see Metoclopramide
Regular insulin, 67
Regurgitation, 113, 357
Relaxation response, 378
Remnant beam, 144
Renal failure, 334
Renal function tests, 250-251, 260
Renal system
    acid-base balance and, 190-191
    anatomy and physiology, 12
    drug excretion, 59
    emergencies of, 330, 334
    emergency patient monitoring, 328-329
    sonographic appearance, 152
    triage, 327
Rennin, 10
Replacement animal, 317, 325
Replication, viral, 264-265
Repolarization, 84
Reproductive system
    anatomy and physiology, 12-14
        avian, 355
    emergencies of, 330, 335
    laboratory animal, 350
    small animal physical examination, 78
Reptile, 224, 359-363
RER; see Rough endoplasmic reticulum
Research, laboratory animals in
    guinea pig, 347
    hamster, 342
    mouse, 339
    rabbit, 345
    rat, 341
Reservoir bag, 185
Residual volume, 11, 17
Resolution, sonographic, 149, 153
Resorption, defined, 124
Respiration
    bandaging assessment, 89
    cardiopulmonary resuscitation, 332

Respiration—cont'd
    physiology, 11
    triage, 327
Respiratory acidosis, 191
Respiratory alkalosis, 191
Respiratory rate, 11
    avian, 356
    feline parturition, 27
    neonatal, 26, 27, 28, 29, 30
    triage, 327
Respiratory system
    acid-base balance and, 190
    anatomy and physiology, 10-12
        avian, 354-355
        circulation, 7-8
        reptilian, 359-360
    disease
        equine, 99-100
        hamster, 344
        mice, 340-341
        rat, 342
    drug therapy, 63-64
    edema, 331
    emergencies of, 329, 330-331
    monitoring
        anesthesia, 187
        emergency patient, 328
    small animal physical examination, 78
    triage, 327
Resting energy requirements, 302
Restraint, 32-47
    avian, 356
    bovine, 39-41
    canine, 33-35
    caprine, 42-43
    electrocardiographic, 85
    equine, 36-39
    feline, 35-36
    ovine, 41-42
    porcine, 43-44
    rabbit, 346
    radiographic, 143
    reptile, 361
Resume, 374
Retained deciduous tooth, 117
Reticular activating system, 7
Reticular connective tissue, 4
Reticulocyte abnormalities, 240
Reticulocyte count, 239
Reticulum, 9
Retina, 15
Retractor, 167-169
Retrobulbar block, 112
Reverberation, sonographic, 151
Rhinitis, 280
Rhinopneumonitis, 98
Rhinotracheitis, 109
Rhizopus, 227
Riboflavin, 298, 321
Ribonucleic acid, 61, 265, 269
Ribosome, 2
Richards forceps, 169
Rickettsia, 81, 291
Right displaced abomasum, 108

Right shift, 247
Ring block, 112
Ring down, sonographic, 152
Ringworm, 289, 350
Rinse bath in film processing, 134
Robamox-V; *see* Amoxicillin
Robert Jones bandage, 89
Rochester-Carmalt forceps, 167
Rochester-Oshner forceps, 167
Rochester-Pean forceps, 167
Rocky Mountain spotted fever, 291
Romanovsky type stain, 245
Romifidine, 178
Rompun; *see* Xylazine
Rongeurs, 169
Root, tooth, 124
Root canal, 124
Rope halter, 40
Rope leash, 34, 36
Rope twitch, 38
Rosine crystals, 237, 238
Rostral, radiographic terminology, 142
Rotating anode, 129
Roto-pro bur, 120
Rough endoplasmic reticulum, 2
Roughages, 316, 324, 325
Rouleaux, 240, 241, 247
Roundworm, 196
Rubbing behavior, 50
Ruby stone, 120
Ruffini endings, 14
Rumen, 9, 108, 313
Rumenotomy, 114
Ruminant
    defined, 17
    dentition, 119
    digestion, 9, 312-318
    diseases of, 107-109
        preventable, 109-110
    drug administration and sample
        collection, 105, 106
    milk sampling, 106-107
    nutrition, 318-320
    parasites, 208-211
    physical examination, 104-105
    surgical procedures, 110-111
    venipuncture, 105-106
Ruminant stomach, 9
Rumping, ovine, 42
Russian tissue forceps, 165

S

Saccharogenic test, 252, 261
Sacral spine, 6
Safety
    dental procedures, 121
    radiographic, 140-142
Saggital, sonographic terminology, 153
Saliva, 124
Salivary amylase, 10
Salmonella
    equine, 96
    fecal culture, 224, 225
    guinea pig, 348

Salmonella—cont'd
   reptile, 362
   zoonosis, 285, 350
Salmonella-Shigella agar, 222
Salt; *see* Sodium
Sample collection; *see* Specimen
   collection
Sanitation, 155-163
Sanitize, defined, 162
SAP; *see* Serum alkaline phosphatase
Saprophyte, 227
Sarcocystis falcatula, 98
Sarcoptes, 202, 217, 218, 288
Sarcosporidia, 108
SC; *see* Subcutaneous
Scabies, 288
Scale film, 136-137
Scaler, 120
Scalpel handle, 169
Scatter radiation, 144
Scavenger system of anesthetic machine,
   185
Scent gland, 42
Schistocyte, 240, 241, 247
Scissors, 164-165
Sclera, 15
Scratching, feline, 50, 55
Screen speed, radiographic, 130-132
Scrub, surgical, 172-173
Scurvy, 348
SD; *see* Sorbitol dehydrogenase
SDA; *see* Sialodacryoadentitis
Seasonally polyestrous, 30
Sebaceous gland, 14
Secondary radiation, 144
Second-degree atrioventricular block, 87
Sector scanner, 149, 153
Sedation, 81, 85
Sedatives, 61-62
Sedimentation rate, 247
Selective media, 221, 222, 229
Selenium, 298, 315, 318-319, 321, 323
Self-retaining forceps, 165, 166
Self-retaining retractor, 167
Semen, 12
   bovine, 28
   canine, 26
   caprine, 28
   equine, 27
   feline, 26
   ovine, 29
   porcine, 30
Semimembranosus, defined, 114
Semitendinosus, defined, 114
Sendai virus, 342
Senn retractor, 167
Senses, 15-16, 354, 359
Separation anxiety, 53
Septic, defined, 336
Septic shock, 332
Septicemia, 362
Sequestration, defined, 337
SER; *see* Smooth endoplasmic reticulum
Serology, 162

Serotonin, 272
Serous, defined, 337
Serum, 250, 261
Serum alkaline phosphatase, 256
Serum amylase, 252
Serum calcium, 258
   milk fever, 107
Serum chloride, 257-258
Serum cholesterol, 257
Serum glucose, 251-252
Serum lipase, 252-253
Serum magnesium, 258
   milk fever, 107
Serum phosphorus, 258
Serum potassium, 257
Serum sodium, 257
Sesamoid bone, 5
Setaria equina, 205
Setting-up, 42, 45
Sex chromosome, 20, 23
Shaping in behavior modification, 52
Sharpening dental instruments, 120-121
Shaving in ultrasound preparation, 152
Sheep
   anesthesia, 112-113
   behavior characteristics, 41
   breeding, reproduction, and neonatal
      care, 29
   castration, 111
   dentition, 119
   digestion, 312-318
   diseases of, 107-109
      preventable, 110
   drug administration and sample col-
      lection, 105, 106
   enzootic abortion, 110
   nutrition, 318-320
   parasites, 208-211
   penis, 13
   physical examination, 104-105
   pregnancy toxemia, 107
   puberty, 29
   restraint and handling, 41-42
   urine specific gravity, 233
   venipuncture, 106
   viral disease, 268
Sheep ked, 211
Sheepdog for restraint, 41
Shepherd's crook, 42, 120
Shigella, 224
Shock, 91, 332, 337
Short bone, 5
Shoulder roll, 39
SI system; *see* Metric system
Sialodacryoadentitis, 342
Sickle scaler, 120
SID; *see* Source image density
Sievert, 141
Silage, 316
Silk suture, 170
Sinus arrhythmia, 86
Sinus bradycardia, 86
Sinus rhythm, 86
Sinus tachycardia, 86

Skeletal muscle, 4, 6
Skeletal system
   anatomy and physiology, 5-6, 78
      avian, 354
      reptilian, 359
Skin
   anatomy and physiology, 14-16
   avian, 354
   reptilian, 359
   scraping for parasitic identification,
      203-218
   small animal physical examination, 77
Slant, 222, 229
Sleeping sickness, 99, 286
Slide preparation, 245
Sling, 90
Slobbers, 348
Small animal medicine, 76-93
   anal sac expression, 87-88
   bandaging, 88-90
   blood collection and transfusion, 81-
      84
   drug administration, 78-79
   electrocardiography, 84-87
   enemas, 88
   fluid therapy, 79-81
   nutrition, 294-311
      basic, 294-295
      critical care, 307-308
      daily energy requirements, 299, 302
      energy-producing nutrients, 295-
         296
      feline lower urinary tract disease,
         306
      life stage requirements, 299-306
      nonenergy-producing nutrients,
         296-299, 300-301
      obesity, 307
      pet food, 308-309
   physical examination, 77-78
Small intestine, 10
Smear, parasitic, 195
Smell, 16
Smooth endoplasmic reticulum, 2
Smooth muscle, 4, 6
Smudge cell, 247
Snake; *see* Reptile
Snap Whole Blood Heartworm Antigen
   Test, 203
Snare, 44
Snuffles, 346
Soap, 158
Social behavior, 49-50, 51
Soda lime canister, 185
Sodium
   nutritional requirements, 299, 314,
      318, 321, 323
   serum, 257, 259
Sodium bicarbonate, 191
Sodium chloride, 83, 223
Sodium thiamylal, 62
Sodium thiopental, 62
Soft tissue
   calcification in guinea pig, 348
   swelling, 330

Software, 369
Soiling, 53-54
Solute, 3, 72
Solution
    calculations, 72-73
    defined, 3, 72
Solvazines; *see* Xylazine
Solvent, 3, 72
Somatic cell, 140
Somatic circulation, 8
Somatic muscle, 6
Somatic nervous system, 6
Somnothane; *see* Halothane
Somnotol; *see* Pentobarbital
Sonolucent sonographic image, 150
Sorbitol dehydrogenase, 256-257
Soremouth, 110
Sound waves, 148
Source image density, 138
Source image distance, 144
Spay hook, 167, 169
Specific gravity, 233
    parasitic examination, 194-195
Specific immunity, 272-273
Specific pathogen free, 351
Specificity, defined, 281
Specimen collection, 223-225
    cellular, 244-245
    laboratory animal
        avian, 356
        gerbil, 345
        guinea pig, 348
        hamster, 343
        mice, 339, 340
        needle sizes and sites, 340
        rabbit, 346
        rat, 342
        reptile, 361
    sample handling, 250
    small animal, 81-84
    urinary, 231-232
    viral, 266
Speculum, 41, 105
Speech, 376
Speed, radiographic, 132, 133, 144
Spencer scissors, 165
Sperm, 12
Spermatozoa
    defined, 30
    in urine, 237
SPF; *see* Specific pathogen free
Spherocyte, 240, 241, 247
Sphincter muscle, 6
Spinal cord, 7
Spine
    bovine regional anesthesia, 112
    enzootic lymphadenitis, 348
    formula for designation, 6
Spin-headed worm, 213
Spleen, 10, 152
Splenectomy, 171
Sponge forceps, 165
Spongy bone, 5
Spontaneous ovulator, 17

Spraying, feline, 54
SQ; *see* Subcutaneous
Squamous cell oral carcinoma, 117
Squamous epithelia, 4
Squeeze chute, 45
Squeeze pen, 43
Staining technique, 245
Stainless steel instruments, 170
Stainless steel suture, 170
Stanchion, 45
Standing heat, 13
Staphylococci, 109, 225
Stationary anode, 128
Status epilepticus, 337
Steam for microbial control, 157,
    160-162
Steam under pressure for microbial
    control, 157
Steatorrhea, 252, 261
Stenotic, defined, 337
Sterilization, 155-163
    in diagnostic microbiology, 221
Sterilize, defined, 162
Stertor, 337
Stock, 38
Stomach
    anatomy and physiology, 9
    ruminant, 313
    sonographic appearance, 152
Stomach bot, 207
Stomach tube, 41, 105, 113
Stomatitis, 117, 362, 363
Stomatocyte, 240, 241
Stool softener, 65
Stored whole blood, 83
Strabismus, 337
Strangles, 99
Stratum corneum, 14
Stratum germinativum, 14
Streaking for isolation, 229
Streptococci
    mastitis, 109
    meningitis, 110
    microbiology identification, 225-226
    strangles, 99
Stresnil, 114
Stress, 378
Stress management, 373
Stressor, 378
Striated muscle, 6
Strongid; *see* Pyrantel tartrate
Strongyloides, 209
Strongylus, 204
Structure mottle, 144
Stupor, 337
Subarachnoid space, 7
Subcutaneous administration, 79, 80
Subgingival curettage, 124
Subject contrast, 144
Subunit vaccine, 278
Successive approximation, 55
Sucking lice, 200, 217
Sucralfate, 65
Sucrase, 10

Suction tip, 169
Sudan Stain, 252
Suicide sac, 3
Sulfa drugs, 60, 61
Sulfonamide, 60
SuperChar; *see* Activated charcoal
Supervisory skills, 370
Suppressor T cell, 273
Supravital staining, 247
Surface sampling, 162
Surgery
    equine, 101-102
    instruments, 164-170
        care of, 170
        forceps, 165-167
        needle holders, 167, 168
        needles and suture material,
            169-170
        orthopedic, 169
        pack preparation, 170-171
        retractors, 167-169
        scissors, 164-165
    operating room, 173-174
    patient preparation, 171-172
    surgical scrub, 172-173
Surgical gut, 169
Surgical milk, 170
Surgical site preparation, 101
Surital; *see* Thiamylal
Suture material, 169-170
SV; *see* Sievert
Swab specimen, 223-224
Swamp fever, 100
Sweat gland, 14
Swine
    anesthesia, 113-114
    behavior characteristics, 43
    breeding, reproduction, and neonatal
        care, 29-30
    castration, 111
    dentition, 119
    diseases of, 107-109
        preventable, 110
    drug administration and sample
        collection, 105, 106
    nutrition, 320-322
    parasites, 212-213
    penis, 13
    physical examination, 104-105
    porcine reproductive and respiratory
        syndrome, 109
    restraint and handling, 43
    urine specific gravity, 233
    venipuncture, 106
    viral disease, 268
Sympathetic nervous system, 6
Synarthrosis, 6
Synovial joint, 6
Syphacia obvelata, 214
Syrian hamster, 342-344
Syringe, 82
Syrup of ipecac, 65
Systematic desensitization in behavior
    modification, 52

Systemic circulation, 8
Systole, 8
Systolic blood pressure, 187

T

T cell, 272-273, 274
T wave, 8, 84, 85
Tablet administration, 78-79
Tachycardia, 86, 87, 192
Tachypnea, 192, 337
Tactile hair, 15
Taenia, 197, 213, 214, 216
Tagamet; *see* Cimetidine
Tail
  bandaging, 90
  as behavior indicator, 37
  bovine
    danger potential, 40
    jacking of, 41
    tying of during laparotomy, 110
    venipuncture, 105-106
Tail docking, 42, 172
Tail tie, 39
Tamponade, 332, 336
Tankage, 325
Tapazole; *see* Methimazol
Tapeworm
  bovine and ovine, 210
  canine and feline, 197-198
  mice and rats, 214-215
  porcine, 213
  zoonosis, 287
Target cell, 241
Task; *see* Organophosphate
Taste, 16
Taurine, 310
Taxonomy, 265-266
TDN; *see* Total digestible nutrient
Teamwork, 370
Tears, 15
  red, 342
Teaser ram, 29
Teat laceration repair, 110
Technique chart, radiographic, 137-140
Teeth; *see* Tooth
Telazol; *see* Tiletamine hydrochloride
Telephone conversation, 368
Telephone system, 369
Temperature
  body; *see* Body temperature
  metric system, 71
  preferred optimal, 360
Terbutaline sulfate, 64
Territory marking, 35, 50, 53
Test cross, 21, 23
Testes, 15
Testicle, 12
Testosterone, 15
Tetanus, 97-98, 109
Tetany, 114
Tetracycline, 59, 60
  dental staining, 117
Tetraparesis, 337
TGC; *see* Time-gain compensation

TGE; *see* Transmissible gastroenteritis
Thalamus, 7
Therabloat; *see* Poloxalene
Therapeutic index, 58-59
Thermionic emission, 144
Thermocouple for sterilization quality
    control, 162
Thermoluminescent dosimeter, 144
Thermometer for sterilization quality
    control, 162
Thiacetarsemide sodium, 66
Thiamin, 298, 321
Thiamylal, 113, 179
Thiazine, 178
Thiobarbiturates, 62, 113, 114, 179
Thioglycollate broth, 222
Thiopental, 113, 179, 180
Third atrioventricular block, 87
Thoracic spine, 6
Thorax bandaging, 89
Threadworm, 205
Thrombocyte, 244; *see also* Platelet
Thrombocytopenia, 247
Thrombocytosis, 247
Thrombosis, 102
Thrombus, 102
Thumb forceps, 165, 166
Thymus, 10
Thyroid gland, 15
Thyroid supplements, 67
Thyroidectomy, 67
Thyrotropic hormone, 15
Thyroxin, 15
TI; *see* Therapeutic index
Tick, 201, 217
Tidal volume, 11, 17, 188
Tiletamine hydrochloride, 62, 178
Time
  management, 372
  metric system, 71
Time-gain compensation, 149
Timer switch in x-ray tube, 129
Tissue, 3-4
Titer, defined, 269
TLI; *see* Trypsin-like immunoreactivity
To-and-Fro system; *see* Rebreathing
    system
Tolazoline, 178
Tolerance, defined, 269, 281
Tong, 411
Tongue examination, 121
Tonsil, 10
Tooth
  anatomy, 118-119
  danger potential, 43
  dental procedures
    instruments, 120-121
    prophy, 121
    radiography, 122-123
    restraint, 38
    safety, 121
  equine, 94-95
  examination, 77, 121
  floating, 95

Tooth—cont'd
  function, 119-120
  interlock, 117
  malocclusions, 116-117
  misdirected, 117
  needle, 43, 45
  numbering, 120
  occlusion, 116-117
  primary, 124
  types, 123
Topical drugs, 68, 79
Torbugesic; *see* Butorphanol
Torbutrol; *see* Butorphanol
Torsion, 337
Tortoiseshell cat, 20-21
Total bilirubin, 258
Total digestible nutrient, 325
Total plasma protein, 80
Total protein, 244
Total serum protein, 254
Toxemia, 348
Toxiband; *see* Activated charcoal
Toxic neutrophil, 243, 247
Toxicity
  avian, 357
  emergencies, 331, 335
  vitamin, 300-301
Toxocara, 196, 287
Toxoplasmosis, 288
TPP; *see* Total plasma protein
Trace minerals, 296, 323
Trachea
  anatomy, 11
  collapsing, 330
Trade name, 58
Tranquazine; *see* Acepromazine
Tranquilizer, 61, 177
Transducer, 148, 153
Transfaunation, 114
Transfusion, blood, 83-84, 190
Transitional epithelia, 4
Translocation in genetics, 22
Transmissible gastroenteritis, 110
Transverse, sonographic terminology,
    153
Trauma
  avian, 357
  canine, 33
  dental, 118
  head, 334
Treat supplementation, 303, 305
Trematode, 198, 210, 218
Treponema hyodysenteriae, 110
Trexan; *see* Naltrexone
Triadan system, 120
Tribrissen; *see* Potentiated sulfa
Trichinella spiralis, 212
Trichomoniasis, 359
Trichophyton, 227, 289
Trichostrongylus axei, 208
Trichostrongylus colubriformis, 208
Trichuris, 196, 209, 212
Triglycerides, 259
Trixacarus caviae, 217

True nucleus, 2-3
Trypsin, 10, 252
Trypsin-like immunoreactivity, 253
Trypticase soy agar, 222
Trypticase soy broth, 222
TSP; *see* Total serum protein
Tube envelope, 128, 129
Tube in diagnostic microbiology, 222, 229
Tube rating chart, 128, 129
Tuberculosis, 285, 292, 357
Tularemia, 285, 350
Tumor; *see* Neoplasia
Tums; *see* Antacids
Tungsten filament, 128
Turgor, defined, 91
Turtle; *see* Reptile
Tushes, 94
Twitch, 38, 45
Tying, equine, 37-38
Tylenol; *see* Acetaminophen
Tympany, 108
Typhoidal, defined, 292
Tyzzer's disease, 341, 345, 346-347

U

Ultrasonic scaler, 120
Ultrasound, 147-154
    for microbial control, 157
    pregnancy diagnosis, 26, 27
Ultraviolet for microbial control, 157
Uncinaria stenocephala, 196
Undulant, defined, 292
United States Army retractor, 167, 168
United States Drug Enforcement
        Administration, 58, 81
Universal F-circuit system, 183
Urea agar slant, 223
Urea nitrogen, 251, 259
Ureter
    anatomy, 12
    rupture, 334
Urethra, 12, 334
Urethrostomy, 172
Uric acid, 238, 259
Urinalysis, 231-237, 238
    chemical constituents, 233-234
    evaluation, 232-233
    microscopic evaluation, 235-237, 238
    specimen collection, 231-232
Urinary bladder, 12
Urinary system; *see* Genitourinary
        system
Urinary tract disease, feline, 306
Urination, 12
Urine
    drug excretion, 59
    output in dehydration, 80
    production, 12
    scent marking, 50
    specimen collection, 224, 339
Urine concentration test, 251
Urine glucose, 251
Urine pH, 233

Urine specific gravity, 233
    dehydration and, 80
Urine urobilinogen, 254
Urinometer, 233
Urobilinogen, 234, 254
Urogram, 337
Uropygial gland, 363
Urticaria, 91, 193, 281, 337
USP; *see* Halothane
Uterine horns, 13
Uterus, 13, 152

V

Vaccination, 67-68
    blood collection, 81
    current trends, 279-280
    difficulties, 278-279
    equine encephalomyelitides, 99
    equine herpes virus, 99
    equine influenza, 100
    immunity and, 277-278
    Potomac horse fever, 96
    precautions, 279
    rabies, 98
    tetanus, 98
Vagina
    anatomy, 13
    specimen collection, 245
Vaginitis, 344
Vagus indigestion, 108
Valium; *see* Diazepam
Vaporized anesthesia, 184-185
Variable expressivity, 19, 23
Vas deferens, 12
Vascular system, 8-9
Vasodilation, 193
Vasodilators, 63
Vasopressin; *see* Antidiuretic hormone
Vasotec; *see* Enalapril maleate
VEE; *see* Venezuelan equine
        encephalomyelitides
Vein, 8
Velocity, sonographic, 148, 153
Velpeau sling, 90
Venezuelan equine encephalomyelitides,
        99, 284
Venipuncture, 105-106
Ventilation
    anesthesia and, 188-189
    physiology, 11
Ventral
    defined, 4
    radiographic terminology, 142
Ventricle, 8
Ventricular fibrillation, 87
Ventricular premature contraction, 87, 91
Ventricular tachycardia, 87
Venule, 8
Verapamil, 62, 63
Verbal communication, 366
Verbrugge forceps, 169
Versed; *see* Midazolam
Vertebral column; *see* Spine
Vesicle, 281

Vetalar; *see* Ketamine
Vial gravitation flotation technique, 194-
        195
Vibriosis, 110
Vicious dog, 33, 34
Viral infection, 263-270
    avian, 358
    classification and identification, 265-
        266
    composition, 263-265
    disabled infectious single-cycle, 279
    hamster, 344
    immunity, 273-274
    prevention, 268
    reptile, 362
    sampling techniques and submission,
        266-268
    zoonosis, 286
Viricidal, defined, 269
Visceral larval migrans, 287
Vision, 15-16
Visual communication, 49
Vitamin nutrition
    bovine, 313
    caprine and ovine, 318-319
    equine, 323
    porcine, 321-322
    small animal, 296-299, 300-301
Vitreous humor, 15
Viviparous, defined, 363
VLM; *see* Visceral larval migrans
Vocal communication, 49
Vocal cord, 11
Volume
    apothecary and household equivalents,
        74
    metric system, 71, 74
Voluntary striated muscle, 6
V-trough, 44
Vulva, 13

W

Warble grubs, 211
Wash bath in film processing, 134
Wasting ketosis, 107
Wasting syndrome, 358
Water, nutritional requirements
    bovine, 315
    caprine and ovine, 318
    equine, 324
    porcine, 320
    small animal, 296
Water deprivation test, 251
Water-soluble vitamins, 296, 300-301
Wavelength, sonographic, 148, 153
Waxy casts, 237
Weaning, 302
WEE; *see* Western equine
        encephalomyelitides
Weight loss, 307
Weight measurement, 74
Weil's disease, 289, 350
Weitlander retractor, 167
Wenckebach atrioventricular block, 87

Western equine encephalomyelitides, 99, 286
Wet tail, 343
Whelping, 30
Whimpering, 49
Whining, 49
Whipworm, 196, 209, 212
White blood cell, 235-236, 242-244
White muscle disease, 110
Whitten effect, 29, 342, 351
Whole blood
   components, 249-250
   transfusion, 83
Win-win conflict resolution, 378
Wire cutting scissors, 165
Wire twister, 169
Wolf teeth, 94
Wool hair, 15
Wound triage, 327
Written communication, 369
Wry mouth, 117

X

X-linked inheritance, 20-21
X-ray, 144; *see also* Radiography
Xyla-ject; *see* Xylazine
Xylazine, 61, 113, 114, 178
Xylocaine; *see* Lidocaine

Y

Yankauer tip, 169
Y-connector, 185
Yeast, 227-228
Yersinia
   fecal culture, 225
   microbiology identification, 226
   zoonosis, 284, 350
Yobine; *see* Yohimbine
Yohimbine, 178

Z

Zantac; *see* Ranitidine
Zero grazing, 108

Zimectrin paste; *see* Ivermectin
Zinc, nutritional requirements
   bovine, 315
   caprine and ovine, 318-319
   equine, 323
   porcine, 321
   small animal n 298
Zolazepam, 62, 177, 178
Zolicef; *see* Cefazolin sodium
Zonary placentation, 30
Zoonosis, 218, 282-293
   bacterial, 283-285
   laboratory animal, 349, 350
   mycotic, 289
   parasitic, 287-288
   viral, 286
Zoonotic, defined, 229
Zygomatic arch, 112